INTRODUCTION TO BIOSTATISTICAL APPLICATIONS IN HEALTH RESEARCH WITH MICROSOFT OFFICE EXCEL® AND R

INTRODUCTION TO BIOSTATISTICAL APPLICATIONS IN HEALTH RESEARCH WITH MICROSOFT OFFICE EXCEL® AND R

Second Edition

ROBERT P. HIRSCH
Foundation for the Advanced Education in the Sciences
Bethesda, MD, USA

WILEY

This second edition first published 2021
© 2021 John Wiley & Sons, Inc.

Edition History
John Wiley and Sons, Inc. (1e, 2016)

Registered Office
John Wiley & Sons, Inc., 111 River Street, Hoboken, NJ 07030, USA

Editorial Office
111 River Street, Hoboken, NJ 07030, USA

For details of our global editorial offices, customer services, and more information about Wiley products visit us at www.wiley.com.

Wiley also publishes its books in a variety of electronic formats and by print-on-demand. Some content that appears in standard print versions of this book may not be available in other formats.

Library of Congress Cataloging-in-Publication Data Applied for:

ISBN 978-1-119-72259-5

Cover image: © (inset figure) Courtesy of Robert P. Hirsch, (background) © iconeer/Getty Images
Cover design by Wiley

Set in 10/12pt, TimesLTStd by SPi Global, Chennai, India.

SKY10024066_011421

To Libby, for her love and support without which I would be lost.

CONTENTS

PREFACE TO FIRST EDITION

Regardless of whether you are a health researcher or someone who wants to understand the health research literature, *Introduction to Biostatistical Applications in Health Research with Excel* will provide you with a basic understanding of the most commonly used statistical methods in health research. The focus of this text is on learning statistical concepts and interpreting the results of performing statistical tests. The text is intended for readers who are not necessarily mathematically minded. To accomplish this, I provide plain language explanations and graphic representations of statistical concepts rather than relying on purely mathematical descriptions that are typical of many statistical texts. Thus, the readers of *Introduction to Biostatistical Applications in Health Research with Excel* can come to understand and appreciate statistical logic with a minimum level of mathematical ability.

This text includes many examples that are patterned after actual analyses of health research data. These examples use two approaches to illustrate statistical principles. Some examples, namely those that illustrate simpler statistical methods, are worked out "by hand" to allow a better understanding of the statistical method. Many of the examples, however, involve statistical methods that would require more complicated calculations that are typically performed by a statistical program. My experience is that little or no understanding of the logic behind these methods is gained by performing these calculations by hand. Instead, we will be learning how to use Excel® to perform these analyses and understand the results.

I believe that health researchers and students of health research will find *Introduction to Biostatistical Applications in Health Research with Excel* to be highly accessible due to its interpretation rather than calculation-oriented presentation.

Also, the overall format of the text is designed so that appropriate statistical methods for a particular set of data can be easily located. The text is divided into four parts. The first of these builds the foundation of statistical logic. The remaining chapters increase in complexity by building on simpler methods. These parts address uni-variable, bivariable, and multivariable analysis respectively. Within each part, there are three chapters. These address methods for continuous, ordinal, and nominal dependent variables. These chapters are oriented to reflect a unique flowchart that is provided in an appendix and in the text. This flowchart serves as a statistical roadmap so that if the reader is able to identify the type of data represented by the dependent variable and independent variable(s) they will be able to select the correct statistical method to analyze their data. At the beginning of each chapter, a continuation of the flowchart reinforces the methods discussed in that chapter and how the statistical methods are selected. I believe that the overall design of this text allows even the most mathematically challenged readers to really under-stand statistical methods used in health research by providing a highly verbal and visual explanation of statistics in a logical progression that builds on itself while also providing the necessary tools in an easily retrievable form.

My principal reason for writing a text using Excel is to provide the reader with access to data analysis without having to depend on a statistical programmer. My reasoning was that Excel is a commonly available program that includes tools needed to perform most statistical analyses.[1] In addition to what is already part of Excel, I am providing BAHR (**B**iostatistical **A**pplications in **H**ealth **R**esearch) programs for Excel that give the reader the ability to perform all of statistical analyses, as well as the data sets used in the examples. These can be found at www .website.com.

I am going to assume that the reader has a basic knowledge of Excel. If you have never used Excel (or other spreadsheet program), you can read the Excel Primer in Appendix D. Even if this is your first time using Excel, I think you will learn very quickly as much as you will need to perform the statistical tests described in this textbook.

One thing you need to do before you start using Excel for statistical analyses is to install two add-ins. These are programs that come with Excel, but they are inactive unless the user activates them. To do this, click on "FILE" on the main menu bar. Then click on "Options" followed by "Add-ins." On the next screen, you will see "Manage": followed by a selection box. Select "Excel Add-ins" and click on "Go ... " This will display a menu that lists the available add-ins. Make sure that there is a check in the boxes for "Solver Add-in and "Analysis Toolpak"[2] Now, you will see a new class in the "DATA" selection from the main menu. That class is called "Analysis."[3] We will be using it soon.

Robert P. Hirsch

---

[1] This is true for most Mac users as well as PC users.

[2] For Mac users, the only add-in available is "Solver Add-in." You can perform the same procedures (and a lot more) by downloading the free version of StatPlus, which can be found on the internet.

[3] For StatPlus, the commands appear in the top menu bar.

PREFACE TO SECOND EDITION

There are a several changes in the second edition. The most obvious is the addition of a thirteenth chapter. This chapter discusses the assumptions that underlie the statistical methods described in Chapters 4–12. In this chapter, you will learn how to identify the assumptions for a particular statistical test and how to evaluate whether the assumptions are satisfied. Further, you will learn what can be done if the assumption is not satisfied.

To further aid in identifying assumptions, Appendix C has been changed. In this appendix, all of the flowcharts are presented. The versions of the flowcharts in Appendix C have added indicators of the assumptions made by each test.

Another change in the second edition is the inclusion of examples in using R to perform the statistical analyses described in Chapters 4–12. R is a free collection of statistical programs, which is gaining in popularity in introductory statistics texts. For the most part, R is an alternative to Excel for analysis, but Excel remains superior for data management. Data sets generated in Excel can be imported into R for analysis there. Appendix E gives a primer for R. There, you will learn how to access R and get it running on your computer as well as some of the basic uses of R.

Provided with this textbook on the companion website is a new version of BAHR programs for Excel. In this new version are new programs for nonparametric analyses, Student–Newman–Keuls tests, and stratified analyses. With these new programs, it is less necessary to perform calculations by hand and, instead, let the computer perform them for us. The methods for perfuming tests by hand are still included in the text for those who find that helps them understand the statistical logic.

At the end of each chapter a chapter summary and exercises from the first edition of the workbook have been added. The answers to the odd exercises appear in Appendix F.

Robert P. Hirsch
Maryland, 2020

ABOUT THE COMPANION WEBSITE

This book is accompanied by a student companion website and an instructor companion website:

www.wiley.com/go/hirsch/healthresearch2e

The student companion website includes

- Workbook
- Datasets
- Excel add-in
- Instructions for installing the add-in

The instructor companion website includes the Solutions Manual.

PART ONE

BASIC CONCEPTS

Statisticians are used to dealing with uncertainty. Even so, there is one fact of which even statisticians are certain: the fact that we, as health researchers and practitioners, are always interested in applying the results of a study to persons, places, and/or times that were not included in the study. Our purpose is to interpret a study's observations as they relate to some larger group. In statistical terms, the larger group is called the **population** and the smaller group is called the **sample**. As we interpret health research data from a particular sample, it is always with the intention of using the sample's observations to draw some conclusion about the population from which that sample was taken.

Since we are always in the position of using a sample to understand the population, it is important that we take samples so that each one is representative of the population. Unfortunately, we do not know how to do that. To appreciate the problem, let us think about a population that we understand completely. For instance, suppose we were to think about a deck of 52 cards. In this "population" there are two characteristics of its members: suit and rank. These characteristics are distributed uniformly among the members of the population so that there are 13 cards in each of 4 suits and each suit has 13 ranks from deuce to ace. Now, thinking of that well-defined population, which five cards would you use to communicate the structure of the population?

Introduction to Biostatistical Applications in Health Research with Microsoft Office Excel® and R,
Second Edition. Robert P. Hirsch.
© 2021 John Wiley & Sons, Inc. Published 2021 by John Wiley & Sons, Inc.
Companion website: www.wiley.com/go/hirsch/healthresearch2e

If you feel frustrated with this question, it is because there is no completely correct answer. Any set of five cards fails to communicate precisely the structure of the deck.

If we are unable to select a representative sample from such a well-defined population, imagine selecting a representative sample from a population that is really of interest to health researchers. It just cannot be done!

Even though we do not know how to make each sample representative of the population, we do know how to make a collection of samples representative of the population. We can do that with the deck of 52 cards by shuffling the deck and dealing several "samples" of 5 cards. In other words, we could let chance determine which members of the population are going to be included in each sample. Any particular hand of five cards might be distinctly unrepresentative of the deck, but if we continued to deal hands of five cards, in the long run those hands would represent the deck. We do the same thing when we take samples from populations as part of research. We let chance determine which members of the population end up in the sample.

It is this principle of **random sampling** that makes it necessary to understand the role of chance when we are interested in interpreting the results of health research. The primary purpose of statistics is to consider how chance influences that interpretation. To be interpreters of health research data, we need to recognize that the samples we examine might, just by chance, be substantially different from the rest of the population. To do this, we need to be comfortable in interpreting the results of statistical analyses. It is the purpose of this text to help you develop that level of comfort.

To understand statistics, we need to understand how chance influences observations in a sample and how the role of chance can be taken into account. Thus, we begin this text by examining the characteristics of chance and how we can use the sample's observations to draw conclusions about the population. First, in Chapter 1, we will look at chance itself to understand how it works. Next, in Chapter 2, we will examine the characteristics of a population to discover how its data can be described. Finally, in Chapter 3, we will concentrate on the sample to see how the sample's observations can be used to describe the population. Once we understand these basic principles, we will be ready to take a look at statistical procedures that are commonly used in health research.

CHAPTER 1

THINKING ABOUT CHANCE

In the introduction to this first part of the text, we learned that chance is used to select samples from the population that are, in the long run, representative of the population from which they came (Figure 1.1). Before we can appreciate how chance influences the composition of those samples, however, we need to understand some things about chance itself. In this chapter, we will look at the basic properties of chance and see how the chances of individual events can be combined to address health issues.

Introduction to Biostatistical Applications in Health Research with Microsoft Office Excel® and R,
Second Edition. Robert P. Hirsch.
© 2021 John Wiley & Sons, Inc. Published 2021 by John Wiley & Sons, Inc.
Companion website: www.wiley.com/go/hirsch/healthresearch2e

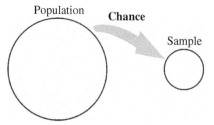

Figure 1.1   Chance determines which data values in the population end up in the sample.

1.1   PROPERTIES OF PROBABILITY

To begin with, we should point out that there are two terms that can be used inter-changeably: **chance** and **probability**. In everyday language, probability (or chance) tells us how many times something happens relative to the number of times it could happen. For example, we might think of the probability that a patient presenting with a sore throat has streptococcal pharyngitis. If we can expect 1 patient to actu-ally have streptococcal pharyngitis out of every 10 patients seen with a sore throat, then the probability of having streptococcal pharyngitis is 0.10. Or equivalently, there is a 10% chance that a person selected at random from among persons with sore throats would have strep throat.

In statistical terminology, the number of times something happens is called its **frequency** and that "something" is called an **event**. The opportunities for an event to occur are called **observations**.[1] When using the concept of probability, we need to understand that there are two possible results for each observation: either the event occurs or the event does not occur. In the previous example, the event was strepto-coccal pharyngitis and the patients seen with a sore throat were the observations.

Everyday language is often cumbersome when discussing issues in statistics. An alternative approach is to examine events and observations graphically. We do this by constructing a **Venn diagram**. In a Venn diagram, we use a rectangle to symbolize all of the observations and a circle to symbolize those observations in which the event occurs. Figure 1.2 is a Venn diagram we could use to think about the probability that a patient with a sore throat has streptococcal pharyngitis.

There are some aspects of observations and events that are evident in a Venn diagram. For instance, we can see that the entire rectangle outside of the circle cor-responds to observations in which the event does not occur. When an event does not occur, we say that the **complement** of the event occurs. In this case, the event is having strep throat and its complement is not having strep throat.

The way a Venn diagram tells us about the magnitude of the probability is by the area of the circle representing the event relative to the area of the entire rectangle. A way we can compare these areas is by creating a **Venn equation**. A Venn equation

---

[1] Statisticians also refer to the opportunity for an event to occur as a **trial**. Since the term *trial* refers to a clinical experiment in health research, we will exclusively use the term *observation* to refer to the opportunity for an event to occur.

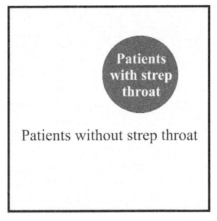

Figure 1.2   An example of a Venn diagram. The rectangular area represents all observations. The circular area represents the observations in which the event occurs. The area within the rectangle but outside of the circle represents those observations in which the event did not occur.

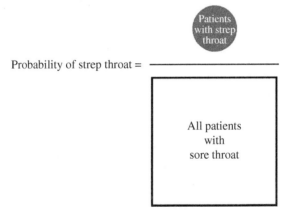

Figure 1.3   A Venn equation illustrating the probability a patient with sore throat has streptococcal pharyngitis.

uses the parts of a Venn diagram in a mathematical equation that shows how the probability of an event is calculated. For the probability that a patient with sore throat has streptococcal pharyngitis, the Venn equation would look like Figure 1.3.

A Venn equation helps us see another property of probabilities that probabilities have a distinct range of possible values. Since an event cannot exist without an observation, the circle can only be as big as the rectangle. In other words, the numerator must be a subset of the denominator. The result of this property is to make the largest possible value for a probability equal to 1 (or 100%). The value of 1 occurs when every observation in the denominator is also an event in the numerator. When the probability of an observation being an event has a value of 1, it is **certain** that the event will occur.

The numerator of a probability contains the number of events. The largest value possible is equal to the number of observations. The smallest value possible is 0. If the numerator of a probability is equal to 0, this implies that none of the observations are events and, therefore, the probability is equal to 0 as well. A probability of 0 indicates that it is **impossible** for an event to occur. A probability can be no smaller than 0 and no larger than 1.[2]

When we want to calculate a probability, it is easier to use some mathematical shorthand. To symbolize a probability, we use a lowercase p followed by a set of parentheses. Within those parentheses, we identify the event addressed by the probability. Then, the equation looks like this:

$$p(\text{event}) = \frac{\text{number of events}}{\text{number of observations}} \tag{1.1}$$

Next, let us take a look at an example that illustrates calculation of a probability and its interpretation.

■ EXAMPLE 1.1

Suppose we did throat cultures for 100 patients who complained of a sore throat and 10 of those cultures were positive for streptococcus. What is the probability a person picked at random would have a positive strep culture?

In this question, a positive strep test is the event and someone with sore throat is an observation. To calculate the probability of a person having a positive strep culture, we can use Equation (1.1).

$$p(\text{event}) = \frac{\text{number of events}}{\text{number of observations}} = \frac{10}{100} = 0.1$$

Thus, there is a probability of 0.1 (or a 10% chance) that a person selected from the group of patients with a sore throat would be positive for streptococcus. ■

A part of the shorthand we use to show how probabilities are calculated concerns the complement of an event (i.e., an observation in which the event does not occur). Rather than inserting the description of the complement of the event within the parentheses, we more often put a bar over the description of the event. So, $p(\overline{\text{event}})$ stands for the probability of the complement of the event occurring (i.e., the probability of the event *not* occurring). For the complement of having strep throat, we could use $p(\overline{\text{strep}})$. There are two properties of a collection of events that an event and its complement always demonstrate. The first is **mutual exclusion**. A collection of events is said to be mutually exclusive if it is impossible for two or more events

---

[2]This range of possible values between 0 and 1 means that a probability is also a proportion.

to occur in a single observation. In this case, it is certainly impossible for a person both to have strep throat and to not have strep throat.

The second property of an event and its complement is that they are **collectively exhaustive**. A collection of events is said to be collectively exhaustive if every observation is certain to consist of at least one of the events. Here, this implies that every person with a sore throat either has or does not have strep throat. Clearly, this is true.

For events that are both mutually exclusive and collectively exhaustive (like an event and its complement), there is a special relationship among the events: the sum of their probabilities is equal to 1. In mathematical language, the relationship between the probability of an event occurring and the probability of the complement of the event occurring is shown in Equation (1.2):

$$p(\text{event}) + p(\overline{\text{event}}) = 1 \qquad (1.2)$$

A little bit of algebra shows us that we can calculate the probability of the complement of an event by subtracting the probability of the event from 1. This is shown in Equation (1.3):

$$p(\overline{\text{event}}) = 1 - p(\text{event}) \qquad (1.3)$$

This relationship can also be described in graphic language as in the Venn equation in Figure 1.4.

So far, we have seen how we can think about probabilities using everyday language, graphic language, and mathematical language. Each one of these ways of examining statistical issues has its own advantages. The sort of things we have

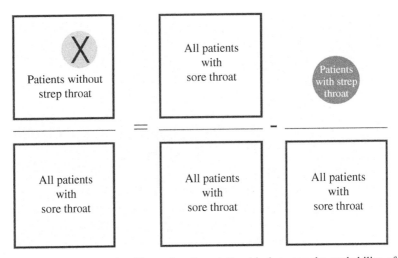

Figure 1.4 A Venn equation illustrating the relationship between the probability of the complement of the event (e.g., not having strep throat) and the probability of the event (e.g., having strep throat).

learned about probability includes the fact that probabilities have a discrete range of possible values ranging from 0 (indicating that the event cannot occur) to 1 (indicating that the event always occurs). Also, we have examined the relationship between an event and its complement. This relationship has two important properties of a collection of events. These properties are mutually exclusive and collectively exhaustive. A collection of events is mutually exclusive if only one of the events can occur in a single observation. To be collectively exhaustive, the collection of events needs to encompass every possibility so that at least one of the events occurs in every observation. Next, we will take a look at other kinds of collections of events.

1.2 COMBINATIONS OF EVENT

There are two ways we might be interested in how two or more events relate to each other. One way is that the events occur together in the same observation. We call this the **intersection** of events. Another way is that at least one event occurs in an observation. We call this the **union** of events.

1.2.1 Intersections

In health research and practice, we are often interested in situations in which more than one event occurs in a single observation. For instance, we might be interested in the relationship between a high-fat diet and development of atherosclerosis. The sorts of people in whom we would be most interested are those who have both of those events, since they are the ones for whom a high-fat diet could have contributed to the risk of disease.

In statistical terminology, we refer to the occurrence of two or more events in a single observation as the intersection of the events. Figure 1.5 illustrates the

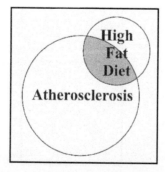

Figure 1.5 Venn diagram illustrating the relationship between a high-fat diet and development of atherosclerosis. The area in which the circles overlap represents those persons who have both a high-fat diet and atherosclerosis.

probabilities of a high-fat diet and atherosclerosis and the intersection of those two events. Their intersection is where the two circles overlap. These are the observations in which a person has both a high-fat diet and atherosclerosis.

The probability of an observation including both events (i.e., the intersection of those events) considers the size of the overlap relative to all the observations. Figure 1.6 shows a Venn equation representing the probability of the intersection of high-fat diet and atherosclerosis.

If we want to calculate the probability of an intersection of events, we use what is called the **multiplication rule**. To see how the multiplication rule works, let us begin with a Venn equation (Figure 1.7).

To the left of the equals sign in the Venn equation in Figure 1.7 is the probability of the intersection of having a high-fat diet and developing atherosclerosis as shown in Figure 1.6. In the numerator of that probability are the persons who had both events. In the denominator are all persons regardless of diet or disease. Immediately to the right of the equals sign is the probability that someone has a high-fat diet. In the numerator of that probability are the persons with a high-fat diet and in the denominator are, as before, all persons regardless of diet or disease.

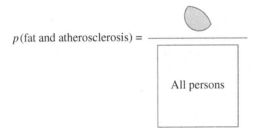

Figure 1.6   Venn equation for the probability that a person has both a high-fat diet (fat) and has atherosclerosis. In the numerator is the area of overlap (intersection) of the two circles in the Venn diagram (Figure 1.5). The denominator represents everyone whether or not they have a high-fat diet or atherosclerosis (i.e., the entire rectangle).

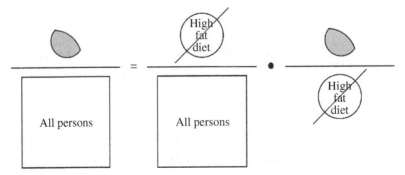

Figure 1.7   Venn equation of the multiplication rule used to calculate the intersection of high-fat diet and atherosclerosis.

The second fraction to the right of the equals sign also is a probability,[3] but it looks different from any probability we have encountered so far. Specifically, it does not include all the observations (represented by the rectangle in a Venn diagram) in its denominator. Rather, it includes only those persons with a high-fat diet in its denominator. This is an example of a very important kind of probability, called a **conditional probability.** A conditional probability tells us the probability of an event occurring given that another event has occurred. In this case, the conditional probability tells us the probability of a person having atherosclerosis given that the person has a high-fat diet.

In mathematical notation, a conditional probability also looks different from other probabilities we have encountered. Equation (1.4) illustrates the mathematical notation for the Venn equation in Figure 1.7.

$$p(A \text{ and } B) = p(A) \cdot p(B \mid A) \tag{1.4}$$

where

$p(A \text{ and } B)$ = probability that an observation will include both event A and event B (i.e., the probability of the intersection of A and B)[4]

$p(A)$ = probability that an observation includes event A (i.e., the unconditional probability of event A)

$p(B \mid A)$ = probability that an observation will include event B given that it includes event A (i.e., a conditional probability of event B)

Or, in terms of a high-fat diet and atherosclerosis,

$$p(\text{fat and atherosclerosis}) = p(\text{fat}) \cdot p(\text{atherosclerosis} \mid \text{fat}) \tag{1.5}$$

From a statistical point of view, it does not matter which event is addressed by the conditional probability.[5] Thus, the probability of the intersection of high-fat diet and atherosclerosis could also be calculated as

$$p(\text{fat and atherosclerosis}) = p(\text{atherosclerosis}) \cdot p(\text{fat} \mid \text{atherosclerosis}) \tag{1.6}$$

---

[3] Recall that, to be a probability, a fraction's numerator must be a subset of its denominator. This is the case here, because those persons with both a high-cholesterol diet and atherosclerosis (the numerator) are all included in the circle representing persons with atherosclerosis (the denominator).

[4] In set notation, this is $p(A \cap B)$.

[5] The way the probability of the intersection is calculated depends only on which probabilities are obtained as part of a particular health research study. If our information about the relationship between the high-fat diet and atherosclerosis comes from a cohort study (a study in which the probability of disease is compared between exposed and unexposed persons), for example, the conditional probability we would measure is the probability of the disease given exposure status. In a case–control study (a study in which the odds of being exposed is compared between persons who have and do not have the disease), however, the conditional probability we measure is the probability of the exposure given the disease status.

In Equations (1.5) and (1.6), we can see that a vertical line is used to separate the two events in the parentheses of a conditional probability. The event to the left of the vertical line is called the **conditional event**. It is the conditional event that the probability addresses. In Equation (1.5), the conditional event is having atherosclerosis, so this conditional probability tells us about the chance that someone has atherosclerosis. The event to the right of the vertical line is called the **conditioning event**. The conditioning event defines the circumstance in which we are interested in the probability of the conditional event. Here, having a high-fat diet is the conditioning event. Thus, Equation (1.5) tells us that we are interested in the probability of having atherosclerosis given (i.e., under the condition) that someone has a high-fat diet.

The reason that conditional probabilities are so important in health research is the fact that they tell us about an important aspect of the relationship between events. Namely, conditional probabilities can be used to see if the occurrence of one event changes the probability of the occurrence of another event. If, for example, we are interested in whether there is this sort of relationship between a high-fat diet and having atherosclerosis, we could compare the conditional probability in Equation (1.5) with the probability that someone has atherosclerosis given that they do not have a high-fat diet (p(atherosclerosis | $\overline{\text{fat}}$)). If those two conditional probabilities have the same value, then we can conclude that a high-fat diet does not influence the chance of having atherosclerosis. In that case, the three probabilities in Equation (1.7) are all equal to the same value.

$$p(\text{atherosclerosis} \mid \text{fat}) = p(\text{atherosclerosis} \mid \overline{\text{fat}}) = p(\text{atherosclersis}) \qquad (1.7)$$

Or, in more general terms,

$$p(B \mid A) = p(B \mid \overline{A}) = p(B) \qquad (1.8)$$

where

$p(B \mid \overline{A})$ = probability that an observation will include event B given that it does not include event A (i.e., another conditional probability of event B)

In statistical terminology, we say two events are **statistically independent** when the probability of one of the events is not affected by occurrence of the other event.[6] In biologic terms, events that are statistically independent cannot have a causal relationship (or any other type of relationship).

---

[6] The term "statistically independent" as statisticians use it can be confusing when we consider the everyday meaning of "independence." If we were to say, for example, that two persons are independent, we are likely to infer that there is no connection between them. This is not what the statistician is implying. Rather, the statistician is saying that you do not need to consider whether or not one event has occurred when addressing the probability of another event. When a statistician implies that there is no overlap between events, the statistician says that they are "mutually exclusive" rather than "statistically independent."

To determine if events are statistically independent, we need to compare only two of the three probabilities in Equation (1.8). If those two probabilities are equal to the same value, then all three probabilities are the same and the conditional and conditioning events are statistically independent. We will take a look at an example of this relationship shortly, but first let us see how conditional probabilities are calculated.

To calculate a conditional probability, we use Equation (1.4) algebraically rearranged as in Equation (1.9).

$$p(B \mid A) = \frac{p(A \text{ and } B)}{p(A)} \tag{1.9}$$

Or, in terms of a high-fat diet and having atherosclerosis,

$$p(\text{atheroslerosis} \mid \text{fat}) = \frac{p(\text{fat and atherosclerosis})}{p(\text{fat})} \tag{1.10}$$

This process of identifying statistical independence is illustrated in Example 1.2.

■ EXAMPLE 1.2

Suppose that, in a particular valley of the Mojave Desert, there are 2,500 residents. Of those 2,500 residents, 625 work for ACME Borax, Inc., a company that recovers chemicals from the brine under a salt flat that covers most of the valley floor. Of the 2,500 residents of the valley, 500 have been diagnosed with leukemia. Of the 500 diagnosed with leukemia, 125 are persons who work for ACME Borax, Inc. Given that information, is working for ACME statistically independent of being diagnosed with leukemia?

First, let us consider the relationship between working for ACME and having leukemia. We are told that 625 persons work for ACME and, of those, 125 have leukemia. From that information, we can calculate the probability of having leukemia under the condition that a person works for ACME using Equation (1.9):

$$p(\text{leukemia} \mid \text{ACME}) = \frac{p(\text{leukemia and ACME})}{p(\text{ACME})} = \frac{125/2{,}500}{625/2{,}500} = 0.2$$

To determine if working for ACME and having leukemia are statistically independent events, we need to compare that conditional probability with either the probability of having leukemia given that a person does not work for ACME or with the overall (i.e., unconditional) probability of having leukemia. The latter probability is

$$p(\text{leukemia}) = \frac{\text{number with leukemia in valley}}{\text{number in valley}} = \frac{500}{2{,}500} = 0.2$$

Since these two probabilities are equal to the same value, we can conclude that working for ACME and having leukemia are statistically independent events. In other words, working for ACME does not change the probability of having leukemia. ■

So far, we have seen that we can use the multiplication rule to calculate the probability of two events occurring in a single observation (i.e., the intersection of those events). To calculate the probability of the intersection of more than two events, we simply include each additional event in the multiplication of conditional probabilities. For each additional event, we include the conditional probability of the event with the conditioning events being all of the events listed previously in the equation. For example, we can calculate the intersection of three events as shown in Equation (1.11).

$$p(A \text{ and } B \text{ and } C) = p(A) \cdot p(B \mid A) \cdot p(C \mid A \text{ and } B) \tag{1.11}$$

where

$p(C \mid A \text{ and } B)$ = probability that an observation will include event C given it includes events A and B (i.e., a conditional probability of event C)

If the events are statistically independent, we can use a simplified version of the multiplication rule. This simplification is to multiply the unconditional probabilities of the events. Equation (1.12) shows the simplified version for the intersection of three events examined in Equation (1.11).

$$p(A \text{ and } B \text{ and } C) = p(A) \cdot p(B) \cdot p(C) \tag{1.12}$$

The reason we can use this simplified version of the multiplication rule is that, by definition, the conditional and unconditional probabilities are the same for statistically independent events (as shown in Equation (1.8)). If the three events are not statistically independent, however, we need to use Equation (1.11) to calculate the intersection of events.

1.2.2 Unions

When our interest is in the probability of any (i.e., 1 or more) of a collection of events occurring in the same observation, we say we are interested in the union of those events. Suppose, for example, we are considering two risk factors for atherosclerosis: high-fat diet and smoking. In that case, we might be interested in calculating the probability a person has at least one of these risk factors (i.e., either high-fat diet or smoking or both high-fat diet and smoking). To illustrate this, let us add smoking to the Venn diagram in Figure 1.5. Then the Venn diagram of all three events will look something like the one in Figure 1.8.

The union of the two risk factors is satisfied if a person either has a high-fat diet or smokes (or both). Thus, the numerator of the probability of the union of those two events includes the part of the Venn diagram covered by either circle.

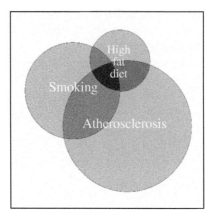

Figure 1.8   Venn diagram showing the relationship between high-fat diet, smoking, and atherosclerosis.

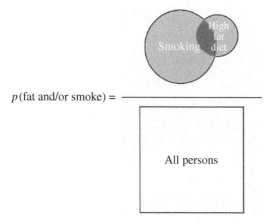

p(fat and/or smoke) =

Figure 1.9   Venn equation showing the probability of the union of smoking and/or high-fat diet

Figure 1.9 shows the Venn equation for the union of smoking and high-fat diet. To calculate the probability of the union of two events, we use the **addition rule**. As the name implies, in the addition rule the probabilities of each of the events are added together.

Since adding the probabilities together includes the intersection of those events twice, the probability of the intersection of the events must be subtracted from the sum. This calculation for the union of smoking and a high-fat diet is illustrated by the Venn equation in Figure 1.10.

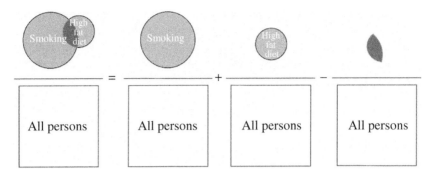

Figure 1.10   Venn equation showing calculation of the union of smoking and a high-fat diet using the addition rule.

In mathematical terms, the calculation of the union of two events is performed as shown in Equation (1.13).

$$p(A \text{ and/or } B) = p(A) + p(B) - p(A \text{ and } B) \qquad (1.13)$$

where

$p(A \text{ and/or } B)$ = probability an observation will include event A and/or event B (i.e., the probability of the union of events A and B)[7]

Now, let us take a look at an example addressing the union of two events.

■ EXAMPLE 1.3

Suppose we are planning a clinical trial of a new live vaccine. In this study, we want to exclude persons who are either pregnant or immunocompromised. Suppose we estimate that the population from which we are planning to take our sample includes 20% of the total number of persons who are pregnant and 10% of the total number of persons who are immunocompromised. If being pregnant and being immunocompromised are statistically independent events, what proportion of our sample will be excluded due to either of these characteristics?

To calculate the probability of the union of two events, we use Equation (1.13). For this application, Equation (1.13) looks like the following:

$$p(\text{preg and/or comp}) = p(\text{preg}) + p(\text{comp}) - p(\text{preg and comp})$$

We know the probability that a person selected at random from the population will be pregnant ($p(\text{preg}) = 0.2$) and the probability that a person selected at random from

---

[7]In set notation, this is $p(A \cup B)$.

the population will be immunocompromised (p(comp) $= 0.1$). We are not given the probability of the intersection of these two events (i.e., the probability a person will be both pregnant and immunocompromised). We are told, however, that these two events are statistically independent. This tells us that we can use the simplified version of the multiplication rule illustrated for three statistically independent events in Equation (1.12). For the two statistically independent events of being pregnant and being immunocompromised, their intersection can be calculated as follows:

$$p(\text{preg and comp}) = p(\text{preg}) \cdot p(\text{comp}) = 0.2 \cdot 0.1 = 0.02$$

Now that we have the probability of the intersection of the two events, we are ready to calculate their union.

$$p(\text{preg and/or comp}) = p(\text{preg}) + p(\text{comp}) - p(\text{preg and comp})$$
$$= 0.2 + 0.1 - 0.02 = 0.28$$

Thus, we can expect that 28% of the persons we select from the population will be excluded from the study because they are either pregnant or immunocompromised (or both). ∎

As with the multiplication rule we used to calculate the probability of the intersection of events, the addition rule for calculation of the probability of the union of events has a simplified version that can be used under a special condition. For the addition rule, the condition is that the events are mutually exclusive. If so, the probability of the union of events can be calculated by simply adding together the probabilities of the events. The intersections of the events do not need to be subtracted from that sum because, by definition, the probability of the intersection of two mutually exclusive events is equal to 0.

1.3 BAYES' THEOREM

Earlier, we learned there are two types of events in a conditional probability: the conditional event(s) and the conditioning event(s). We also learned that these types of events have very different roles in a conditional probability. The conditional event is the event for which the probability is calculated (i.e., conditional probabilities tell us the chance of the conditional event occurring). All of the characteristics of unconditional probabilities (those discussed at the beginning of this chapter) apply to the conditional event. For instance, the probability of the complement of the conditional event is found by subtracting the conditional probability from 1 (see Equation (1.3)). Equation (1.14) shows that relationship for conditional probabilities:

$$p(\overline{A} \mid B) = 1 - p(A \mid B) \tag{1.14}$$

The conditioning event defines the condition under which we are interested in the probability of the conditional event. None of the characteristics of unconditional probabilities discussed at the beginning of this chapter apply to the conditioning event. For example, we cannot find the probability of the conditional event given that the conditioning event does not occur by subtracting from 1 the conditional probability given that the conditioning event occurs. Equation (1.15) shows this inequality in mathematical notation:

$$p(A \mid \overline{B}) \neq 1 - p(A \mid B) \qquad (1.15)$$

So, there are important differences in the way conditional and conditioning events affect interpretation of conditional probabilities. Under most circumstances, we need to only keep these differences in mind. Under some circumstances, however, the conditional probabilities we know something about have the conditional and conditioning events reversed relative to our interest. Examples of such "backward" conditional probabilities are the sensitivity and specificity of a diagnostic test. Sensitivity tells us the probability that a person with a particular disease (D) will have a positive test result (T). Specificity tells us the probability that a person without that disease $(\overline{D})$ will have a negative test result $(\overline{T})$. In mathematic notation, Equations (1.16) and (1.17) describe the sensitivity and specificity of a diagnostic test.

$$\text{Sensitivity} = p(T \mid D) \qquad (1.16)$$

$$\text{Specificity} = p(\overline{T} \mid \overline{D}) \qquad (1.17)$$

Since the conditioning event is having the disease, sensitivity can only be interpreted for those persons known to have the disease. Likewise, specificity can only be interpreted for those persons known not to have the disease. When a diagnostic test is used, however, it is not known whether or not the person has the disease. What is known is whether the test has a positive or negative result. To interpret a diagnostic test, we need to interchange the conditional and conditioning events in sensitivity and specificity.[8] The way we do this is by using **Bayes' theorem**. Equation (1.18) shows Bayes' theorem in general terms.

$$p(B \mid A) = \frac{p(B) \cdot p(A \mid B)}{[p(B) \cdot p(A \mid B)] + [p(\overline{B}) \cdot p(A \mid \overline{B})]} \qquad (1.18)$$

where

$p(B \mid A) = $ probability of event B occurring given event A has occurred

$p(B) = $ unconditional probability of event B occurring

---

[8] Since sensitivity and specificity are "backward" conditional probabilities, you might wonder why we use them to address the performance of a diagnostic test. The reason is the way studies examine diagnostic tests. In one study, the test is used on persons with the disease. That study estimates sensitivity. In another study, the test is used on persons without the disease. That study estimates specificity.

$p(A \mid B)$ = probability of event A occurring given event B has occurred

$p(\overline{B})$ = unconditional probability of event B not occurring

$p(A \mid \overline{B})$ = probability of event A occurring given event B has not occurred.

Example 1.4 applies Bayes' theorem to sensitivity and specificity.

■ EXAMPLE 1.4

Suppose we are screening a particular population for cervical cancer. In that population, 1 out of 1,000 women has cervical cancer. The diagnostic test we use for screening has a sensitivity of 0.9 and a specificity of 0.7. What is the probability a person with a positive test result really has cervical cancer?

To begin with, let us take a look at the information we have. Knowing that 1 out of 1,000 women in the population have cervical cancer tells us that the probability that any particular woman has cervical cancer is 0.001. A sensitivity of 0.9 implies that a person with cervical cancer has a 90% chance of having a positive test result and a specificity of 0.7 implies that a person without cervical cancer has a 70% chance of having a negative test result. In mathematic notation, we know

$$p(D) = 0.001$$

$$p(T \mid D) = 0.9$$

$$p(\overline{T} \mid \overline{D}) = 0.7$$

Our interest is in the probability of a person with a positive test result has cervical cancer. At first this sounds like the sensitivity, but it is not the same thing. In sensitivity, our interest is confined to people who have the disease. To interpret a positive test result, however, we need to confine our interest to persons with a positive result. Thus, our interest is in the same events that make up sensitivity, but with the conditional and conditioning events transposed. We can transpose conditional and conditioning events by using Bayes' theorem (from Equation (1.18)).

$$p(D \mid T) = \frac{p(D) \cdot p(T \mid D)}{[p(D) \cdot p(T \mid D)] + [p(\overline{D}) \cdot p(T \mid \overline{D})]}$$

$$= \frac{0.001 \cdot 0.9}{[0.001 \cdot 0.9] + [(1 - 0.001) \cdot (1 - 0.7)]} = 0.003$$

So, the probability that a woman with a positive test result has cervical cancer is 0.003. You might be surprised that this probability is so low. The principal reason for this is the fact that cervical cancer occurs in only 1 out of 1,000 women. Among women with a positive test result, this changes to 3 out of 1,000. So, the chance of cervical cancer is three times as great among women with a positive test result, but it is still a low probability (i.e., 0.003). Bayes' theorem has helped us to appreciate the meaning of a positive test result when the diagnostic test is used for screening this population. ■

Now that we have an understanding of probabilities, we are ready to apply what we have learned to the process of taking samples from populations. In the next chapter, we will begin doing this by focusing on populations.

CHAPTER SUMMARY

In Chapter 1, we learned that probabilities are useful in thinking about events (things that occur or characteristics that exist) relative to observations (opportunities for things to occur or characteristics to exist). When thinking about probabilities, we use literary, graphic, or mathematic language. In literary language, a probability is the frequency of events relative to the number of observations. In graphic language, we use Venn diagrams to think about probabilities. In Venn diagrams, a circular area usually represents occurrences of the event and a rectangle represents the observations. Then, the probability of the event is reflected by the area of the circle relative to the area of the rectangle. Mathematically, probabilities are proportions, because the number of events is part of the number of observations.

Regardless of which language we use to think about probabilities, we notice that probabilities have certain properties. One of these is that a probability must have a value within the range of 0 to 1. A probability of 0 tells us that the event never occurs. A probability of 1 tells us that the event always occurs. Probabilities between 0 and 1 tell us that the event sometimes occurs.

In addition to thinking about single events, we can use probabilities to think about collections of events. The first collection of events considered in Chapter 1 includes the event and its complement. The complement of an event includes everything that could happen in an observation except the event. Events and their complements always have two characteristics. One is that they are always collectively exhaustive. Events are collectively exhaustive when at least one of the events must occur in every observation. Another characteristic of events and their complements is that they are mutually exclusive. Being mutually exclusive means that, at most, only one of the events can occur in a particular observation.

We can have collections of events other than just a particular event and its complement. Other collections of events might be collectively exhaustive and/or mutually exclusive. An event and its complement, however, are always collectively exhaustive and mutually exclusive.

With other collections of events, we can be interested in two types of relationships of the events. These are the intersection and the union of those events. In an intersection of events, we are interested in those observations in which all of the events occur. In a union of events, we are interested in those observations in which at least one of the events occurs.

When we are interested in the intersection of events, we can use the multiplication rule to calculate the probability of the intersection of events. There are two versions of the multiplication rule. The simplified version involves multiplying the probabilities of each event together. This simplified version is appropriate if the events are statistically independent (from each other). That is, if the probability of each event is the same regardless of whether the other event(s) occur(s). The full version of the multiplication rule uses conditional probabilities.

Many of the probabilities we encounter in health research and practice are conditional probabilities. What distinguishes conditional probabilities from other probabilities is the fact that conditional probabilities address a subset of the observations, rather than all of the observations. That subset of observations is specified by the conditioning event(s). The event(s) addressed by the conditional probability is specified by the conditional event(s). If events are statistically independent, then the probability of the conditional event occurring is the same regardless of whether the conditioning event occurs.

When we are interested in the union of events, we use the addition rule to calculate the probability of the union. There are two versions of the addition rule. In the simplified version, the probabilities of the events in the union are added together. This simplified version of the addition rule can be used when the events are mutually exclusive. If the events are not mutually exclusive, the probabilities of their intersections need to be taken into account.

The conditional and conditioning events in conditional probabilities have very different functions. A conditional probability addresses the probability that the conditional event(s) will occur under the assumption that the conditioning event(s) has occurred. Often, we find we are interested in the probability that the conditioning event will occur assuming the conditional event has occurred. One example of this situation is the relationship among the probabilities used in interpreting diagnostic tests. Tests are characterized by their sensitivities and specificities. The conditioning events in sensitivity and specificity are whether or not a person has the disease. To interpret the result of a diagnostic test, however, we want to consider the probability that a person has the disease. In other words, we want to change whether someone has the disease from being the conditioning event to be the conditional event. The way in which we exchange conditional and conditioning events is by using Bayes' theorem.

EXERCISES

1.1. In a particular high school, 40 of the 200 graduating seniors report they have had unprotected sexual intercourse and 100 of the 200 graduating seniors report they have tried smoking marijuana at least once during high school. Further, 30 of the 100 graduating seniors who report they have tried smoking marijuana have also had unprotected sexual intercourse. Based on that information, which of the following is the best description of the relationship between having unprotected sexual intercourse and smoking marijuana?

   A. Having unprotected sexual intercourse and smoking marijuana are not statistically independent, but they are mutually exclusive.

B. Having unprotected sexual intercourse and smoking marijuana are statistically independent, but they are not mutually exclusive.

C. Having unprotected sexual intercourse and smoking marijuana are both statistically independent and mutually exclusive.

D. Having unprotected sexual intercourse and smoking marijuana are neither statistically independent nor mutually exclusive.

E. There is not enough information given here to determine statistical independence and mutual exclusion of having unprotected sexual intercourse and smoking marijuana.

1.2. Suppose 25% of the children in a certain elementary school developed nausea and vomiting following a holiday party. None of the children who drank the apple cider at that party became ill. Based on that information, which of the following is the best description of the relationship between becoming ill and drinking apple cider at the party?

A. Becoming ill and drinking cider are not statistically independent but they are mutually exclusive.

B. Becoming ill and drinking cider are statistically independent but they are not mutually exclusive.

C. Becoming ill and drinking cider are both statistically independent and mutually exclusive.

D. Becoming ill and drinking cider are neither statistically independent nor mutually exclusive.

E. There is not enough information given here to determine statistical independence and mutual exclusion of becoming ill and drinking cider.

1.3. In a particular population, 30% of the people smoke cigarettes and 10% of the people have chronic obstructive pulmonary disease (COPD). If having COPD is independent of smoking, what percent of the population would you expect to find who smoke and also have COPD?

A. 0%

B. 3%

C. 10%

D. 30%

E. 40%

1.4. In a particular population, 5% of the infants have a low birthweight (<2,500 gm) and 60% of the mothers have at least 16 years of education. If having a mother with at least 16 years of education and having a low birthweight are statistically independent, which of the following is closest to the percentage of infants who have a mother with at least 16 years of education and who have a low birthweight?

A. 0%

B. 3%

C. 6%

D. 30%

E. 40%

1.5. Suppose in a population of 10,000 persons, 5,000 smoke cigarettes and 7,500 have a high-fat diet. Further, suppose that among the 5,000 persons who smoke cigarettes there are 3,000 who are also among the 7,500 who have a high-fat diet. Based on that information, which of the following is closest to the percentage of persons in the population who smoke cigarettes and/or have a high-fat diet?

A. 38%

B. 50%

C. 75%

D. 95%

E. 125%

1.6. In a particular population, 60% of infants receive only their mother's breast milk, 20% receive only commercial infant formula, and 20% receive both. What is the chance that a particular infant selected randomly would receive breast milk and/or formula?

A. 0%

B. 20%

C. 80%

D. 100%

E. 120%

1.7. Suppose we are interested in the efficacy of a new treatment for anemia. To investigate this treatment, we randomly assign 50 persons with anemia to receive the new treatment and 50 persons with anemia to receive the standard treatment. Among those 100 persons, suppose 60% are cured. If there is no association between treatment and the chance of being cured, what percentage of the persons who received the new treatment would we expect to be cured?

A. 0%

B. 30%

C. 36%

D. 50%

E. 60%

1.8. In a certain industry, 20% of the workers develop liver disease and 40% develop respiratory disease. If there is no association between developing liver disease and developing respiratory disease, what percentage of the workers who develop liver disease would we expect to also develop respiratory disease?

A. 8%

B. 20%

C. 40%

D. 52%

E. 60%

CHAPTER 2

DESCRIBING DISTRIBUTIONS

The purpose of research is to describe a population. In a very general sense, what we want to do is to describe the **distribution** of data in the population (Figure 2.1). A distribution of data tells us not only which data values exist in a population but also how frequently each value occurs. In this chapter, we will take a look at the distribution of data in the population and see how we can use knowledge of that distribution to take chance into account.

Introduction to Biostatistical Applications in Health Research with Microsoft Office Excel® and R,
Second Edition. Robert P. Hirsch.
© 2021 John Wiley & Sons, Inc. Published 2021 by John Wiley & Sons, Inc.
Companion website: www.wiley.com/go/hirsch/healthresearch2e

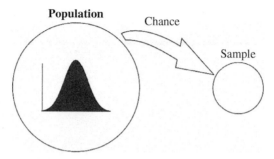

Figure 2.1 Our purpose in research is to describe distributions of data in a population.

2.1 TYPES OF DATA

One of the things that determines the distribution of data in the population is the type of data it describes. For our purpose, there are three types of data: continuous, ordinal, and nominal. An important part of understanding statistical methods is being able to distinguish these three types of data, so we will begin thinking about distributions by describing these three types of data.

Continuous data have a large number of possible values,[1] which are evenly spaced. By "evenly spaced" we mean that a change in value of one unit is the same regardless of where in the range of possible values that the change occurs. Examples of continuous data include age, weight, blood pressure, and pH.

Ordinal data have values that can be ordered,[2] but the values are not considered to be evenly spaced. In fact, any intrinsic spacing between values is ignored when we consider the data to be ordinal. Examples of ordinal data include the number of persons in a household, patient satisfaction scores, and stages of disease.

Nominal data differ from ordinal data in that they cannot be ordered in any relevant way. Also included as nominal data are any data that have only two possible values. Examples of nominal data include gender, race, disease status (e.g., active vs. in remission), and country of origin.

There are two ways we describe the distribution of data in a population. One way is to describe that distribution graphically. The other is to describe them mathematically.[3] We will begin with the graphic approach.

---

[1] The formal definition of continuous data states that these data have an infinite number of possible values. In practice, however, we are able to measure only a finite number of possible values. Recognition of this fact allows us to analyze data that do not really have an infinite number of possible values (like the number of hairs on your head) as though they were continuous.

[2] For a statistician to consider a set of data to be ordered, the data must consist of a minimum of three different values. As a result, data with only two possible values are considered to be nominal data.

[3] A third way we might try to describe distributions is in literary language. For example, we could say that a distribution is a symmetric bell-shaped curve.

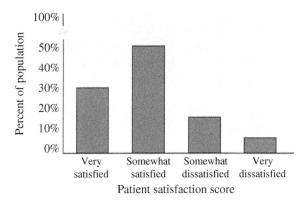

Figure 2.2   A bar graph of the distribution of patient satisfaction scores.

2.2 DESCRIBING DISTRIBUTIONS GRAPHICALLY

The types of graphs we use can be separated into two groups. One group is for **continuous data**. The other is for either ordinal or nominal data, both of which are considered to be **discrete data**. First, we will look at graphing discrete data, since the options for discrete data are more limited than the options for continuous data.

2.2.1   Graphing Discrete Data

For discrete data, we usually describe the distribution graphically by using a **bar graph**. In a bar graph, data values are listed on the horizontal axis and how frequently each value occurs is indicated by the vertical axis. Figure 2.2 illustrates a distribution of ordinal data arranged in a bar graph.

Next, let us take a look at an example that illustrates how a bar graph is constructed to describe discrete data graphically.

■ **EXAMPLE 2.1**

In the United States, the ABO blood group phenotypes occur with percentages approximately equal to the values in the following table:

Phenotype	Percent
O	45
A	40
B	10
AB	5

Let us describe these data graphically as a bar graph.

These are nominal data, because they describe categories that cannot be ordered in any relevant way. When drawing a graph of nominal data, there is no prescribed order for the bars. The table lists the phenotypes in order of decreasing percentages. The following bar graph is organized in the same way.

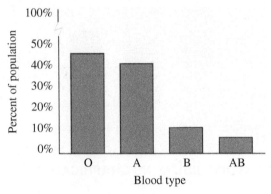

Excel and R can be used to construct a bar graph. The next example illustrates the construction of a bar graph for the data in Example 2.1 using Excel and R.

■ EXAMPLE 2.2

Many kinds of graphs can be constructed in Excel. Most of them can be found under the INSERT tab.[4] The graph most similar to the bar graph is called a **column chart** in Excel. To create a bar graph, select the data and then select a column chart.

This is the column chart we obtain for the data in Example 2.1:

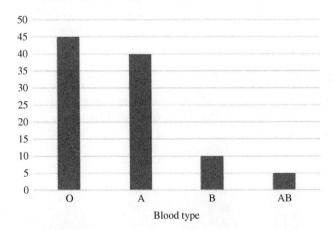

---

[4]Mac users use the "Chart" tab.

That bar graph is acceptable for personal use, but axis titles and an informative chart title need to be included. To change the chart title, double click on the default title. To create axis titles, click on the DESIGN tab under CHART TOOLS. Then expand Add Chart Element and select Axis titles. The following is an example of adding titles:

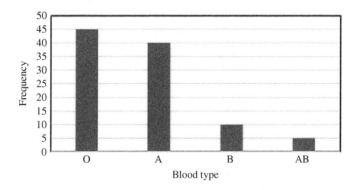

A bar graph can also be constructed in R. To do that, we first create a table. The easiest way to create a table is to copy it from Excel. First, create a table of blood types in Excel and copy it to the clipboard.[5] Then, create the table in R with the following command:

>PHENOTYPE <- read.table("clipboard")

Then, create the bar graph, enter the following command:

>barplot(table(PHENOTYPE))

This results in the following bar graph:

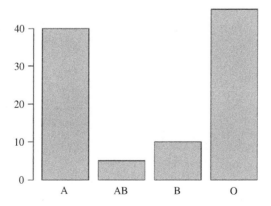

[5] Another way to import an Excel spreadsheet into R is described in Appendix E.

To this, we can add axis labels.

>barplot(table(PHENOTYPE),xlab="Blood Type",ylab="Frequency")

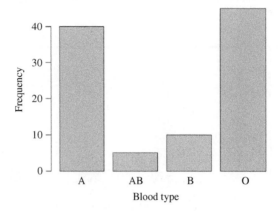

■

2.2.2 Graphing Continuous Data

If we were to use a bar graph to display continuous data, we would need to have a very large number of bars if each bar represented a single data value.[6] Instead, we use a **histogram** to display the distribution of continuous data. In a histogram,

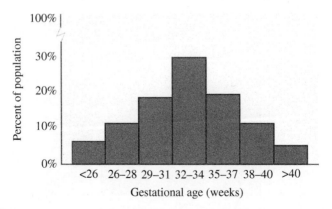

Figure 2.3 Histogram illustrating the distribution of gestational ages in a population.

[6]Theoretically, there are an infinite number of possible values for continuous data. This implies that we would need to have an infinite number of bars if each bar represented a single data value.

each bar represents an interval of data values rather than a single value. Also, we remind ourselves that the bars in a histogram represent a continuum of data, rather than discrete values, by drawing the bars so that they touch each other.[7] Figure 2.3 illustrates a distribution of continuous data displayed in a histogram.

In the next example, we will see how a histogram is constructed from continuous data values.

■ EXAMPLE 2.3

Suppose we were to measure changes in serum cholesterol levels before and after one month on a low-fat diet for 11 patients newly diagnosed with hypercholesterolemia. Imagine the following are the values we observe when the serum cholesterol levels after the diet are subtracted from the serum cholesterol levels before the diet: 10, 42, −5, 9, −2, 0, 16, 28, 4, 5, and 3 mg/dL. Let us graphically describe these data as a histogram.

To construct a histogram, we need to define the intervals of values that will correspond to each bar. There are two aspects of these intervals that we need to consider. First, we need to decide how wide the intervals will be. The fewer the data values we will graph, the larger the intervals need to be to give an impression of the shape of the distribution (otherwise, many bars would be missing since the interval includes no observations). Next, we need to decide where to begin the first interval. This choice can also change the appearance of the histogram, especially if there are few data values.

For this histogram, let us use 10 mg/dL for the width of the intervals. This will give us 5 bars representing these 11 data values. If we were to start the first interval at −10 mg/dL, we would get the following histogram:

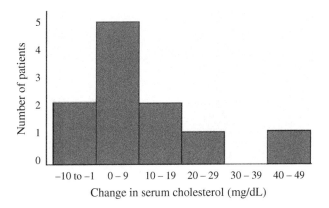

---

[7] You can make bars in a column chart touch by right clicking on one of the bars and selecting "Format Data Series." Then set "Gap Width" to zero.

On the other hand, if we were to start the first interval at −5 mg/dL, we would get the following histogram:

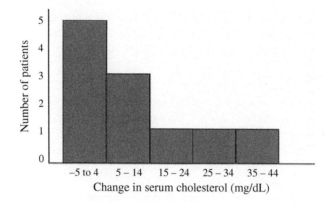

Both of these histograms are correct. Even so, they give a somewhat different impression about the shape of the distribution. As the number of bars in the histogram increases, the choice of where to begin the first interval has less effect on the histogram's shape.

With Excel, we can construct a histogram using "Data Analysis." Excel also gives us the option of defining the ranges of data ("**bins**") or it will make its own selection. Histograms can be found in the "DATA" tab under "Data Analysis." To create Excel's version of a histogram, select the "Histogram" analysis tool in "Data Analysis." You need to select the "Chart" option in the "Histogram" dialog box to have it create a graph.

If we use Excel to create a histogram for these data, we get the following output:

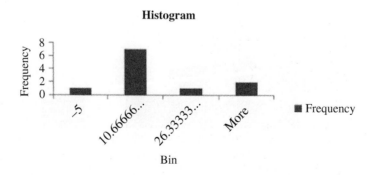

Unfortunately, Excel fails to create a true histogram with the bars touching, but we can still use it to graphically examine continuous data. The "bins" are the upper limits of the data intervals that define each bar. The way Excel has decided to create the bins, its histogram is most like the first one we constructed in this example.

In R, we can create a histogram from a vector of changes in serum cholesterol (named CHGCHOL)[8] as follows:

>hist(CHGCHOL)

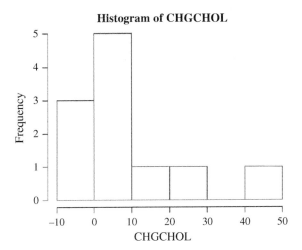

Histogram of CHGCHOL

There are many other ways continuous data can be described graphically. One that has been commonly used in statistical analysis software is the **stem-and-leaf plot**.[9]

The stem-and-leaf plot is similar to a histogram, but with two differences. The first difference is that the data values are listed vertically, instead of horizontally as in a histogram. The second difference is that a stem-and-leaf plot displays all of the data values in addition to the frequency of data in specified intervals as in a histogram. Thus, the stem-and-leaf plot provides more information about the data than does the histogram.

The first step in constructing a stem-and-leaf plot is to define the intervals of data that will be used. To define those intervals, we consider all but the right-most digit in each data value. For example, a data value of 2.5 could be assigned to the interval that includes values from 2.0 to 2.9.[10] These groups make up the "stem" of a stem-and-leaf plot. This is the same process that we use to begin construction of a histogram, but a stem-and-leaf plot represents groups as separate rows in a table instead of bars in a graph. The next step in developing a stem-and-leaf plot is to

[8] See Appendix E to learn how to create such a dataset in R.
[9] The reason the stem-and-leaf plot is a popular choice in statistical analysis software has its origin in the days when computer output was limited to typing ASCII characters. These are the only characters needed to produce a stem-and-leaf plot.
[10] If there are more than a few data values to be plotted, intervals can represent a smaller range of values. For instance, one interval might include values from 2.0 to 2.4 and another interval might include values from 2.5 to 2.9.

represent each data value in a particular row according to the value of the right-most digit (these are the "leaves").

This sounds confusing, but it will be clearer when we look at an example of a stem-and-leaf plot (Example 2.4).

■ EXAMPLE 2.4

In Example 2.3, we constructed a histogram to describe changes in serum cholesterol levels before and after one month on a low-fat diet for 11 patients newly diagnosed with hypercholesterolemia. The differences in serum cholesterol levels were 10, 42, 5, 9, −2, 0, 16, 28, 4 −5, and 3 mg/dL. Let us graphically describe these data using a stem-and-leaf plot.

To begin with, let us sort the data by decreasing numeric magnitude and then separate the right-most digits from the other digits. If there is only one digit in a data value, the other digit is represented by 0 (or 0 when the data are negative).

Data Value	Other Digits	Right-Most Digit
42	4	2
28	2	8
16	1	6
10	1	0
9	0	9
5	0	5
4	0	4
3	0	3
0	0	0
−2	−0	2
−5	−0	5

Next, we create groups according to the value of the "other" digits. Each possible value for these "other" digits is included, even if there are no data values observed in that interval.

Stem	Leaves
4	2
3	
2	8
1	06
0	03459
−0	25

This is a stem-and-leaf plot for the data in Example 2.3. The number of right-most digits in each group tells us how frequently data values occur in that group. This is the same information we get when we use a histogram to describe continuous data graphically. With a stem-and-leaf plot, however, the "bars" extend horizontally instead of vertically (compare this plot with the first histogram in Example 2.3). In addition, the value of the right-most digit is listed in a stem-and-leaf plot, telling us the actual numeric data value.   ■

Another way to describe a distribution of continuous data graphically is by using a line instead of bars to represent the frequency with which data values occur. This type of graph is called a **frequency polygon**. To begin thinking about a frequency polygon, we can think about a histogram with a line connecting the middle of the upper extreme of each bar. Each of the bars in a histogram represents an interval of continuous data. If we have lots of data values (as in a population), we can make each bar represent a narrower interval of values. The result will be that the number of bars in the histogram will increase and the width of each bar will decrease. Also, as the number of bars increases, the line representing these bars becomes smoother. Figure 2.4 shows this process.

Now, if we were to imagine making each of the bars represent a single data value, the histogram would consist of an infinite number of infinitely narrow bars. When that happens, the bars in the histogram disappear, leaving just the line that traces the tops of all of the bars, creating a frequency polygon. Figure 2.5 illustrates a frequency polygon.

So, one of the ways we can think about distributions of data in the population is graphically. Next, we will see how these distributions can be represented mathematically.

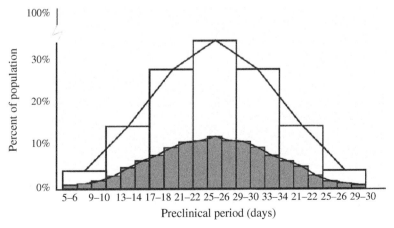

Figure 2.4   Smoothing of the line connecting the upper midpoints of each bar as the interval represented by each bar decreases and the number of bars increases.

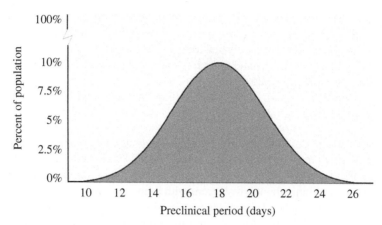

Figure 2.5 A frequency polygon representing the distribution of preclinical periods (continuous data) for a hypothetical disease.

2.3 DESCRIBING DISTRIBUTIONS MATHEMATICALLY

An advantage of a frequency polygon is that the line can be described mathematically as well as graphically. We will not be looking at the actual mathematical formulas for distributions. Instead, we will identify a distribution by naming it and by providing the details needed so that one particular distribution is described.

In Figure 2.5, we see a symmetric bell-shaped curve that is very commonly used by statisticians to take chance into account. This is a **Gaussian distribution**.[11] When we name our distribution a Gaussian distribution, the statistician thinks of a mathematical equation that can be used to calculate probabilities of getting various data values from the population.

Naming the distribution a Gaussian distribution, however, is not enough to allow the statistician to calculate probabilities. The problem is that there are lots of different Gaussian distributions. These distributions differ according to where they are centered on the continuum of data values and according to how spread out they are around their center. If we specify these two characteristics, we can describe one unique Gaussian distribution completely.

The characteristics that mathematically describe a particular distribution are called **parameters** of the distribution. A Gaussian distribution has two parameters. One is a parameter of **location** that tells us where the distribution is centered. The other is a parameter of **dispersion** that tells us how spread out the data values are. If we want to describe a particular Gaussian distribution, we need to provide numeric values for these two parameters.

---

[11] The Gaussian distribution is also called the **normal distribution**.

2.3.1 Parameter of Location

The parameter that tells us where a Gaussian distribution is centered on the continuum of possible values is the **mean**. Figure 2.6 shows Gaussian distributions that have different means.

The mean is probably the most often used and best understood value we calculate from a distribution of data. Even so, if asked to define the mean of a population, you would probably rely on a mathematical definition. Specifically, you would (most likely) suggest that a population's mean is the sum of all data values divided by the number of data values in the population. In mathematical language, the mean of the population's distribution of data is represented as shown in Equation (2.1):

$$\mu = \frac{\sum Y_i}{N} \tag{2.1}$$

where

μ = mean of the distribution of data in the population (symbolized with the Greek letter "mu")

N = number of data values in the population

$\sum Y_i$ = sum ($\sum$) of the individual data values (Y_i) in the population

Another way to understand the mean of a distribution of data, however, is by imagining the distribution to be a three-dimensional object instead of a two-dimensional one. Then the mean can be thought of as the center of gravity

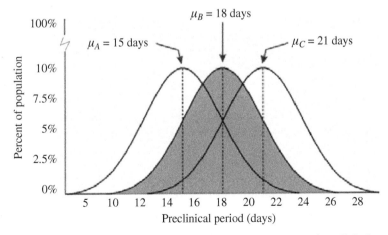

Figure 2.6 Three frequency polygons representing the distributions of preclinical periods for a hypothetical disease in three populations (*A*, *B*, and *C*), each of which has a different mean.

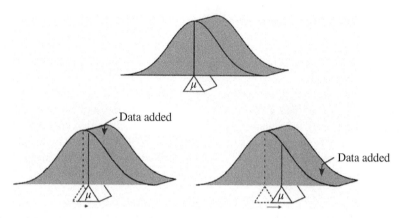

Figure 2.7 Illustration of the mean being the center of gravity of a distribution of data. Like a center of gravity, the position of the mean is affected more by data added farther from it than it is by data added closer to it.

of the distribution. In other words, the mean is the point in a distribution at which the distribution "balances" (there is an equal "weight" of data above and below the mean). Adding data values just above the mean will cause the mean to shift slightly to the right, whereas adding data far above the mean will cause the mean to shift substantially to the right. This conceptualization of the mean is illustrated in Figure 2.7.

Although the mean of a distribution of continuous data is the parameter of location that is used in the mathematical description of the Gaussian distribution, there are other ways the location of a distribution can be represented. The most commonly used alternative to the mean is the **median**. The median is the physical center (rather than the center of gravity) of a distribution. That is to say, the median is selected so that half of the data values are greater than the median and half are less than the median.[12] Extreme observations cause the median to move in the direction of the observation, but, unlike the mean, the amount the median moves is the same regardless of whether the observations added are close to or far from the median. Thus, the median is less affected by the addition of extreme data values than is the mean.

For a symmetric distribution (e.g., a Gaussian distribution), the mean and the median are equal. When a distribution is asymmetric (i.e., **skewed**), the mean will be closer to the extreme data values than will the median. This is illustrated in Figure 2.8.

Another measure of location is the **mode**. The mode is the most frequently occurring data value. An advantage of the mode is that it can be determined for nominal data. It is not used in health research as a measure of location for distributions of continuous or ordinal data, because it communicates so little information about the location of a distribution of data.

---

[12]The median can be used to specify the location of ordinal data, but it is not a parameter, since it does not fit into a mathematical representation of the distribution the way the mean does.

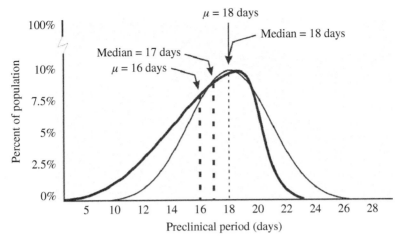

Figure 2.8 Relationship between the mean and the median. For a symmetric distribution (lighter), the mean and the median are equal to the same value. For a skewed distribution (darker), the mean is closer to the most extreme values than is the median.

Now, let us take a look at an example (Example 2.5) in which we will calculate and compare the mean and median of a skewed distribution.

■ EXAMPLE 2.5

In Examples 2.3 and 2.4, we looked at the change in serum cholesterol levels for 11 persons on a low-fat diet. Now, let us use these same data to calculate the mean and the median change in serum cholesterol as if those persons made up the entire population. To calculate the mean, we use Equation (2.1)

$$\mu = \frac{\sum Y_i}{N} = \frac{10 + 42 + 5 + \cdots + 4 - 5 + 3}{11} = \frac{110}{11} = 10 \,\mathrm{mg/dL}$$

To find the median, we begin by arranging the observations in order of numeric magnitude:

Order	1	2	3	4	5	**6**	7	8	9	10	11
Value	−5	−2	0	3	4	**5**	9	10	16	28	42

When there is an odd number of data values, the median is the middle value.[13] Here, we have 11 data values, so the median is the sixth largest value. This is the

---

[13] The median is easiest to calculate for an odd number of data values for which there is one, and only one middle value. That is to say, when there are no other values equal to the middle value. For instance, suppose that the fifth largest data value in Example 2.5 was also equal to 5 mg/dL. If that were the case, 5 mg/dL is not really the median value, since there are four values below it and five values above

median since there are five values above it and five values below it. In this case, the median of the changes in serum cholesterol levels is equal to 5 mg/dL (in bold).

In this example, the mean (10 mg/dL) is considerably larger than the median (5 mg/dL). This implies that the distribution of data values is asymmetric with a few extreme (in this case, higher) data values that affect the mean more than the median. In Example 2.3, we constructed a histogram for these data. From the histogram, it is clear that the distribution has that kind of asymmetry.

Here, we have an odd number of data values, so the median is the number in the middle. When there is an even number of data values, we usually say that the median is equal to the mean of the two numbers in the middle. For instance, suppose that we have data from a 12th person and that person's change in serum cholesterol is greater than 9 mg/dL (for the median, it does not matter how much greater). Then, the median would be the mean of 5 and 9 mg/dL as follows:

$$\text{Median} = \frac{5 + 9}{2} = 7 \text{ mg/dL} \qquad \blacksquare$$

The median can also be called the **50th percentile**. Percentiles tell us what percentage of the data values occurs before a particular datum. Two other useful percentiles are the **25th percentile** and the **75th percentile**. These designate the first and last quarters of the data values.

If a distribution is symmetric, the median will be equidistant from the 25th and 75th percentiles. This relationship is sometimes examined graphically in a **box and whisker plot**. The "box" represents the 25th and 75th percentiles (the **interquartile range**). Within this box, the median is represented as a vertical line. The symmetry of a distribution is reflected by the degree to which the median falls equidistant from the limits of the box. The "whiskers" are lines extending from the two vertical sides of the box. The length of these lines can be used to represent a number of different

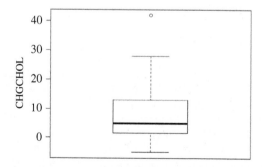

Figure 2.9   Box and whisker plot of the change in serum cholesterol from R.

it. Unfortunately, statisticians do not agree as to what should be done to find the median in this case. Fortunately, the different methods for determining the median in this circumstance give us values for those that are usually close to each other in numeric magnitude.

aspects of the data. Frequently, the lengths of the two lines represent the range of the data values. R provides a box and whisker plot in response to the "boxplot()" command. Figure 2.9 shows a boxplot from R. By default, in R the whiskers extend to the extreme data point that is no more than 1.5 times the interquartile range. The extreme data value beyond 1.5 times the interquartile range (42) is indicated by a small circle.

Both the mean and the median are measures of location, but it is the mean that is used to describe the location of a Gaussian distribution since it fits into the mathematical description of that distribution. Next, we will take a look at ways we can describe the dispersion of a distribution of continuous data.

2.3.2 Parameter of Dispersion

For data from a Gaussian distribution, even after the location of the distribution has been specified using the mean, there are still an infinite number of possible distributions with that same mean. These distributions differ in how much the data vary from the mean. Figure 2.10 illustrates Gaussian distributions with the same mean, but with different dispersions around the mean.

Graphically, we can see that the farther the data values in a distribution are, on the average, from the mean of the distribution, the more the dispersion. To describe the average distance between data values and the mean, we might use Equation (2.1), substituting differences between the data values and the mean for the data values in the numerator of that equation. Then, we could calculate the mean distance between the data values and the mean. This modification of Equation (2.1) is shown in Equation (2.2):

$$\text{Mean difference from the mean} = \frac{\sum Y_i - \mu}{N} \qquad (2.2)$$

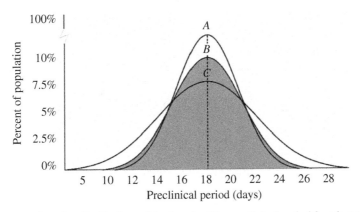

Figure 2.10 Gaussian distributions of the length of the preclinical period for a hypothetical disease in each of three populations. All three populations in this figure have the same mean, but they have different dispersions of preclinical periods. Preclinical periods in population A are the least dispersed and preclinical periods in population C are the most dispersed.

One surprising feature of Equation (2.2) is that it is always equal to 0, regardless of how dispersed the data values are! This is because the mean is the "center of gravity" of a distribution, and thus there is an equal "weight" of data on either side of the mean. In other words, the sum of the positive differences from the mean will always be exactly equal to the sum of the negative differences.[14] To make Equation (2.2) useful as a measure of the amount of dispersion in a distribution of continuous data, we need to keep the negative differences from canceling the positive differences. The way statisticians do this is by squaring the differences between each data value and the mean before adding them up.[15] Equation (2.3) illustrates this calculation:

$$\sigma^2 = \frac{\sum (Y_i - \mu)^2}{N} \tag{2.3}$$

where

σ^2 = variance of the distribution of data in the population (symbolized by the Greek letter "sigma" squared)

Y_i = a data value

μ = mean of the distribution of data in the population

N = number of data values in the population

The value calculated in Equation (2.3) is the parameter of dispersion for the Gaussian distribution. It is called the **variance** of the distribution and we symbolize it using the Greek letter sigma squared (σ^2). The reason that we use a squared sigma is to remind us that the units of measurement for the variance are the square of the units for the data. Thus, the variances of the distributions in Figure 2.10 have days^2 as their units of measurement.

To express the dispersion of a distribution in the same units in which the data are measured, we often take the square root of the variance as the value that describes the dispersion of a distribution of continuous data. The square root of the variance is called the **standard deviation**. The relationship between the variance and the standard deviation is illustrated in Equation (2.4):

$$\sigma = \sqrt{\sigma^2} = \sqrt{\frac{\sum (Y_i - \mu)^2}{N}} \tag{2.4}$$

where

σ = the standard deviation of the distribution of data in the population (symbolized with the Greek letter "sigma")

σ^2 = the variance of the distribution of data in the population

---

[14] This is true whether or not the distribution is symmetrical.

[15] Statisticians often use this solution of squaring to deal with negative values. We will encounter this several times in the remaining chapters of this text.

Y_i = a data value

μ = the mean of the distribution of data in the population

N = the number of data values in the population

Except that the variance has squared units of measure and the standard deviation has the same units of measure as do the data, there is no difference between the two. When asked "What is the measure of dispersion of a Gaussian distribution?" we can respond with either the variance or the standard deviation. Both are correct.[16]

Now, let us take a look at an example (Example 2.6) in which we determine the variance and the standard deviation of a distribution of data.

◼ EXAMPLE 2.6

In Examples 2.2 through 2.4, we looked at the change in serum cholesterol levels for 11 persons on a low-fat diet. In Example 2.4, we found that the mean change in serum cholesterol is equal to 10 mg/dL. Now, let us use these same data to calculate the variance and standard deviation of change in serum cholesterol for that group of 11 patients as if those persons made up the entire population.

To calculate the variance, we use Equation (2.3). To prepare for that calculation, it is easier to keep track of things if we arrange the data in a table. Also, it is helpful to use the table to calculate the values we will use in the numerator of Equation (2.3).

Patient	Y_i	$Y_i - \mu$	$(Y_i - \mu)^2$
TY	10	0	0
HT	42	32	1,024
IO	5	−5	25
SO	9	−1	1
IM	−2	−12	144
SU	0	−10	100
RC	16	6	36
EH	28	18	324
AF	4	−6	36
LU	−5	−15	225
LN	3	−7	49
Total	110	0	1,964

Notice that one of the columns we have included in the table gives the differences between each data value and the mean of all of the data. As implied by Equation (2.2), this adds up to 0. Including this column in our calculations can help us check for calculation errors.

[16] In fact, both the variance and the standard deviation appear in the mathematical formula for the Gaussian distribution.

Now, let us calculate the variance of these data using Equation (2.3):

$$\sigma^2 = \frac{\sum (Y_i - \mu)^2}{N} = \frac{1{,}964}{11} = 178.5 \text{ mg/dL}^2$$

Also, we can use Equation (2.4) to calculate the standard deviation of changes in serum cholesterol among these 11 patients:

$$\sigma = \sqrt{\sigma^2} = \sqrt{178.5} = 13.4 \text{ mg/dL}$$

Thus, we can say that the average squared difference between all of the data values and the mean is equal to 178.5 mg/dL^2, or we could express the dispersion of changes in serum cholesterol in mg/dL by saying that the standard deviation is equal to 13.4 mg/dL.   ■

The variance (or the standard deviation) is the parameter of dispersion for the Gaussian distribution. There are other ways we might express dispersion, however, even if they are not parameters of the Gaussian distribution. One example is the **range**. The range is the difference between the lowest and the highest data values. The range, however, has limits as a measure of dispersion of the distribution of data in the population. The primary reason for this is that the range uses a very limited amount of information about the distribution; it reflects the relationship between only two data values (i.e., the lowest and the highest values). The dispersion of all of the remaining data values does not affect the value of the range. This feature makes the range incapable of reflecting other aspects of dispersion. For example, Figure 2.11 illustrates how two distributions can have the same range, but be substantially different in their amount of dispersion.

Another characteristic of the range that diminishes its usefulness as a measure of dispersion is the fact that it is influenced by the number of data values in the distribution.[17] The reason for this is the fact that the most extreme data values are usually the most infrequently occurring values. As the number of data values in a distribution increases, it becomes more likely that the distribution will include those extreme values. Thus, we can expect to see the values of the range increase as the number of data values increases, even if there is no change in the variance and standard deviation of the distribution.

There is another measure of dispersion that is related to the range, but that is not influenced by the number of data values in the distribution. This measure of dispersion is the interquartile range. A quartile consists of one-quarter of the data values. To calculate the interquartile range, the distribution is first divided in half by determining the median. Then, the median of each half is used to separate the entire

---

[17]We usually think of populations as having a very large number of data values (i.e., N is a very large number). In large populations, this is not an important problem. In smaller populations and especially in samples from populations, this can seriously affect the usefulness of the range as a measure of dispersion.

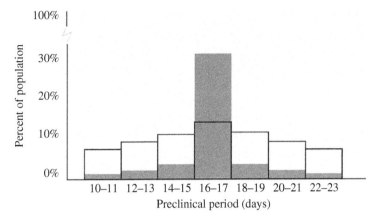

Figure 2.11   Histograms of two distributions with the same range, but different variances. The distribution represented by the shaded bars has very little dispersion, since most of the persons have a preclinical period between 16 and 17 days. The distribution represented by unfilled bars, however, has quite a bit of dispersion, since there are a substantial number of persons with preclinical periods throughout the entire range of values.

distribution into four equal parts. The interquartile range is the distance between the extremes of the middle two quartiles (the 25th and 75th percentiles), which delineates the middle half of the distribution.

We will see how to calculate an interquartile range shortly, but first let us consider how to interpret it. Probably the easiest way to interpret the interquartile range is to relate it to the standard deviation. If we were to multiply the interquartile range from a Gaussian distribution by 2/3, it would be equal to the standard deviation of that distribution.[18] For distributions that are not Gaussian, two-thirds of the interquartile range will be somewhat smaller than the standard deviation of the distribution. Calculation of the standard deviation is illustrated in Equation (2.5).

$$\sigma = \frac{2}{3} \cdot \text{IQR} \qquad (2.5)$$

where

σ = standard deviation of a Gaussian distribution

IQR = interquartile range of a Gaussian distribution

So, when we are comfortable with the concept of a standard deviation, it is only a small step to become comfortable with the interquartile range. The next example (Example 2.7) illustrates calculation and interpretation of an interquartile range.

---

[18]This comes from considering that, in a Gaussian distribution, an interval of one standard deviation beyond the mean accounts for one-third of the data values (we will see this later in this chapter) and that the interquartile range accounts for half of the data values. Thus, the interquartile range is equal to 1/2 divided by 1/3 standard deviations.

■ EXAMPLE 2.7

In Examples 2.2 through 2.6, we looked at changes in serum cholesterol levels before and after one month on a low-fat diet for 11 patients newly diagnosed with hypercholesterolemia. The following are the changes in serum cholesterol levels when serum cholesterol after the diet is subtracted from serum cholesterol before the diet: 10, 42, 5, 9, −2, 0, 16, 28, 4, −5, and 3 mg/dL. Now, let us determine the interquartile range of the changes in serum cholesterol for that group of 11 patients.

To begin with, we need to arrange the data in order of numeric magnitude and determine the median, just as we did in Example 2.5:

Order	1	2	3	4	5	**6**	7	8	9	10	11
Value	−5	−2	0	3	4	**5**	9	10	16	28	42

To find the interquartile range, we find the median of each half of the distribution separated by the median of the entire distribution. The median is part of both halves, so there are an even number of data values in each half. The medians of those halves are the mean of the two middle values. For the lower half, the median is the mean of 0 and 3 or 1.5. For the upper half, the median is the mean of 10 and 16 or 13.

So, the median of the lower half is equal to 1.5 and the median of the upper half is equal to 13. We have now divided the distribution of data into four equal parts (i.e., having the same number of data values).

The interquartile range is the difference between the data values that separate the two extreme quartiles (i.e., Q1 and Q4). In this case, the difference is equal to
13 − 1.5=11.5.

To interpret the interquartile range, we can calculate the corresponding standard deviation by using Equation (2.5).

$$\sigma = \frac{2}{3} \cdot \text{IQR} = \frac{2}{3} \cdot 11.5 = 7.7 \, \text{mg/dL}$$

For a Gaussian distribution, the standard deviation calculated using the interquartile range will be equal to the standard deviation calculated using Equation (2.4). In this case, the standard deviation calculated from the interquartile range (7.7 mg/dL) is smaller than the value we calculated using Equation (2.4) in Example 2.6 (13.4 mg/dL). The reason for this is that the distribution of these data is not really a Gaussian distribution. In fact, it is asymmetric. This can be seen in the histograms in Example 2.3.   ■

The relationship between the standard deviation and the interquartile range is similar to the relationship between the mean and the median. Both the mean and the standard deviation are influenced by how far away data values are. The interquartile range is like the median in that it is influenced only by the direction of data values relative to the measurement and not by how extreme these data values are. Thus, two-thirds of the interquartile range is a better estimate of the standard deviation when the data include extreme values that might not be part of the same distribution. We will consider this further in Chapter 3 when we estimate the standard deviation of the distribution of the data in the population from the sample's observations.

These parameters can be calculated in Excel using either functions or "Data Analysis." The next example shows how to obtain these parameters using functions and how they can be obtained in R.

■ EXAMPLE 2.8

Let us use Excel functions to calculate the mean, median, variance, standard deviation, range, and interquartile range for the data from Example 2.6.

	A B	C	D	E
1	CHOL			
2	10			
3	42			
4	5			
5	9			
6	−2			
7	0			
8	16			
9	28			
10	4			
11	−5			
12	3			
13	10	=average(a2:a12)		Mean
14	5	=median(a2:12)		Median
15	178.5455	=varp(a2:a12)		Population's variance
16	13.36209	=stdevp(a2:a12)		Population's standard deviation
17	−5	=min(a2:a12)		Minimum value
18	42	=max(a2:a12)		Maximum value
19	47	=a18-a17		Range
20	1.5	=quartile(a2:a12,1)		25th percentile
21	13	=quartile(a2:a12,3)		75th percentile
22	11.5	=a21-a20		Interquartile range

The data and results of calculations are in column A. Column C shows the formula used to perform each calculation and column E provides the name of the value calculated.

If we compare the Excel calculations to the ones obtained by hand in previous examples, we find that they are the same.

To get some of this same information in R, we use the summary command.
>summary(CHGCHOL)

```
Min. 1st Qu.  Median   Mean 3rd Qu.   Max.
-5.0     1.5     5.0   10.0    13.0   42.0
```

These values agree with those from Excel and our calculations.   ■

2.4   TAKING CHANCE INTO ACCOUNT

Once we are able to describe the distribution of data, we can calculate probabilities that certain data values in the population will be selected to be part of the sample. The way we do this is very similar to the way probabilities are calculated from a Venn diagram. Namely, the probability of certain data values being selected is equal to the part of the distribution that corresponds to those data values divided by the entire distribution. Figure 2.12 illustrates this process.

In Figure 2.12, an interval of values (i.e., 22 days or more), rather than a single data value (e.g., exactly 22 days), is addressed in the probability. This will always be the case when we are thinking about distributions of continuous data. The reason for this is that there are so many possible values for continuous data (theoretically, an infinite number) that the probability of any single value is virtually 0.

The mathematical method for calculating areas in sections of curves involves calculus (namely, integration of the mathematical equation describing the distribution). Fortunately, we do not need to do this calculus ourselves! Instead, we use a statistical table that tells us the result of integrating a Gaussian distribution. Our only task is to change our distribution so that it is on the same scale as the distribution described in Table B.1 (in Appendix B).

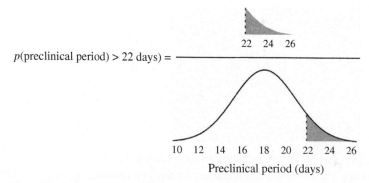

Figure 2.12   Venn equation illustrating the probability of selecting a person with a preclinical period equal to or greater than 22 days; this equation compares the part of the distribution that corresponds to 22 days or more to the entire distribution.

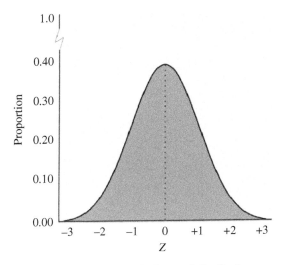

Figure 2.13 The standard normal distribution.

2.4.1 Standard Normal Distribution

There are several standard distributions we will encounter as we examine various statistical procedures. The first of these is the **standard normal distribution**. The standard normal distribution is a Gaussian distribution that has a mean equal to 0 and a standard deviation equal to 1. When data values are converted to that scale (i.e., $\mu = 0$ and $\sigma = 1$), we call these converted data values **standard normal deviates** and symbolize them with the letter z (instead of Y). Figure 2.13 shows the standard normal distribution.

To use the standard normal distribution, we need to convert our data from their original scale to the standard normal scale. As it turns out, this conversion is rather straightforward. To change the scale so that it has a mean of 0, we subtract the mean from each of the data values. To change the scale so that it has a standard deviation of 1, we divide by the standard deviation of the data measured on the original scale. Equation (2.6) shows how we can convert a particular data value from its original scale to the standard normal scale.

$$z = \frac{Y_i - \mu}{\sigma} \tag{2.6}$$

where

$z =$ standard normal deviate (**z-value**) that represents the data value Y_i

$Y_i =$ data value on the original scale

$\mu =$ mean of the distribution of Y_i

$\sigma =$ standard deviation of the distribution of Y_i

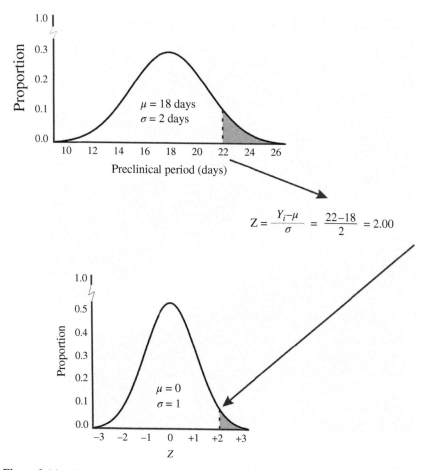

Figure 2.14 Conversion of a preclinical period of 22 days on the data's original scale (i.e., days) to a value of 2.00 on the standard normal scale involves subtraction of the mean from the original distribution and division by the standard deviation of that same distribution.

This process of converting a value from its original scale to the standard normal scale is illustrated graphically in Figure 2.14.

Now, let us take a look at an example of how we can convert data values from their original scale to the standard normal scale.

■ **EXAMPLE 2.9**

Imagine that the incubation period for *Salmonella*-induced gastroenteritis has a Gaussian distribution with a mean of 25 h and a standard deviation of 6 h. Suppose we are interested in examining students in a university 35 h after they were exposed to *Salmonella*. If we are interested in the probability of selecting an infected person with an incubation period greater than 35 h (i.e., they will be asymptomatic at 35 h), we can use the standard normal distribution to calculate that probability. In preparation, let us determine what value on the standard normal scale would correspond to 35 h on the original scale.

In this problem, we are provided with the following information summarized using the corresponding mathematic symbols:

$$\mu = 25 \text{ h} \qquad \sigma = 6 \text{ h} \qquad Y_i = 35 \text{ h}$$

To convert 35 h to the standard normal scale, we use Equation (2.6):

$$z = \frac{Y_i - \mu}{\sigma} = \frac{35 - 25}{6} = 1.67$$

So, 35 h on a scale that has a mean of 25 h and a standard deviation of 6 h is equal to 1.67 on the standard normal scale.   ■

The purpose of converting data to the standard normal scale is to enable us to use a table or a program to determine the probability of selecting certain intervals of data values. Table B.1 (in Appendix B) gives us probabilities for standard normal deviates. The values on the margins of that table are the standard normal deviates. Units and tenths of a standard normal deviate are listed on the left margin and hundredths are listed on the top margin. In the body of the table are the probabilities. Specifically, these are the probabilities of selecting by chance the corresponding standard normal deviate or a larger standard normal deviate.[19] Since our data value

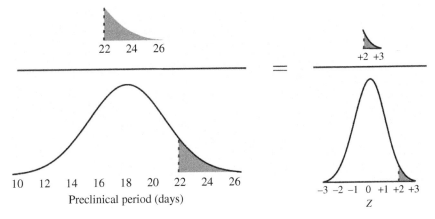

Figure 2.15   The probability of selecting a preclinical period equal to or greater than 22 days is the same as the probability of selecting corresponding standard normal deviates from the standard normal distribution (a standard normal deviate equal to or greater than 2.00).

---

[19] These are also interpreted as the probability of selecting a larger standard normal deviate (i.e., excluding the specific standard normal deviate). The reason that the same probability is used regardless of whether or not the specific value is included is that the probability of selecting any single value from a distribution of continuous values is virtually 0.

is represented by a standard normal deviate, the probability of selecting by chance the standard normal deviate or a larger value is the same as the probability of selecting by chance the data value or a larger value. This principle is illustrated graphically in Figure 2.15, and mathematically in Equation (2.7) for the data in Figure 2.14.

$$p(\text{preclinical period} \geq 22 \text{ days}) = p(z \geq 2.00) \tag{2.7}$$

Now, let us take a look at an example of using the standard normal table (Table B.1) to find a probability for an interval of data values.

■ EXAMPLE 2.10

In Example 2.9, we considered a Gaussian distribution of incubation periods with a mean of 25 h and a standard deviation of 6 h. In this example, we were interested in the probability of selecting someone from the population with an incubation period equal to or greater than 35 h. To prepare to calculate that probability, we determined that a standard normal deviate of 1.67 on the standard normal scale corresponds to 35 h on the original scale. Now, let us determine the probability associated with those values.

Turn to Table B.1 and find the row that corresponds to the units and tenths of the standard normal deviate (1.6) and the column that corresponds to the hundredths of the standard normal deviate (7). Where that row and column intersect is the probability of selecting, by chance, a standard normal deviate equal to or greater than 1.67. This probability is equal to 0.0475. This process can be illustrated graphically as follows:

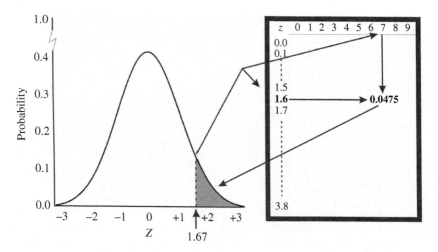

Now, we use the principle illustrated in Figure 2.4 and Equation (2.7) to determine the probability of an exposed person having an incubation period greater than 35 h. Since 1.67 on the standard normal scale is the same as 35 h on the original scale, we can conclude that the probability of selecting someone with an incubation period greater than 35 h is also equal to 0.0475.

$$p(\text{incubation period} > 35 \text{ h}) = p(z > 1.67) = 0.0475$$

This tells us that almost 5% of the persons in this population who are infected with *Salmonella* will be asymptomatic 35 h postexposure.   ■

Table B.1 consists of probabilities of selecting a standard normal deviate equal to or greater than values that range from 0 to 3.89. All of these values are positive. If the data value that we want to convert to the standard normal scale is smaller than the mean on the original scale, Equation (2.6) will result in a negative standard normal deviate. This is not a problem, since the standard normal distribution is symmetric around its mean of 0. Instead, we can find the probability of obtaining the absolute value[20] of the standard normal deviate and interpret that probability as the chance of obtaining the negative standard normal deviate or less. The next example illustrates how this is done.

■ EXAMPLE 2.11

In Examples 2.9 and 2.10, we considered that the incubation period for *Salmonella*-induced gastroenteritis has a Gaussian distribution with a mean of 25 h and a standard deviation of 6 h. In these examples, we were interested in selecting a person with an incubation period greater than 35 h. Now, let us determine the chance of selecting a person with an incubation period of less than 12 h.

The information provided in this example is the same as that provided in Example 2.9, except for the data value we need to convert to a standard normal deviate. Thus, we can use Equation (2.6) as we did in the previous example, substituting 12 h for 35 h.

$$z = \frac{Y_i - \mu}{\sigma} = \frac{12 - 25}{6} = -2.17$$

To find the probability associated with −2.17, we look for the absolute value of −2.17 (i.e., 2.17), since negative values do not appear in Table B.1. From the table, we learn that the chance of selecting a standard normal deviate of 2.17 or more is equal to 0.0150. Since the standard normal distribution is symmetric around 0, we can conclude that the probability of selecting a standard normal deviate equal to 2.17 or less is also equal to 0.0150.

Another way we can interpret a standard normal deviate is to use Excel or R to calculate the probability of obtaining a particular z-value. In Excel, the function to use is "=norm.s.dist (z,true). In R, we use the pnorm(z) command. These

---

[20]In other words, we change negative values to positive values.

give us the probability of obtaining the specified z-value or less. For $z = 2.17$, the probability is 0.984997. This agrees with what we found from Table B1, but gives us better precision (i.e., more than two decimal places). When using this function, however, we need to keep in mind that it gives the probability of the specified standard normal deviate or less. So, if we are to use it to determine the probability of a particular z-value or more, we have to subtract the result of using the function from 1. For example, a z-value of 2.17 gives us 0.984997. This is the complement of the probability of 2.17 or more. Subtracting that probability from 1 gives us 0.015003. ∎

Often, we are interested in the probability of obtaining a data value either equal to or greater than a particular value or equal to or less than another particular value.[21] Such a probability is called a **two-sided** or **two-tailed** probability. This term comes from our reference to extreme values in a distribution as being in the "tail" of that distribution.[22] To calculate a two-tailed probability, we just need to recall from Chapter 1 how to calculate the probability of the union of two events. We do this by using the addition rule.[23] Figure 2.16 shows this calculation as a Venn equation, and Equation (2.8) shows it in mathematical language.

$$p(Y \leq Y_{\text{smaller}} \text{ and/or } Y \geq Y_{\text{larger}}) = p(Y \leq Y_{\text{smaller}}) + p(Y \geq Y_{\text{larger}}) \qquad (2.8)$$

where

$p(Y \leq Y_{\text{smaller}}$
  and/or $=$ probability of getting a data value either less than or equal to
$Y \geq Y_{\text{larger}})$
  one particular value (Y_{smaller}) or greater than or equal to another particular value (Y_{larger}). This is a two-tailed probability

$p(Y \leq Y_{\text{smaller}}) =$ probability of getting a data value equal to or less than a particular value(Y_{smaller}). This is a one-tailed probability

$p(Y \geq Y_{\text{larger}}) =$ probability of getting a data value equal to or greater than a particular value (Y_{larger}). This is a one-tailed probability

$Y_{\text{smaller}} =$ smaller of two particular data values

$Y_{\text{larger}} =$ larger of two particular data values

---

[21] For example, we might be interested in a clinical measurement that has abnormal values both above and below the range of normal results. Blood pressure is such a measurement. If someone has a blood pressure within the range of normal, we say that they are "normotensive." A person who has a blood pressure below the range of normal is "hypotensive" and a person who has a blood pressure above the range of normal is "hypertensive." Then, we might be interested in the probability that someone selected at random from the population would be either hypotensive or hypertensive.

[22] Consequentially, the probability of data values in a single interval in either tail of a distribution is called a **one-tailed** probability

[23] We use the simplified version of the addition rule for this calculation since the probability of getting a value in one tail is mutually exclusive of the probability of getting a value in the other tail.

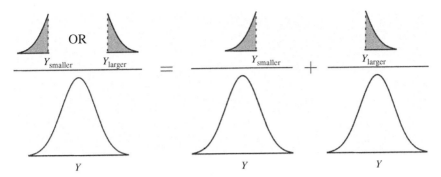

Figure 2.16 Venn equation showing how the addition rule is used to calculate a two-tailed probability.

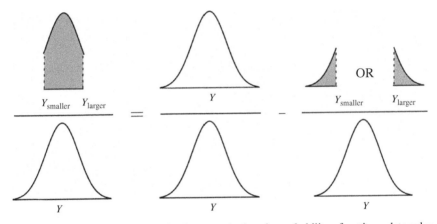

Figure 2.17 Venn equation showing how to calculate the probability of getting a data value from an interval in the center of the distribution.

Another probability in which we are often interested is the probability of getting a data value between two particular values (i.e., in the middle of the distribution). To determine this probability, we begin by calculating the probability of getting a data value in the tails of the distribution (i.e., those values that are excluded from the part for which we want to calculate a probability). These tails are the complement of the values in the middle in which we are interested. In Chapter 1, we learned that we can calculate the probability of the complement by subtracting the probability of the event from 1 (see Equation (1.3)). Figure 2.17 shows this principle applied to a distribution of data, and Equation (2.9) shows it in mathematical language:

$$p(Y_{smaller} \leq Y \leq Y_{larger}) = 1 - p(Y \leq Y_{smaller} \text{ and/or } Y \geq Y_{larger}) \qquad (2.9)$$

where

$$p(Y_{smaller} \le Y \le Y_{larger}) = \text{probability of getting a data value between two particular values } (Y_{smaller} \text{ and } Y_{larger})$$

Now, let us take a look at an example that shows how to calculate these probabilities.

■ EXAMPLE 2.12

In the previous examples, we have been considering that the preclinical period for *Salmonella*-induced gastroenteritis has a Gaussian distribution with a mean of 25 h and a standard deviation of 6 h. In Example 2.10, we calculated the probability of selecting a person with an incubation period equal to or greater than 35 h. This probability is equal to 0.0475. In Example 2.11, we calculated the probability of selecting a person with an incubation period equal to or less than 12 h. This probability is equal to 0.0150. Now, let us determine the chance of selecting a person with an incubation period between 12 and 35 h.

This example asks us to calculate the probability of getting a data value in the middle of the distribution. To calculate this probability, we begin by calculating the probability of its complement: the probability of getting a value from either tail of the distribution. To find that probability, we use Equation (2.8):

$$p(Y \le Y_{smaller} \text{ and/or } Y \ge Y_{larger}) = p(Y \le Y_{smaller}) + p(Y \ge Y_{larger})$$
$$= 0.0475 + 0.0150 = 0.0625$$

Next, we calculate the probability of the complement of getting a value from either tail of the distribution as shown in Equation (2.9):

$$p(Y_{smaller} \le Y \le Y_{larger}) = 1 - p(Y \le Y_{smaller} \text{ and/or } Y \ge Y_{larger}) = 1 - 0.0625$$
$$= 0.9375$$

Thus, there is a probability of 0.9375 that a person selected at random from the population would have an incubation period between 12 and 35 h. ■

Table B.1 can be used to determine the probability associated with any standard normal deviate between the values of 0 and 3.89,[24] but there are a few values that are helpful to emphasize. The numeric magnitude of a standard normal deviate tells us how many multiples of the standard deviation a data value is away from the mean. Understanding this fact allows us to interpret means and standard deviations reported in the health research literature. For instance, if the distribution of

---

[24]The probability associated with higher z-values is very small, so they are not included in Table B.1.

data is a Gaussian distribution, the mean ± one standard deviation includes about two-thirds of all the data values in the distribution.[25] Likewise, the mean ± two standard deviations include about 95% of the data values in the distribution.[26] This

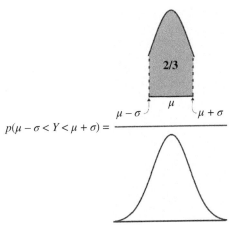

$$p(\mu - \sigma < Y < \mu + \sigma) = \underline{\hspace{4cm}}$$

Figure 2.18   Approximately two-thirds of all data values in a Gaussian distribution are in the interval specified by the mean ± one standard deviation.

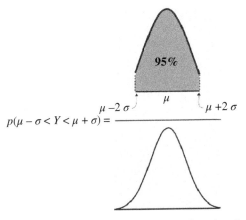

$$p(\mu - \sigma < Y < \mu + \sigma) = \underline{\hspace{4cm}}$$

Figure 2.19   Approximately 95% of all data values in a Gaussian distribution are in the interval specified by the mean ± two standard deviations.

[25]From Table B.1, we find that a standard normal deviate of one corresponds to a probability of 0.1587 in one tail of the distribution. Thus, the mean ± one standard deviation includes 1 −(0.1587 +0.1587) = 0.6826 or 68.26% of all the data values in the distribution.
[26]More precisely, the mean ± two standard deviations includes 95.44% of the data values in the distribution.

relationship between the standard deviation and the proportion of data values in a Gaussian distribution[27] is illustrated in Figures 2.18 and 2.19.

Now, let us take a look at an example of how we can use these relationships to interpret the results of health research.

■ **EXAMPLE 2.13**

In a research article reporting the result of a study of determinants of gestational age at birth (*N Engl J Med* 1998;339:1434–1439), the following means and standard deviations appear in a table:

Number of Infants	Gestational Age (Weeks)
Singleton	39.2 (±1.9)*
Twins	35.8 (±3.2)
Higher order	32.2 (±3.3)

*Mean ± SD.

Based on this information, let us compare the distributions of gestational age in the population for each of these three groups.

From the means and standard deviations of gestational age, we can specify an interval of data values that will include a given percentage of all data values in a Gaussian distribution. To include two-thirds of all births, we take the mean gestational age and add and subtract the standard deviation. To include 95% of all births, we take the mean and add and subtract two standard deviations. The following table summarizes these calculations:

Number of Infants	Gestational Age (Weeks)	Two-Thirds of All Births	95% of All Births
Singleton	39.2 (±1.9)	37.3–41.1	35.4–43.0
Twins	35.8 (±3.2)	32.6–39.0	29.4–42.2
Higher order	32.2 (±3.3)	28.9–35.5	25.6–38.8

From these intervals, we can get an idea of how the distributions would appear. ■

Use of integers as multiples of the standard deviation to specify a certain proportion of the population's data is an approximation. This approach is useful when

[27]If the distribution of data is not a Gaussian distribution, these percentages will be smaller. The lower limits of these percentages are 0% for the mean ± one standard deviation and 75% for the mean ± two standard deviations regardless of the type of distribution.

we want to calculate an interval of data values in our head. If we want to be more precise, however, we can use the table of standard normal deviates (Table B.1) to find the exact multiple of the standard deviation that specifies a certain proportion of a Gaussian distribution. To do this, we look for one-half of the complement of the proportion of data values in the body of the table. For instance, if we were interested in the central 95% of the data values in a Gaussian distribution, we would look in Table B.1 to find the standard normal deviate that corresponds to a probability of 0.0250 [=(1 − 0.95)/2]. This standard normal deviate is equal to 1.96. So, a more precise interval of data values corresponds to the mean ± 1.96 times the standard deviation. For the gestational ages of singleton births in Example 2.13, the precise interval that includes 95% of the data values goes from 35.5 to 42.9 weeks. This exact interval is just slightly narrower than the approximate interval determined in Example 2.13 (35.4–43.0 weeks).

In this chapter, we have looked at the distribution of data in the population and we have seen how understanding that distribution allows us to determine the effect of chance on selecting individuals from the population. In the next chapter, we will examine the ways we can use the sample's observations to describe the distribution of data in the population.

CHAPTER SUMMARY

In Chapter 2, we encounter distributions of data. A distribution of data is a description of how frequently various data values occur. In health research, we are interested in describing the distribution of data in the population. There are three ways we can do this. We can use literary language, graphic language, or mathematic language.

In literary language, we can describe a distribution of data by reporting which data values occur most frequently, less frequently, and least frequently. A literary description of a distribution of data is relatively easy to construct, but it leaves out quite a bit of detail about the distribution.

A better way to describe a distribution of data is using graphic language. There are several ways we can graphically describe a distribution; five of which are introduced in Chapter 2. These are a bar graph, a histogram, a stem-and-leaf plot, a box-and-whisker plot, and a frequency polygon.

A bar graph is used to describe distributions of discrete data. Discrete data include ordinal and nominal data. Ordinal data are values that can be ordered in a meaningful way, but the spacing between the data values is not considered. Nominal data are values that describe groups that cannot be ordered in a meaningful way.

A bar graph has data values on the horizontal axis and either the frequency, proportion, or percent of each of the data values on the vertical axis. A bar is drawn for each data value, the height of which corresponds to the frequency, proportion, or percent of data values in the population equal to that specific value.

A histogram is used to describe continuous data. Continuous data have a large number of possible ordered values that are evenly spaced.

A histogram is similar to a bar graph in that data values are on the horizontal axis; frequency, proportion, or percent is on vertical axis; and bars of various heights are used to represent the occurrence of the corresponding data values. There are two differences between a bar graph and a histogram. First, the bars in a histogram touch each other while there are spaces between the bars in a bar graph. This distinction reflects the differences between discrete data, in which there are spaces between data values and continuous data, in which (theoretically) there are no spaces between values.

The second distinction between a bar graph and a histogram is that the data values in a bar graph are specific values, while data values in a histogram are represented by intervals of values. This distinction is due to the fact that there are (theoretically) an infinite number of possible values for continuous data. If there are an infinite number of possible values, then the probability associated with any single value is essentially equal to 0. To have nonzero probabilities for continuous data, we need to think of intervals of values.

When we use histograms to describe a distribution of data, we need to decide how narrow the intervals will be. The narrower the intervals, the greater is the number of bars. As we approach an infinite number of bars that are infinitely narrow, the bars disappear. Then, we are left with just the tops of the bars that have the appearance of a line instead of a collection of bars. When we reach this point, we call the graph a frequency polygon.

The third graphic approach to describing distributions of data considered in this chapter is the stem-and-leaf plot. A stem-and-leaf plot is similar to a histogram, but it is easier to construct, especially when we graph relatively few data values. To begin, we put the left digit(s) for each value in a column. These are called the stem. Each of the components of the stem is like an interval of values in a histogram. Then, we list in a row following each component of the stem the right-most digit for each of the values that have that particular set of numbers to the left. These right-most digits are called the leaves. The result is like a histogram in which the number of leaves corresponds to the height of a bar in a histogram.

A box-and-whisker plot is especially useful for visualizing the symmetry of a distribution. The box represents the interquartile range and the whiskers represent the range of the data.

Most often, we use a mathematic description of the distribution of data in the population. To describe a distribution mathematically, we must first state the type of distribution and then, provide values for the parameters of the distribution. Parameters are numbers that designate a specific distribution of the stated type.

The type of distribution we considered, using the mathematic approach, was the Gaussian (or normal) distribution. The Gaussian distribution is a symmetric bell-shaped distribution. To specify a particular Gaussian distribution, we need to provide numeric values for two parameters. One parameter describes the location of the distribution in a continuum of values. The other parameter describes how dispersed the data are around that location.

The parameter of location for a Gaussian distribution is the mean. The mean can be thought of as the center of gravity of a distribution that reflects not only on which side of a distribution data values occur, but also how far away they are from the middle of the distribution. This is in contrast to the median, which reflects only on which side of the distribution data values occur.

The parameter of dispersion for a Gaussian distribution is the variance (or its square root: the standard deviation). The variance can be thought of as the mean of the squared differences between the data values and the mean of the distribution.

Once we can describe the distribution of data in the population, we can begin thinking about the role of chance in selecting a sample from that population. There are two ways we might do this. One of these is based on a graphic description of the distribution. The other is based on a mathematic description of the distribution.

The graphic approach is related to Venn diagrams and Venn equations examined in Chapter 1. Instead of a rectangle, all possible observations are represented by the entire distribution. For the events, we use the portion(s) of the distribution that corresponds to the values for which the probability is being calculated.

For the mathematic approach, we use the mathematic description of the distribution and the values of the parameters to calculate probabilities. Rather than do this for each distribution, these calculations have been performed for us and tabulated for standard distributions (see Appendix B). One of the standard distributions that can be used for a Gaussian distribution is called the standard normal distribution.

The standard normal distribution is a Gaussian distribution with a mean equal to 0 and a standard deviation equal to 1. When we want to calculate a probability for a datum from a Gaussian distribution, we can convert the mean of the distribution to a mean of 0 by subtracting the actual mean from each data value. Then, we can convert the standard deviation to a value of 1 by dividing the difference between the mean and a data value by the actual standard deviation. We call the result a standard normal deviate or a z-value.

This process of converting a datum to a z-value determines what value on the standard normal scale corresponds to a particular value on the original scale. Then, we can determine the probability of an interval of values defined by that datum by determining the probability of an interval of values defined by the corresponding z-value. To determine the probability for an interval of values defined by a z-value, we use a statistical table.

A statistical table for the standard normal distribution appears in Table B.1 of the textbook. Table B.1 gives us the probabilities of getting a data value in an interval equal to the specific z-value or greater. This is called the upper tail of the distribution. In the standard normal distribution, the upper half of the distribution corresponds to positive z-values. The lower half of the distribution does not appear in Table B.1, but the standard normal distribution is a symmetric distribution centered on 0, so what is true for a positive value or more is the same as what is true for a negative value or less. To find probabilities for intervals of values in the middle of the standard normal distribution, we determine the probabilities for the tails excluded by the interval and subtract the probability from 1.

EXERCISES

2.1. In a particular population, the mean birth weight is equal to 3,500 gm and the standard deviation of birth weights is equal to 800 gm. Given that information, and assuming that birth weight has a Gaussian distribution, which of the following is closest to the probability that an infant selected randomly will weigh between 3000 and 4000 gm?

   A. 0.2676

   B. 0.4648

   C. 0.5352

   D. 0.7324

   E. 0.9175

2.2. Suppose we are interested in the length of gestation among live births in a particular population. If the mean gestation period is equal to 38 weeks and the standard deviation is equal to 1 week, and if we assume the distribution of gestational age is a Gaussian distribution, which of the following is closest to the probability that any given pregnancy will last longer than 38 weeks?

   A. 0.0228

   B. 0.0456

   C. 0.5000

   D. 0.9544

   E. 0.9772

2.3. In a particular population, the mean age is 45 years and the variance of age is equal to 225 years^2. Given that information, and assuming age has a Gaussian distribution, what is the probability a person selected randomly will be between 30 and 60 years of age?

   A. 0

   B. 0.1587

   C. 0.3174

   D. 0.6826

   E. 0.8413

2.4. The mean systolic blood pressure in a particular population is 130 mmHg and has a standard deviation of 20 mmHg. Hypertension is considered severe if a patient has a systolic blood pressure equal to or greater than 180 mmHg. Given that information, and assuming that the distribution of systolic blood pressures is a Gaussian distribution, what percent of the population would have severe hypertension?

A. 0.6%

B. 2.0%

C. 6.0%

D. 17.1%

E. 20.2%

2.5. Consider a population in which the mean systolic blood pressure is 130 mmHg with a standard deviation of 20 mmHg. People with systolic blood pressure between 140 and 180 mmHg are considered to have mild to moderate hypertension. Given that information, and assuming that the distribution of systolic blood pressures is a Gaussian distribution, what percent of the population would have mild to moderate hypertension?

A. 3.0%

B. 3.3%

C. 30.2%

D. 43.8%

E. 67.1%

2.6. Consider a population in which the mean systolic blood pressure is 130 mmHg with a standard deviation of 20 mmHg. People with systolic blood pressure below 90 mmHg are considered to have hypotension. Given that information, and assuming that the distribution of systolic blood pressures is a Gaussian distribution, what percent of the population would have hypotension?

A. 2.3%

B. 4.6%

C. 24.3%

D. 45.4%

E. 47.7%

CHAPTER 3

EXAMINING SAMPLES

Any sample consists of a subset of the data in a population. Our task is to examine the observations in the sample and, as a result of that examination, draw conclusions about the distribution of data in the population. We do this by using two approaches (Figure 3.1). One approach is to use the data in the sample to come up with a good guess about the numeric value of a parameter of the distribution of data in the population. This approach is called **estimation**. Another is to use the data in the sample to test a hypothesis about a parameter of the distribution of data in a population. This

Introduction to Biostatistical Applications in Health Research with Microsoft Office Excel® and R,
Second Edition. Robert P. Hirsch.
© 2021 John Wiley & Sons, Inc. Published 2021 by John Wiley & Sons, Inc.
Companion website: www.wiley.com/go/hirsch/healthresearch2e

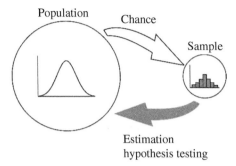

Estimation
hypothesis testing

Figure 3.1   The sample's observations are used to make estimates or test hypotheses about the distribution of data in a population.

approach is called **hypothesis testing**. In this chapter, we will see how those two approaches allow us to draw conclusions about a population by examining a sample.

3.1   NATURE OF SAMPLES

As we prepare to make a transition from thinking about a population to examining a sample, it is important that we make clear the distinction between the population and the sample. Conceptually, the population is the group about which we would like to draw a conclusion, but which we can never actually examine.[1] The sample, on the other hand, is the group that we examine, but we are not satisfied simply describing the results of that examination. Instead, we are interested in applying the results of examining the sample to our understanding about the population.

This distinction between the population and the sample is sufficiently meaningful that statisticians have a number of conventions they use when referring to each of these groups. Those conventions are summarized in Table 3.1.

Usually in statistics we assume the sample has been selected by chance from the population. This is called **probability sampling**. If every element of the population has the same chance of being selected to be included in the sample, the type of probability sampling is called **simple random sampling**. If, on the other hand, some elements have a different chance of being selected to be included in the sample, we call the type of probability sampling **stratified random sampling**.

Now that the distinction between the population and the sample has been clarified, we are ready to discover how the sample's observations can be used to draw conclusions about the population.

---

[1] In health research, the population has three dimensions: person, place, and time. It is the dimension of time that makes it impossible to examine the entire population. The other dimensions make it highly unlikely, but not impossible.

TABLE 3.1. Conventions Used to Distinguish between the Population and the Sample

Population	Sample
Data are the values in the population	**Observations** are those data values selected to be included in the sample
Parameters are the numeric values that mathematically define the distribution of data in the population (e.g., mean and variance). We never know the actual value of a parameter	**Estimates** are the values calculated from the sample's observations that are used to guess at the value of the population's parameters
Greek letters are used to symbolize the population's parameters in mathematic equations	**English letters** are used to symbolize the sample's estimates in mathematic equations
N symbolizes the number of data values in the population	n Symbolizes the number of observations in the sample

3.2 ESTIMATION

The purpose of estimation is to make a good guess at the value of a parameter in the population. There are two kinds of estimates that we can make from the sample's observations. A **point estimate** is the single best guess about the value of the population's parameter. The trouble with point estimates is that they have a low probability of being exactly equal in value to the population's parameter.[2] To make an estimate that has a good chance of being equal to the population's parameter, we need to use an interval of values, rather than a single value.[3] Such an estimate is called an **interval estimate** or a **confidence interval**.

3.2.1 Point Estimates

In Chapter 2, we learned that we need two parameters to mathematically describe a distribution of continuous data.[4] These are the mean and the variance (or standard deviation). In developing point estimates, we use the sample's observations to calculate the most likely values for those parameters in the population. One feature

---

[2] Recall from Chapter 2 that the probability of any particular value from a continuum is virtually 0 because of the large number of possible values in the denominator of that probability.

[3] It was this principle that led us to calculate probabilities for intervals of data values, instead of for specific data values, in Chapter 2.

[4] In the introductory chapters of this book, we are confining our interest to distributions of continuous data. Later, we will see how these principles apply to distributions of other types of data.

these estimates must have is that they must be equal, on the average, to the parameter they estimate. This implies that, if we took lots of samples from the population, the mean of all the estimates would be equal to the population's parameter.[5] Such an estimate is said to be **unbiased**. Every estimate we calculate from the sample's observations must be an unbiased estimate of the population's parameter, or it is not an accurate reflection of the parameter, even on the average.

The first method of calculating an estimate we consider when searching for an unbiased estimate is one in which the same calculations are performed on the sample's observations as would be performed to calculate the population's parameter. For instance, Equation (2.1) illustrates how the mean of the population's data would be calculated if we knew the values of all of those data. Equation (3.1) shows that the same calculation is performed on the sample's observations.

$$\overline{Y} = \frac{\sum Y_i}{n} \tag{3.1}$$

where

$\overline{Y}$ = mean of the observations in the sample (called "Y bar")

$\sum Y_i$ = sum of the individual data values in the sample

n = number of observations in the sample

Before we go further, we need to make a distinction between equations for the population's data and equations for the sample's observations. To do this, we need to confess that we can never know all of the data in the population. If we cannot know all the data in the population, we cannot calculate the population's parameters. Thus, Equation (2.1) describes a concept, not a calculation. On the other hand, we do know all the observations in the sample. So, we can do the calculation described in Equation (3.1).

The value calculated in Equation (3.1) is the mean of the sample's observations. More importantly, it is an unbiased estimate of the mean of the population's data. In other words, the mean of the sample's observations is, on the average, equal to the mean of the population's data. Equation (3.2) shows this important relationship in mathematical notation:

$$\mu \triangleq \overline{Y} = \frac{\sum Y_i}{n} \tag{3.2}$$

where

μ = mean of the data in the population

$\triangleq$ = is estimated by

$\overline{Y}$ = mean of the observations in the sample (called "Y bar")

---

[5]This requirement stems from the use of chance to select the members of the population who will be part of the sample. This strategy results in samples that are representative of the population only on the average. Any particular sample's estimate, however, is unlikely to be exactly equal to the population's parameter.

Estimating the variance of the distribution of data in the population is a little more complicated than estimating the mean. If we were to use the same calculations on the sample's observations that we used to define the population's variance (Equation (2.3)), we would get a biased estimate of the population's variance. This is because the variance of the sample's observations is systematically smaller than the population's variance.

The reason for this bias is that the most extreme data values (i.e., those that are farthest from the mean) occur very infrequently in the population. As a result, it is very unlikely that these extreme data values will be included among the sample's observations. These extreme data values, however, have the greatest impact on the numeric magnitude of the variance. Since samples systematically exclude these influential values, the sample's variance systematically underestimates the population's variance.[6] This bias is illustrated in Equation (3.3):

$$\sigma^2 > \frac{\sum (Y_i - \overline{Y})^2}{n} \tag{3.3}$$

where
> = is greater than
σ^2 = variance of the distribution of data in the population

To calculate an unbiased estimate of the population's variance, we need to make a change in Equation (3.3), which will increase the numeric value of the sample's estimate of the population's variance. Also, we want that change to have more impact on the estimate of the variance from smaller samples than from larger samples. The reason for this is that as the size of the sample increases, the probability of including extreme values in the sample also increases. Thus, the larger the sample, the less biased the estimate shown in Equation (3.3). To accomplish both of these goals, we subtract 1 from the number of observations in the sample in the denominator of Equation (3.3) to provide an unbiased estimate of the population's variance. Equation (3.4) illustrates that unbiased estimate of the population's variance:

$$\sigma^2 \triangleq s^2 = \frac{\sum (Y_i - \overline{Y})^2}{n - 1} \tag{3.4}$$

where
σ^2 = population's variance of distribution of data
s^2 = sample's estimate of the population's variance

At first, the choice to subtract 1 from the number of observations in the sample in calculation of the variance's estimate might seem arbitrary, but it is not. Instead, $n - 1$ reflects the amount of information available in the sample for estimation of the variance (called the "**degrees of freedom**"). Since we need at least two observations

---

[6]This bias does not affect the sample's estimate of the mean since missing extreme data values above and below the population mean are balanced and, thus, cancel each other. In the variance, however, squaring the differences between the data values and the mean prevents canceling of negative and positive effects.

to observe dispersion, the amount of information in the sample that can be used to estimate the variance is equal to $n - 1$ instead of n.

Now, let us take a look at an example of point estimation.

■ EXAMPLE 3.1

Suppose that we are interested in the efficacy of a new topical treatment for glaucoma. To investigate this efficacy, we identify nine persons with elevated intraocular pressure. Each of these nine persons is randomly assigned to use the new treatment in one eye and the standard treatment in the other eye. After one week of treatment, the difference in intraocular pressure between the two eyes (ΔIOP) is measured for each person (mmHg). Suppose that we observed the following results:

Patient	ΔIOP
TH	3
IS	0
MA	3
KE	2
SM	−3
ES	11
OH	1
AP	6
PY	4
Total	27

From those observations, let us calculate unbiased estimates of the population's parameters.

To begin with, we need to estimate the mean difference in intraocular pressure. To calculate this estimate, we use Equation (3.2):

$$\mu \triangleq \overline{Y} = \frac{\sum Y_i}{n} = \frac{27}{9} = 3 \, \text{mmHg}$$

Thus, our best guess of the mean of the distribution of data in the population is 3 mmHg.

Next, we will use Equation (3.4) to calculate an estimate of the population's variance. In preparation for that calculation, we need to calculate the squared differences between each of the observations and the estimated mean. The following table shows those calculations.

Patient	ΔIOP	$Y_i - \bar{Y}$	$(Y_i - \bar{Y})^2$
TH	3	0	0
IS	0	-3	9
MA	3	0	0
KE	2	-1	1
SM	-3	-6	36
ES	11	8	64
OH	1	-2	4
AP	6	3	9
PY	4	1	1
Total	27	0	124

Now, we are ready to use Equation (3.4) to calculate the sample's estimate of the population's variance.

$$\sigma^2 \triangleq s^2 = \frac{\sum (Y_i - \bar{Y})^2}{n - 1} = \frac{124}{9 - 1} = 15.5 \text{ mmHg}^2$$

So, an unbiased estimate of the population's variance is equal to 15.5 mmHg^2. If we prefer, we can estimate the standard deviation by taking the square root of the variance estimate:

$$s = \sqrt{s^2} = \sqrt{15.5 \text{ mmHg}^2} = 3.94 \text{ mmHg}$$

■

If we had used Equation (3.3) instead of Equation (3.4) to calculate the variance estimate in Example 3.1, we would have gotten (124/9 =) 13.8 mmHg^2 for the variance estimate, which corresponds to a standard deviation of 3.71 mmHg. These values are both less than those we calculated (15.5 mmHg^2 and 3.94 mmHg, respectively). Since they underestimate the population's parameters, they are biased estimates. The degree of bias observed for that sample of nine patients is equal to 0.23 mmHg (3.94–3.71) for the standard deviation. If the sample were bigger, the magnitude of this bias would be smaller.

Since there is no distinction between the method of calculation of the population's mean and calculation of the sample's estimate of the mean, we use the same function for both in Excel. There is, however, a distinction in the calculation of the sample's estimate of the population's variance or standard deviation. This means that we need to use a different function for sample's estimates of those parameters. The next example illustrates these differences.

■ **EXAMPLE 3.2**

In Example 3.1, we were interested in the efficacy of a new topical treatment for glaucoma and measured the difference in intraocular pressure between the two eyes (ΔIOP) for each of nine persons. The following are the results we obtain when we analyze these data in Excel:

	A	B	C		D	E
1	ΔIOP					
2	3					
3	0					
4	3					
5	2					
6	−3					
7	11					
8	1					
9	6					
10	4					
11	3		= average(A2:A10)			Population's mean or the sample's estimate of the population's mean
12	13.77778		= varp(A2:A10)			Population's variance
13	15.5		= var.s(A2:A10)			Sample's estimate of the population's variance
14	3.711843		= stdevp(A2:A10			Population's standard deviation
15	3.937004		= stdev.s(A2:A10)			Sample's estimate of the population's standard deviation

These values are consistent with those we obtained when we calculated them manually.

In *R*, you get the mean with the mean() command, the sample's estimate of the variance with the var() command, and the sample's estimate of the standard deviation with the sd() command. These give you the same values as given by Excel. *R* does not provide the population's values. ■

Even though these point estimates are equal to the population's parameters on the average, any particular point estimate (i.e., from a particular sample) is probably not exactly equal to its corresponding parameter. The problem is that we use chance to determine the composition of a sample and point estimates do not take that role of chance into account. Interval estimates, on the other hand, reflect this role of

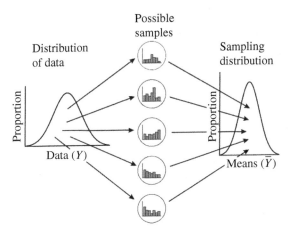

Figure 3.2 The sampling distribution shows estimates of the mean from all possible samples with n observations.

chance. We will see how to calculate interval estimates later in this chapter, but first we need to think in depth about how chance affects a sample's estimate.

3.2.2 The Sampling Distribution

In Chapter 2, we looked at the distribution of data in the population and used that distribution to address the probability that certain members of the population would be selected for inclusion in the sample. Thus, we were interested in the role of chance as it affects individuals. Now, we have a different focus. Instead of the effect of chance on individuals, we are interested in the effect of chance on estimates.

Although these two roles of chance are related, it makes it easier for us to understand statistical procedures if we think of a different distribution for each. To take chance into account for individuals in the population, we use the distribution of data. To take chance into account for estimates of the population's parameters, we use a distribution called the **sampling distribution**. In a sampling distribution, we look at the frequency of different estimates that we could obtain if we were to take all possible samples with n observations from the population. Figure 3.2 illustrates the origin of the sampling distribution for estimates of the mean from a distribution of continuous data.

It is the sampling distribution that tells us about the role of chance in getting particular estimates of a population's parameter. Clearly, this is an important distribution to understand. Unfortunately, the sampling distribution has a characteristic that sometimes acts as an impediment to understanding. That is, the sampling distribution does not really exist, except as a mathematical construct of the distribution of data. For the sampling distribution to be an entity in and of itself, we would have to take all possible samples of a given size from the population and estimate the mean from the observations in each sample. In truth, we take only a single sample from which we calculate a single estimate of the mean. Even so, the sampling distribution represents the mathematical effect of chance on estimates (e.g., of the mean) and, thus, allows us to think of that role of chance graphically, instead of mathematically.

In Figure 3.2, both the distribution of data and the sampling distribution are represented as Gaussian distributions. To use the standard normal distribution to calculate the probability of obtaining a particular data value (via the distribution of data) or a particular estimate of the mean (via the sampling distribution), we need to assume that the corresponding distribution is a Gaussian distribution. For the distribution of data, this is an uncomfortable assumption. Most distributions of biologic and physical data are asymmetric and, therefore, not Gaussian distributions.[7] This fact limits the usefulness of the methods described in Chapter 2, at least when applied to distributions of data.

This same limitation does not apply to sampling distributions, however. This is because sampling distributions (for estimates of a parameter of location like the mean) tend to be Gaussian, even if the data from which the sample was taken is not Gaussian. This tendency of sampling distributions to be Gaussian is addressed by what is called the "**central limit theorem**."

According to the central limit theorem, the distributions of estimates of a parameter of location (e.g., the mean) will always be Gaussian if the data themselves have a Gaussian distribution. The central limit theorem goes on to state that sampling distributions, regardless of the distribution of data, tend to be Gaussian with that tendency increasing as the size of the samples increase. By the time we consider samples with about 30 observations or more, the sampling distribution will be Gaussian regardless of the shape of the distribution of data. Figure 3.3 illustrates the central limit theorem by showing the results of a computer simulation of the sampling process with various sample's sizes.

If the sampling distribution is a Gaussian distribution, we need to provide estimates for its mean and variance (or standard deviation) if we want to calculate probabilities of obtaining certain estimates of the mean. Of these two, the mean of the sampling distribution is the easier to determine. To see how the mean of a sampling distribution is determined, recall that the definition of an unbiased estimate states that unbiased estimates are equal to the population's parameters, on the average. This is reflected in the sampling distribution by the mean of that distribution being equal to the population's parameter being estimated. Thus, the mean of the sampling distribution of estimates of the mean in the population is equal to the population's mean. This is illustrated in Equation (3.5):

$$\mu_{\overline{Y}} = \mu \triangleq \overline{Y} \tag{3.5}$$

---

[7]The most common distribution of natural data is called the log-normal distribution. The log-normal distribution has a Gaussian distribution of the logarithms of the data values. This is the reason we often analyze data on a log scale.

where

$\mu_{\bar{Y}}$ = mean of the distribution of estimates of the mean (i.e., the sampling distribution)

μ = mean of the distribution of data

$\bar{Y}$ = sample's estimate of the mean of the distribution of data

The variance of the sampling distribution is only a little more complicated to understand than is the mean of that distribution. There are two things that affect the variability of estimates. One of them is the variability of the data. The greater the dispersion of the data values, the more variability we expect to see among estimates of the mean. The other is the size of the sample. The larger the sample, the less variability we expect to see among estimates of the mean.

To understand why the size of the samples affects the variability among estimates of the mean, imagine what happens to the estimate of the mean when an extreme data value is included in the sample. If the sample consists of few other observations, the extreme value will result in an estimate of the mean that is far from the actual mean in the population. If the sample consists of many observations however, the influence of that extreme data value will be diminished by less extreme values and even some extreme observations in the opposite direction.[8]

Thus, there are two things that influence the dispersion of the sampling distribution: the variance of the distribution of data and the number of observations in the

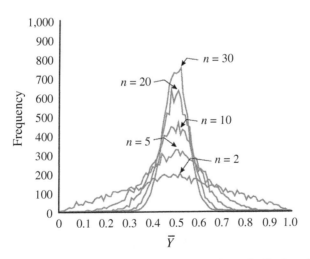

Figure 3.3 Computer simulation of sampling from a uniform distribution of data (i.e., a distribution in which all data values occur with the same frequency) to illustrate the tendency of the sampling distribution for estimates of the mean to be Gaussian, with that tendency increasing as the size of the sample increases.

[8] A way to think about this process of estimating a mean is to imagine it as a process of "buffering" data values. In this analogy, we can think of the observations close to the mean as reducing the impact of extreme observations in the sample.

sample. Equation (3.6) shows this relationship in mathematical language:

$$\sigma_{\bar{Y}}^2 = \frac{\sigma^2}{n} \triangleq \frac{s^2}{n}$$

(3.6)

where

$\sigma_{\bar{Y}}^2$ = variance of the distribution of estimates of the mean (i.e., the sampling distribution)

σ^2 = variance of the distribution of data in the population

s^2 = sample's estimate of the variance of the distribution of data

n = sample's size

If we were to take the square root of the variance of the sampling distribution, the result would be the standard deviation of that distribution. To help us keep the sampling distribution and the distribution of data distinct, however, we give a special name to the standard deviation of the sampling distribution. It is called the **standard error**. Equation (3.7) shows the standard error in the population and how its estimate is calculated from the sample's observations:

$$\sigma_{\bar{Y}} = \sqrt{\frac{\sigma^2}{n}} \triangleq s_{\bar{Y}} = \sqrt{\frac{s^2}{n}} \text{ or } \frac{s}{\sqrt{n}}$$

(3.7)

where

$\sigma_{\bar{Y}}$ = standard error (i.e., the standard deviation of the sampling distribution) in the population

$s_{\bar{Y}}$ = sample's estimate of the standard error

s^2 = sample's estimate of the variance of the distribution of data

n = sample's size

The next example illustrates the way the standard error is estimated from the sample's observations.

■ EXAMPLE 3.3

In Example 3.1, we looked at a study of the efficacy of a new topical treatment for glaucoma and observed the difference in intraocular pressure between the two eyes for each of nine persons. From those observations, we calculated estimates of the parameters of the population's distribution of data. In that example, we estimated the mean to be equal to 3 mmHg and the variance to be equal to 15.5 mmHg². Now, let us use these same data to estimate the parameters of the sampling distribution.

As stated in Equation (3.5), the mean of the sampling distribution is the same as the mean of the distribution of data. Thus, the sample's estimate of the mean of the sampling distribution is equal to the sample's estimate of the mean of the distribution of data. In Example 3.1, we calculated that estimate and found it to be equal to 3 mmHg.

To calculate the estimate of the standard error, we use Equation (3.7):

$$\sigma_{\bar{Y}} \triangleq \sqrt{\frac{s^2}{n}} = \sqrt{\frac{15.5}{9}} = 1.31 \text{ mmHg}$$

Thus, the estimates of the parameters of the sampling distribution are 3 mmHg for the mean and 1.31 mmHg for the standard error. ∎

Excel can calculate the standard error for us as shown in the next example.

■ EXAMPLE 3.4

In Example 3.1, we were interested in the efficacy of a new topical treatment for glaucoma. In Excel, we need to calculate or estimate the standard deviation and divide by the sample's size to obtain the standard error. The following are the results we obtain when we use Excel to calculate the standard error.

	A	B C	D E
1	ΔIOP		
2	3		
3	0		
4	3		
5	2		
6	−3		
7	11		
8	1		
9	6		
10	4		
11	9	= count(A2:A10)	Sample's size
12	3.711843	= stdevp(A2:A10)	Population's standard deviation
13	1.237281	= A12/sqrt(A11)	Population's standard error
14	3.937004	= stdev.s(A2:A10)	Sample's estimate of the population's standard deviation
15	1.312335	= A14/sqrt(A11)	Sample's estimate of the population's standard error

These values are consistent with those we obtained when we calculated them manually.

R does not calculate the standard error. Rather, the standard error has to be calculated from the standard deviation and the sample's size.

> sd(CHGIOP)/sqrt(9)

∎

Now that we are aware of the sampling distribution and familiar with its parameters, we are ready to address the influence of chance on estimates of the population's mean.

3.2.3 Interval Estimates

The idea behind interval estimation is to calculate an interval of values to estimate the population's parameter with a specified level of confidence that the population's parameter is included within the interval. The interval we calculate is usually centered on the point estimate, our best single-value guess at the value of the parameter. The result is called a **two-sided confidence interval**.[9]

How wide we make the confidence interval depends on two things. First, the width of the interval reflects our desired level of confidence that the population's parameter is included in the interval. To have a higher level of confidence, a wider interval is required.[10]

Second, the width of the interval is affected by the precision with which we can estimate the population's parameter from the sample's observations. That precision is reflected by the standard error. As the standard error decreases, so does the width of the interval estimate. The standard error can be decreased in two ways. One way is by decreasing the variance of the distribution of data (σ^2). That is to say, the more precisely the data are measured, the more precisely the mean is estimated. The other way is by increasing the size of the sample. The larger the sample, the more precise the estimate of the mean from that sample's observations.

Calculation of the limits of the interval estimate is similar to calculation of the interval of data values that correspond to a given percentage of a Gaussian distribution we discussed at the end of Chapter 2. There is an important difference between limits of the interval estimate and the limits of the interval that corresponds to a given proportion of the distribution of data. That is, the limits of the interval estimate are calculated from the sampling distribution, while the interval of data values is calculated from the distribution of data. There are two implications of that difference. First, we use the standard error instead of the standard deviation when calculating an interval estimate. Second, we are assured by the central limit theorem that it is appropriate to use methods based on Gaussian distributions as long as the size of the sample is not too small.

In Chapter 2, we looked at both an approximate method and an exact method for calculating the interval of data values. The approximate method presented looks at interval multipliers of the standard deviation to determine the data interval that corresponds to a particular proportion of all the data values. This approximate method

---

[9]If we were to allow one of the limits of the interval estimate to be equal to infinity, we would create a **one-sided** confidence interval. A one-sided confidence interval is not centered on the point estimate, making it more difficult to interpret. We will not consider further one-sided confidence intervals in this text.

[10]The extremes for the level of confidence are 0 and 100%. At a 0% level of confidence, we are certain that the population's parameter is not included in the interval. A 0% interval is equal to the point estimate. At a 100% level of confidence, we are certain that the population's parameter is included in the interval. A 100% interval includes all possible values for the parameter (e.g., $-\infty$ to $+\infty$).

is useful when interpreting means and standard deviations tabulated in a research article. That application was demonstrated in Example 2.14.

We can use a similar method to calculate an approximate interval estimate of the mean. When calculating an interval for means, rather than for data, it is multiples of the standard error we use, instead of the standard deviation. This is because the interval for means is calculated from the sampling distribution instead of the distribution of data. The next example shows how this can be done for tabulated means and standard errors from a research article.

■ EXAMPLE 3.5

In a study of 53 patients with renal disease (*N Engl J Med* 1998; 339:1364–1370), the mean blood pressure during the winter months was reported as "153 (±3)" mmHg for systolic pressure and "82 (±2)" mmHg for diastolic pressure. The text of this report tells us that the numbers in parentheses are the corresponding standard errors. Let us use the approximate method to interpret these results.

When we used the approximate method to interpret standard deviations in Example 2.10, we calculated intervals centered on the mean and having limits of either one standard deviation or two standard deviations on either side of the mean. These intervals encompass about two-thirds and about 95% of the data in a Gaussian distribution of data, respectively. If we were to calculate those same intervals, but with multiples of the standard error instead of the standard deviation, the intervals would include about two-thirds and about 95% of the possible estimates of the mean in a Gaussian sampling distribution. The following table shows the approximate confidence intervals we obtain using the information provided in this research article:

Measurement	Mean (mmHg)	SE (mmHg)	±1SE (mmHg)	±2SE (mmHg)
Systolic blood pressure	153	3	150–156	147–159
Diastolic blood pressure	82	2	80–84	78–86

These intervals give us an idea of how different the means would be if we were to take several samples from the population. For systolic blood pressure, about 95% of the means would be in the 12 mmHg interval between 147 and 159 mmHg. Similarly, 95% of mean diastolic blood pressure values would be in the 8 mmHg interval between 78 and 86 mmHg. These intervals reflect the precision with which we are able to estimate the means.   ■

The approximate method of calculating an interval estimate is appropriate when we are performing an informal interpretation of health research data. If we are using interval estimates in a formal interpretation (i.e., in writing a research article or making a presentation), however, we should use the exact method to calculate interval estimates. The exact method involves a standard normal deviate[11] that corresponds to one-half of the complement of the level of confidence we desire. For a 95% confidence interval, the standard normal deviate would correspond to 2.5% (or a proportion of 0.025). Equation (3.8) illustrates how that exact method is used to calculate an interval centered on the point estimate of the mean:

$$\mu \triangleq \overline{Y} \pm (z_{\alpha/2} \cdot \sigma_{\overline{Y}}) \tag{3.8}$$

where

μ = population's mean

$\overline{Y}$ = sample's estimate of the population's mean

α = complement of the degree of confidence desired (e.g., if we want a 95% confidence level, $\alpha = 1 - 0.95 = 0.05$)

$z_{\alpha/2}$ = a standard normal deviate that corresponds to a probability of one-half the complement of the degree of confidence we desire in one tail of the standard normal distribution

$\sigma_{\overline{Y}}$ = standard error (i.e., the standard deviation of the sampling distribution) in the population

Now, let us take a look at an example using this method to calculate an interval estimate.

■ EXAMPLE 3.6

In Example 3.5, we calculated approximate interval estimates for mean systolic and diastolic blood pressures during the winter months among 53 persons with renal disease. Now, we will use the exact method to calculate 95% two-sided interval estimates for those means.

To calculate an exact interval estimate, we use Equation (3.8). In this equation, we need a standard normal deviate that corresponds to one-half of the complement of the degree of confidence we desire. In this case, we are going to calculate a 95% confidence interval, so α is equal to $1 - 0.95 = 0.05$. Since this will be a two-sided interval estimate, we need to find a standard normal deviate that corresponds to half of α ($0.05/2 = 0.025$) in the upper tail of the standard normal distribution. From Table B.1, we find that standard normal deviate by finding a probability of 0.0250 in the body of the table. That probability corresponds to the row headed by "1.9" and the column headed by "6." So, the standard normal deviate that corresponds to a probability of 0.025 is equal to 1.96. With that value and the estimates of the standard errors from Example 3.5, we obtain the following 95%, two-sided confidence intervals for the results reported in this research article.

---

[11] Note that we are assuming we know the value of the population's standard error. In Chapter 4, we will deal with the more likely circumstance that we are only estimating the standard error.

Measurement	Mean (mmHg)	SE (mmHg)	±1.96SE (mmHg)
Systolic blood pressure	153	3	147.1–158.9
Diastolic blood pressure	82	2	78.1–85.9

These confidence intervals are close to the approximate intervals using two standard errors on either side of the mean. Even so, we should use this exact method to calculate intervals we intend to publish. ■

Excel has a function that can help with these confidence intervals. It calculates the width of the interval. In other words, it provides a value that we subtract and add to the mean to reflect the level of confidence and the precision of the estimate. This is illustrated in the next example.

■ EXAMPLE 3.7

In Example 3.1, we were interested in the efficacy of a new topical treatment for glaucoma. Let us use Excel to calculate a 95%, two-sided confidence for the estimate of the mean. If we do that, we get the following results:

	A	B C		D E
1	ΔIOP			
2	3			
3	0			
4	3			
5	2			
6	−3			
7	11			
8	1			
9	6			
10	4			
11	9	= count(A2:A10)		Sample's size
12	3	= average(a2:a10)		Sample's estimate of the mean
13	3.937004	=stdev.s(A2:A10)		Sample's estimate of the population's standard deviation
14	2.572129	= confidence.norm (0.05,A13,A11)		Width of 95% confidence interval
15	0.427871	= A12 − A14		Lower limit of 95% confidence interval for the mean
16	5.572129	= A12 + A14		Upper limit of 95% confidence interval for the mean

These values are consistent with those we obtained when we calculated them manually. ■

Interval estimation is one way we can take into account the role of chance in determining the composition of our sample. In this approach, we calculate an interval centered on the sample's estimate of the population's parameter. The width of this interval determines the level of confidence we can have that the population's parameter is, in fact, included in the interval. Also influencing the width of the interval is the precision of the estimate. Another way we can take the role of chance into account in determining the composition of our sample is through the process of hypothesis testing. This is the next topic we will consider in this chapter.

3.3   HYPOTHESIS TESTING

There are four steps in the process of statistical hypothesis testing. The first step is to formulate the hypothesis about the nature of the population that will be tested. Next, we take a sample from the population. Then, we calculate the probability of getting that sample if the hypothesis were true. In the final step, we reject the hypothesis as a description of the population if the probability of getting that sample assuming that the hypothesis was true is sufficiently small. These steps are illustrated in Figure 3.4.

The first step in statistical hypothesis testing is to formulate the hypothesis to be tested. At this point, no data have been collected from the population. Thus, the hypothesis to be tested is not in any way influenced by the sample's observations. Instead, the hypothesis is a tentative description of the population that might be changed after the data are collected and analyzed.

The hypothesis to be tested has to satisfy two requirements. First, the hypothesis must describe a condition that is interesting to test. Second, the hypothesis must make a specific statement about the population. For instance, if the hypothesis addresses the population's mean, the hypothesis must suggest a single numeric value for that mean. The types of hypotheses that satisfy both of these requirements are usually statements about the population that suggest that there are no relationships between measurements. In such a circumstance, differences are equal to 0, ratios are equal to 1, and nothing changes in relation to anything else. Because of this characteristic, the hypothesis that we test is called the **null hypothesis** and is identified by the symbol H_0. The next example illustrates how the null hypothesis is formulated.

■ EXAMPLE 3.8

In Example 3.1, we were interested in the efficacy of a new topical medication that is intended to lower intraocular pressure. The study that was performed involved nine patients with ocular hypertension. Each of those patients was randomly assigned to use the new medication in one eye and the standard treatment in the other eye. After one week of treatment, the difference in intraocular pressure between the two eyes was measured. Now, let us develop the null hypothesis that we could test in this study that would address the efficacy of the new medication.

The reason we are doing this study is because we think that there will be a difference between the intraocular pressures in each person's eyes. This is the hypothesis that motivated us to perform the study, but it cannot be used as the null hypothesis. The reason is that this hypothesis does not make a specific statement about the population (i.e., it does not provide a single numeric value for the mean difference in intraocular pressure). For a hypothesis to be testable, it must make a specific statement about the population.

Instead of testing the hypothesis that motivated the study, we can use its denial (i.e., the complement of that hypothesis) since it provides a specific value for the population's mean, namely zero. Thus, the null hypothesis that we will test is that the mean difference in intraocular pressure between each person's eyes is equal to 0 in the population. Mathematically, the null hypothesis is given as

$$H_0 : \mu_0 = 0$$

where μ_0 is the value of the population's mean difference according to the null hypothesis. ∎

Quite a bit of what we do when analyzing data is to accomplish the third step of hypothesis testing. In this step, we calculate the probability of getting an estimate (e.g., of the mean) at least as far from the hypothesized value as the sample's estimate assuming the null hypothesis is true. This probability is called the **P-value**. The P-value is a conditional probability in which the conditional event is obtaining an estimate at least as extreme as the sample's estimate and the conditioning event is the null hypothesis being true.[12] Equation (3.9) illustrates the P-value in

(1) Formulate hypothesis

(2) Take sample from population

(3) Calculate probability of getting an estimate as far from the hypothesized value as the sample's estimate if the hypothesis were true

(4) If probability is small, reject hypothesis

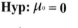 **Hyp:** $\mu_0 = 0$

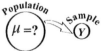

$$P(\text{estimate} \geq \overline{Y} \mid \mu = 0)$$

 Hyp $\mu = 0$

Figure 3.4   Steps in testing a statistical hypothesis.

[12] It is the need to calculate the P-value that requires a null hypothesis to make a specific statement about the population. It would be extremely complicated, if even possible in practice, to calculate a P-value for a null hypothesis that includes more than one value.

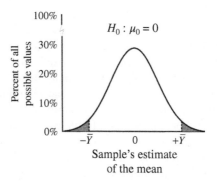

Figure 3.5 The sampling distribution as defined by the null hypothesis (i.e., the "null distribution"). $\bar{Y}$ is the absolute value of the point estimate obtained in the sample.

mathematic language (we will also look at the P-value graphically in a moment):

$$P\text{-value} = p(\text{estimate} \geq \bar{Y} \mid H_0 \text{ true}) \qquad (3.9)$$

Calculation of a P-value is similar to calculation of the probability of selecting persons from the population within an interval of data values, as we did in Chapter 2 (Equation (2.7)). There are three differences, however, between calculation of the probability of obtaining an interval of data values and calculation of a P-value. One difference is that, in hypothesis testing, the population's mean is taken to be equal to the specific value stated in the null hypothesis, rather than the population's actual value. Thus, we think of the sampling distribution defined by the null hypothesis, instead of the actual sampling distribution. The sampling distribution representing the null hypothesis being true is called the **null distribution**. Figure 3.5 illustrates the null distribution when the null hypothesis states that the mean is equal to 0.

The second difference is that calculation of a P-value involves the sampling distribution, rather than the distribution of data. Thus, the standard deviation used in calculation of a P-value is the standard deviation of the sampling distribution (i.e., the standard error). Equation (3.10) illustrates how a standard normal deviate can be calculated as part of the process of determining a P-value:

$$z = \frac{\bar{Y} - \mu_0}{\sigma_{\bar{Y}}} \qquad (3.10)$$

where

z = standard normal deviate that corresponds to the sample's estimate of the population's mean

$\bar{Y}$ = sample's estimate of the population's mean

μ_0 = value of the population's mean stated in the null hypothesis

$\sigma_{\bar{Y}}$ = standard deviation of the sampling distribution (i.e., the standard error)

The third difference is that the P-value is almost always calculated by considering both tails of the sampling distribution. This implies that the P-value is the

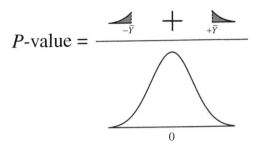

$$P\text{-value} = \frac{\begin{array}{c}\underset{-\bar{Y}}{\blacktriangle} + \underset{+\bar{Y}}{\blacktriangleright}\end{array}}{\underset{0}{\bigwedge}}$$

Figure 3.6   Calculation of a *P*-value from the null distribution. $\bar{Y}$ is the absolute value of the point estimate obtained in the sample.

probability of getting a sample with an estimate at least as far from the value in the null hypothesis, without specifying on which side of that value the sample's estimate ($\bar{Y}$) occurs. We will consider this issue further, but first let us take a look at Figure 3.6 which illustrates the *P*-value in graphic language.

Now, let us take a look at an example of how to calculate the *P*-value.

■ EXAMPLE 3.9

In Example 3.8, we were interested in the efficacy of a new topical treatment for ocular hypertension. In that example, we considered the null hypothesis that the mean difference in intraocular pressure between a person's eyes is equal to 0 in the population. In Example 3.1, we found that the mean difference in intraocular pressure is equal to 3 mmHg for these nine patients. In Example 3.3, we calculated the standard error for the mean difference in intraocular pressure and found it to be equal to 1.31 mmHg. Now, let us assume that the population's standard error is equal to our estimate and calculate the *P*-value that we can use to test the null hypothesis that the mean difference in intraocular pressures between each person's eyes is equal to 0 in the population.

P-values are determined from the sampling distribution, so we will use Equation (3.10) to calculate the standard normal deviate that will represent the observed mean difference in the standard normal distribution:

$$z = \frac{\bar{Y} - \mu_0}{\sigma_{\bar{Y}}} = \frac{3 - 0}{1.31} = 2.29$$

So, a standard normal deviate of 2.29 corresponds to a sample's mean of 3 mmHg if the mean difference in the population is really equal to 0 (i.e., if the null hypothesis were true). In Table B.1, we find that a standard normal deviate of 2.29 or greater corresponds to a probability of 0.0110. If we confine our interest to means above 0, the *P*-value would be equal to 0.0110. If we were interested in means that are at least as far away from 0 as 3 mmHg in either direction, the *P*-value would be equal to 0.0110 for means greater than 0 plus 0.0110 for means less than 0. In that case, the *P*-value is equal to 0.0220.

The following is a graphic illustration of how this *P*-value is calculated. First, the sample's estimate of the mean change in intraocular pressure is converted from its original scale.

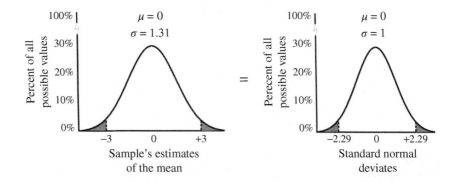

Then, the probability of obtaining the corresponding standard normal deviate (2.29) or a larger value is determined by looking up 2.29 in Table B.1. This probability is equal to 0.0110. Finally, the *P*-value is calculated as follows:

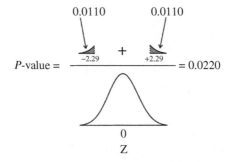

The final step in testing a statistical hypothesis is to stop believing in the null hypothesis if the *P*-value is small enough. This is called "rejecting" the null hypothesis. When we reject the null hypothesis, we say that the result is **statistically significant**.

To reject the null hypothesis, we need to decide how small the *P*-value needs to be to doubt the veracity of the null hypothesis. Usually, we consider a *P*-value equal to or less than 0.05 to be small enough to reject the null hypothesis. Thus, in Example 3.9, obtaining a *P*-value of 0.0220, we would conclude that the null hypothesis is not true. That is to say, we would reject the null hypothesis.

When we reject the null hypothesis, something else happens automatically: we believe that a second hypothesis is true. This second hypothesis is called the **alternative hypothesis**. Since our belief in the alternative hypothesis occurs only by the process of eliminating the null hypothesis, the alternative hypothesis must include all possibilities for the population that are not included in the null hypothesis.[13] So, if the null hypothesis states that the population's mean is equal to 0, the alternative hypothesis is that the population's mean is not equal to 0.

An alternative hypothesis that includes values on both sides of the value in the null hypothesis is called a **two-sided** alternative hypothesis. It is when we have a two-sided alternative hypothesis that the P-value is calculated from both tails of the sampling distribution. A **one-sided** alternative hypothesis, however, includes values on only one side of the value in the null hypothesis and the corresponding P-value is calculated only from the single tail of the sampling distribution on that same side of the value in the null hypothesis.

Virtually all alternative hypotheses should be two-sided. To use a one-sided alternative hypothesis, it must be impossible for the population's value to occur on the other side of the null value.[14] This is rarely true, so all of the alternative hypotheses we will consider in this text are two-sided.

At the final step in the process of hypothesis testing we can reject the null hypothesis if the P-value is sufficiently small (i.e., $P \leq 0.05$). If the P-value is not small enough to reject the null hypothesis (i.e., $P > 0.05$), however, we do not accept the null hypothesis as being true. Instead, we avoid drawing a conclusion about the null hypothesis when it cannot be rejected. The statistical terminology we use when the P-value is too large to reject the null hypothesis is to say that we "fail to reject" the null hypothesis.

To understand why we "fail to reject" rather than "accept" the null hypothesis, we need to consider the potential errors that we might make when we are testing a null hypothesis. There are two types of errors possible. A **type I error** occurs when the null hypothesis is true, but we mistakenly reject it. A **type II error** occurs when the null hypothesis is false, but we wrongly accept it. Those errors are illustrated in Table 3.2. The probability of making a type I error is symbolized by the Greek letter α (alpha). Equation (3.11) illustrates α in mathematical language:

$$\alpha = p(\text{type I error}) = p(\text{reject } H_0 \mid H_0 \text{ true}) \qquad (3.11)$$

and Figure 3.7 illustrates α graphically.

The value of α is chosen when we decide how small a P-value must be before we reject the null hypothesis. If we use the conventional value of 0.05, the probability of making a type I error is then also equal to 0.05 (i.e., $\alpha = 0.05$). Thus, the probability of making a type I error is known and it is considered to be sufficiently small to justify rejection of the null hypothesis when the P-value is equal to or less than α. When the alternative hypothesis is two-sided, the value of α is evenly divided

---

[13]In statistical terms, the null hypothesis and the alternative hypothesis are a collectively exhaustive set.
[14]The reason that it must be *impossible* for the population's value to occur on the other side of the value in the null hypothesis to use a one-sided alternative hypothesis is because the alternative hypothesis is embraced through the process of elimination once the null hypothesis is rejected. For a one-sided alternative hypothesis to be appropriate, values on the other side of the null value must be eliminated by a process other than rejection of the null hypothesis.

TABLE 3.2. There are Four Possible Results in the Process of Hypothesis Testing*

		Conclusion	
		Accept H_0	Reject H_0
Truth	H_0 true	Correct	Type I error
	H_0 false	Type II error	Correct

[a] In two of these four possible results, our conclusion is incorrect.

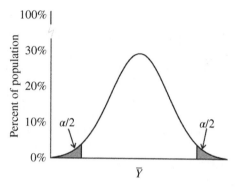

Figure 3.7   The value of α is split between the two tails of the sampling distribution corresponding to the null hypothesis when the alternative hypothesis is two-sided.

between both tails of the sampling distribution as defined in the null hypothesis. Figure 3.7 illustrates α when the alternative hypothesis is two-sided.

The next example shows how we use the value of α to draw a conclusion about the null hypothesis.

■ EXAMPLE 3.10

In Example 3.9, we calculated a P-value of 0.0220 when testing the null hypothesis that the mean difference in intraocular pressures between the two eyes of each patient (one treated with new medication) is equal to 0 in the population. If we are willing to take a risk of 0.05 of making a type I error, what is the best conclusion to draw?

By saying that we are willing to take a 0.05 risk of making a type I error, we are saying that the value of α is 0.05. If the P-value is equal to or less than the value of α, we can reject the null hypothesis. In this case, the P-value is less than 0.05, so we can reject the null hypothesis that the mean difference in intraocular pressures is equal to 0 in the population. Then, through the process of elimination, we can accept the alternative hypothesis. The two-sided alternative hypothesis is that the mean difference in intraocular pressures is not equal to 0 in the population. The biologic interpretation is that the new medication makes a difference in intraocular pressure. ∎

The probability of making a type II error is symbolized by the Greek letter β (beta). Equation (3.12) illustrates β in mathematical language:

$$\beta = p(\text{type II error}) = p(\text{accept } H_0 \mid H_0 \text{ false}) \tag{3.12}$$

The probability of making a type II error is based on the assumption that the null hypothesis is false and, therefore, that the alternative hypothesis is true. Since the alternative hypothesis does not provide a specific value for the population's parameter, it is essentially impossible to calculate the probability of making a type II error. This inability to determine the probability of making a type II error makes statisticians uneasy. We do not mind taking a chance of being wrong, as long as we know the magnitude of the risk, but we do not know the risk of making a type II error. One way to avoid the risk of making a type II error is to never conclude that the null hypothesis is true. Illustrated in Table 3.3, that strategy eliminates the left-hand column of the table, including the situation in which we can make a type II error. When we say that we "fail to reject" the null hypothesis, what we are really saying is that we refuse to draw a conclusion about the null hypothesis, since to do so would involve the risk of making a type II error.

3.3.1   Relationship Between Interval Estimation and Hypothesis Testing

In this chapter, two methods have been described that take the role of chance into account in selecting the sample from the population: interval estimation and hypothesis testing. Since it is the same role of chance these two methods take into account, you might expect the methods to be related to each other. In fact, the method of calculating a confidence interval and the method of testing a hypothesis we have

TABLE 3.3. Avoiding a Type II Error by Not Accepting the Null Hypothesis as True When It Cannot be Rejected

		Conclusion	
		Accept H_0	Reject H_0
Truth	H_0 True	~~Correct~~	**Type I error**
	H_0 False	~~Type II error~~	Correct

considered are algebraically identical.[15] From a mathematical point of view, it does not really matter which approach we use. We can calculate a confidence interval if we know the P-value of the sample's estimate or we can test a hypothesis if we know the limits of the confidence interval. The latter is the easier of the two. To test a null hypothesis using a confidence interval, we decide whether the value in the null hypothesis is included within the confidence interval. To be included in the interval, the null value must be greater than the lower limit and less than the upper limit. If the null value is included in the confidence interval, we would fail to reject the null hypothesis with α equal to the complement of the degree of confidence that the interval reflects (i.e., $\alpha = 0.05$ for a 95% confidence interval). If, on the other hand, the value in the null hypothesis is either equal to or less than the lower limit or it is equal to or greater than the upper limit, we can reject the null hypothesis with that same value of α. This method of interpreting a confidence interval is illustrated in the next example.

■ EXAMPLE 3.11

In Example 3.10, we tested the null hypothesis that the mean difference in intraocular pressures between a patient's eyes was equal to 0 for a group of nine patients when the two eyes were treated with different topical medications. Now, let us suppose that we were to take chance into account by calculating a 95% confidence interval. What conclusion could we draw about the null hypothesis by examining the confidence interval?

Using Equation (3.8) and the standard error of 1.31 mmHg calculated in Example 3.3, we get the following 95%, two-sided confidence interval for the mean difference in intraocular pressure:

$$\mu \triangleq \overline{Y} \pm (z_{\alpha/2} \cdot \sigma_{\overline{Y}}) = 3 \pm (1.96 \cdot 1.31) = 0.4 - 5.6 \, \text{mmHg}$$

Now, we can test the null hypothesis that the mean difference in intraocular pressures is equal to 0 in the population by determining whether or not 0 is included in the confidence interval. Since 0 is less than the lower limit of the confidence interval, we can reject the null hypothesis that the mean difference is equal to 0. Biologically, the new medication makes a difference in intraocular pressure. This is the same conclusion we drew in Example 3.10.   ■

In these first three chapters, we have examined the logical basis for what we do and say about statistical analysis of health research data. For the next nine chapters, we will discover the methods themselves, when they should be used, and how to interpret their results.

---

[15]This is true for all methods we will discuss for continuous data. It is almost true for the methods we will discuss for nominal data. We will consider this distinction further in Chapter .

CHAPTER SUMMARY

In Chapter 3, we learned how to draw inferences about the population by examining a sample's observations. There are two processes that we can use. The first of these is estimation. In the process of estimation, the goal is to guess about the value of a parameter in the population. There are two kinds of estimates we use. One of those is a point estimate. A point estimate is a single number that is our best guess at the value of the parameter. The problem with point estimates is that they have a very low chance of being exactly equal to the population's parameter. This is because there are so many possible values that the probability for any single value is close to 0.

The other kind of estimate is an interval estimate, which is also known as a confidence interval. It differs from a point estimate in that an interval estimate implies that the population's parameter lies within an interval of values. The width of an interval estimate determines the level of confidence we can have that the population's parameter is included in the interval. The most commonly used interval estimate gives us 95% confidence that the parameter is included. In addition to the selected level of confidence, the width of an interval estimate is affected by the precision with which we can estimate the parameter. The greater the precision, the narrower the interval.

The second process we can use to draw inferences about the population by examining a sample is statistical hypothesis testing. In statistical hypothesis testing, we begin with a hypothesis that makes a specific statement about the population. This hypothesis is called the null hypothesis. It is so named because a specific statement that has a relevant biologic interpretation usually says that nothing is different. The next step is to take a sample from the population. It is important to note, in statistical hypothesis testing, the hypothesis comes before the data are collected.

Most of the "work" in statistical hypothesis testing involves calculations necessary to determine the P-value. A P-value is a conditional probability. The conditional event is getting a sample at least as different from what the null hypothesis states as the sample we observed. The conditioning event is that the null hypothesis is true. It is important not to get these events interchanged. A P-value does not tell us the probability that the null hypothesis is true. Instead, the P-value assumes that it is true.

The final step in hypothesis testing is deciding what to conclude. Our conclusion depends on how the numeric magnitude of the P-value compares to some preselected value called alpha (α). The most usual value of alpha is 0.05. If the P-value is less than or equal to alpha, we reject the null hypothesis. That is to say, we conclude that the null hypothesis is not a true statement about the population.

When we reject the null hypothesis, we automatically accept the alternative hypothesis as true. The alternative hypothesis is not tested. It is considered to be true whenever the null hypothesis is considered to be false. For this to work, the null and alternative hypotheses must cover all possibilities for the population. Keeping this in mind is important when choosing between a two-sided (in which differences from the null hypothesis can occur in both directions) and a one-sided (in which differences from the null hypothesis can occur in only one direction) alternative hypothesis. Most often, two-sided alternative hypotheses are the appropriate choice.

There are two kinds of errors that can be made in hypothesis testing. A type I error occurs when the null hypothesis is rejected but it is, in fact, true. The chance of making a type I error is determined by the choice of the value of alpha. If alpha is equal to 0.05, there is a 0.05 chance of making a type I error. A type II error occurs when the null hypothesis is accepted as true but it is, in fact, false. We do not know the probability of making a type II error, since the alternative hypothesis does not make a specific statement about the population. Because we do not know the chance of making a type II error, we avoid any opportunity for this type of error to occur. We do this by refusing to conclude that the null hypothesis is true. When the *P*-value is larger than alpha, we do not accept the null hypothesis as being true. Instead, we refrain from drawing a conclusion about the null hypothesis. This is often referred to as "failing to reject" the null hypothesis.

Both interval estimation and hypothesis testing take into account the role of chance in selecting a sample from the population. In Chapter 2, we considered this role of chance in selecting an individual from the population by using the distribution of data. When we are taking the role of chance on the entire sample, we use a different distribution. This distribution is called the sampling distribution. It is the distribution of estimates from all possible samples of a given size.

An important feature of the sampling distribution is that is tends to be a Gaussian distribution, even if the distribution of data is not a Gaussian distribution. This is especially true of sampling distributions of estimates of parameters of location from larger samples. This principle is called the central limit theorem. It is because of the central limit theorem that many of the statistical procedures commonly used in analyzing health research data are based on Gaussian distributions.

The parameters of the sampling distribution are related to the parameters of the distribution of data. The means of the two distributions are equal to the same value. This will always be the case for any unbiased estimate. An unbiased estimate is equal to the population's parameter, on the average. This is reflected in the sampling distribution by having the mean equal to the parameter that is being estimated (i.e., mean of the distribution of data).

The variances and standard deviations of the sampling distribution and distribution of data are related, but not equal to the same value. The sampling distribution is less dispersed than is the distribution of data. The reason for this is that the impact of extreme data values in a sample is offset by less extreme data values. Thus, estimates of the mean have less variation than do the data. How much less, depends on the number of observations in the sample. The greater the number of observations, the less variable the estimates. To emphasize the difference in dispersion between the sampling distribution and the distribution of data, the standard deviation of the sampling distribution is usually called the standard error.

Both interval estimation and hypothesis testing use the sampling distribution to take into account the role of chance in selecting a sample from the population. In hypothesis testing, it is the sampling distribution that is used to calculate a P-value. In interval estimation, it is the standard error of the sampling distribution that is used to represent the precision with which the parameter has been estimated. Although these sound like different processes, they are really just mirror images of the same logical procedure. If a null hypothesis is rejected, the null value will be outside the limits of the confidence interval.[16] If the null value is inside the confidence interval, the null hypothesis would not be rejected. This relationship allows us to use confidence intervals to test null hypotheses.

EXERCISES

3.1. Suppose we were to take a sample of 10 births from a given population and determine the gestational ages (in days) at birth. Imagine that we observe the following results: 266, 267, 256, 259, 261, 255, 270, 271, 269, 266. Create an Excel dataset using those observations. What is the point estimate of the mean gestational age in the population from which this sample was drawn?

    A. 220

    B. 225

    C. 255

    D. 264

    E. 306

3.2. Suppose we were to take a sample of 10 births from a given population and determine the gestational ages (in days) at birth. Imagine that we observe the following results: 266, 267, 256, 259, 261, 255, 270, 271, 269, 266. Create an Excel dataset using those observations. What is the sample's estimate of the standard deviation of gestational age in the population from which this sample was drawn?

    A. 2.6

    B. 3.1

    C. 3.4

    D. 4.3

    E. 5.8

3.3. Suppose we are interested in diastolic blood pressure (dbp) among persons in a particular population. To investigate this, we take a sample of nine persons from the population and measure their dbp. Imagine we obtain the following

---

[16]Being exactly equal to the limit of a confidence interval is considered to be outside the interval.

results 75, 80, 81, 72, 85, 88, 91, 87, 88. Create an Excel dataset using those observations. Which of the following is closest to the sample's estimate of the variance of diastolic blood pressure values?

A. 6.4

B. 17.5

C. 41.5

D. 74.7

E. 83.0

3.4. Suppose we take a sample of 36 persons from a particular population and measure their body weight. Then, we give each person a one-month's supply of appetite suppressants. At the end of the month, we weigh each person again and subtract their new weight from their first weight. Suppose we observe a mean difference in weight equal to 10 kg and we know the variance of differences in weight in the population is equal to $900 \, kg^2$. Which of the following is closest to the interval of values within which we have 95% confidence that the population's mean lies?

A. 0.0–20.0

B. 0.2–19.8

C. 2.3–17.7

D. 5.0–15.0

E. 8.0–12.0

3.5. Suppose we were to conduct a study in which 16 persons with hypothyroidism were given two medications in a random order. In this study, we measure thyroid-stimulating hormone (TSH) after the participants had taken each of the medications for a week. Suppose we observe that the mean difference in TSH levels was equal to 20 mg/dL and we know the standard deviation of differences between TSH levels is equal to 60 mg/dL in the population. Which of the following is closest to the value that reflects the precision with which we will be able to estimate the mean from that sample's observations (i.e., the standard error)?

A. 1.9

B. 3.7

C. 5.0

D. 7.7

E. 15.0

3.6. Suppose we were to conduct a study in which 16 persons with hypothyroidism were given two medications in a random order. In this study, we measure TSH after the participants had taken each of the medications for a week. Suppose we estimate the mean difference in TSH levels to be equal to 20 mg/dL and we estimate the standard deviation of differences between TSH levels to be equal to 60 mg/dL. What is the best null hypothesis to test about the mean difference in the population?

A. $\mu = 0$

B. $\mu > 0$

C. $\mu < 0$

D. $\mu \neq 0$

E. $\mu = ?$

3.7. Suppose we were to conduct a study in which 16 persons with hypothyroidism were given two medications in a random order. In this study, we measure TSH after the participants had taken each of the medications for a week. Suppose we estimate the mean difference in TSH levels to be equal to 20 mg/dL and we estimate the standard deviation of differences between TSH levels to be equal to 60 mg/dL. What is the best alternative hypothesis to consider about the mean difference in the population?

A. $\mu = 0$

B. $\mu > 0$

C. $\mu < 0$

D. $\mu \neq 0$

E. $\mu = ?$

3.8. Suppose we were to conduct a study in which 16 persons with hypothyroidism were given two medications in a random order. In this study, we measure TSH after the participants had taken each of the medications for a week. Suppose we estimate the mean difference in TSH levels to be equal to 20 mg/dL and we estimate the standard deviation of differences between TSH levels to be equal to 60 mg/dL. Test the appropriate null hypothesis allowing a 5% chance of making a type I error. Which of the following is the best conclusion to draw?

A. Reject the null hypothesis

B. Accept the null hypothesis

C. Fail to reject the null hypothesis

D. Fail to accept the null hypothesis

E. Hypothesis testing is not appropriate for these data

3.9. Suppose we take a sample of 36 persons from a particular population and measure their body weight. Then, we give each person a one-month's supply of appetite suppressants. At the end of the month, we weigh each person again and subtract their new weight from their first weight. Suppose we observe a mean difference in weight equal to 10 kg and calculate a 95% confidence interval for the estimate that ranges from 0.2 to 19.8 kg. Which of the following are the best null and alternative hypotheses to test about the mean difference in the population?

A. H_0: $\mu = 0$ and H_A: $\mu = 0$

B. H_0: $\mu \neq 0$ and H_A: $\mu = 0$

C. H_0: $\mu = 0$ and H_A: $\mu \neq 0$

D. H_0: $\mu = 0$ and H_A: $\mu > 0$

E. H_0: $\mu = 0$ and H_A: $\mu < 0$

3.10. Suppose we take a sample of 36 persons from a particular population and measure their body weight. Then, we give each person a one-month's supply of appetite suppressants. At the end of the month, we weigh each person again and subtract their new weight from their first weight. Suppose we observe a mean difference in weight equal to 10 kg and calculate a 95% confidence interval for that estimate that ranges from 0.2 to 19.8 kg. Which of the following is the best conclusion to draw if we were to test the null hypothesis that the mean difference in weight is equal to 0 in the population?

A. Reject both the null and alternative hypotheses

B. Accept both the null and alternative null hypotheses

C. Reject the null hypothesis and accept the alternative hypothesis

D. Accept the null hypothesis and reject the alternative hypothesis

E. It is best not to draw a conclusion about the null and alternative hypotheses from these observations

PART TWO

UNIVARIABLE ANALYSES

In Part One, we examined three basic principles of statistics. First, we found out how chance works. Next, we considered different ways in which a population's data can be described. Finally, we learned how a sample's observations can be used to describe the population's data. Now that we understand these basic principles, we are ready to learn about the actual methods that are used to analyze data encountered in health research.

The organization of the remainder of this text is designed to reflect how a statistician selects an appropriate method to analyze a particular set of data. There are two reasons the text is organized in this way. First, this organization helps us to see how different statistical methods fit together. As you read the remaining chapters, you should get the impression that statistical methods share the same logical framework. Second, this organization will assist you when using this text as a reference. When you are ready to analyze your own data or interpret the results of someone else's analysis, you can use Flowchart 1 to find the chapter that discusses the statistical procedure that is most commonly used to analyze a particular set of data. Before we talk about specific statistical methods, however, we need to take a look at how a statistician thinks when faced with data to analyze.

As part of the process of research, the researcher records data. These data, however, are not necessarily used in statistical analyses in the same form that they are recorded. Statisticians think of the collection of data to be used in a statistical

Introduction to Biostatistical Applications in Health Research with Microsoft Office Excel® and R,
Second Edition. Robert P. Hirsch.
© 2021 John Wiley & Sons, Inc. Published 2021 by John Wiley & Sons, Inc.
Companion website: www.wiley.com/go/hirsch/healthresearch2e

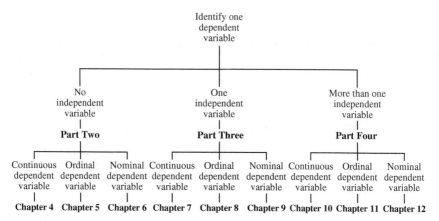

FLOWCHART 1   The process a statistician uses to begin selecting a statistical method and how that process relates to the structure of this textbook.

procedure a little bit differently than the collection of data that are recorded by the researcher. Rather than data, statisticians think about **variables**. Variables represent the researcher's data in the mathematics of statistical methods.

Variables have two characteristics. The first of these characteristics is determined by the type of data the variable represents. For continuous or ordinal data, corresponding variables represent those data just as they were observed. Thus, there is a one-to-one correspondence between continuous or ordinal data recorded by the researcher and continuous or ordinal variables analyzed by the statistician.

Nominal data, however, are a little bit different. In statistical procedures, nominal variables are limited to a dichotomous (yes/no) classification that indicates the presence or absence of a condition. Nominal data with only two categories, such as gender, can be expressed by one nominal variable. Here, we might use a nominal variable indicating the presence or absence of, say, being female. For nominal data consisting of more than two categories, on the other hand, more than one nominal variable is needed to represent those data. It is important to appreciate this relationship, since different statistical methods are designed to analyze different numbers of variables.

As an example of the relationship between nominal data and nominal variables, let us consider race as a characteristic that we might measure with four categories: black, Asian, white, and other. In this case, we need to create three nominal variables to indicate a person's race. The first variable might indicate the presence or absence of being black, the second variable might indicate the presence or absence of being Asian, and the third variable might indicate the presence or absence of being white. Notice that we do not need a fourth variable to indicate the presence or absence of being a member of a race included in the category called "other," for anyone who is not black, Asian, or white *must* be a member of one of the other races. In general, if nominal data contain k categories, then $k - 1$ nominal variables will be used in statistical procedures to represent these k categories.

The second characteristic of variables is determined by their function in the statistical analysis. A variable can serve either of two functions. The first function is to represent the data of primary interest to the researcher. This is the variable for which estimates are to be made or hypotheses are to be tested. We call the variable that represents the data of primary interest the **dependent variable**. For illustration, let us say that we are interested in the effect of some intervention on serum lipid levels. Here, it is of primary interest to make estimates or test hypotheses about serum lipid levels; therefore, the dependent variable should represent some measure of the lipid level.

Most often in health research, a single statistical analysis will involve only one dependent variable. If a set of research observations includes more than one collection of data for which an estimate will be made or a hypothesis will be tested, the usual approach is to conduct more than one analysis, each involving one of the variables of primary interest as the dependent variable. For instance, if we have several different measurements of serum lipids (e.g., high-density lipoprotein (HDL), low-density lipoprotein (LDL), and total cholesterol), the usual approach to analyze these observations would be to examine each of the serum lipid measurements in a separate statistical analysis.[1]

The second function of variables in statistical analysis is to specify conditions under which estimates will be made or a hypothesis will be tested for the dependent variable. Variables that serve this function are known as **independent variables**. In our example of a study of an intervention to affect serum lipid levels, an independent variable would tell us whether or not a particular patient received the intervention. In other words, we are interested in comparing serum lipid levels between persons who received and persons who did not receive the intervention. Therefore, the independent variable indicating the presence or absence of the intervention defines the conditions under which we wish to examine the dependent variable. Other independent variables we might have included in this example are age and gender. Our reason for including age and gender in our analysis is probably because we like to take into account (or control for) their effect on serum lipid levels. The way in which we can control for characteristics when analyzing data is to include the variables representing those characteristics in the analysis. A role of independent variables is to control for their effect.

A key to understanding how statisticians think is by understanding variables. Once we are comfortable with the variables, we are ready to see the way a statistician begins to select a statistical method to analyze a particular set of data. The following flowchart illustrates that process:

---

[1] Procedures for analyzing a single dependent variable are collectively called **univariate** methods. Statistical procedures that involve more than one dependent variable are collectively called **multivariate** methods. Multivariate methods are rarely encountered in the health research literature except in those areas of research that overlap social or behavioral sciences. Multivariate methods will not be discussed in this text.

Flowchart 1 not only summarizes the way a statistician begins to select an appropriate statistical method but also outlines the organization of the next nine chapters of this book. Inspection of this flowchart reveals that the next three parts of the book are characterized by the number of independent variables involved in the analysis. Thus, in Part Two we will be interested in analyzing a dependent variable without any independent variables. Methods used to examine sets of observations containing a dependent variable and no independent variables are known as **univariable** methods, hence the name of Part Two is "Univariable Analyses." Having no independent variables in an analysis implies that there are no special conditions under which we are interested in making an estimate or testing a hypothesis about the dependent variable. Instead, we are interested in the dependent variable in general.

In Part Three, we will discuss **bivariable** methods in which we have one dependent variable and one independent variable. In bivariable analysis, there are special conditions under which we are interested in examining the dependent variable. In Part Four, the conditions under which we are interested in the dependent variable can be rather complex due to **multivariable** statistical methods that are used to analyze the dependent variable and more than one independent variable.[2]

As you examine the chapters within the next three parts of this book, you will notice that each part contains three chapters that correspond to the three types of data that can be represented by the dependent variable. In selecting an analytic approach, the statistician determines the number of variables, identifies dependent and independent variables, and classifies the type of data contained in the dependent variable.

Each chapter in the remaining parts also begins with another component of the flowchart. These flowcharts are extensions of one we have just examined. The flowcharts at the beginning of these chapters will help us choose a particular method of analysis for a set of data. They will summarize the issues we have to consider in choosing a statistical procedure. In each chapter, you will find a discussion of how to evaluate these issues.

Following any branch of the flowchart to its end will reveal the name of a standard distribution or statistical approach that is appropriate for either interval estimation or statistical hypothesis testing on the corresponding data set. In Chapter 3, we learned that estimation and hypothesis testing are closely related processes. In this text, we will discuss these procedures mostly from the point of view of statistical hypothesis testing. By this choice, we do not mean to imply that hypothesis testing is the only, or even the better, way to evaluate a data set. It is, however, the more commonly encountered approach in the health research literature.

---

[2]Notice a subtle distinction in terminology here. Multi**variable** methods are appropriate for three or more variables, while multi**variate** methods are appropriate for more than one dependent variable. The root "variable" refers to the number of variables without regard to their function. The root "variate" refers only to the number of dependent variables. A very common mistake and source of confusion in statistical terminology that you will find in the health research literature is a reference to a statistical procedure that examines one dependent variable and more than one independent variable as a multivariate rather than a multivariable procedure.

CHAPTER 4

UNIVARIABLE ANALYSIS OF A CONTINUOUS DEPENDENT VARIABLE

In this chapter we will take a look at the appropriate way to analyze a continuous dependent variable with no independent variables. That approach is summarized in Flowchart 2, which is a continuation of Flowchart 1.

In Chapter 2, we learned that continuous data are most often assumed to come from a distribution that can be described, at least in part, by two parameters: the mean (μ) and the variance (σ^2).[1] Although estimation and hypothesis testing for continuous data can focus on either parameter, we are almost always concerned

---

[1] This is not the same as assuming that the distribution of data is a Gaussian distribution, or any other particular type of distribution. Rather, this only assumes that the mean and variance help to characterize the distribution.

Introduction to Biostatistical Applications in Health Research with Microsoft Office Excel® and R,
Second Edition. Robert P. Hirsch.
© 2021 John Wiley & Sons, Inc. Published 2021 by John Wiley & Sons, Inc.
Companion website: www.wiley.com/go/hirsch/healthresearch2e

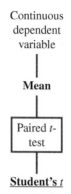

FLOWCHART 2   Flowchart showing univariable analysis of a continuous dependent variable. The point estimate that is most often used to describe the dependent variable (the mean) is in bold. The common name of the statistical test (paired *t*-test) is enclosed in a box. The standard distribution used in interval estimation and hypothesis testing is in bold and underlined.

with estimating or testing a hypothesis about the mean.[2] In Chapter 3, we examined procedures for estimation and hypothesis testing for the mean when we have a single dependent variable and no independent variables. Specifically, these procedures involved conversion of the sample's estimate of the population's mean to the standard normal scale by subtracting the hypothesized population's mean (μ_0) from the sample's mean ($\bar{Y}$) and dividing by the standard error ($\sigma_{\bar{Y}}$). This is a relatively straightforward procedure. Unfortunately, it is a little bit too simple to be entirely appropriate when analyzing real data.

To understand why the method described in Chapter 3 is not the method we should use to analyze a continuous dependent variable, let us take a moment to review what it is that we are doing when we perform statistical procedures on a mean observed in a sample. The sample that we have observed is only one of many possible samples we could have obtained from the population. Therefore, the mean we have calculated from our sample is only one of many possible means. We assume that chance, and only chance, determines which of all of the possible means we have actually observed in our sample. Regardless of whether we are interested in estimation or hypothesis testing, the purpose of the statistical procedure that we apply to our sample's observations is to take this influence of chance in estimation of the mean into account.

The method of converting a sample's mean to the standard normal scale appropriately reflects the influence of chance on estimation of the population's mean, but it overlooks another effect of chance. To see this other effect, let us reexamine the method we used to convert the sample's mean to the standard normal scale in

---

[2] In Chapter 2, we found out that the mean is a parameter of location of a distribution of continuous data. Most statistical methods used to analyze health research data address measures of location.

Chapter 3 (Equation (3.10)).

$$z = \frac{\overline{Y} - \mu_0}{\sigma_{\overline{Y}}} \qquad (4.1)$$

where

z = a standard normal deviate (i.e., a value from the standard normal distribution)
$\overline{Y}$ = the sample's estimate of the mean of the distribution of data
μ_0 = the value of the population's mean according to the null hypothesis (H_0)
$\sigma_{\overline{Y}}$ = the population's value of the standard error of the mean

Notice that the denominator of Equation (4.1) consists of the population's standard error. To include the population's standard error in that calculation, we need to assume that we know the variance of the distribution of data in the population (σ^2). Since we cannot observe the entire population, we cannot know the population's variance exactly. Rather, we estimate the population's variance from the sample's observations. To reflect that estimation, the right-hand part of Equation (4.1) becomes

$$\frac{\overline{Y} - \mu_0}{s_{\overline{Y}}} \qquad (4.2)$$

where

$s_{\overline{Y}}$ = the sample's estimate of the standard error of the mean

Now that we are realistic about what we know and what we have to estimate, we realize there are two independent parameters we are estimating from the sample's observations: the mean and the variance. Conversion of the sample's mean to the standard normal scale allows us to take into account the effect of chance in estimating the population's mean. It does not, however, allow us to take into account the way chance influences our estimate of the population's variance as well. To take into account the influence of chance in estimating the population's variance, we need to use a different standard distribution. **Student's *t*-distribution** allows us to take into account the independent roles of chance in estimating both the mean and the variance.

4.1   STUDENT'S *T*-DISTRIBUTION

Student's *t*-distribution, like the standard normal distribution, is a **standard distribution**. By this, we imply that values from Student's *t*-distribution and their associated probabilities appear in a table (or can be calculated using Excel or R) that we can use to convert observed values to take into account the role of chance in selecting the sample. We do not assume that the population's distribution of means from all possible samples of a certain size (i.e., the sampling distribution for the mean) is shaped like Student's t-distribution. Rather, we continue to assume that the population's distribution of all possible estimates of the mean is a Gaussian distribution.[3]

In Chapter 3, we converted the sample's mean to the standard normal scale to avoid having to use calculus to calculate probabilities. This is also an advantage of converting to Student's t-scale. Conversion to Student's t-scale provides an additional advantage we will examine in a moment. First, let us see how to convert observed values to t-values.

Recall that the standard normal distribution is a Gaussian distribution with a mean equal to 0 and a variance equal to 1. Student's t-distribution also has a mean equal to 0 and a variance equal to 1. Therefore, conversion of the sample's mean to a value in Student's t-distribution is accomplished in exactly the same way as is conversion to the standard normal distribution. Specifically, we subtract the population's mean from the sample's mean and divide by the standard error. This is illustrated in Equation (4.3).

$$t = \frac{\overline{Y} - \mu_0}{s_{\overline{Y}}} \tag{4.3}$$

where

$t =$ Student's t-value that corresponds to the sample's mean

The calculation to the right of the equal sign in Equation (4.3) is identical to the calculation of a standard normal deviate in Equation (4.2). Student's t-distribution is not, however, the same as the standard normal distribution. What distinguishes them from each other is that Student's t-distribution has three, rather than two, parameters. That is to say, three summary measures are needed to fully characterize Student's t-distribution mathematically. In addition to a mean and variance (as with the standard normal distribution), Student's t-distribution has a third parameter called **degrees of freedom**.

As we said earlier, our interest in Student's t-distribution is to take into account the fact that we are estimating the population's variance, as well as the population's mean, from our sample's observations. Degrees of freedom reflect the amount of information a sample contains for estimation of the population's variance. At first, we might suppose that the amount of information in a sample to estimate the population's variance is the same as the number of observations in that sample. This is almost correct. Actually, the amount of information in a sample that can be used to estimate the population's variance in a univariable sample is equal to the number of observations in the sample minus 1. A way to think about degrees of freedom is that they are equal to 1 when we have the smallest possible sample that allows the variance to be estimated. We cannot estimate the variance from a single observation,

---

[3]Because of the central limit theorem (Chapter 3), we are comfortable in making this assumption for the distribution of estimates of the mean, as long as the sample's size is not too small.

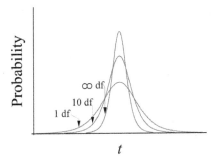

Figure 4.1   Student's *t*-distribution. The dispersion of Student's *t*-distribution decreases as the degrees of freedom increase. When the degrees of freedom are equal to infinity, Student's *t*-distribution is the same as the standard normal distribution.

since the variation for a single observation is always equal to 0. Thus, the smallest sample that will allow estimation of the variance has two observations.

Figure 4.1 shows Student's *t*-distribution for a few different values of degrees of freedom. Notice that the distribution becomes less dispersed or spread out as the degrees of freedom increase. Since degrees of freedom reflect how much information a sample contains to estimate the population's variance, they reflect the influence of chance in estimating the variance. The larger a sample's size, the more degrees of freedom it contains. As the degrees of freedom increase, there is less influence of chance on a variance estimate. Degrees of freedom in Student's *t*-distribution cause us to "penalize" ourselves for our uncertainty in estimation of the population's variance: The larger our sample's size, the less the penalty.

For a moment, let us consider an extreme value for degrees of freedom. Suppose we had an infinitely large sample. Then, we would have infinite degrees of freedom and, thus, an infinite amount of information to estimate the variance. Student's *t*-distribution with an infinite number of degrees of freedom is exactly the same as the standard normal distribution. When we think about it, that makes good sense. If we have an infinitely large sample, then we have, in fact, observed the entire population. If we observe the entire population, we are certain that our estimate of the population's variance is exactly equal to the population's variance. Therefore, we need not penalize ourselves and we can use the standard normal distribution. In practice, this is never the case. With large samples, however, the penalty for uncertainty in estimation of the variance is very small.[4]

Student's *t*-distribution is the first of several distributions that we will encounter in this text, which are related to the standard normal distribution. These distributions are members of the **Gaussian family** of distributions. This and other members of the Gaussian family and their relationships to each other appear in Appendix C. One characteristic that we will discover about all members of the Gaussian family

[4]When the degrees of freedom are equal to 60 (corresponding to a sample size of 61 in the current application) the *t*-value is equal to 2.00, which is quite close to 1.96.

except the standard normal distribution is that degrees of freedom is 1 (or more) of their parameters. In each case, degrees of freedom will be used to reflect the amount of information in a sample. Thus, understanding degrees of freedom is an important step in understanding many statistical procedures.

Table B.2 presents values from Student's t-distribution and their corresponding probabilities. This table has a format that is substantially different from the format of the table presenting values from the standard normal distribution (Table B.1). In Table B.2, the probabilities associated with different Student's t-values appear in the top row. In that row are two lines of probabilities. The top line of probabilities (labeled "$\alpha(2)$") tells us that the probability is split evenly between the two tails of Student's t-distribution. The bottom line of probabilities (labeled "$\alpha(1)$") tells us the probability in the upper tail of Student's t-distribution. This bottom line of probabilities is similar to the probabilities associated with standard normal deviates in Table B.1.

In the body of Table B.2 are Student's t-values that correspond to the probabilities in the top row of the table. In the left-most column of Table B.2 are the degrees of freedom. Notice that the degrees of freedom in the left-most column go up to infinity (∞). When the sample has infinite degrees of freedom, we are certain we have estimated the variance correctly. Now, take a look at the t-values in that last row. The value that corresponds to infinite degrees of freedom and an α of 0.05 split between the two tails of Student's t-distribution is equal to 1.96. If this number sounds familiar, it is because 1.96 is the standard normal deviate that corresponds to an α of 0.05 split between the two tails of the standard normal distribution!

4.2 INTERVAL ESTIMATION

We can use Student's t-distribution in hypothesis testing or interval estimation for a mean from a univariable sample of continuous data. Let us first consider interval estimation. We calculate a two-sided confidence interval for the population's mean in the same way we did using the standard normal distribution (see Equation (3.8)). Now, however, we recognize that we should use a t-value with $n - 1$ degrees of freedom rather than a standard normal deviate. Equation (4.4) shows how a two-sided confidence interval is calculated using Student's t-distribution.

$$\mu \triangleq \overline{Y} \pm (t_{\alpha/2} \cdot s_{\overline{Y}}) \tag{4.4}$$

where

$t_{\alpha/2}$ = t-value that corresponds to α split between the two tails of Student's t-distribution

Now, let us take a look at an example that compares confidence intervals calculated with a standard normal deviate to confidence intervals calculated with a t-value.

■ EXAMPLE 4.1

In Example 3.6, we calculated 95% two-sided confidence intervals for the mean systolic and diastolic blood pressures during the winter months among 53 patients with renal disease. In that example, we used a standard normal deviate to represent the level of confidence. That approach assumes we know the value of the population's variances. Now, let us recalculate those confidence intervals recognizing that the variances have been estimated from the sample's observations.

In Example 3.6, the confidence interval for mean systolic blood pressure ranged from 147.1 to 158.9 mmHg and the confidence interval for mean diastolic blood pressure ranged from 78.1 to 85.9 mmHg. These calculations used a standard normal deviate of 1.96 to represent the role of chance in deriving those estimates. Now, we will recalculate those confidence intervals, recognizing that the variances have been estimated from the sample's observations and taking into account the independent roles of chance in estimating the means and the variances of blood pressure values. For both intervals, the t-value we will use to represent 95% confidence is found from Table B.2 by selecting the column that corresponds to an α of 0.05 split between the two tails of Student's t-distribution and the row that corresponds to $53 - 1 = 52$ degrees of freedom. Since 52 degrees of freedom is not listed in Table B.2, we can use the next lower number of degrees of freedom that is listed.[5] This value is 50 degrees of freedom.

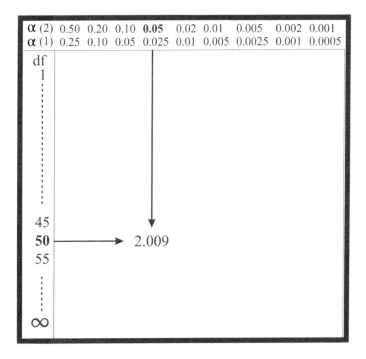

Thus, the *t*-value we will use in our calculations is equal to 2.009. With that information, we are ready to use Equation (4.4) to calculate confidence intervals for systolic and diastolic blood pressures.

$$\mu_{SBP} \triangleq \overline{Y} \pm (t_{\alpha/2} \cdot s_{\overline{Y}}) = 153 \pm (2.009 \cdot 3) = 147.0 - 59.0 \, \text{mmHg}$$

$$\mu_{DBP} \triangleq \overline{Y} \pm (t_{\alpha/2} \cdot s_{\overline{Y}}) = 82 \pm (2.009 \cdot 2) = 78.0 - 86.0 \, \text{mmHg}$$

Notice that both of these confidence intervals are slightly wider than the confidence intervals we calculated in Example 3.4 (147.1–158.9 mmHg for systolic blood pressure [SBP] and 78.1–85.9 mmHg for diastolic blood pressure [DBP]). The reason for this is that we are now taking into account the additional role of chance in estimating the variances. Since these intervals reflect a greater role of chance, they have to be wider to represent the same level of confidence that they include the population's means. With 50 degrees of freedom, the increase in the width of the confidence intervals is small. If we had fewer observations and, therefore, fewer degrees of freedom, there would be a larger increase in the width of the confidence intervals to reflect the greater role of chance in estimating the variances.   ∎

We can calculate the confidence interval more precisely using Excel. The next example illustrates that application.

■ EXAMPLE 4.2

Let us use Excel to calculate 95% two-sided confidence intervals for the mean systolic and diastolic blood pressures during the winter months among 53 patients with renal disease. In Excel, we use a function called "confidence.t." The information passed to that function includes α, the sample's estimate of the standard deviation, and *n*. Since the information available to us includes the standard error, not the standard deviation, we need to have Excel calculate the standard deviation from the standard error.

The Excel output for this problem looks different from the output we have seen before. This is so because we are given estimates, rather than data.

	A	B	C	D	E	F
1		SBP	DBP			
2						
3	mean	153	82			
4	SE	3	2			
5	SD	21.84032967	14.56021978		=B3*sqrt(53)	=C3*sqrt(53)
6	95% interval width	6.019940415	4.01329361		=confidence.t(0.05,B4,53)	=confidence.t(0.05,C4,53)
7	Lower Limit	146.9800596	77.98670639		=B2-B5	=C2-C5
8	Upper Limit	159.0199404	86.01329361		=B2+B5	=C2+C5

Except for the number of decimal places, these results are the same as those obtained in Example 4.1. ■

4.3 HYPOTHESIS TESTING

Recall from Chapter 3 that statistical hypothesis testing involves testing a specific condition for the population's parameter described in the null hypothesis. For most univariable samples, it is difficult to imagine what value we should hypothesize for the population. For instance, consider Examples 4.1 and 4.2. In these examples, we examined systolic and diastolic blood pressure measurements taken on patients with renal disease. Our objective was to calculate an interval estimate for the mean systolic and mean diastolic blood pressure values in the population from which those patients were selected for observation. This is a logical way to take chance into account for those data. It is difficult to imagine, however, what hypothesis might be tested using those same observations.

To perform statistical hypothesis testing, we need to state a specific value for the population's mean. Often, with univariable samples, there is no hypothetical value that has biologic relevance. For this reason, interval estimation is more commonly used than hypothesis testing for univariable samples.

There is, nevertheless, one kind of univariable sample in which hypothesis testing makes sense. This is when we have a **paired sample**. The most common type of paired sample is when we take two measurements of the same characteristic under different conditions for each subject.[6] Example 3.1 illustrates such a paired sample for a continuous dependent variable. There, each patient's intraocular pressure was measured twice: once in the eye receiving the new treatment, and once in the eye receiving the conventional treatment. The dependent variable that is examined using statistical hypothesis testing in that case represents the differences in intraocular pressure measurements between these two eyes. Since each patient has only one difference, this is a univariable sample.[7] The sensible null hypothesis for such a paired sample is that the mean difference is equal to 0, indicating that the measurements are the same under the two conditions.

---

[6]Less commonly, we might see paired samples in which similar, but not identical, individuals are compared with one another. For example, a paired sample might consist of individuals compared with their siblings.

[7]A legitimate paired sample will allow a particular individual to be compared to one, and only one, other individual. Groups that are balanced according to some characteristic, but in which individual members of every pair cannot be identified are called **group-** (or **frequency-**) matched samples. It is not appropriate to use univariable methods to compare group-matched samples.

To perform statistical hypothesis testing on the mean from a univariable sample, we convert the sample's mean to a Student's t-statistic using the method in Equation (4.3). The next example illustrates such a hypothesis test.

■ EXAMPLE 4.3

In Example 3.1, we considered the mean difference in intraocular pressure in a group of nine patients who received a new medication in one eye and the standard treatment in the other eye. In Example 3.9, we tested the null hypothesis that the mean difference in intraocular pressure is equal to 0 in the population by using the standard normal distribution to determine the P-value. Now, let us recognize that the variance of differences in intraocular pressure is unknown and, thus, must be estimated from the sample's observations. What effect does this additional role of chance have on the results of testing that null hypothesis?

In Example 3.4, the sample's estimate of the population's variance in intraocular pressure was 15.5 mmHg and the standard error was found to be equal to 1.31 mmHg. Recognizing that this standard error was calculated from an estimate of the standard deviation rather than from the actual standard deviation does not change the value of the standard error. Therefore, we use that same standard error in Equation (4.3) to calculate the t-value that corresponds to a mean change in the difference in intraocular pressure of 3 mmHg.

$$t = \frac{\overline{Y} - \mu_0}{s_{\overline{Y}}} = \frac{3 - 0}{1.31} = 2.29$$

Thus, a t-value of 2.29 corresponds to a mean difference in intraocular pressure of 3 mmHg. This is the same as the standard normal deviate calculated in Example 3.9. Recognizing that the variance is estimated from the sample's observations does not change the result of the calculation. Instead, it is the interpretation of that result that changes. In Example 3.9, we used Table B.1 to get a P-value of 0.0220. Now, we need to use Table B.2 to find the P-value that reflects the independent roles of chance in estimating the variance as well as the mean. To find that P-value, we look for 2.29 in the row of the table that corresponds to $9 - 1 = 8$ degrees of freedom.

When we go to Table B.2 to find a t-value of 2.29 in the row that corresponds to 8 degrees of freedom, we find that a t-value of 1.860 corresponds to a probability of 0.10 split between the two tails of Student's t-distribution and a t-value of 2.306 corresponds to a probability of 0.05 split between the two tails of that distribution.

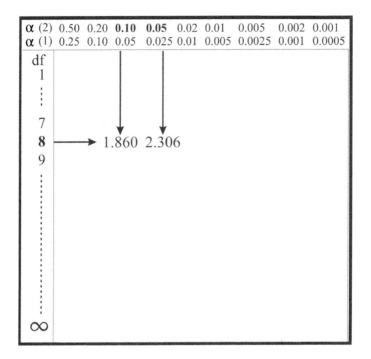

α (2)	0.50	0.20	**0.10**	**0.05**	0.02	0.01	0.005	0.002	0.001
α (1)	0.25	0.10	0.05	0.025	0.01	0.005	0.0025	0.001	0.0005
df									
1									
⋮									
7									
8			1.860	2.306					
9									
⋮									
∞									

Since 2.29 occurs between these two probabilities, we can express the P-value as being less than 0.10, but greater than 0.05. In mathematical shorthand, that P-value is

$0.10 > P > 0.05$ Even though we do not know the exact value of the P-value from Table B.2, we do know that it is greater than 0.05. Thus, we cannot reject the null hypothesis that the mean change in intraocular pressure is equal to 0 in the population. Instead, we fail to reject that null hypothesis.

The effect of recognizing the additional role of chance in estimating the variance of changes in intraocular pressure has altered our conclusion about the null hypothesis, since the P-value is now greater than 0.05. It will not always be the case that the conclusion we can draw will be different using these two approaches, but recognizing the additional role of chance in estimating the variance of dependent variable values will always result in a higher P-value. ∎

Example 4.3 showed how we could perform the paired t-test by hand. Going through those calculations can be helpful in understanding this statistical method, but when analyzing real data, we will probably use a computer program to do the calculations for us. In Excel, the paired t-test can be performed using the function "t.test" or by using the "*t*-Test: Paired Two Sample for Means" analysis tool in Data Analysis. For either of these, the data have to be presented as two measurements, rather than the difference between the measurements. The next example illustrates the use of the *t*-test function[8] and a paired *t*-test in R.

■ EXAMPLE 4.4

In Example 4.3, we performed a paired *t*-test on a set of data from a study in which we looked at the difference between intraocular pressures in both eyes for a sample of nine persons. Let us now examine these data in more detail. Rather than as a difference between two measurements, the data are of the two measurements themselves. Even so, we are still testing the null hypothesis that the mean difference is equal to 0 in the population.

The following output is the result of analyzing these data using Excel:

	A	B	C	D	E	F
1	IOP OS*	IOP OD	ΔIOP		*P*-value	
2	23	20	3		0.051586	=t.test(A2:A10,B2:B10,2,1.)
3	21	21	0			
4	20	17	3			
5	24	22	2			
6	18	21	-3			
7	27	16	11			
8	28	27	1			
9	25	19	6			
10	23	19	4			
11	*OS refers to the left eye and OD refers to the right eye.					

The *P*-value calculated in Excel (0.051586) is greater than 0.05, so we fail to reject the null hypothesis that the mean difference is equal to 0 in the population. This is the same conclusion we obtained in Example 4.3.

In R, we can perform a paired *t*-test and calculate a confidence interval using the t.test() command. The input for the t.test() command is the difference between the two measurements.

```
>t.test(CHGIOP)
```

```
One Sample t-test

data: CHGIOP
t = 2.286, df = 8, p-value = 0.05159
```

---

[8]Do not let the references to "Variable 1" and "Variable 2" in the Data Analysis approach mislead you. There is only one variable: the difference between the two measurements.

```
alternative hypothesis: true mean is not equal to 0
95 percent confidence interval:
 -0.02624912 6.02624912
sample estimates:
mean of x
 3
```

The result of the hypothesis test is identical to the result we got from Excel. In addition, R gives us a 95% confidence interval for the mean and its point estimate. ■

Now, we are ready to go on to the next chapter, which examines univariable analysis of an ordinal dependent variable.

CHAPTER SUMMARY

In Chapter 4, we begin investigating the statistical procedures that are actually used to analyze health research data. Up to this point, we have been studying the principles of statistical logic, but using simplified methods. This was to prevent us from being encumbered with too many issues all at once so we could focus on the principles relative to the mean. Beginning in this chapter, that changes.

The most important simplification made in previous chapters was the assumption that the variance of the distribution of data in the population is known. This was so we could assume that chance had an effect on our estimate of the mean, but not on our estimate of the variance. This allowed us to see how we can take chance into account for the estimate of the mean without being concerned about the independent role of chance on the estimate of the variance. Now it is time to recognize that there are two, independent, roles of chance when we are calculating confidence intervals or testing hypotheses about a mean.

The standard normal distribution we used in Chapters 2 and 3 appropriately takes chance into account for individuals and for estimates of the mean, but it does nothing about the role of chance in estimating the variance. The standard distribution that takes both of those effects of chance simultaneously is Student's t-distribution. That distribution takes the role of chance in estimating the mean into account exactly the way the standard normal distribution does. In addition, Student's t-distribution takes into account the role of chance in estimating the variance. It does this by adding a third parameter called "degrees of freedom."

When a sample is very large, the influence of chance on the estimate of the variance is small. In that circumstance, Student's t-distribution is almost identical to the standard normal distribution.[9] As the sample becomes smaller, Student's t-distribution becomes more dispersed (i.e., spread out) than would be the standard normal distribution with the same variance. This increased dispersion is the

---

[9] In fact, when the sample is infinitely large, Student's t and the standard normal distributions are identical.

effect of chance on the estimate of the variance. It causes confidence intervals to be wider and P-values to be larger. This reflects our uncertainty about the value of the variance.

The third parameter, degrees of freedom, reflects how much information a sample contains that can be used to estimate the variance. These are the same degrees of freedom we used in Chapter 3 in the denominator of the variance estimate to make it unbiased. For a univariable sample, those degrees of freedom are equal to the sample's size minus 1.

Other than the fact that we are using Student's t-distribution instead of the standard normal distribution, the methods we use to calculate confidence intervals and test hypotheses are the same as in Chapter 3.

EXERCISES

4.1. Suppose we take a sample of 36 persons from a particular population and measure their body weights. Then, we give each person a one-month's supply of appetite suppressants. At the end of the month, we weigh each person again and subtract their new weight from their first weight. Suppose we observe a mean difference in weight equal to 10 kg and we estimate the variance of differences in weight in the population to be 900 kg. Which of the following is closest to the interval of values within which we have 95% confidence that the population's mean lies?

A. −32.2 to 51.8

B. −0.2 to 20.2

C. 0.0 to 20.0

D. 0.2 to 20.2

E. 2.3 to 17.7

4.2. Suppose we take a sample of 36 persons from a particular population and measure their body weights. Then, we give each person a one-month's supply of appetite suppressants. At the end of the month, we weigh each person again and subtract their new weight from their first weight. Suppose we observe a mean difference in weight equal to 10 kg and that we estimate the variance of differences in weight in the population to be 900 kg^2. Test the null hypothesis that the difference in weight is equal to 0 in the population versus the alternative hypothesis that it is not equal to 0. If you allow a 5% risk of making a type I error, which of the following is the best conclusion to draw?

A. Reject both the null and alternative hypotheses

B. Accept both the null and alternative hypotheses

C. Reject the null hypothesis and accept the alternative hypothesis

D. Accept the null hypothesis and reject the alternative hypothesis

E. It is best not to draw a conclusion about the null and alternative hypotheses from these observations

4.3. Suppose we were to conduct a study in which 16 persons with hypothyroidism were given two medications in a random order. In this study, we measure thyroid-stimulating hormone (TSH) after the participants had taken each of the medications for a week. Suppose we estimate the mean difference in TSH levels to be equal to 20 mg/dL and we estimate the standard deviation of differences between TSH levels to be equal to 60 mg/dL. Test the null hypothesis that the mean difference is equal to 0 in the population versus the alternative hypothesis that the mean difference is not equal to 0. If you allow a 5% risk of making a type I error, which of the following is the best conclusion to draw?

A. Reject both the null and alternative hypotheses

B. Accept both the null and alternative hypotheses

C. Reject the null hypothesis and accept the alternative hypothesis

D. Accept the null hypothesis and reject the alternative hypothesis

E. It is best not to draw a conclusion about the null and alternative hypotheses from these observations

4.4. Suppose we were to conduct a study in which 16 persons with hypothyroidism were given 2 medications in a random order. In this study, we measure TSH after the participants had taken each of the medications for a week. Suppose we estimate the mean difference in TSH levels to be equal to 20 mg/dL and we estimate the standard deviation of differences between TSH levels to be equal to 60 mg/dL. What is an interval within which we are 95% confident that the mean difference in the population is included?

A. −88.2 to 147.0

B. −12.0 to 52.0

C. −9.4 to 49.4

D. −5.1 to 36.4

E. 0.0 to 40.0

4.5. We are interested in the effect of a vegetarian diet on blood urea nitrogen (BUN). To investigate this, we select 12 graduate students who have been eating an omnivorous diet all of their lives. We determine their BUN and ask them to follow a vegetarian diet for 28 days. Then, we measure their BUN again and subtract this second measurement from the initial measurement. Suppose we observe a mean difference of 4 mg/dL and estimate the standard deviation of the differences to be equal to 8 mg/dL. Which of the following is an interval of values within which we can be 95% confident that the population's mean is included?

    A. −1.1 to 9.1

    B. −0.1 to 8.9

    C. 0.0 to 8.0

    D. 0.6 to 7.4

    E. 1.2 to 6.8

4.6. We are interested in the effect of a vegetarian diet on BUN. To investigate this, we select 12 graduate students who have been eating an omnivorous diet all of their lives. We determine their BUN and ask them to follow a vegetarian diet for 28 days. Then, we measure their BUN again and subtract this second measurement from the initial measurement. Suppose we observe a difference of 4 mg/dL and estimate the standard deviation of the differences equal to 8 mg/dL. Test the null hypothesis that the difference in BUN is equal to 0 in the population versus the alternative hypothesis that the difference is not equal to 0. If you allow a 5% chance of making a type I error, which of the following is the best conclusion to draw?

    A. Reject both the null and alternative hypotheses

    B. Accept both the null and alternative hypotheses

    C. Reject the null hypothesis and accept the alternative hypothesis

    D. Accept the null hypothesis and reject the alternative hypothesis

    E. It is best not to draw a conclusion about the null and alternative hypotheses from these observations

4.7. Patients on a particular treatment often suffer from anemia. To counter this effect, we think that these patients might be helped if they were given folic acid. To evaluate this, we identify 21 patients on the treatment who have been diagnosed with anemia and measure their hematocrit. Then, we give these patients supplemental folic acid for a period of 14 days. Then, we measure their hematocrit again and subtract this second measurement from the initial measurement. Suppose we observe a mean difference between these two hematocrit determinations of −5%. Also suppose that we estimate the standard deviation of differences in hematocrit measurements to be equal to 10%. Based on that information, test the null hypothesis that the mean difference in hematocrit is equal to 0 in the population versus the alternative hypothesis that it is not equal to 0. If we were to allow a 5% chance of making a type I error, which of the following would be the best conclusion to draw?

    A. Reject both the null and alternative hypotheses

    B. Accept both the null and alternative hypotheses

    C. Reject the null hypothesis and accept the alternative hypothesis

    D. Accept the null hypothesis and reject the alternative hypothesis

    E. It is best not to draw a conclusion about the null and alternative hypotheses from these observations

4.8. Patients on a particular treatment often suffer from anemia. To counter this effect, we think that these patients might be helped if they were given folic acid. To evaluate this, we identify 21 patients on the treatment who have been diagnosed with anemia and measure their hematocrit. Then, we give these patients supplemental folic acid for a period of 14 days. Then, we measure their hematocrit again and subtract this second measurement from the initial measurement. Suppose we observe a mean difference between these two hematocrit determinations of −5%. Also suppose we estimate the standard deviation of differences in hematocrit measurements to be equal to 10%. Based on that information, which of the following is an interval of mean differences in hematocrit within which we can be 95% confident that the population's value occurs?

A. −9.6 to −0.4

B. −9.6 to 0.4

C. −0.4 to 9.6

D. 0.0 to 9.6

E. 0.4 to 9.6

CHAPTER 5

UNIVARIABLE ANALYSIS OF AN ORDINAL DEPENDENT VARIABLE

We learned in Chapter 2 that ordinal data can differ from continuous data in that ordinal data are not necessarily evenly spaced. There are some types of information in health research that are naturally measured on an ordinal scale. For example, the original Bethesda system for cervical cytology included four stages of epithelial cell abnormalities on a Pap smear. These are atypical squamous cells of undetermined significance (ASCUS), low-grade squamous intraepithelial lesion (LSIL), high-grade squamous intraepithelial lesion (HSIL), and squamous cell carcinoma. These data have both characteristics of ordinal data. They have a small number of possible values (i.e., four) and we are unable to say that the spacing between each stage is the same (i.e., the "distance" between ASCUS and LSIL is not the same as the "distance" between LSIL and HSIL).

Introduction to Biostatistical Applications in Health Research with Microsoft Office Excel® and R,
Second Edition. Robert P. Hirsch.
© 2021 John Wiley & Sons, Inc. Published 2021 by John Wiley & Sons, Inc.
Companion website: www.wiley.com/go/hirsch/healthresearch2e

5.1   NONPARAMETRIC METHODS

Statistical methods for ordinal dependent variables can be used to analyze data that naturally occur on an ordinal scale, but this is not the most common use of these methods. Rather, these statistical procedures are used more often to analyze continuous data that have been converted to an ordinal scale. When these methods are used in that way, we refer to them as **nonparametric** methods.

Nonparametric methods are an alternative to statistical methods designed for continuous data. Thus, the statistical procedures we will encounter in chapters addressing ordinal dependent variables will have parallel procedures for continuous dependent variables. In Chapter 4, we discussed the paired t-test. In this chapter, we will discuss the **Wilcoxon signed-rank test** (Flowchart 3). The Wilcoxon signed-rank test is the nonparametric parallel to the paired t-test.

Given the relationship between statistical methods for continuous and ordinal dependent variables, we need to think about which of the two approaches is the more appropriate one under a specific set of conditions. The distinction is based on assumptions made about the sampling distribution. When we analyze continuous data represented by a continuous dependent variable, we take into account the effect of chance on the estimate of the mean by considering the sampling distribution for the mean. Statistical methods for continuous dependent variables assume that the sampling distribution is a Gaussian distribution. We learned in Chapter 3 that the sampling distribution for the mean tends to be a Gaussian distribution with that tendency increasing as the size of the samples increases. We know this is true from the central limit theorem.

When a sample of continuous data contains few observations, the sampling distribution for the mean depends on the distribution of data to be a Gaussian distribution. If the distribution of data in such a small sample does not appear to be a Gaussian

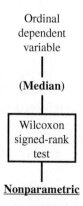

Ordinal
dependent
variable

(Median)

Wilcoxon
signed-rank
test

<u>Nonparametric</u>

FLOWCHART 3   Flowchart showing univariable analysis of an ordinal dependent variable. The point estimate that is most often used to describe the dependent variable (the median) is in bold. The common name of the statistical test (Wilcoxon signed-rank test) is enclosed in a box. The general procedure that is used to test hypotheses and calculate confidence intervals (nonparametric) is in bold and underlined.

distribution, we become concerned about the assumption that the sampling distribution is a Gaussian distribution. One solution to this problem is to represent those continuous data with an ordinal dependent variable instead of with a continuous dependent variable. Distributions of ordinal data do not have parameters as do distributions of continuous data (i.e., the mean and variance). Without a parameter to estimate, there is no sampling distribution to take into account the role of chance. Without a sampling distribution, there is no assumption that the distribution is a Gaussian distribution. Thus, statistical methods designed for ordinal dependent variables can be used to analyze continuous data converted to an ordinal scale to avoid this assumption of a Gaussian sampling distribution.

The first step in using a nonparametric test on continuous data involves conversion of the data to an ordinal scale. This conversion is accomplished by representing the continuous data by their **relative ranks**. What ranking accomplishes is to maintain the order of numeric magnitude without the information about how far apart data values are from one another. The particular rules for ranking differ somewhat depending on the particular test that will be performed, but there are two rules that are consistent for all nonparametric tests. The first rule is that rank 1 is assigned to the smallest data value and that the ranks increase as the numeric magnitude of the data increases. The second rule tells us how to assign ranks to data that are of the same numeric magnitude on the continuous scale. In this case, we give all of these data values the same rank and that rank is equal to the mean of the ranks they would have been assigned if they were of different numeric magnitudes. This sounds a bit complicated, but it is easier to see how this works by examining an example.

■ EXAMPLE 5.1

In Example 3.1 we examined data from nine persons with elevated intraocular pressure. Each of these persons was randomly assigned to use a new topical treatment for glaucoma in one eye and a standard topical treatment in the other eye. After one week of treatment, the difference in intraocular pressure (ΔIOP) between the two eyes was measured for each person. The following results were observed:

Patient	ΔIOP
TH	3
IS	0
MA	3
KE	2
SM	−3
ES	11
OH	1
AP	6
PY	4

Now, let us convert these continuous data to an ordinal scale by ranking.

The smallest data value is a difference in intraocular pressure of -3 mmHg for patient SM, so we will give this data value rank 1. Then we assign the next higher rank to the next higher data value. In this set of data, two patients had a difference in intraocular pressure of 3 mmHg. If they had different numeric magnitudes, they would be assigned the ranks of 5 and 6. Because they are equal to the same value, we assign the average of those ranks to both data values:

Patient	ΔIOP	Rank
TH	3	5.5
IS	0	2
MA	3	5.5
KE	2	4
SM	-3	1
ES	11	9
OH	1	3
AP	6	8
PY	4	7

■

Excel can be used to convert data values to relative ranks. A function called "rank .avg" creates ranks using the ranking method assumed by nonparametric methods. The following example illustrates the use of that function.

■ EXAMPLE 5.2

The following results are observed when using the rank.avg function on Excel to prepare data for a nonparametric analysis.

	A	B	C	D
1	ΔIOP	Rank		
2	3	5.5		=rank.avg(A2,A$2:A$10,1)
3	0	2		=rank.avg(A3,A$2:A$10,1)
4	3	5.5		=rank.avg(A4,A$2:A$10,1)
5	2	4		=rank.avg(A5,A$2:A$10,1)
6	-3	1		=rank.avg(A6,A$2:A$10,1)
7	11	9		=rank.avg(A7,A$2:A$10,1)
8	1	3		=rank.avg(A8,A$2:A$10,1)
9	6	8		=rank.avg(A9,A$2:A$10,1)
10	4	7		=rank.avg(A10,A$2:A$10,1)

These are the same ranks as those assigned in Example 5.1.   ■

Thus, we might want to analyze continuous data by converting these continuous data to an ordinal scale. When continuous data are converted to an ordinal scale, we do not have to make the assumption that the estimates from all possible samples have a Gaussian distribution (i.e., the sampling distribution is Gaussian). It is important to remember, however, that nonparametric methods are not completely free of assumptions. Regardless of the statistical method we use, we always assume that, at the minimum, dependent variable values were obtained by a random sample of the population of interest (as discussed in Chapter 2).[1]

5.2 ESTIMATION

Unlike distributions of continuous (or nominal) data, distributions of ordinal data do not have parameters that mathematically describe them. Even so, there are numbers we can use to summarize data on an ordinal scale. To be appropriate for data on an ordinal scale, summary values must not be influenced by how far apart data values are.

Recall from Chapter 2 that mean is the parameter of location we use for data on a continuous scale. That mean is the "center of gravity" of the distribution. By calling the mean the center of gravity of the distribution, we recognize that the mean is affected by the numeric distance between data values. Thus, the mean would not be an appropriate way to summarize ordinal data.

In that same chapter, we encountered another measure of location of a distribution: the **median**. The median is the "physical center" of a distribution of data rather than its center of gravity. By physical center, we imply that half of the data values occur on either side of the median. How far away these data values are from each other does not change the median. Thus, median is an appropriate measure to summarize the location of a distribution of ordinal data.

In addition to the point estimate of the median, it is also possible for us to take chance into account by calculating an interval estimate for the median. This is not something that Excel provides us, so it must be calculated by hand. This is done by calculating the ranks of the limits of the confidence interval. The ranks associated with 90, 95, and 99% confidence intervals for samples with 7–40 observations are given in Table B.11. The next example demonstrates how this table is used to determine a confidence interval for a median.

■ EXAMPLE 5.3

In Example 2.2, we looked at the change in serum cholesterol levels for 11 persons on a low-fat diet. These data values are 10, 42, 5, 9, −2, 0, 16, 28, 4, −5, and 3 mg/dL. In Example 2.4, we calculated the median of these data and found it to be equal to 5 mg/dL. Now, let us determine a 95% confidence interval for the estimate of the median.

---

[1] In Chapter 13, we will learn of other assumptions of nonparametric methods.

First, we need to rank these data. This was done in Example 2.4 to calculate the median. These ranks are as follows:

Rank	1	2	3	4	5	6	7	8	9	10	11
Value	−5	−2	0	3	4	5	9	10	16	28	42

Next, we look at Table B.11 and determine which ranks correspond to the limits of a 95% confidence interval when we have a sample of 11 observations. To do this, we find 11 in the left-most column and 95% in the top row. Where they intersect, we find that the lower limit has a rank of 2 and the upper limit has a rank of 10. The data value with a rank of 2 is equal to −2 mg/dL. The data value with a rank of 10 is equal to 28 mg/dL. Thus, the 95% confidence interval for the estimate of the median is equal to −2 to 28 g/dL.   ∎

5.3   WILCOXON SIGNED-RANK TEST

We learned in Chapter 3 that the first step in statistical hypothesis testing is to formulate the hypothesis to be tested (i.e., the null hypothesis). So far in this text, all of the null hypotheses we have encountered have made specific statements about the population's parameter. Since a distribution of ordinal data has no parameters, we need to think about a different sort of null hypothesis. In Chapter 4, the null hypothesis addressed by the paired t-test was that the mean difference is equal to 0 in the population. The Wilcoxon signed-rank test is the nonparametric equivalent to the paired t-test. The null hypothesis tested in the Wilcoxon signed-rank test is that a balance of ranks exists between positive and negative differences. This nonparametric null hypothesis makes a specific statement about the ordinal data, but it does that without referring to a parameter.

The first step in all nonparametric procedures is to assign relative ranks to each of the data values. Each nonparametric procedure has its own particular way in which this ranking is done. In the Wilcoxon signed-rank test we rank the **absolute value** of the differences rather than the differences themselves. Also, data values of 0 are not ranked at all.[2] The next example shows how this method of ranking data is performed.

∎ EXAMPLE 5.4

In Example 5.1 we examined data taken from nine persons with elevated intraocular pressure. In that example we ranked these data so that the negative data values had

---

[2]The purpose of the Wilcoxon signed-rank test is to compare positive differences with negative differences. Data of 0 provide no information about this balance.

the lowest ranks. Now, let us rank the absolute value of these data in preparation for performing the Wilcoxon signed-rank test.

First, we record the absolute value for each data value and then rank these absolute values. This process is summarized in the following table:

Patient	ΔIOP	|ΔIOP|	Rank
TH	3	3	4
IS	0	–	–
MA	3	3	4
KE	2	2	2
SM	−3	3	4
ES	11	11	8
OH	1	1	1
AP	6	6	7
PY	4	4	6

After ranks have been assigned, we then separate those ranks according to the original sign of the data on the continuous scale. Then, we add up the ranks that correspond to positive data values (T_+) and those that correspond to negative data values (T_-). These two sums of ranks are the results of the Wilcoxon signed-rank test (Equations (5.1) and (5.2)):

$$T_+ = \sum \text{Ranks of positive differences} \qquad (5.1)$$

$$T_- = \sum \text{Ranks of negative differences} \qquad (5.2)$$

Which data values are negative and which are positive is entirely arbitrary. In the example we have been discussing, the sign of a difference in IOP depends on whether the pressure in the eye that received the new treatment is subtracted from the pressure in the eye that received the standard treatment or vice versa. We only need to select one of the two sums of ranks to compare with values in a table of Wilcoxon signed-rank test statistics. For a two-sided alternative hypothesis, we choose the sum of the ranks that is smaller of the two.[3]

The table we use to test the null hypothesis in the Wilcoxon signed-rank test is Table B.3. If we take a look at Table B.3, we find a structure somewhat like the structure of the table for the paired t-test (Table B.2). Across the top of Table B.3, we see one- and two-sided values of α similar to those in Table B.2. Down the left-most column of Table B.3 is the number of observations in the sample. This is not too

---

[3] If we are interested in a one-tailed test, the choice of which of the two statistics to compare to a value in the table (Table B.3) is determined by which of the two statistics the alternative hypothesis implies will be the smaller.

different from the degrees of freedom in the left-most column of Table B.2. There is, however, one important difference between these two tables. In Table B.2, Student's t-values get bigger as the value of α (and, therefore, the P-value) gets smaller, but in Table B.3 the opposite is true. Table B.3 is the only table we will use in which α and the P-value get smaller as the test statistic gets smaller. This is something we need to keep in mind when using Table B.3.

Now, let us take a look at an example of how the Wilcoxon signed-rank test statistic is calculated and compared with values in the corresponding table.

■ EXAMPLE 5.5

In Example 5.4, we ranked data taken from nine persons with elevated intraocular pressure using the method of ranking required by the Wilcoxon signed-rank test. Now, let us calculate the Wilcoxon signed-rank test statistic for these data and draw a conclusion about the null hypothesis that there is a balance of negative and positive differences in IOP in the population. To draw that conclusion, let us use $\alpha = 0.05$.

Only one of the differences in IOP is negative. That is the difference for patient SM. All the rest of the (nonzero) differences are positive. Thus, we find the following sums of ranks using Equations (5.1) and (5.2):

$$T_+ = \sum \text{Ranks of positive differences} = 4 + 4 + 2 + 8 + 1 + 7 + 6 = 32$$

$$T_- = \sum \text{Ranks of negative differences} = 4$$

Since the sum of the negative difference ranks (4) is smaller than the sum of the positive difference ranks (32), it is the former that we compare with values in Table B.3. In the left-most column of Table B.3, we need to find the number of observations in the sample. This number of observations includes only those without differences equal to 0. In this sample, therefore, the number of nonzero observations is 8. If we look in that row of the table, we find that our calculated value of 4 occurs between the values of 3 (corresponding to an α of 0.05) and 5 (corresponding to an α of 0.1). Thus, the P-value is less than 0.1 and greater than 0.05. Since this is greater than α of 0.05, we fail to reject the null hypothesis.   ■

Example 5.5 shows how the Wilcoxon signed-rank test can be performed manually. This test, like other nonparametric tests, is relatively easy to calculate manually, or by using Excel to create ranks and do the math. There are no built-in functions in Excel that help us perform the Wilcoxon signed-rank test, other than rank.avg. The BAHR program "Nonparametric" can perform a Wilcoxon Sign-Rank test and R can perform the Wilcoxon signed-rank test from the differences between measurements. The next example shows this test in Excel and R.

■ EXAMPLE 5.6

In Excel, the BAHR program "Nonparametric" can perform the Wilcoxon Signed-Rank test. The following is output from that program.

	Wilcoxon Signed-Rank Test					
Statistic =	4	$z =$	1.970073	P-value =		0.04883
Warning: Sample too small for normal approximation						
Use Table B.3						

In R, the Wilcoxon signed-rank test is performed by using the wilcox.test() command. For the difference in intraocular pressure from Example 3.1, we get the following results.

>wilcox.test(CHGIOP)

```
Wilcoxon signed rank test with continuity correction

data: CHGIOP
V = 32, p-value = 0.05747
alternative hypothesis: true location is not equal to 0
```

The P-value from the R analysis is larger than the P-value from Excel. The reason for this is that by default R uses a continuity correction. If we were to ask R not to use a continuity correction, we would get the same P-value that we got from Excel.

```
Wilcoxon signed rank test

data: CHGIOP
V = 32, p-value = 0.04883
alternative hypothesis: true location is not equal to 0
```

Excel and R give us approximate P-values. That approximation is best when the sample contains at least 10 observations. We can ask R to calculate an exact P-value as follows:

>wilcox.test(CHGIOP, exact=TRUE)

We cannot do that in this case, since R cannot calculate an exact P-value when there are tied ranks or zeros. ■

5.4   STATISTICAL POWER OF NONPARAMETRIC TESTS

We have learned in this chapter that continuous data can be converted to an ordinal scale to circumvent some of the assumptions required for the analysis of continuous dependent variables. We also learned that information about the distance between data values is lost when continuous data are converted to an ordinal scale. We gain flexibility by performing such a conversion, but we must pay a price. The resultant loss of information can mean a loss of statistical power which, in turn, implies a greater chance of failing to reject a false null hypothesis.

Loss of power occurs when the assumptions required by a statistical procedure for a continuous dependent variable are satisfied, but instead we choose to convert our continuous data to an ordinal scale for analysis. In other words, it occurs when it would have been appropriate to use a statistical procedure designed for a continuous dependent variable, but we used a nonparametric procedure instead.

The decision about whether or not to convert data to another scale is a common one in analysis of health research data. Unfortunately, it is not often an easy decision to make. In this text we will look only at the loss of power that can occur when we make an incorrect decision. One way to examine power is by considering P-values. The greater the power of a statistical procedure, the smaller the P-value will be.[4] To examine this loss of power for the intraocular pressure data we have been using in our examples, let us look at the P-values: the P-value for the Wilcoxon signed-rank test is 0.0547 (from Example 5.5), whereas the P-value for the paired t-test is 0.0516 (from Example 4.3). Since the nonparametric test has a higher P-value, a larger difference in intraocular pressures would be required to reject the null hypothesis. Using either P-value we fail to reject the null hypothesis. Here, as well as in most instances, the loss of statistical power due to use of a nonparametric test will be small[5] and will not often affect the conclusion we draw in statistical hypothesis testing.

In the next chapter, we will encounter the last of the univariable statistical methods: those designed to analyze a nominal dependent variable.

CHAPTER SUMMARY

To perform statistical analysis of ordinal dependent variables, the values of those variables are converted into relative ranks. This is done regardless of whether the variables are from data that naturally occur on an ordinal scale or from continuous data that we wish to convert to an ordinal scale. Such a conversion of continuous data to ranks is done to allow statistical analysis without assuming that the distribution of estimates from all possible samples is a Gaussian distribution.

---

[4]We can think of the P-value as the minimum value we could have used for α in an analysis and still have rejected the null hypothesis.

[5]Some nonparametric tests are associated with a substantial loss of power, but they are not commonly used (for the very reason that they have low statistical power). The nonparametric tests that are described in this text are among the most powerful nonparametric tests available.

Conversion of data to ranks can be accomplished by assigning the rank of one to the smallest value, two to the next larger value, and so on. Observations that have the same value, called tied observations, are assigned the mean of the ranks they would have received if they were given separate ranks.

Estimation of parameters of a population's distribution is not relevant for ordinal dependent variables since no particular distribution is assumed. This lack of assumptions concerning distributions and parameters has led to procedures for ordinal data being referred to as distribution-free or nonparametric procedures. Even so, the median and the interquartile range can be determined from ordinal data and used as estimators of the population's values, even though they are not parameters.[6]

The most common method for performing statistical hypothesis testing on a single ordinal variable is the Wilcoxon signed-rank test. The test statistics for that procedure are the sum of the ranks for the negative differences and the sum of the ranks for the positive differences between paired observations. Unlike for other test statistics, we reject the null hypothesis if the calculated Wilcoxon signed-rank test statistic is equal to or smaller than the value in the table. For a two-tailed test, we calculate both the sum of the negative ranks and the sum of the positive ranks and choose the smaller of the two. A one-tailed test uses either the sum of the positive ranks or the sum of the negative ranks. Which of the two sums is used depends on the alternative hypothesis. Specifically, the appropriate test statistic is the sum that is assumed, according to the alternative hypothesis, to be the smaller of the two sums.

When continuous data are converted to an ordinal scale for statistical analysis, we are able to circumvent certain assumptions about the distribution of estimates derived from all possible samples. We cannot, however, ignore the assumption that dependent variable values are randomly selected from the population.

As a result of this conversion to an ordinal scale, we have the potential for losing statistical power. That is to say, it can become more difficult to reject a false null hypothesis. This loss of statistical power occurs when the assumptions of the statistical procedure for continuous data are not violated, but the data are analyzed as if they were ordinal. The loss of power is usually small and usually has no effect on the conclusions we draw in hypothesis testing.

EXERCISES

5.1. Patients on a particular treatment often suffer from anemia. To counter this effect, we think that these patients might be helped if they were given folic acid. To evaluate this, we identify eight patients on the treatment who have been diagnosed with anemia and measure their hematocrit. Then, we give these patients supplemental folic acid for a period of 14 days. Then, we measure their hematocrit again and subtract this second measurement from the initial measurement. Suppose that we observe the following differences: −0.2, 0.5, 0.8, −1.3, −1.4, −5.4, −9.7, −18.2. Create an Excel or R dataset from those values.

---

[6]Parameters are used in the mathematic description of a distribution. There is no distribution in nonparametric analysis.

Using those data, and without assuming a Gaussian sampling distribution, test the null hypothesis that there is a balance of increases and decreases in hematocrit versus the alternative hypothesis that there is not a balance. If you were to allow a 5% chance of making a type I error, which of the following is the best conclusion to draw?

A. Accept both the null and alternative hypotheses

B. Reject both the null and alternative hypotheses

C. Reject the null hypothesis and accept the alternative hypothesis

D. Accept the null hypothesis and reject the alternative hypothesis

E. It is best not to draw a conclusion about the null and alternative hypotheses from these observations

5.2. Patients on a particular treatment often suffer from anemia. To counter this effect, we think that these patients might be helped if they were given folic acid. To evaluate this, we identify eight patients on the treatment who have been diagnosed with anemia and measure their hematocrit. Then, we give these patients supplemental folic acid for a period of 14 days. Then, we measure their hematocrit again and subtract this second measurement from the initial measurement. Suppose that we observe the following differences: -0.2, 0.5, 0.8, -1.3, -1.4, -5.4, -9.7, -18.2. Create an Excel or R dataset from those values. Calculate the median of those values. Which of the following is closest to that median?

A. -4.36

B. -1.35

C. 0

D. 1.35

E. 4.36

5.3. Suppose we are interested in a new treatment for arthritis pain. To evaluate this new treatment, we give it to 100 arthritis patients and ask them to use it for two weeks. At the end of that time, we ask them whether or not their level of pain improved, worsened, or did not change. Suppose that we make the observations in the following table.

Response	Number of Patients
Very much improved	26
Somewhat improved	32
No change	27
Somewhat worse	12
Very much worse	3

Calculate the median of those values. Which of the following is closest to that median?

A. Very much improved

B. Somewhat improved

C. No change

D. Somewhat worse

E. Very much worse

5.4. Suppose we are interested in a new treatment for arthritis pain. To evaluate this new treatment, we give it to 100 arthritis patients and ask them to use it for two weeks. At the end of that time, we ask them whether or not their level of pain improved, worsened, or did not change. Suppose that we make the observations in the following table.

Response	Number of Patients
Very much improved	26
Somewhat improved	32
No change	27
Somewhat worse	12
Very much worse	3

Test the null hypothesis that there was no change in the level of pain versus the alternative hypothesis that there was a change. If you allow a 5% chance of making a type I error, which of the following is the best conclusion to draw?

A. Accept both the null and alternative hypotheses

B. Reject both the null and alternative hypotheses

C. Reject the null hypothesis and accept the alternative hypothesis

D. Accept the null hypothesis and reject the alternative hypothesis

E. It is best not to draw a conclusion about the null and alternative hypotheses from these observations

CHAPTER 6

UNIVARIABLE ANALYSIS OF A NOMINAL DEPENDENT VARIABLE

Much of the data we encounter in health research are measured on a nominal scale.[1] We learned in the introduction to Part Two that a nominal variable consists of dichotomous (yes/no) information. For an individual, a nominal variable indicates

[1] Continuous or ordinal data can also be converted to a nominal scale. If this is done, information is lost and the chance of making a type II error increases.

Introduction to Biostatistical Applications in Health Research with Microsoft Office Excel® and R,
Second Edition. Robert P. Hirsch.
© 2021 John Wiley & Sons, Inc. Published 2021 by John Wiley & Sons, Inc.
Companion website: www.wiley.com/go/hirsch/healthresearch2e

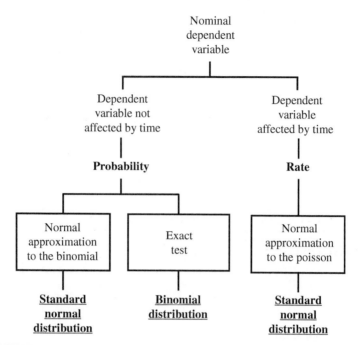

FLOWCHART 4 Flowchart showing univariable analysis of a nominal dependent variable. The point estimates that are most often used to describe the dependent variable (either a probability or a rate) are in bold. The common names of statistical tests are enclosed in boxes. The standard distributions that are used to test hypotheses and calculate confidence intervals are in bold and underlined.

either the presence or absence of some characteristic (e.g., female gender) or the occurrence or nonoccurrence of some event (e.g., death). When information is combined for several individuals, however, nominal dependent variables are often summarized as probabilities or rates. In this chapter we will see how to estimate probabilities and rates and how we can take into account the role of chance on these estimates (Flowchart 4).

6.1 DISTRIBUTION OF NOMINAL DATA

A distribution of nominal data that are represented by a single nominal variable (i.e., having two possible values) can be represented graphically as shown in Figure 6.1. To completely describe this distribution of data, we need only a single parameter. The most commonly used parameter is the probability of the event or characteristic. That probability is considered to reflect the location of the distribution of nominal data. There is no need for a second parameter (like variance for a distribution of

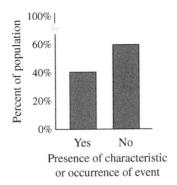

Figure 6.1 Distribution of nominal data with two possible conditions: the presence or absence of a characteristic or the occurrence or nonoccurrence of an event.

continuous data). Once you know the probability of the event, you know everything you need to describe or draw the distribution of nominal data. For the distribution in Figure 6.1, the probability of the event or characteristic is equal to 0.4. We know that is the case, since 40% of the population has the event or characteristic and 60% do not have the event or characteristic.

When we talked about the parameters of a distribution of continuous data in Chapter 2, we used Greek letters to represent the population's parameters. We continue with this convention when discussing about the parameter of a distribution of nominal data. For the probability of the event, we use the Greek letter theta (θ).

Equation (6.1) illustrates how we would calculate θ if we were able to observe the entire population.

$$\theta = \frac{\lambda}{N} \qquad (6.1)$$

where

θ = (theta) the probability of an event or characteristic in the population

λ = (lambda) the number of events or persons with the characteristic in the population

N = total number of persons in the population

6.2 POINT ESTIMATES

When calculating estimates of the population's parameters, we use English, rather than Greek letters. Equation (6.2) illustrates in mathematical language the sample's estimate of the population's probability of the event or characteristic.

$$\theta \triangleq p = \frac{a}{n} \qquad (6.2)$$

where

   p = probability of the event or characteristic in the sample

   a = number of events or persons with the characteristic in the sample

   n = total number of persons in the sample

6.2.1 Probabilities

Equation (6.2) shows how to calculate the point estimate for the probability in the population. In addition to this general formula for a probability, there are two special probabilities that we use in health research, especially when the event of interest is having a particular disease. These special probabilities are called **prevalence** and **risk**.

In its most common form, prevalence is the probability that someone in a population has a particular disease at a particular point in time.[2] It is estimated from the sample's observations by dividing the number of persons in the sample with the disease by the total number of persons in the sample (Equation (6.3)).

$$\text{Prevalence} = \frac{\text{Number of persons with the disease at time } t}{\text{Total number of persons}} \qquad (6.3)$$

Risk is the probability that a person will develop a particular disease over a specified period of time. It is estimated from the sample's observations by dividing the number of persons in a sample that develop the disease over the time period by the total number of disease-free persons in the sample at the beginning of the time period (Equation (6.4)). The number of disease-free persons in a sample at the beginning of a time period is called the number "at risk."

$$\text{Risk}_{\Delta t} = \frac{\text{Number of persons developing the disease over } \Delta t}{\text{Total number of disease-free persons at } t = 0} \qquad (6.4)$$

Both prevalence and risk are probabilities with properties just like those described for probabilities in Chapter 1. For example, prevalence or risk can have any value between 0 and 1. The distinction between prevalence and risk is that prevalence addresses the proportion of persons with a characteristic at a point in time while risk addresses the proportion of persons who develop a disease over a specified period of time. This is an important distinction, for prevalence can be estimated from a single examination of a sample, while estimation of risk involves an examination to determine which persons do and do not have the characteristic and a second examination after a period of time to discover how many persons have developed the characteristic during the time interval. This distinction is illustrated in the next example.

---

[2]More precisely, this is called a point prevalence.

■ **EXAMPLE 6.1**

Suppose we are interested in the probability of retinopathy among diabetics. At one point in time, we examine 500 persons with diabetes and find 6 persons who have diabetic retinopathy. Five years later, we reexamine the 494 persons who did not have retinopathy at the initial examination and find that 68 have developed retinopathy during the five-year period of time. From these observations, let us estimate the prevalence and risk of diabetic retinopathy in the population from which these persons were sampled.

There are two different points in time for which we could estimate the prevalence of retinopathy. One of these is at the time of the initial examination. At that point in time, 6 out of the 500 persons examined had retinopathy. Thus, the prevalence of retinopathy at the first examination is calculated using Equation (6.3) as follows:

$$\text{Prevalence} = \frac{\text{Number of persons with the disease at intial examination}}{\text{Total number of persons}}$$

$$= \frac{6}{500} = 0.012$$

We can also estimate the prevalence of retinopathy at the time of the final examination. At that time, the original 6 persons who had retinopathy at the initial examination still have retinopathy plus an additional 68 people have developed retinopathy during the five-year time period. Thus, the prevalence of retinopathy at the final examination is (using Equation (6.3))

$$\text{Prevalence} = \frac{\text{Number of persons with the disease at final examination}}{\text{Total number of persons}}$$

$$= \frac{6 + 68}{500} = 0.148$$

Although we can estimate two different prevalences of retinopathy (corresponding to the time of each of the two examinations), we can estimate only one risk. Since risk, in this example, is the probability of developing diabetic retinopathy over a five-year time period, our interest is confined to persons who do not have retinopathy at the beginning of the time period. If the person already has retinopathy, that person is not "at risk" of developing retinopathy.

The purpose of the first examination is to identify the persons who already have retinopathy. In this case, six persons were found to have retinopathy at the first examination. Thus, the number of persons "at risk" of developing retinopathy was $500 - 6 = 494$.

The purpose of the second examination is to find out how many of the 494 persons without retinopathy at the beginning of the five-year period developed that condition over the five-year period. Thus, our estimate of the five-year risk of diabetic retinopathy is (using Equation (6.4)):

$$\text{Risk}_{\Delta t} = \frac{\text{Number of persons developing the disease over the five-year period}}{\text{Total number of disease-free persons at the beginning of the five-year period}}$$

$$= \frac{68}{500 - 6} = 0.138$$

∎

6.2.2   Rates

Although the most commonly used parameter for a distribution of nominal data is the probability of the event or condition, there is one circumstance in which a probability may not be the best choice. That is when the likelihood of seeing the event represented by the nominal dependent variable is affected by time. To be affected by time, a nominal dependent variable has to meet two criteria.

The first criterion for being affected by time is that the event represented by the nominal dependent variable is more likely to be observed longer the period of time spent looking for it. In Example 6.1, the event was development of retinopathy. That event satisfies this first criterion for being affected by time. The longer the period of time, the more new cases of retinopathy we would expect to observe. In health research, most events in which we are interested meet this first criterion for being affected by time.

The second criterion for a nominal dependent variable being affected by time is that different persons in a study must be followed for different periods of time. In Example 6.1, everyone who was at risk for developing retinopathy was followed for five years. Thus, this second criterion is not met in Example 6.1, and we need not consider the nominal dependent variable to be affected by time. For this reason, it is appropriate for us to describe the development of retinopathy using risk. It would not have been appropriate to use risk, however, if some people were not followed for the entire five-year period.

There are two ways in which persons in a study might be followed for different periods of time. One of these is due to persons withdrawing from a study before its planned end. To statisticians, the term "withdrawing" subsumes all reasons that a person might not be examined at the end of a period of follow-up. One of these reasons might be that the person chooses not to be examined, but it also includes the person moving or even dying before the end of the study.

Alternatively, individuals may be followed for different periods of time if they entered a study at different times. It is not unusual in health research to take a long period of time to find a sufficient number of persons who are eligible to be in the study. In this case, there is a period during which persons are recruited into the study. This feature of a study is called **staggered admission** and is a very common feature of clinical trials.

The reason that staggered admission causes different individuals to be followed for different periods of time is that follow-up usually ends for everyone in the study at the same point in time, regardless of when they were recruited. So, those persons

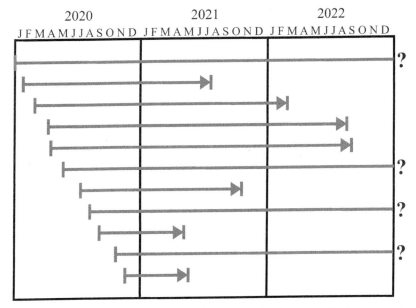

Figure 6.2 Staggered admission of 11 subjects during the first year of a three-year study. ⊢ Indicates the time at which the individual entered the study (and consequently, the time at which follow-up began), ▶ indicates follow-up ending because of occurrence of the event of interest, and **?** indicates end of follow-up without the event (because the study was concluded). Staggered admission is a feature of studies that can result in a nominal dependent variable being affected by time.

who entered the study later are followed for a shorter period of time than individuals who entered the study earlier. In Example 6.1, we could have staggered admission, and, thus, different periods of follow-up for different persons. This could be a result of the admission criterion of being a newly diagnosed diabetic. If that were the case, we would need to have a period of time over which we were watching for newly diagnosed diabetics. Figure 6.2 shows a pattern of staggered admission that would lead to a nominal dependent variable affected by time if the event is more likely to be observed the longer we look for it.

In Figure 6.2, there are four persons who have question marks on the outside of the time chart. For these persons, the study ended before they were observed to have the outcome. These are called **censored** observations. As the name implies, we do not know when or if these persons would have the event. Censored observations are a common feature of a nominal dependent variable affected by time.

When a nominal dependent variable is affected by time, we usually describe the nominal dependent variable using a rate instead of a probability.[3] Probabilities and

---

[3]In Chapter 12, we will look at life-table analysis. It is a statistical method that allows us to estimate probabilities from a nominal dependent variable affected by time.

rates differ according to the information that is used in their denominators. For a probability, the denominator reflects the number of persons who are candidates for having the event. For a rate, the denominator reflects the number of persons as well as how long each person was followed, waiting for the event.

Having time in the denominator of a rate gives it 1/time as its units of measure. Probabilities, on the other hand, have no units of measure. Having time in the denominator of a rate also changes the range of possible values. In Chapter 1, we learned that a probability can have any value between 0 and 1. A rate, on the other hand, can have any value between 0 and infinity.[4]

When we are interested in the rate of disease occurrence, we use a special name for the rate at which new cases appear in a population. We call this rate the **incidence** of the disease. Equation (6.5) shows how an incidence is calculated:

$$\text{Incidence} = \frac{\text{Number of new cases of disease}}{\sum\limits_{i=1}^{n}(\text{Time of follow-up for the } i\text{th person})} \tag{6.5}$$

where

$$\sum\limits_{i=1}^{n} = \text{sum of values (e.g., follow-up times) for individuals from the first individual}$$

$(i = 1)$ to the nth individual

There are two ways in which we commonly calculate the follow-up time used in the denominator of a rate. The best way is to simply add up each person's individual follow-up time. A person's follow-up time begins when he or she enters the study. It ends either when the person has the event or when the person is no longer followed. The other way to calculate follow-up time is to assume that follow-up ended half-way between the time that the person was last seen without the event and the time at which the person either had the event or disappeared. This way of estimating follow-up time is called the **actuarial method**. The actuarial method is used only when we do not know the actual time follow-up ends, but we are able to identify two points in time between which follow-up ended. The next example illustrates both methods of determining follow-up time.

■ EXAMPLE 6.2

Suppose that Figure 6.2 shows the results of following 11 individuals for up to three years looking for the development of retinopathy at monthly examinations. The following table shows, for each of these 11 persons, the month at which follow-up began, when it ended, and whether or not the person had the event.

---

[4]One way to think of the reason for this is to realize that the denominator of an incidence can be infinitely small if we express the incidence in an infinitely long period of time. For instance, one person-year is equal to 0.1 person-decades or 0.001 person-millennia.

Patient	Date Began	Date Ended	Event?
TH	1/20	12/22	No
IS	2/20	8/21	Yes
JU	3/20	3/22	Yes
ST	4/20	8/22	Yes
GE	4/20	9/22	Yes
TS	5/20	12/22	No
BE	7/20	11/21	Yes
TT	8/20	12/22	No
ER	9/20	5/21	Yes
DU	10/20	12/22	No
DE	11/20	6/21	Yes
Total			7 events

Now, let us estimate the incidence of retinopathy using the actuarial method to approximate the total follow-up time.

In this set of data, we know the month during which each individual had the event, but we do not know exactly when it occurred. When this is the case, we need to make an assumption about the time at which the event occurred. The assumption in the actuarial method is that, on the average, events occur in the middle of the time period between examinations. To reflect this assumption, we allow each person who had the event to contribute to the overall follow-up time only half of the time (in this case, half-a-month) from the examination at which they first had the event and the previous examination. The following table shows those data as they would appear if the actuarial method were used to determine the length of follow-up:

Patient	Date Began	Follow-Up Date Ended	Follow-Up Length (Months)	Event?
TH	1/20	12/22	36	No
IS	2/20	8/21	$18 + 1/2 = 18.5$	Yes
JU	3/20	3/22	$24 + 1/2 = 24.5$	Yes
ST	4/20	8/22	$28 + 1/2 = 28.5$	Yes
GE	4/20	9/22	$29 + 1/2 = 29.5$	Yes
TS	5/20	12/22	32	No
BE	7/20	11/21	$16 + 1/2 = 16.5$	Yes
TT	8/20	12/22	29	No
ER	9/20	5/21	$8 + 1/2 = 8.5$	Yes
DU	10/20	12/22	27	No
DE	11/20	6/21	$7 + 1/2 = 7.5$	Yes
Total			257.5	7 events

The total follow-up time, using the actuarial method, is equal to 257.5 months (or 257.5/12 = 21.5 years). Notice how the follow-up time for those individuals who had the event is reduced by half-a-month. This represents the assumption that, in the actuarial method, persons who had the event had it at the middle of the time between examinations, on the average. With that information and the fact that seven persons developed retinopathy, we can use Equation (6.5) to calculate the estimated incidence.

$$\text{Incidence} = \frac{\text{Number of new cases of disease}}{\sum_{i=1}^{n}(\text{Time of follow-up for the } i\text{th person})}$$

$$= \frac{7}{257.5/12} = \frac{7}{21.5} = 0.33 \text{ per year}$$

∎

Prevalence, risk, and incidence are measurements of disease frequency. Most of the diseases of interest to health researchers are rare. Therefore, values of prevalence, risk, and incidence are generally small numbers. For instance, the prevalence of pancreatic cancer in the United States in 1999 was about 0.00008. To keep us from having to deal with all the zeros in these small numbers, prevalence and risk are often presented as a larger number times 10^{-5} (number of cases per 10^5 persons)[5] and incidence is frequently given as a larger number times 10^{-5} years (number of cases per 10^5 person-years). In the case of pancreatic cancer, we would report that the prevalence is equal to 8×10^{-5} (or 8 cases per 10^5 persons). For more common diseases, prevalence and risk are usually expressed as a percentage (i.e., prevalence $\times$ 100%). For example, the prevalence of heart disease among women in the United States is about 0.29 or 29%. Since incidence has the unit 1/time, it cannot be expressed as a percentage.

6.3 SAMPLING DISTRIBUTIONS

To take chance into account, we need to consider the sampling distribution for estimates of the probability or the rate of occurrence of an event in the population. To begin with, let us consider a nominal dependent variable represented by the probability of the event. Later, we will discuss the sampling distribution for the rate of an event.

When we discussed the sampling distribution for estimates of the mean of a distribution of continuous data, we assumed that the sampling distribution is a Gaussian distribution. We are comfortable with that assumption if the sample is not too small; since the central limit theorem tells us that sampling distributions for estimates of the mean tend to be Gaussian distributions, with that tendency increasing as the size of the samples increases. The sampling distribution for estimates of the

---

[5]This is known as scientific notation. 10^{-5} is equal to 1 over 10 to the 5th power or 1/100,000. 10^5 is equal to 10 to the 5th power or 100,000.

probability of an event (θ), however, is not assumed to be a Gaussian distribution. Instead, the sampling distribution for estimates of θ is a **binomial distribution**.[6]

6.3.1 Binomial Distribution

The binomial distribution is different from the Gaussian distribution in three ways. First, the binomial distribution is a discrete, rather than continuous, distribution. This is because there are a limited number of possible estimates of θ from samples of a given size. For instance, samples with 20 observations must provide 1 of 21 different estimates. This limited number of estimates is due to the fact that the numerator of an estimate of the probability of the event must be an integer (i.e., a whole number) between 0 and the total number of observations. There are 21 integers in the interval from 0 to 20.

Recognition of the binomial distribution as a discrete distribution is reflected in the way in which binomial distributions are presented graphically. Recall from Chapter 2 that bar graphs are used for discrete data. Figure 6.3 shows a bar graph for a binomial sampling distribution.

The second way the binomial distribution is different from the Gaussian distribution is that the binomial distribution has a discrete range of possible values, whereas the Gaussian distribution has (theoretically) an infinite range of possible values. The reason that this distinction is important is that a distribution with a discrete range of possible values is symmetric only when its parameter is in the middle of that range. In Figure 6.3, θ is equal to 0.5, which is in the middle of the

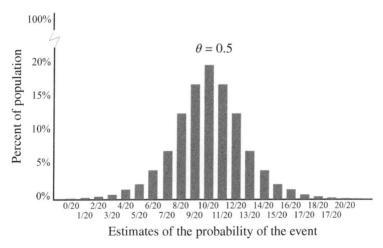

Figure 6.3 A graphic representation of the binomial sampling distribution for estimates of θ from all possible samples with 20 observations when the population's value of θ is equal to 0.5.

---

[6]This is not an assumption, but rather a statement of fact. The sampling distribution for estimates of θ will always be a binomial distribution.

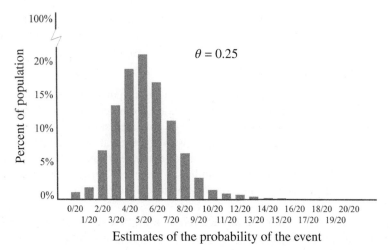

Figure 6.4   A graphic representation of the binomial sampling distribution for estimates of θ from all possible samples with 20 observations when the population's value of θ is equal to 0.25.

range of possible values for a probability (i.e., 0–1). Consequently, the binomial distribution in Figure 6.3 is symmetric. If we were to change the value of θ to some other value, however, the binomial distribution would no longer be symmetric. Figure 6.4 shows a binomial distribution for 20 observations and with θ equal to 0.25. This distribution is asymmetric.

The third way the binomial distribution is different from the Gaussian distribution is in the number of parameters that are needed to mathematically define those distributions. A Gaussian distribution is defined by two parameters: the mean and the variance (or standard deviation). A particular binomial distribution, on the other hand, requires only one parameter to distinguish it from other binomial distributions. This single parameter is θ, the probability of the event in the population.[7] θ is analogous to the mean of a Gaussian distribution.[8]

Thus, we think of θ as a parameter of location of the binomial distribution. This parameter of location is the only value needed to identify a particular binomial distribution.

Statistical methods that address the binomial distribution itself are called **exact methods**. These methods are computationally cumbersome and, as a result, are not often the way we analyze a nominal dependent variable.[9] More frequently, we use methods that are based on a **normal approximation**. In a normal approximation, we recognize that probabilities calculated using the actual sampling distribution for

[7] θ is the parameter of the distribution of nominal data (Figure 6.1) as well as the binomial sampling distribution.

[8] If we were to represent the occurrence of the event with the number 1 and the nonoccurrence of the event with 0, the mean of those values would be equal to θ.

[9] With the fast computers we use today, this really is not a good excuse for using a method other than an exact method. Even so, changing the way in which researchers traditionally analyze data is a slow process.

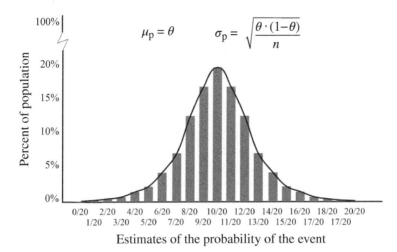

Figure 6.5 When the normal approximation to the binomial is used to take into account the role of chance in estimating θ e think of the sampling distribution as being approximated by a Gaussian distribution.

a parameter of a nominal dependent variable are, under certain circumstances, not very different from probabilities calculated assuming a Gaussian sampling distribution. When that is the case, we can use statistical methods based on a Gaussian sampling distribution to take into account the role of chance in estimating θ from the sample's observations (Figure 6.5).

We are comfortable with a normal approximation when the sample is not too small. For a symmetric binomial distribution, samples of 10 or more observations can be analyzed using the normal approximation. For an asymmetric binomial distribution, the sample's size needs to be larger than 10 observations. How much larger depends on the degree of asymmetry. The rule of thumb we use is that at least five events and at least five nonevents are required to use the normal approximation to the binomial distribution. If, for example, θ is equal to 0.10, then the minimum number of observations required to use the normal approximation is 50. Among the 50 persons, 5 would have the event (since the probability of having the event is 0.1) and 45 would not have the event.

In a normal approximation to the binomial distribution, we think about the binomial sampling distribution as if it were a Gaussian sampling distribution. If the sampling distribution were a Gaussian distribution, we would need two parameters to mathematically define that sampling distribution: a mean and a standard error.

The ways in which we would calculate these parameters, if we observed the entire population, are shown in Equations (6.6) and (6.7).

$$\mu_p = \theta \qquad (6.6)$$

$$\sigma_p = \sqrt{\frac{\theta \cdot (1 - \theta)}{n}} \qquad (6.7)$$

where

μ_p = mean of the sampling distribution for estimates of θ when the normal approximation to the binomial is used to take chance into account

σ_p = standard error for estimates of θ when the normal approximation to the binomial is used to take chance into account

Equations (6.6) and (6.7) suggest that the sampling distribution has two parameters, but a closer look at these equations reveals only a single parameter: θ. For any particular value of the mean (θ), there is only one standard error possible, since the standard error is simply an algebraic function of θ. This is unlike the standard error for estimates of the mean for continuous data. For a particular value of the mean of a distribution of continuous data, the variance and, hence, the standard error for the sampling distribution for that mean can be equal to any value. Thus, we say that there is an independent role of chance in estimating the variance of a distribution of continuous data. There is not, however, an independent role of chance in estimating a variance of a distribution of nominal data. With nominal data, there is one, and only one, possible value for the variance with any particular value of θ.

The independent role of chance in estimating the variance of a distribution of continuous data is the reason that Student's t-distribution was used in Chapter 4. Student's t-distribution takes into account this independent role of chance by using degrees of freedom to reflect how much information the sample contains that can be used to estimate the variance. Since there is no independent role of chance in estimating the variance when we are using a normal approximation for a nominal dependent variable, we do not use Student's t-distribution. Instead, we use the standard normal distribution when we are performing a normal approximation.

The sampling distribution for an estimate of a probability is a binomial distribution. When a nominal dependent variable is represented as a rate, however, we cannot use the binomial distribution. The problem is that the binomial distribution takes chance into account for estimates that can range from 0 to 1 and that have no unit of measure. Rates have 0 as their lower bound, but rates have no upper bound. Rates also have 1/time as their units of measure. Thus, to take chance into account for estimates of the rate of an event, we need to use a different sampling distribution.

6.3.2 Poisson Distribution

The problem with rates stems from the fact that time is in their denominators. The solution to this problem is to use a sampling distribution that is not affected by what is in the denominator. The **Poisson distribution**[10] is the sampling distribution

---

[10]We always capitalize "Poisson," since this is the name of the French mathematician who derived this distribution.

we use most often to take into account the role of chance in estimating a rate. The parameter of a Poisson distribution is the number of events. That is to say, the parameter is the numerator of the rate. We symbolize this parameter with the Greek letter lambda (λ).[11] This is the same as the numerator of θ in Equation (6.1). The point estimate of λ calculated from the sample's observations is symbolized with the letter a. This is the same as the numerator of p in Equation (6.2).

$$\lambda \triangleq a \qquad (6.8)$$

To take the role of chance into account when estimating the rate at which events occur, we can perform an exact procedure that uses the Poisson distribution itself or we can use a normal approximation to the Poisson distribution. The same reason that motivated us to use the normal approximation to the binomial distribution also motivates us to use the normal approximation to the Poisson distribution. Namely, normal approximations are computationally less complicated.

Since the Poisson distribution has no upper bound, the Poisson distribution tends to be very asymmetric. Figure 6.6 shows an example of the Poisson distribution.

If we were to use a normal approximation for the Poisson distribution shown in Figure 6.6, we would need to have a relatively large sample to overcome the asymmetry of the distribution. Instead, what we do is use a **transformation** for the

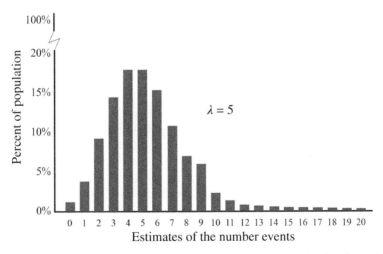

Figure 6.6 A graphic representation of the Poisson sampling distribution for estimates of λ from all possible samples with 20 observations when the population's value of λ is equal to 5.

---

[11] The Poisson distribution can also be used as a sampling distribution for probabilities of rare events, but when performing normal approximations, it is better to use the binomial distribution for probabilities.

number of events and, then, do a normal approximation for the transformed number of events. What statisticians mean by a transformation is performing a mathematical operation on dependent variable values or estimates so that they are easier to use in statistical analyses. The transformation we use for the estimate of the number of events in the normal approximation to the Poisson distribution is the **square root transformation**.

The way this transformation works is that we take the square root of the number of events and perform our statistical analysis on that transformed value. Then, after the statistical analysis is complete, the results of the analysis are changed back to the original scale by squaring the estimates. We will see how this works later, but for now, let us take a look at the parameters we use when performing a normal approximation to the Poisson distribution.

The mean and standard error of the sampling distribution for the square root of the number of events are illustrated in Equations (6.9) and (6.10).

$$\mu_{\sqrt{a}} = \sqrt{\lambda} \tag{6.9}$$

$$\sigma_{\sqrt{a}} = \frac{1}{2} \tag{6.10}$$

where

$\mu_{\sqrt{a}}$ = mean of the sampling distribution for estimates of the square root of λ when the normal approximation to the Poisson is used to take chance into account

$\sigma_{\sqrt{a}}$ = standard error for estimates of the square root of λ when the normal approximation to the Poisson is used to take chance into account

As in estimation of the parameters in the normal approximation to the binomial (Equations (6.6) and (6.7)), estimation of the parameters in the normal approximation to the Poisson involves only a single role of chance. That role is the effect of chance on estimation of the mean of the distribution. When we discussed the normal approximation to the binomial, we found that there was no independent role of chance for estimation of the variance, since the variance was merely an algebraic form of the mean of the distribution (Equation (6.7)). In the normal approximation to the Poisson, the lack of an independent role of chance in estimating the variance is even clearer than it was in the normal approximation to the binomial. In the normal approximation to the Poisson, the variance is equal to a constant and, thus, requires no estimation at all.

Now that we are familiar with the sampling distributions for the normal approximations to the binomial and Poisson distributions, we are ready to see how we can use these sampling distributions to take chance into account through the processes of interval estimation and hypothesis testing.

6.4   INTERVAL ESTIMATION

In Chapter 3, we used the standard normal distribution to calculate a confidence interval for the mean of a distribution of continuous data. This method is not appropriate for a continuous dependent variable, but it is appropriate for calculating a confidence interval for the probability of an event, since there is no independent role of chance in estimating the variance of a distribution of nominal data. Equation (6.11) shows how a two-sided confidence interval for θ is calculated in the normal approximation to the binomial.

$$\theta \triangleq p \pm \left(z_{\alpha/2} \cdot \sqrt{\frac{\theta \cdot (1-\theta)}{n}} \right) \triangleq p \pm \left(z_{\alpha/2} \cdot \sqrt{\frac{p \cdot (1-p)}{n}} \right) \qquad (6.11)$$

The standard error in Equation (6.11) is a little different from the standard error in Equation (6.7). Equation (6.7) uses the population's value of θ instead of the sample's estimate (p) to calculate the standard error. When we are calculating a confidence interval from the sample's observations, we do not know the value of θ. Our best guess for the value of θ is the point estimate (p). Thus, Equation (6.11) uses p instead of θ in the standard error.

Now, let us take a look at an example of how we calculate a confidence interval for the probability of an event represented by a nominal dependent variable.

■ EXAMPLE 6.3

In Example 6.1, we estimated the five-year risk of developing retinopathy to be equal to 0.138 from a group of 494 persons without retinopathy at the beginning of the five-year follow-up period. Now, let us calculate a 95%, two-sided confidence interval for that risk.

To calculate that confidence interval, we use Equation (6.11):

$$\theta \triangleq p \pm \left(z_{\alpha/2} \cdot \sqrt{\frac{p \cdot (1-p)}{n}} \right) = 0.138 \pm \left(1.96 \cdot \sqrt{\frac{0.138 \cdot (1-0.138)}{494}} \right)$$

$$= 0.108 - 0.168$$

Thus, we can have 95% confidence that the actual five-year risk of developing retinopathy in the population is between 0.108 and 0.168.   ■

As we found out earlier in this chapter, normal approximations are used to analyze a nominal dependent variable because exact methods involve cumbersome calculations. If we are calculating a confidence interval by hand, the normal approximation is easier. However, the difficulty of the calculation is not an issue when the computer is doing the calculating.

In Excel, we can calculate an exact confidence interval for a proportion. The next example shows how this can be done.

■ EXAMPLE 6.4

In Example 6.1, we estimated the five-year risk of developing retinopathy to be equal to 0.138 from a group of 494 persons without retinopathy at the beginning of the five-year period of follow-up, 68 of whom developed retinopathy. In Example 6.3, we used a normal approximation to calculate a 95%, two-sided confidence interval for the risk. Now, let us calculate an exact 95% confidence interval.

What makes a method an exact method is when the actual sampling distribution is used to calculate the estimates. For a proportion, the actual sampling distribution is the binomial distribution. In Excel, the BINOM.DIST function can be used to calculate the probability of obtaining a given number of events or more for a particular sample size and a particular θ. To find the exact confidence intervals, we want to find what values of θ correspond to the upper $1 - \alpha/2$ of the binomial distribution for the lower limit and the lower $\alpha/2$ for the upper limit. The "Binomial CI" BAHR[12] program does this in Excel:

Exact binomial 95% confidence interval				
$p =$	0.138	$n =$	494	$a =$ 68.172
		Limits		
	Lower		Upper	
	0.108784		0.171632	

We can also calculate an exact binomial confidence interval in R. This is demonstrated in Example 6.7 later in this chapter ■

Using a normal approximation to calculate a confidence interval for the rate at which events occur involves three steps, but we can perform all three of these steps using a single equation. Equations (6.12) and (6.13) show the first two steps in deriving Equation (6.14). In practice, we perform all three of these steps in the single calculation illustrated in Equation (6.14).

The first step in this process is to calculate a confidence interval for the square root of the number of events. This step is shown in Equation (6.12):

$$\sqrt{\lambda} \triangleq \sqrt{a} \pm \left(z_{\alpha/2} \cdot \frac{1}{2} \right) \tag{6.12}$$

In the next step, we change the limits of that confidence interval from the square root of the number of events to the number of events by squaring the limits. Equation (6.13) shows how Equation (6.12) changes to reflect this step:

$$\lambda \triangleq \left[\sqrt{a} \pm \left(z_{\alpha/2} \cdot \frac{1}{2} \right) \right]^2 \tag{6.13}$$

---

[12]Biostatistical Analysis in Health Research. These are the Excel programs supplied with this textbook.

Finally, we change the limits of that confidence interval so that they reflect the rate at which new events are occurring by dividing the limits by the total time of follow-up in the sample.

$$\text{Incidence} \triangleq \frac{[\sqrt{a} \pm (z_{\alpha/2} \cdot 1/2)]^2}{\displaystyle\sum_{i=1}^{n} \text{Length of follow-up for the } i\text{th person}} \tag{6.14}$$

Equation (6.14) includes all three steps in a single equation. In the next example, we will take a look at how we can use Equation (6.14) to calculate an interval estimate for a rate.

■ EXAMPLE 6.5

In Example 6.2, we considered the results of 11 persons followed for up to three years looking for the development of diabetic retinopathy. Among these 11 persons, 7 developed retinopathies during the follow-up period. The total time of follow-up for the 11 persons was 21.5 years. Using that information, we estimated in Example 6.2 that the incidence of retinopathy in the population is equal to 0.32 cases per person-year. Now, let us calculate a 95%, two-sided confidence interval for the incidence of retinopathy in the population.

We calculate the confidence interval for a rate by using Equation (6.14):

$$\text{Incidence} \triangleq \frac{[\sqrt{a} \pm (z_{\alpha/2} \cdot 1/2)]^2}{\displaystyle\sum_{i=1}^{n} \text{Length of follow-up for the } i\text{th person}}$$

$$= \frac{[\sqrt{7} \pm (1.96 \cdot 1/2)]^2}{21.5} = 0.13 - 0.60 \text{ per year}$$

Thus, we have 95% confidence that the incidence of retinopathy in the population is between 0.13 and 0.60 new cases per person-year. ■

6.5 HYPOTHESIS TESTING

In Chapter 3, we learned that using hypothesis testing as a way to take the role of chance into account depends on our ability to formulate a testable null hypothesis. A testable null hypothesis is one that makes a specific statement about the population, and that is also an interesting hypothesis to test. Often, this cannot be done for a univariable sample. In Chapter 4, we learned that a univariable sample with a continuous dependent variable is a candidate for hypothesis testing if the data are from a paired study. For mean differences, it makes sense to test the null hypothesis that the mean difference between two measurements for each individual is equal to 0. Otherwise, taking chance into account for a univariable sample of a continuous dependent variable is limited to interval estimation.

For the same reasons, we usually take chance into account by calculating a confidence interval when the dependent variable in a univariable data set represents nominal data. There is one exception. This is when each person in the study is exposed to both of the two nominal categories represented by the nominal dependent variable and the one considered to be "better" for each individual is recorded. Studies of this type are called **preference studies**. In a preference study, each person selects the nominal category he or she prefers more. Then, the data are summarized by determining the proportion of persons preferring a particular category.

The null hypothesis in a preference study is that half of the persons will choose a particular category (i.e., H_0: $\theta = 0.5$). This null hypothesis is the same as saying that there is no overall preference for either of the two categories. To test this null hypothesis, we can use either an exact test or a normal approximation. If offered the results of both, the exact test is the better method. If we are performing the calculation by hand, however, the normal approximation is easier.

For the normal approximation, the observed proportion preferring a selected category is converted to a standard normal deviate using Equation (6.15).

$$z = \frac{p - \theta_0}{\sqrt{\frac{\theta_0 \cdot (1-\theta_0)}{n}}} = \frac{p - 0.5}{\sqrt{\frac{0.5 \cdot (1-0.5)}{n}}} \tag{6.15}$$

where

θ_0 = proportion of persons preferring a particular category of the nominal dependent variable according to the null hypothesis. In a preference study, this proportion is equal to 0.5

In Equation (6.15), the value of θ used in the calculation of standard error is the value stated in the null hypothesis. The reason for this is that, when we are preparing to calculate P-values, we assume that the null hypothesis is true (see Equation (3.10)). Since the standard error in the normal approximation to the binomial is an algebraic function of θ, the value of that standard error reflects the value of θ in the null hypothesis rather than the observed probability of preferring a particular category. Thus, the standard error in hypothesis testing (Equation (6.15)) is different from the standard error in interval estimation (Equation (6.11)).

The next example illustrates a preference study and how the null hypothesis can be tested using the normal approximation to the binomial.

■ EXAMPLE 6.6

Suppose we are interested in comparing two antinausea medications (called "A" and "B"). To make this comparison, we randomly assign one of the medications to 12 persons who have chronic nausea to use on that day. Then, they are instructed to use the other medication on another day. Suppose that 8 of the 12 persons reported better control of nausea with medication "A." From these observations, let us test the null hypothesis that, in the population, there is no preference for either of the medications, versus the alternative hypothesis that there is a preference. In testing this null hypothesis, we will allow a 5% chance of making a type I error (i.e., $\alpha = 0.05$).

The null hypothesis that there is no preference for either of the two medications in the population is the same as saying that half of the persons in the population would prefer medication "A" and the other half of the persons in the population would prefer medication "B." In terms of the parameter of a distribution of nominal data (θ), the null hypothesis is

$$H_0 : \theta = 0.5$$

To test this null hypothesis using the normal approximation to the binomial, we need to have at least five events (preferring "A") and five nonevents (preferring "B"). In this sample, there are eight persons preferring "A" and four persons preferring "B." At first, this might seem to be insufficient to permit us to use the normal approximation, since there are only four persons preferring "B." However, when using hypothesis testing, we think about how many persons would prefer "B" if the null hypothesis were true. The null hypothesis tells us that half of the individuals prefer "B" (and the other half prefer "A"). With a sample of 12, we would expect 6 persons preferring each medication. This is sufficient to use the normal approximation.

Having decided to use the normal approximation to the binomial, we use Equation (6.15) to convert the observed proportion preferring "A" (8/12 = 0.67) into a standard normal deviate (i.e., a z-value).

$$z = \frac{p - \theta_0}{\sqrt{\frac{\theta_0 \cdot (1-\theta_0)}{n}}} = \frac{0.67 - 0.5}{\sqrt{\frac{0.5 \cdot (1-0.5)}{12}}} = 1.15$$

If we look up 1.15 in Table B.1, we find that it is associated with a probability in the upper tail of the standard normal distribution equal to 0.1251. Since the alternative hypothesis (i.e., that there is a preference) is two-sided, we need to double that probability to get the P-value. Thus, the P-value is equal to 0.2502. Since this is larger than α (0.05), we fail to reject the null hypothesis (i.e., we cannot draw a conclusion about the null hypothesis from this sample). From a biologic perspective, we cannot conclude that one medication is preferred over the other.[13]   ∎

The confidence interval and hypothesis test for the binomial distribution we have examined are based on a normal approximation. Using R, we can get an exact

---

[13] It is important to keep in mind that this is not the same as saying that there is no preference. To conclude that there is no preference would be to accept the null hypothesis as true. We do not accept null hypotheses as being true so that we can avoid type II errors. This is discussed in Chapter 3.

confidence interval and P-value. We do that with the binom.test(a,n) command. The next example shows the exact result for a binomial distribution.

■ EXAMPLE 6.7

In Example 6.6, we considered an experiment in which 12 persons were given 2 antinausea medications (A and B) and asked to choose which seemed to provide the greater relief. Of those 12, 8 chose medication A. Let us use R to test the hypothesis that there is no preference in the population versus the alternative that there is a preference.

>binom.test(8,12)

```
Exact binomial test

data: 8 and 12
number of successes = 8, number of trials = 12, p-value = 0.3877
alternative hypothesis: true probability of success is not equal to 0.5
95 percent confidence interval:
 0.3488755 0.9007539
sample estimates:
probability of success
 0.6666667
```

Since the P-value (0.3877) is greater than 0.05, we fail to reject the null hypothesis. This conclusion is consistent with what we concluded using the normal approximation in Example 6.6.[14]   ■

Taking chance into account for an estimate of the rate at which events occur is limited to interval estimation. The reason for this limitation is that it is impossible to formulate a testable null hypothesis for a rate. This is because we cannot select a specific value for a rate that is biologically interesting to test. Even so, R provides us with a command that performs an exact test for the Poisson distribution. This is not useful to test a null hypothesis, but it also calculates an exact confidence interval for a rate. The next example illustrates that calculation in R.

■ EXAMPLE 6.8

In Example 6.5, we calculated a confidence interval for rate at which people develop diabetic retinopathy using a normal approximation. In that example, 11 persons were followed for a total of 21.5 years during which 7 persons developed retinopathy. Let us use R to calculate an exact 95% confidence interval for the rate at which diabetic retinopathy occurs in the population.

The R command poisson.test(a,t) is used to calculate this confidence interval.

---

[14]The P-value from the exact test is larger than the P-value from the normal approximation. This will always be the case. The P-values would be closer together if we had used a continuity correction in the normal approximation.

```
>poisson.test(7,21.5)

Exact Poisson test

data: 7 time base: 21.5
number of events = 7, time base = 21.5, p-value = 0.0005088
alternative hypothesis: true event rate is not equal to 1
95 percent confidence interval:
 0.1309006 0.6708221
sample estimates:
event rate
 0.3255814
```

That event rate and confidence interval are consistent with those found in Example 6.5. The small difference in the upper limits of the confidence interval is due to the fact that Example 6.5 provides an approximate interval while this example provides an exact interval. ∎

Now we have completed our look at univariable analysis. We are ready to begin Part Three of this text, which addresses bivariable analyses.

CHAPTER SUMMARY

Nominal data can be summarized by probabilities or by rates. Two special types of probabilities we encounter in health research are prevalence and risk. Prevalence of a disease is the probability that an individual chosen at random from a population will have that particular disease. Risk is the probability that a disease-free individual in the population will develop the disease during a specified period of time.

Rates are different from probabilities in that rates contain a measure of time in their denominator. The most commonly used rate in health research is the incidence of disease. Incidence is the number of cases of disease that develop per unit of person-time (e.g., per person-year).

Estimates of probabilities and rates do not come from Gaussian distributions. Instead, they come from either binomial (for probabilities) or Poisson (for rates) distributions. Interval estimation and hypothesis testing for probabilities and rates are usually accomplished using a normal approximation. A normal approximation means that the distribution of estimates is close to a Gaussian distribution. The justification for using a Gaussian distribution for interval estimation and hypothesis testing on probabilities and rates is that, like means of continuous data, estimates of probabilities and rates from all possible samples tend to come from binomial or Poisson distributions similar to a Gaussian distribution, especially when the sample's sizes are large (this is an application of the central limit theorem).

Standard errors for probabilities and rates are different from standard errors for continuous data. For probabilities, the standard error is a function of the probability itself. For rates, the standard error is a constant. This means that we do not have an independent role of chance in estimating a variance. Since we do not have to make a separate estimate of the variance of data in the population (as we do for continuous data), we do not have to use Student's t distribution to take into account errors in estimating that variance. Rather, normal approximations to the binomial and Poisson distributions use the standard normal distribution.

As with other univariable analyses, statistical hypothesis testing on a single nominal dependent variable is less often of interest than is estimation. A reason for this preference for estimation is the difficulty in formulating an appropriate null hypothesis. When such a null hypothesis can be constructed, however, we can use the normal approximation to the binomial or Poisson distributions to test it. A special case of hypothesis testing for probabilities is the preference test. This is a paired study in which each individual is given a choice of two things and chooses the one she prefers. The null hypothesis is that the probability of preferring one of the choices will be equal to 0.5 (which means there is no preference). The alternative hypothesis is the probability of preferring one of the choices is not equal to 0.5.

EXERCISES

6.1. Suppose we are interested in the risk of peripheral neuropathy among persons with diabetes. To study this relationship, we identify 100 persons with a history of diabetes. At an initial examination, 3 of those 100 persons were found to have peripheral neuropathy. Five years later, the group was reexamined, and 12 additional persons were found to have peripheral neuropathy. Based on that information, which of the following is the prevalence of peripheral neuropathy in this group of 100 patients at the end of the five-year study?

    A. 0.03

    B. 0.07

    C. 0.12

    D. 0.15

    E. 0.17

6.2. Suppose we are interested in the proportion of persons who work for a specific industry who develop chronic obstructive pulmonary disease (COPD). To investigate this relationship, we examine 150 new employees and find that 10 already have COPD. Then, we examine those same 150 persons after they have worked in the industry for 10 years and find 28 new cases of COPD. Which of the following is closest to the point estimate of prevalence of COPD among employees in this industry at the time of the last examination?

    A. 0.19

    B. 0.20

    C. 0.22

D. 0.25

E. 0.31

6.3. Suppose we are interested in the proportion of persons who work for a specific industry who develop COPD. To investigate this relationship, we examine 150 new employees and find that 10 already have COPD. Then, we examine those same 150 persons after they have worked in the industry for 10 years and find 28 new cases of COPD. Which of the following is the 10-year risk of developing COPD among employees in this industry?

A. 0.19

B. 0.20

C. 0.22

D. 0.25

E. 0.31

6.4. Suppose we are interested in the risk of peripheral neuropathy among persons with diabetes. To study this relationship, we identify 100 persons with a history of diabetes. At an initial examination, 3 of those 100 persons were found to have peripheral neuropathy. Five years later, the group was reexamined, and 12 additional persons were found to have peripheral neuropathy. Based on that information, which of the following is closest to the five-year risk of peripheral neuropathy in this group of patients?

A. 0.03

B. 0.07

C. 0.12

D. 0.15

E. 0.17

6.5. Suppose we are interested in the risk of peripheral neuropathy among persons with diabetes. To study this relationship, we identify 100 persons with a history of diabetes. At an initial examination, 3 of those 100 persons were found to have peripheral neuropathy. Five years later, the group was reexamined, and 12 additional persons were found to have peripheral neuropathy. Based on that information, calculate an interval of risk estimates within which we can be 95% confident that the five-year risk of neuropathy in the population occurs. Which of the following is closest to the limits of that interval?

A. 0.02–0.22

B. 0.04–0.17

C. 0.06–0.19

D. 0.08–0.17

E. 0.10–0.13

6.6. Suppose we are interested in the proportion of persons who work for a specific industry who develop COPD. To investigate this relationship, we examine 150 new employees and find that 10 already have COPD. Then, we examine those same 150 persons after they have worked in the industry for 10 years and find 28 new cases of COPD. Which of the following is closest to the interval estimate for the prevalence of COPD among employees in this industry at the time of the last examination within which we are 95% confident that the population's value is included?

A. 0.18–0.32
B. 0.21–0.29
C. 0.23–0.28
D. 0.24–0.26
E. 0.25–0.26

6.7. Suppose we are interested in the proportion of persons who work for a specific industry who develop COPD. To investigate this relationship, we examine 150 new employees and find that 10 already have COPD. Then, we examine those same 150 persons after they have worked in the industry for 10 years and find 28 new cases of COPD. Which of the following is closest to the incidence of COPD among employees in this industry?

A. 0.014 per year
B. 0.020 per year
C. 0.022 per year
D. 0.032 per year
E. 0.042 per year

6.8. Suppose we are interested in the risk of peripheral neuropathy among persons with diabetes. To study this relationship, we identify 100 persons with a history of diabetes. At an initial examination, 3 of those 100 persons were found to have peripheral neuropathy. Five years later, the group was reexamined, and 12 additional persons were found to have peripheral neuropathy. Based on that information, which of the following is closest to the incidence of peripheral neuropathy in this group of patients?

A. 0.025 per year
B. 0.026 per year
C. 0.027 per year
D. 0.029 per year
E. 0.032 per year

6.9. Suppose we are interested in the risk of peripheral neuropathy among persons with diabetes. To study this relationship, we identify 100 persons with a history of diabetes. At an initial examination, 3 of those 100 persons were found to have peripheral neuropathy. Five years later, the group was reexamined, and 12 additional persons were found to have peripheral neuropathy. Based on that information, calculate an interval of incidence estimates within which we can be 95% confident that the incidence of neuropathy in the population occurs. Which of the following is closest to the limits of that interval?

A. 0.0–0.112 per year

B. 0.001–0.056 per year

C. 0.010–0.045 per year

D. 0.014–0.043 per year

E. 0.008–0.048 per year

6.10. Suppose we are interested in the proportion of persons who work for a specific industry who develop COPD. To investigate this relationship, we examine 150 new employees and find that 10 already have COPD. Then, we examine those same 150 persons after they have worked in the industry for 10 years and find 28 new cases of COPD. Which of the following is closest to the interval estimate for the incidence of COPD among employees in this industry within which we are 95% confident that the population's value is included?

A. 0.015–0.031 per year

B. 0.017–0.049 per year

C. 0.020–0.041 per year

D. 0.022–0.044 per year

E. 0.025–0.030 per year

PART THREE

BIVARIABLE ANALYSES

In the introduction to Part Two, we learned that variables serve either of two functions. One function is to represent the data of primary interest. This function is served by the dependent variable. To identify the dependent variable, we ask ourselves, "For which data do we want to make an estimate or test a hypothesis?" The answer to this question identifies the data represented by the dependent variable. Every set of data must have some of the data values represented by the dependent variable.[1]

The other function served by variables is to specify the conditions under which we are interested in examining the dependent variable. This function is served by the independent variable(s). It is not necessary that a set of data has some of its data values represented by an independent variable. In univariable analyses (the subject of Part Two), there are no independent variables. This implies that there are no special conditions under which we are interested in examining the dependent variable in univariable analysis. Instead, we are interested in making estimates of or testing hypotheses about the dependent variable in general. This situation changes in bivariable analyses.

---

[1] If a set of data does not have some of its data values represented by a dependent variable, the implication is that there are no data for which we are interested in calculating an estimate or testing a hypothesis. In this case, we do not need statistical analyses.

Introduction to Biostatistical Applications in Health Research with Microsoft Office Excel® and R,
Second Edition. Robert P. Hirsch.
© 2021 John Wiley & Sons, Inc. Published 2021 by John Wiley & Sons, Inc.
Companion website: www.wiley.com/go/hirsch/healthresearch2e

In bivariable analyses, we have conditions that define our interest in examining the dependent variable. The nature of these conditions is determined by the type of data represented by the independent variable. In most cases, independent variables represent either continuous or nominal data.

When an independent variable represents continuous data, dependent variable values are arrayed along the continuum of independent variable values. As an example, suppose we are interested in the ability of various dosages of a medication to lower diastolic blood pressure. In this case, the decrease in diastolic blood pressure is represented by the dependent variable and dose is represented by a continuous independent variable. Our interest in the decrease in diastolic blood pressure is how the dependent variable values are arrayed throughout the continuum of doses.

There are two aspects of the relationship between a dependent variable and a continuous independent variable that might be of interest. One of these is the strength of the association between the dependent and independent variables. In the example, the strength of the association between the dose of a medication and the decrease in diastolic blood pressure would reflect how consistently the decrease in diastolic blood pressure changes as the dose changes.

Another aspect of the relationship between a dependent variable and a continuous independent variable that might be of interest is the ability to estimate dependent variable values that correspond to particular values of the continuous independent variable. In the example, we would be interested in this aspect of the relationship if we wanted to be able to calculate the decrease in the diastolic blood pressure we would expect to observe if a person were given a particular dose of the medication.

When an independent variable represents nominal data, the nominal independent variable values divide the dependent variable values into two groups. Our interest, then, is to compare estimates of or test hypotheses about the parameters in these two groups. As an example, suppose we are interested in the change in diastolic blood pressure between persons who received a new medication and persons who received standard therapy. The value of the nominal independent variable, in this case, indicates which treatment a person received.

The type of data represented by the independent variable helps to determine the statistical method that is appropriate to analyze those data. In each of the three chapters in Part Three of this book, the continuation of the flowchart will begin by deciding the type of data represented by the independent variable.

CHAPTER 7

BIVARIABLE ANALYSIS OF A CONTINUOUS DEPENDENT VARIABLE

As shown in Flowchart 5, bivariable analysis of a continuous dependent variable can involve an independent variable that represents either continuous data or nominal data. We will begin by considering a bivariable data set in which both the dependent and independent variables represent continuous data.

7.1 CONTINUOUS INDEPENDENT VARIABLE

When the independent variable represents continuous data, the effect is to array dependent variable values along the continuum of independent variable values.

Introduction to Biostatistical Applications in Health Research with Microsoft Office Excel® and R,
Second Edition. Robert P. Hirsch.
© 2021 John Wiley & Sons, Inc. Published 2021 by John Wiley & Sons, Inc.
Companion website: www.wiley.com/go/hirsch/healthresearch2e

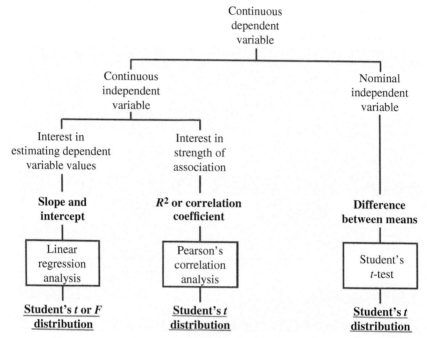

FLOWCHART 5 Flowchart showing bivariable analysis of a continuous dependent variable. The point estimate that is most often used to describe the dependent variable is in bold. The common name of the statistical test is enclosed in a box. The standard distributions that are used to test hypotheses and calculate confidence intervals are in bold and underlined.

This is easiest to appreciate if we examine the relationship between these variables graphically. The type of graph we use to look at this relationship is called a **scatter plot**. Figure 7.1 illustrates a scatter plot:

The convention we use in drawing a scatter plot is to put the independent variable values on the horizontal axis (the **abscissa**) and the dependent variable values on the vertical axis (the **ordinate**). These are also called the **X-axis** and the **Y-axis**, respectively. They are named so because we represent independent variable values with the letter X and dependent variable values with the letter Y.

Examination of the scatter plot tells us a number of things about the relationship between dietary sodium intake and mean arterial blood pressure. For one thing, we can see that the numeric magnitude of blood pressure increases as dietary sodium intake increases. We call this a **direct association**, when both variables change in the same direction. An **inverse association** occurs when values of the dependent variable decrease in numeric magnitude as values of the independent variable increase. For example, we would expect to observe an inverse association between the dose of an antihypertensive medication (the independent variable) and mean arterial pressure (the dependent variable). In that case, the mean arterial pressure would decrease as the dose of the medication increases.

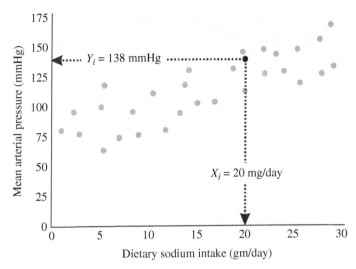

Figure 7.1 Scatter plot showing the relationship between dietary sodium intake (the independent variable) and mean arterial blood pressure (the dependent variable). Each point in the scatter plot tells us the value of both of these variables for an individual. For example, the indicated point corresponds to a dietary sodium intake of 20 gm/day and a mean arterial pressure of 138 mmHg.

7.1.1 Regression Analysis

Another thing we can do with continuous data in a scatter plot is to estimate the value of the dependent variable that, on the average, is associated with a particular value of the independent variable. When we are interested in estimating values of the dependent variable that correspond to specific values of the independent variable, we are interested in performing a **regression analysis**.[1]

There are two ways we can do a regression analysis. One of these is a graphic approach and the other is a mathematic approach. In the graphic approach, the scatter plot is used to estimate dependent variable values. For example, we might be interested in using the data in Figure 7.1 to determine the most likely mean arterial pressure for a person with a particular dietary sodium intake level of, say, 15 gm/day. Figure 7.2 shows us how we might use the scatter plot to make that estimate.

7.1.1.1 *Linear Regression Equation.* Estimating values of the dependent variable that correspond to a particular value of the independent variable can be more precise if we use a mathematical approach instead of a graphical approach. To use the mathematical approach, we need to select a mathematical equation that

---

[1] When referring to the estimation of dependent variable values in regression analysis, statisticians often use the term "predict" rather than "estimate." This implies that there is a difference between estimating dependent variable values in regression analysis and estimating other parameters. There is no difference.

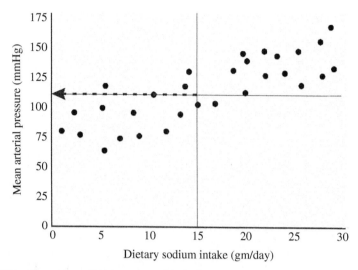

Figure 7.2   Illustration of how a scatter plot can be used to estimate the value of the dependent variable that is associated (on the average) with a particular value of the independent variable. First, a vertical line is drawn to represent the value of the independent variable. Then, a horizontal line is drawn to represent where the vertical line crosses the data points. That horizontal line corresponds to the dependent variable value. In this case, the mean arterial blood pressure associated with a dietary sodium intake of 15 gm/day is estimated to be approximately 110 mmHg.

represents the relationship between the dependent and independent variables. Most often, the mathematical equation we use is for a straight line. Thus, it is called a **linear regression** equation. Equation (7.1) shows the equation for a straight-line relationship between a continuous dependent variable and a continuous independent variable in the population.[2]

$$\mu_{Y|X} = \alpha + (\beta \cdot X_i) \tag{7.1}$$

where

$\mu_{Y|X}$ = mean of the dependent variable corresponding to a particular value of the independent variable (X_i)

α = value of the dependent variable in the population (on the average) when the independent variable is equal to 0. It is called the **intercept** of the straight-line equation

---

[2]In statistics, we use symbols in the equation for a straight line differently from the equation we learned in algebra. In algebra, the equation for a straight line was $y = mx + b$. In the statistical equation, α is used in place of b and β is used in place of m.

β = amount that the dependent variable value in the population changes (on the average) when the independent variable value is increased by one unit. It is called the **slope** of the straight-line equation

X_i = a particular value of the independent variable

The statistical equation for a straight line probably looks different from what you might have expected. For one thing, Greek letters are used for the slope (β) and intercept (α). The reason for this is that Equation (7.1) represents the straight line relationship in the population and, following the usual convention, we use Greek letters to represent the population's parameters. Even more surprising might be the use of $\mu_{Y|X}$ to represent the dependent variable. As we know from Chapter 2, the Greek letter μ is used to represent the mean of the dependent variable values in the population. It represents the same thing here, except that instead of a single mean, the dependent variable has different values for its mean corresponding to different values of the independent variable. The implication is that, in the population, there is a distribution of dependent variable values for each specific value of the independent variable and that $\mu_{Y|X}$ is the mean of each of these distributions. Figure 7.3 illustrates the population's regression line and the distributions of dependent variable values corresponding to each value of the independent variable.

Figure 7.3 also illustrates the way the slope (β) and the intercept (α) mathematically describe the regression line. The slope indicates how quickly and in which direction values of the dependent variable change as the value of the independent

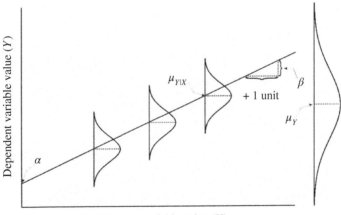

Figure 7.3   The regression line in the population indicating the slope (β), the intercept (α), and the mean of dependent variable values corresponding to a specific value of the independent variable ($\mu_{Y|X}$). The small Gaussian distributions on the regression line correspond to the distribution of dependent variable values that occur in persons with a particular independent variable value. The large Gaussian distribution to the right of the regression line corresponds to the distribution of dependent variable values for all values of the independent variable.

variable increases. The numeric magnitude of the slope tells us how many units the dependent variable changes for a one-unit increase in the numeric magnitude of the independent variable. A slope with a value that is greater than 0 (i.e., a positive value) indicates that the dependent variable values increase as values of the independent variable increase. Thus, a positive slope indicates a direct association. In contrast, a slope with a value less than 0 indicates that dependent variable values decrease as the value of the independent variable increases. Thus, a negative slope indicates an inverse association. The intercept reflects the elevation of the regression line, specifically by indicating the mean of the dependent variable values that correspond to an independent variable value of 0.[3]

Equation (7.1) illustrates the regression equation in the population. In practice, we use our sample's observations to estimate those parameters. Equation (7.2) shows the regression equation estimated from the sample's observations.

$$\mu_{Y|X} \triangleq \widehat{Y}_i = a + (b \cdot X_i) \tag{7.2}$$

where

$\mu_{Y|X}$ = mean of the dependent variable in the population corresponding to a particular value of the independent variable (X_i)

$\widehat{Y}_i$ = estimated value of the dependent variable corresponding to a particular value of the independent variable (X_i)

a = sample's estimate of the intercept of the regression line

b = sample's estimate of the slope of the regression line

X_i = a particular value of the independent variable

With the addition of $\widehat{Y}_i$ in Equation (7.2), we now have three ways to think about dependent variable values in a sample. First, we can think of the dependent variable values that are actually observed in the sample. We use Y_i to symbolize these observed dependent variable values. Second, we can summarize all of the dependent variable values in the sample by referring to the mean of these values. We use $\overline{Y}$ to symbolize that mean. To these, we add $\widehat{Y}_i$, which is the estimated value of the dependent variable that we obtain by using a particular independent variable value in the regression equation (Equation (7.2)). Figure 7.4 illustrates these three dependent variable values on a scatter plot.

7.1.1.2 *Estimation of the Slope and Intercept.* If we were to draw a straight line on a scatter plot to represent the relationship between the dependent and independent variables, we would draw that line to accomplish two things. First, we would want to draw a line in a way that the differences between observed and estimated values of the dependent variable balance (i.e., so that positive differences were equal to the negative differences). Second, we would draw the line in a way that would minimize the differences between the observed and estimated values of the dependent variable.

---

[3]Thus, we could symbolize the intercept as $\mu_{Y|X=0}$ instead of α.

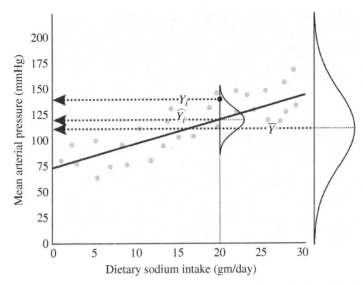

Figure 7.4 Scatter plot showing the relationship among an observed value of the dependent variable ($Y_i = 138$ mmHg), an estimated value ($\widehat{Y}_i$), and the mean of the dependent variable ($\overline{Y}$). The small Gaussian distribution corresponds to the distribution of dependent variable values that occur in persons with a dietary sodium intake of 20 gm/day. The large Gaussian distribution corresponds to the distribution of dependent variable values for all values of the independent variable.

The mathematical procedure we use to estimate the slope and the intercept is based on those same two criteria. Mathematically, the way we represent these criteria is by using a method that minimizes the sum of the squared differences between the observed and estimated values of the dependent variable.[4] The value we want to minimize is illustrated in Equation (7.3).

$$\sum (Y_i - \widehat{Y}_i)^2 \tag{7.3}$$

where

Y_i = a particular observed value of the dependent variable

$\widehat{Y}_i$ = estimated value of the dependent variable corresponding to a particular value of the independent variable

Estimates of the slope and intercept that are calculated in a way that minimizes the sum of the squared differences in Equation (7.3) are called **least squares**

[4] In the first criterion, we draw a regression line, so positive and negative differences are balanced. If those differences are balanced, then the sum of these differences will be equal to 0. Thus, in the mathematical approach, we need to square each of the differences so they do not add up to 0.

estimates.[5] The least squares method we use to estimate the slope of the regression equation is illustrated in Equation (7.4).

$$\beta \triangleq b = \frac{\frac{\sum (Y_i - \overline{Y}) \cdot (X_i - \overline{X})}{n-1}}{s_X^2} \tag{7.4}$$

where

β = slope of the regression line in the population

b = sample's estimate of the population's slope

Y_i = a particular observed value of the dependent variable

$\overline{Y}$ = sample's mean of the dependent variable

X_i = a particular observed value of the independent variable

$\overline{X}$ = sample's mean of the independent variable

n = number of observations in the sample

s_X^2 = sample's estimate of the variance of independent variable values.

In the numerator of Equation (7.4) is the **sum of cross products** $\sum (Y_i - \overline{Y}) \cdot (X_i - \overline{X})$ divided by the degrees of freedom $(n - 1)$. This value is the sample's estimate of the **covariance**. The covariance tells us the degree to which the dependent and independent variables vary relative to each other.[6]

To estimate the intercept of the regression line, we use the estimate of the slope obtained in Equation (7.4) and the fact that every least squares regression line will pass through the point corresponding to the means of the dependent and independent variables. At that point, the regression equation can be written as

$$\overline{Y} = a + (b \cdot \overline{X}) \tag{7.5}$$

where

$\overline{Y}$ = mean of the dependent variable values in the sample

a = sample's estimate of intercept of the regression line

b = sample's estimate of the slope of the regression line (from Equation (7.4))

$\overline{X}$ = mean of the independent variable values in the sample

[5] The method of least squares is one of two logical approaches we use to calculate estimates in statistics. The method of least squares is the more commonly used approach. The other approach, called the method of maximum likelihood, is used most often in multivariable analysis of a nominal dependent variable. We will discuss that approach in Chapter 12.

[6] Variance tells us how values of a variable vary among themselves by adding up the squared differences between each of the data values and the mean. Covariance tells us how values of the dependent variable vary with values of the independent variable. We can think of covariance as being like a combination of the variances of the dependent and independent variables in that covariance adds up the difference of each dependent variable value from its mean multiplied by the corresponding difference of the independent variable value from its mean.

The only term in Equation (7.5) that has not yet been estimated from the sample's observations is the intercept of the regression equation. Thus, we can estimate the intercept by algebraically rearranging Equation (7.5). The calculation is illustrated in Equation (7.6).

$$\alpha \triangleq a = \overline{Y} - (b \cdot \overline{X}) \tag{7.6}$$

where

α = intercept of the regression line in the population

Now, let us take a look at an example showing how we can estimate the slope and intercept of a regression equation from a sample's observations.

■ **EXAMPLE 7.1**

The data in the following table were used to draw the scatter plots in Figures 7.1, 7.2, and 7.4:

Patient	Dietary Sodium (X_i) (gm/day)	Arterial Pressure (Y_i) (mmHg)
TH	1.0	78
ER	2.3	93
EI	2.9	75
SN	5.2	97
OT	5.4	62
HI	5.5	115
NG	7.0	72
ON	8.4	93
EA	9.0	74
RT	10.5	108
HL	11.8	78
IK	13.3	92
EA	13.8	115
NI	14.2	127
CE	15.1	100
RE	16.9	101
GR	18.8	128
ES	19.8	142
SI	20.0	110
ON	20.2	136
TO	22.0	144
CH	22.1	124
EE	23.3	140
RS	24.1	126

Patient	Dietary Sodium (X_i) (gm/day)	Arterial Pressure (Y_i) (mmHg)
TA	25.5	144
TI	25.8	116
ST	27.8	152
IC	28.0	124
IA	28.9	164
NS	29.2	130

Let us use these data to estimate the parameters of a straight line that can be used, in turn, to estimate mean arterial pressure corresponding to particular levels of dietary sodium intake.

To prepare, we make the calculations appearing in the following table:

Patient	X_i	Y_i	$X_i - \overline{X}$	$(X_i - \overline{X})^2$	$Y_i - \overline{Y}$	$(Y_i - \overline{Y}) \cdot (X_i - \overline{X})$
TH	1.0	78	−14.93	222.81	−34	507.50
ER	2.3	93	−13.63	185.69	−19	258.91c
EI	2.9	75	−13.03	169.69	−37	481.99
SN	5.2	97	−10.73	115.06	−15	160.90
OT	5.4	62	−10.53	110.81	−50	526.33
HI	5.5	115	−10.43	108.72	3	−31.28
NG	7.0	72	−8.93	79.69	−40	357.07
ON	8.4	93	−7.53	56.65	−19	143.01
EA	9.0	74	−6.93	47.98	−38	263.21
RT	10.5	108	−5.43	29.45	−4	21.71
HL	11.8	78	−4.13	17.03	−34	140.31
IK	13.3	92	−2.63	6.90	−20	52.53
EA	13.8	115	−2.13	4.52	3	−6.38
NI	14.2	127	−1.73	2.98	15	−25.90
CE	15.1	100	−0.83	0.68	−12	9.92
RE	16.9	101	0.97	0.95	−11	−10.71
GR	18.8	128	2.87	8.26	16	45.97
ES	19.8	142	3.87	15.00	30	116.20
SI	20.0	110	4.07	16.59	−2	−8.15
ON	20.2	136	4.27	18.26	24	102.56
TO	22.0	144	6.07	36.89	32	194.35
CH	22.1	124	6.17	38.11	12	74.08
EE	23.3	140	7.37	54.37	28	206.45
RS	24.1	126	8.17	66.80	14	114.43
TA	25.5	144	9.57	91.65	32	306.35
TI	25.8	116	9.87	97.48	4	39.49
ST	27.8	152	11.87	140.98	40	474.93
IC	28.0	124	12.07	145.77	12	144.88

Patient	X_i	Y_i	$X_i - \bar{X}$	$(X_i - \bar{X})^2$	$Y_i - \bar{Y}$	$(Y_i - \bar{Y}) \cdot (X_i - \bar{X})$
IA	28.9	164	12.97	168.31	52	674.61
NS	29.2	130	13.27	176.18	18	238.92
Total	477.8	3,360	0.00	2,234.24	0	5,574.19

Now we are ready to calculate the estimates of the slope and the intercept of the regression equation, describing the relationship between dietary sodium intake and mean arterial pressure. First, we estimate the slope using Equation (7.4) and the values from the previous table.

$$\beta \triangleq b = \frac{\frac{\sum(Y_i - \bar{Y}) \cdot (X_i - \bar{X})}{n-1}}{s_X^2} = \frac{\frac{\sum(Y_i - \bar{Y}) \cdot (X_i - \bar{X})}{n-1}}{\frac{\sum(X_i - \bar{X})^2}{n-1}} = \frac{\frac{5,574.19}{30-1}}{\frac{2,234.24}{30-1}}$$

$$= 2.49 \text{ mmHg/gm/day}$$

Next, we use Equation (7.6) to estimate the intercept of the regression equation:

$$\alpha \triangleq a = \bar{Y} - (b \cdot \bar{X}) = \frac{\sum Y_i}{n} - \left(b \cdot \frac{\sum X_i}{n}\right) = \frac{3,360}{30} - \left(2.49 \cdot \frac{447.8}{30}\right)$$

$$= 112 - (2.49 \cdot 15.9) = 72.3 \text{ mmHg}$$

Thus, the regression equation is

$$\hat{Y} = a + (b \cdot X) = 72.3 + (2.49 \cdot X)$$

This regression equation can be used to estimate dependent variable values associated with particular values of the independent variable. For instance, suppose we want to estimate the mean arterial blood pressure associated with a dietary sodium intake of 15 gm/day. Using that value of the independent variable in the regression equation allows us to make the following estimate.

$$\hat{Y} = a + (b \cdot X) = 72.3 + (2.49 \cdot 15) = 109.7 \text{ mmHg}$$

So, on the average we expect persons with a dietary sodium intake of 15 gm/day to have a mean arterial blood pressure of 109.7 mmHg. This is consistent with the corresponding values from the graphic approach to estimation of dependent variable values (Figure 7.2). ∎

Even though it is not very difficult to perform a regression analysis by hand, you will probably never do that. All statistical programs that deal with data can do this for you. In Excel, there are functions that calculate the slope ("=SLOPE") and intercept ("=INTERCEPT"). In R, the slope and intercept are estimated by the "lm(DV~IV,data)" command.[7] Use of these functions is illustrated in the next example.

[7] lm standards for "linear model."

■ EXAMPLE 7.2

The following Excel output demonstrates estimation of the slope and intercept.

	A	B	C	D
1	Dietary	Arterial		
2	Sodium (X_i)	Pressure (Y_i)		
3	1	78		
4	2.3	93		
5	2.9	75		
6	5.2	97		
7	5.4	62		
8	5.5	115		
9	7	72		
10	8.4	93		
11	9	74		
12	10.5	108		
13	11.8	78		
14	13.3	92		
15	13.8	115		
16	14.2	127		
17	15.1	100		
18	16.9	101		
19	18.8	128		
20	19.8	142		
21	20	110		
22	20.2	136		
23	22	144		
24	22.1	124		
25	23.3	140		
26	24.1	126		
27	25.5	144		
28	25.8	116		
29	27.8	152		
30	28	124		
31	28.9	164		
32	29.2	130		
33	Slope =	2.49489908		=slope(B3:B32,A3:A32)
34	Intercept =	72.2645739		=intercept(B3:B32,A3:A32)

In R, we get the following output by using the "lm(DV~IV,data)" command:

>lm(ARTPRESS~SODIUM,Example7_1)

```
Call:
lm(formula = ARTPRESS ~ SODIUM, data = Example7_1)

Coefficients:
(Intercept) SODIUM
 72.265 2.495
```

■

7.1.1.3 *Taking Chance into Account for the Slope and Intercept.* Now that we know how to calculate and interpret estimates of the slope and the intercept, we are almost ready to see how we can take chance into account for those estimates. There is one thing, however, that we need to consider first. That is the way in which we can think about variation of continuous dependent variable values now that we have an independent variable.

There are two ways we can think of the variation of dependent variable values. One way is regardless of the value of the independent variable (i.e., without taking that independent variable's value into account). This is the **univariable variance** of the dependent variable and it is the same as the variance we first encountered in Chapter 2 (Equation (2.3)). In bivariable analysis, this univariable variance is symbolized as s_Y^2 to distinguish the variance of the dependent variable from the variance of the independent variable (s_X^2). The population's value of this univariable variance of the dependent variable is illustrated in Equation (7.7).

$$\sigma_Y^2 = \frac{\sum (Y_i - \mu_Y)^2}{N} \tag{7.7}$$

where

σ_Y^2 = variance of the distribution of dependent variable values in the population (same as σ^2 in Equation (2.3))

Y_i = a value of the dependent variable

μ_Y = mean of the distribution of dependent variable values in the population (same as μ in Equation (2.3))

N = number of data values in the population

The other way to think about variation in dependent variable values is to consider only those dependent variable values that correspond to a particular value of the independent variable. $\sigma_{Y|X}^2$ is the way in which we symbolize that variance. Equation (7.8) illustrates that variance mathematically.

$$\sigma_{Y|X}^2 = \frac{\sum (Y_i - \mu_{Y|X})^2}{N} \tag{7.8}$$

where

$\sigma_{Y|X}^2$ = variance of the distribution of dependent variable values in the population that corresponds to a particular value of the independent variable (X)

$\mu_{Y|X}$ = mean of the distribution of dependent variable values in the population that corresponds to a particular value of the independent variable (X)

This is the **bivariable variance** of the dependent variable. When we want to take chance into account for estimates we have made in a bivariable analysis, it is the bivariable variance we use to represent variation in dependent variable values. Figure 7.5 indicates the distributions of dependent variable values that are addressed by these two measures of variation.

Equations (7.7) and (7.8) as well as Figure 7.5 illustrate the population's values of the univariable and bivariable variance of dependent variable values. In practice, these are unknown and must be estimated from the sample's observations. We saw how this is done for the univariable variance in Chapter 3 (Equation (3.4)). In regression, however, we use some new terms to refer to variance estimates and the values from which they are calculated.

Understanding bivariable (and multivariable) analysis of a continuous dependent variable is easier if we take some time to learn these new terms. First, there is a new term for the variance estimate itself. It is called a **mean square**. To refer to the univariable variance estimate in particular, we use the term "**total mean square**."

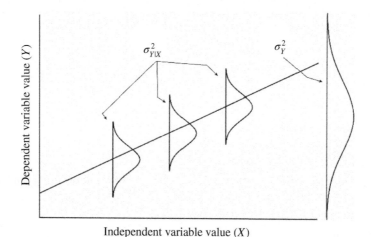

Figure 7.5   The Gaussian distributions on the regression line correspond to values of the dependent variable that occur in persons with a particular value of the independent variable. The variance of these distributions is called the variance of Y "given X," and is symbolized as $\sigma_{Y|X}^2$. The large Gaussian distribution to the right of the regression line corresponds to the distribution of dependent variable values for all values of the independent variable. Its variance is symbolized as σ_Y^2.

The total mean square is calculated by dividing the **total sum of squares** by the **total degrees of freedom**. Equation (7.9) shows how these new terms relate to the sample's estimate of the univariable variance of dependent variable values (i.e., the total mean square).

$$\sigma_Y^2 \triangleq s_Y^2 = \frac{\sum (Y_i - \overline{Y})^2}{n - 1} = \frac{\text{Total sum of squares}}{\text{Total degrees of freedom}} = \text{Total mean square} \quad (7.9)$$

where

s_Y^2 = sample's estimate of the variance of the distribution of dependent variable values

Y_i = a value of the dependent variable observed in the sample

$\overline{Y}$ = sample's estimate of the mean of the dependent variable values in the population

n = number of observations in the sample

The sample's estimate of the bivariable variance of dependent variable values is called the **"residual" mean square**.[8] Equation (7.10) shows how the estimate of the bivariable variance of dependent variable values (i.e., the residual mean square) is calculated.

$$\sigma_{Y|X}^2 \triangleq s_{Y|X}^2 = \frac{\sum (Y_i - \widehat{Y}_i)^2}{n - 2} = \frac{\text{Residual sum of squares}}{\text{Residual degrees of freedom}}$$

$$= \text{Residual mean square} \quad (7.10)$$

where

$s_{Y|X}^2$ = sample's estimate of the variance of the distribution of dependent variable values that corresponds to a particular value of the independent variable

$\widehat{Y}_i$ = estimated value of the mean of dependent variable values that corresponds to a particular value of the independent variable

Notice that the residual degrees of freedom in Equation (7.10) are equal to $n - 2$ instead of $n - 1$, as used in estimating the univariable variance. The reason for this difference is that at least two observations are required to estimate the univariable variance, but at least three observations are required to estimate the bivariable variance. This is because the residual mean square reflects how observed values of the dependent variable differ from values estimated from the regression equation. If the sample contained only two observations, the regression line would go through both points corresponding to the two observations and, thus, the two points would show no variation from the regression line.

---

[8]The residual mean square is often called the "error mean square" in textbooks. Here, we will use "residual mean square" to be consistent with the terminology used in Excel and to use more descriptive terminology.

Let us take another look at the residual sum of squares in the numerator of Equation (7.10). This is the same as the value in Equation (7.3). It is this value that is minimized in the process of least squares estimation. Thus, the method of least squares as used in estimating the parameters of the regression equation has the effect of minimizing the bivariable variance of dependent variable values.

Now, we are ready to take into account the role of chance in estimating the slope and the intercept. First, we must think about the sampling distributions for estimates of the slope and the intercept. As with the sampling distribution for estimates of the mean, the sampling distributions for the slope and the intercept tell us about probabilities associated with various estimates of those parameters. Fortunately, as with the sampling distribution of estimates of the mean, the sampling distributions for the slope and intercept are also influenced by the central limit theorem.[9] This implies that we can use the same sort of approach to take chance into account for the slope and intercept as we used for the mean. Namely, we can test a null hypothesis or calculate a confidence interval for either the slope or the intercept by using Student's t-distribution in the same way we used it for the mean in Chapter 4 (Equation (4.3)).

The following equations illustrate how we can test the null hypothesis that the population's slope (Equation (7.11)) or that the population's intercept (Equation (7.12)) is equal to a specific value.

$$t = \frac{b - \beta_0}{s_b} \tag{7.11}$$

where

t = Student's t-value that corresponds to the sample's estimate of the slope

b = sample's estimate of the slope

β_0 = slope of the regression line in the population according to the null hypothesis

s_b = standard error for estimates of the slope

$$t = \frac{a - \alpha_0}{s_a} \tag{7.12}$$

where

t = Student's t-value that corresponds to the sample's estimate of the intercept

a = sample's estimate of the intercept

α_0 = intercept of the regression line in the population according to the null hypothesis

s_a = standard error for estimates of the intercept

To calculate a confidence interval for the slope or intercept, we use the same sort of calculations we used to calculate a confidence interval for the mean in Chapter 4

---

[9] Recall that the central limit theorem states that a sampling distribution tends to be a Gaussian distribution with that tendency increasing as the size of the sample increases.

(Equation (4.4)). The following equations show how that calculation applies to the estimate of the slope (Equation (7.13)) and to the estimate of the intercept (Equation (7.14)).

$$\beta \triangleq b \pm (t_{\alpha/2} \cdot s_b) \tag{7.13}$$

where

$t_{\alpha/2}$ = Student's t-value with $n - 2$ degrees of freedom that corresponds to α split between the two tails of Student's t-distribution

$$\alpha \triangleq a \pm (t_{\alpha/2} \cdot s_a) \tag{7.14}$$

In practice, a computer will calculate the standard errors for the intercept and the slope for us, so we are seldom in the position of having to calculate these standard errors by hand. It is helpful to our understanding of precision in regression analysis, however, to take a look at the way we could calculate the standard error if it were not supplied by a computer program. Equation (7.15) shows the standard error for estimates of the slope.[10]

$$\sigma_b \triangleq s_b = \sqrt{\frac{s_{Y|X}^2}{\sum (X_i - \overline{X})^2}} \tag{7.15}$$

where

s_b = standard error for estimates of the slope

$s_{Y|X}^2$ = sample's estimate of the variance of dependent variable values (i.e., the residual mean square)

$\sum (X_i - \overline{X})^2$ = sum of squares for the independent variable

Notice in Equation (7.15) that the standard error for estimates of the slope is influenced by the dispersions of both the dependent and independent variables. The dispersion of dependent variable values is represented by the residual mean square. As the dispersion of dependent variable values increases, the residual mean square increases and, consequently the standard error for estimates of the slope increases, indicating a decrease in the precision with which we estimate the population's slope from the sample's observations. This relationship makes sense: as the variability of the data increases, the precision with which we estimate the slope decreases.[11]

Now, take a look at how dispersion of independent variable values influences the standard error of the slope. That dispersion is represented by the sum of squares of the independent variable values in the sample. The surprising part is that the sum of squares of the independent variable is in the denominator of the standard

---

[10]The standard error for estimates of the intercept contains the residual mean square and the sum of squares for the independent variable, as well as other information.

[11]Precision of an estimate is equal to the inverse of the variance of the estimate (i.e., the inverse of the square of the standard error).

error. That implies that the precision with which we estimate the slope increases as the dispersion of independent variable values in the sample increases. This is the opposite of the effect of the dispersion of dependent variable values.

Although we might find this relationship surprising, it makes sense as we consider it more carefully. This increase in precision of the estimate of the slope, which occurs with an increase in the dispersion of independent variable values, is reflecting the same logic we would use when selecting two points through which we draw a straight line. In that case, we know that our ability to precisely draw a line increases as the two points we use to draw it become further apart. This influence of the dispersion of independent variable values on the standard error of the slope is a mathematical representation of that same logical process.

In the next example, we will calculate the standard error for the estimate of the slope and see how we can use that standard error to calculate a confidence interval.

■ **EXAMPLE 7.3**

Let us use the data in Example 7.1 to calculate a 95%, two-sided confidence interval for the slope of the regression equation describing the relationship between dietary sodium intake and mean arterial blood pressure.

The point estimate of the slope, calculated in Example 7.1, is 2.49 mmHg/gm/day. Before we can calculate a confidence interval for the slope, we need to calculate its standard error. To do that, we need to know the sum of squares for the independent variable. In Example 7.1, the sum of squares for dietary sodium intake (the independent variable) was found to be equal to 2,234.24 gm/day^2.

Also needed to calculate the standard error of the slope is the residual mean square (i.e., the sample's estimate of the variance of dependent variable values corresponding to a particular value of the independent variable). Equation (7.10) shows us that the residual mean square is equal to the residual sum of squares divided by the residual degrees of freedom. The residual degrees of freedom are equal to $n - 2$, or in this case, $30 - 2 = 28$. The residual sum of squares is calculated by estimating the dependent variable value corresponding to each observed value of the independent variable ($\hat{Y}_i$), subtracting that estimated value from the observed value of the dependent variable (Y_i), and adding up the squares of those differences. These calculations are summarized in the following table:

Patient	X_i	Y_i	$\hat{Y}_i$	$(Y_i - \hat{Y}_i)$	$(Y_i - \hat{Y}_i)^2$
TH	1.0	78	74.8	3.2	10.5
ER	2.3	93	78.0	15.0	224.9
EI	2.9	75	79.5	−4.5	20.2
SN	5.2	97	85.2	11.8	138.3
OT	5.4	62	85.7	−23.7	563.4
HI	5.5	115	86.0	29.0	841.8
NG	7.0	72	89.7	−17.7	314.3

Patient	X_i	Y_i	$\hat{Y}_i$	$(Y_i - \hat{Y}_i)$	$(Y_i - \hat{Y}_i)^2$
ON	8.4	93	93.2	−0.2	0.0
EA	9.0	74	94.7	−20.7	429.3
RT	10.5	108	98.5	9.5	90.9
HL	11.8	78	101.7	−23.7	561.9
IK	13.3	92	105.4	−13.4	180.8
EA	13.8	115	106.7	8.3	69.0
NI	14.2	127	107.7	19.3	372.8
CE	15.1	100	109.9	−9.9	98.8
RE	16.9	101	114.4	−13.4	180.3
GR	18.8	128	119.2	8.8	78.0
ES	20.0	110	122.2	−12.2	147.9
SI	19.8	142	121.7	20.3	413.6
ON	20.2	136	122.7	13.3	177.9
TO	22.0	144	127.2	16.8	283.8
CH	22.1	124	127.4	−3.4	11.6
EE	23.3	140	130.4	9.6	92.2
RS	24.1	126	132.4	−6.4	40.9
TA	25.5	144	135.9	8.1	65.9
TI	25.8	116	136.6	−20.6	425.7
ST	27.8	152	141.6	10.4	107.7
IC	28.0	124	142.1	−18.1	328.4
IA	28.9	164	144.4	19.6	385.4
NS	29.2	130	145.1	−15.1	228.5
Total	477.8	3,360			6,884.9

Using the residual sum of squares from the table (6,884.9 mmHg^2), we calculate the residual mean square by using Equation (7.10):

$$s_{Y|X}^2 = \frac{\sum (Y_i - \hat{Y}_i)^2}{n - 2} = \frac{6,884.9}{30 - 2} = 245.9 \text{ mmHg}^2$$

Next, we use Equation (7.15) to calculate the standard error for the estimate of the slope:

$$s_b = \sqrt{\frac{s_{Y|X}^2}{\sum (X_i - \overline{X})^2}} = \sqrt{\frac{245.9}{2,234.24}} = 0.33 \text{ mmHg/g/day}$$

Now, we are ready to calculate the 95%, two-sided interval estimate for the slope. To perform this calculation, we use Equation (7.13).

$$\beta \triangleq b \pm (t_{\alpha/2} \cdot s_b) = 2.49 \pm (2.048 \cdot 0.33) = 1.82 \text{ to } 3.17 \text{ mmHg/g/day}$$

Thus, we are 95% confident that the population's slope is between 1.82 and 3.17 mmHg/gm/day. ∎

Although these standard errors are not difficult to calculate, in practice we will use a computer to calculate them. In Excel, these standard errors are part of the output from the "Regression" analysis tool under "Data Analysis" in the "Data" tab. In R, these standard errors are part of the output from the "summary(lm(DV~IV,data))" command. The next example demonstrates how to obtain these standard errors in Excel and R as well as calculate confidence intervals and test hypotheses about the slope and intercept.

■ **EXAMPLE 7.4**

Let us use the "Regression" analysis tool in "Data Analysis" in Excel to analyze the dietary sodium/arterial blood pressure data as arrayed in Example 7.2.

First, let us take a look at the "Regression" dialog box with the values we would need to analyze these data.

With these values, we get the following output:

SUMMARY OUTPUT

Regression statistics	
Multiple R	0.817842418
R square	0.668866221
Adjusted r square	0.657040015
Standard error	15.68089549
Observations	30

ANOVA

	df	SS	MS	F	Significance F
Regression	1	13,907.06647	13,907.06647	56.55796954	3.4273E–08
Residual	28	6,884.933533	245.8904833		
Total	29	20,792			

	Coefficients	Standard error	t stat	P-value	Lower 95%	Upper 95%
Intercept	72.26457394	6.009401951	12.02525219	1.41763E–12	59.95487207	84.57427582
X variable 1	2.494899083	0.331746293	7.520503277	3.4273E–08	1.815347607	3.174450558

The last table in this output contains the information in which we are interested. The intercept and slope are in the rows of that table headed by "Intercept" and "X Variable 1," respectively. The point estimates are in the column labeled "Coefficients." The standard errors of these estimates appear in the next column. The standard error of the slope is the same as calculated by hand in Example 7.3. The next two columns test the null hypotheses that the intercept and the slope are equal to 0 in the population. Since both P-values are less than 0.05, we can reject both hypotheses. Finally, this table provides us with 95% confidence intervals for the intercept and the slope. These results are the same as, but showing greater precision than, the results we obtained in Examples 7.1 through 7.3.

Next, let us examine the output from the "summary(lm(DV~IV,data))" command.

>summary(lm(ARTPRESS~SODIUM,Example7_1))

```
Call:
lm(formula = ARTPRESS ~ SODIUM, data = Example7_1)

Residuals:
 Min 1Q Median 3Q Max
-23.737 -13.442 1.509 11.416 29.014

Coefficients:
 Estimate Std. Error t value Pr(>|t|)
(Intercept) 72.2646 6.0094 12.025 1.42e-12 ***
```

```
SODIUM 2.4949 0.3317 7.521 3.43e-08 ***
---
Signif. codes: 0 '***' 0.001 '**' 0.01 '*' 0.05 '.' 0.1 ' ' 1

Residual standard error: 15.68 on 28 degrees of freedom
Multiple R-squared: 0.6689, Adjusted R-squared: 0.657
F-statistic: 56.56 on 1 and 28 DF, p-value: 3.427e-08
```

The table in the middle of this output with the label "Coefficients:" contains the information in which we are interested. This table provides us with the point estimates of the intercept and slope (labeled with the name of the independent variable) as well as their standard errors. Unlike Excel, R does not provide us with the confidence intervals. Instead, we need to use Equation (7.13). ∎

7.1.1.4   *The F-Ratio.*

So far, we have taken chance into account by considering sampling distributions for the slope and intercept and using Student's t-distribution to test a hypothesis or to calculate a confidence interval. These procedures are the same as other procedures we have used to take chance into account for a continuous dependent variable in that they involve examination of the sample's estimate of a particular parameter in the population. There is another approach to examining the relationship between a continuous dependent variable and a continuous independent variable, however. This approach is to examine the amount of variation in dependent variable values that is explained by the association with the independent variable.

Earlier, we distinguished between the univariable variation of dependent variable values (called the "total" variation) and the bivariable variation of dependent variable value (called the "residual" variation). Actually, there is another way to think about the bivariable variation of a continuous dependent variable. The "residual" variation is the variation in dependent variable values that is "left over" after we have used the regression equation to estimate the dependent variable values that correspond to particular values of the independent variable. The other way we can think about the bivariable variation of dependent variable values is to consider the variation that is "explained" by using the regression equation to estimate dependent variable values. The "explained" variation is called the **regression** variation. The actual amount of explained variation is called the **regression sum of squares** and the average explained variation is called the **regression mean square**. As with the total and residual mean squares, the regression mean square is calculated by dividing the regression sum of squares by the regression degrees of freedom, as shown in Equation (7.16).

$$\text{Regression mean square} = \frac{\text{Regression sum of squares}}{\text{Regression degrees of freedom}} = \frac{\sum (\hat{Y}_i - \overline{Y})^2}{1}$$

(7.16)

Let us take a moment to examine Equation (7.16). Perhaps the first thing you will notice is that the regression degrees of freedom is equal to 1. Actually, the regression degrees of freedom is equal to the number of independent variables that are used to estimate values of the dependent variable. In bivariable regression analysis, we have one independent variable. Thus, the regression degrees of freedom is equal to 1 in bivariable analyses.[12]

Another interesting aspect of Equation (7.16) is that the regression sum of squares, unlike the total and residual sums of squares, does not consider the observed values of the dependent variable (Y_i). Instead, it includes the estimated values of the dependent variable values variable ($\widehat{Y}_i$) and the mean of the dependent variable ($\overline{Y}$). The mean of the dependent variable can be considered the estimate of the dependent variable we would use if we did not know about the relationship between the dependent and independent variables. The estimated values of the dependent variable, on the other hand, are the values we use to estimate the dependent variable values when we take into account this relationship with the independent variable. Thus, the regression sum of squares compares bivariable estimates ($\widehat{Y}_i$) with the univariable estimate ($\overline{Y}$) for the dependent variable.[13] The bigger this difference, the more variability of the dependent variable is explained by the relationship with the independent variable.

To interpret the numeric magnitude of the regression mean square as a reflection of how well the independent variable explains the variation of the dependent variable, we need to consider what we would expect to see if there were no relationships between those variables in the population. Since chance influences the selection of dependent variable values, we would expect to observe some apparent explained variation in the sample, even when the independent variable does not explain any variation of the dependent variable in the population. How much apparent explained variation we observe in a sample depends on how much variation there is among dependent variable values in the population. The more variation in dependent variable values, the greater the apparent explained variation we can expect to see in a sample due to chance alone. Thus, we would expect to see, on the average, the regression mean square (the average explained variation) equal to the residual mean square (the average unexplained variation) in samples from a population within which there is no association between the variables.

So, one way we can examine the relationship between a continuous dependent variable and a continuous independent variable is to compare the regression mean square with the residual mean square. The way we compare mean squares is by examining their ratio.[14] The result is called an **F-ratio**. Equation (7.17) illustrates calculation of the F-ratio in regression analysis.

$$F = \frac{\text{Regression mean square}}{\text{Residual mean square}} \qquad (7.17)$$

---

[12] The regression degrees of freedom will no longer be equal to one in multivariable regression analysis, since in multivariable regression analysis, by definition, we have more than one independent variable to estimate dependent variable values.

[13] Another way to calculate the regression sum of squares is to subtract the residual sum of squares from the total sum of squares. This also works with degrees of freedom. Namely, the residual degrees of freedom added to the regression degrees of freedom equal the total degrees of freedom. It does not work, however, to add the residual mean square to the regression mean square to get the total mean square.

[14] When comparing the regression mean square to the residual mean square, we always put the regression mean square in the numerator of the ratio and the residual mean square in the denominator of the ratio.

If the independent variable does not help to estimate dependent variable values, we expect that the F-ratio will be equal to one (on the average) in the sample. If the independent variable does help to estimate dependent variable values, the F-ratio will be greater than one, indicating that more variation in the dependent variable is explained by the independent variable than can be attributed to chance.

We interpret the numeric magnitude of the F-ratio by testing the **omnibus null hypothesis**. The omnibus null hypothesis states that the independent variable does not help estimate dependent variable values. When the omnibus null hypothesis is true, the F-ratio will be equal to 1 (on the average). When the omnibus null hypothesis is not true, the F-ratio will be greater than 1.[15] The larger the F-ratio, the less likely it is that the omnibus null hypothesis is true.

To test the omnibus null hypothesis, we can compare the F-ratio calculated from the sample's observations with the value in a table of the F-distribution. In this text, the F-distribution is described in Table B.4.

The F-distribution is a member of the Gaussian family of distributions. It comes from Student's t-distribution with two features that distinguish it from Student's t. First, there are no negative values in the F-distribution. This is an important feature of the F-distribution because it is impossible for an F-ratio to be negative.[16] To get rid of negative numbers as we go from Student's t-distribution to the F-distribution, we use the same old trick statisticians use so often to get rid of negative values: we square t-values to get F-values.

In addition, a second parameter is added to the t-distribution to make it the F-distribution. This parameter is called "degrees of freedom," but it is not the same as the parameter called "degrees of freedom" that was added to the standard normal distribution to create Student's t-distribution. The degrees of freedom that is a parameter of Student's t-distribution takes into account the role of chance in estimating the variance of dependent variable values. This same number of degrees of freedom is also associated with the residual mean square in the F-distribution. Since the residual mean square is always in the denominator of the F-ratio, it is called the **denominator degrees of freedom**.

The degrees of freedom added as a parameter to create the F-distribution is the degrees of freedom associated with the regression mean square. Recall from our introduction to the regression mean square that the regression degrees of freedom tell us how many independent variables are used to estimate dependent variable values. In bivariable regression analysis, we have only one independent variable, so the regression degrees of freedom is equal to 1. Since the regression mean square is always in the numerator of the F-ratio, this number of degrees of freedom is called the **numerator degrees of freedom**. The next example illustrates how we can use the F-ratio to examine the relationship between a continuous dependent variable and a continuous independent variable.

---

[15]When we are using the F-ratio to test the omnibus null hypothesis, we use an F-*value* that corresponds to all of α in the upper tail. That is because the alternative hypothesis for the F-ratio is one-sided; if F is not equal to 1, it must be greater than 1, at least on the average (an F-ratio in a particular sample can be less than 1, but this is considered to be a reflection of the null hypothesis).

[16]For the F-ratio to be negative, one of the mean squares would need to be negative. Remember that mean square is another name for a variance estimate. Variances are always positive.

■ **EXAMPLE 7.5**

Let us use the F-ratio to examine the relationship between dietary sodium intake and mean arterial blood pressure as reflected by the data in Example 7.1. We do that by testing the omnibus null hypothesis that knowing dietary sodium intake does not help to estimate mean arterial blood pressure.

To calculate the F-ratio, we need to know the values of the residual mean square and of the regression mean square. In Example 7.3, the residual mean square was found to be equal to 245.9 mmHg^2. To calculate the regression mean square, we need the mean of the dependent variable (Y). The following table summarizes these to compare the estimated values of the dependent variable (Y_i from Example 7.3) with comparisons:

Patient	X_i	Y_i	$\widehat{Y}_i$	$(\widehat{Y}_i - \overline{Y})$	$(\widehat{Y}_i - \overline{Y})^2$
TH	1.0	78	74.8	−37.2	1,386.9
ER	2.3	93	78.0	−34.0	1,155.8
EI	2.9	75	79.5	−32.5	1,056.3
SN	5.2	97	85.2	−26.8	716.2
OT	5.4	62	85.7	−26.3	689.7
HI	5.5	115	86.0	−26.0	676.7
NG	7.0	72	89.7	−22.3	496.0
ON	8.4	93	93.2	−18.8	352.6
EA	9.0	74	94.7	−17.3	298.6
RT	10.5	108	98.5	−13.5	183.3
HL	11.8	78	101.7	−10.3	106.0
IK	13.3	92	105.4	−6.6	42.9
EA	13.8	115	106.7	−5.3	28.2
NI	14.2	127	107.7	−4.3	18.6
CE	15.1	100	109.9	−2.1	4.3
RE	16.9	101	114.4	2.4	5.9
GR	18.8	128	119.2	7.2	51.4
ES	19.8	142	121.7	9.7	93.4
SI	20.0	110	122.2	10.2	103.3
ON	20.2	136	122.7	10.7	113.7
TO	22.0	144	127.2	15.2	229.6
CH	22.1	124	127.4	15.4	237.2
EE	23.3	140	130.4	18.4	338.4
RS	24.1	126	132.4	20.4	415.8
TA	25.5	144	135.9	23.9	570.5
TI	25.8	116	136.6	24.6	606.8
ST	27.8	152	141.6	29.6	877.5
IC	28.0	124	142.1	30.1	907.3
IA	28.9	164	144.4	32.4	1,047.6
NS	29.2	130	145.1	33.1	1,096.6
Total	477.8	3,360		0.0	13,907.1

Using the regression sum of squares from this table ($13,907.1\ \text{mmHg}^2$), we calculate the regression mean square by using Equation (7.16).

$$\text{Regression mean square} = \frac{\sum(\hat{Y}_i - \overline{Y})^2}{1} = \frac{13,907.1}{1} = 13,907.1\ \text{mmHg}^2$$

Next, we use Equation (7.17) to calculate the F-ratio:

$$F = \frac{\text{Regression mean square}}{\text{Residual mean square}} = \frac{13,907.1}{245.9} = 56.6$$

Thus, the F-ratio that represents the regression mean square relative to the residual mean square is equal to 56.6. That F-ratio has 1 degree of freedom in the numerator and 28 $(30 - 2)$ degrees of freedom in the denominator.

To interpret the F-ratio, we need to compare it with values in the table for the F-distribution. The F-distribution is in Table B.4, which includes many pages of tables, each page corresponding to the number of degrees of freedom in the numerator of the F-ratio. In this case, the regression degrees of freedom is equal to 1, so it is the first page of the F-distribution that is used in bivariable regression analysis. In this table, we look for the F-value in the body of the table that corresponds to 28 denominator degrees of freedom and an α equal to 0.05.

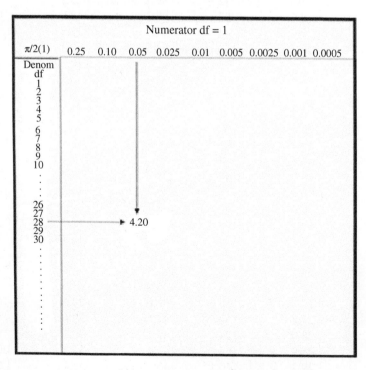

In Table B.4, we find that an F-ratio of 4.20 is associated with 1 degree of freedom in the numerator, 28 degrees of freedom in the denominator, and an α of 0.05. This is the **critical value** to which we need to compare our calculated F-ratio (56.6).[17] Since the calculated value is larger than the critical value, we reject the omnibus null hypothesis and, through the process of elimination, accept the alternative hypothesis that states that knowing dietary sodium intake (the independent variable) helps to estimate mean arterial blood pressure (the dependent variable).   ∎

We can also test the omnibus null hypothesis in Excel and R. The information about the omnibus null hypothesis is in the second table labeled "ANOVA" of our output from the "Regression" analysis tool in Excel. In R, the F-ratio and its corresponding P-value are at the bottom of the output. Go back to Example 7.4 and compare the results from Excel and R with the results in Example 7.5.

We find in Example 7.5 that we are able to reject the omnibus null hypothesis that the independent variable does not help estimate dependent variable values. With that in mind, let us take a moment to imagine what the population's regression line looks like when the omnibus null hypothesis is true. If knowing the value of the independent variable does not help to estimate dependent variable values, the implication is that the same value of the dependent variable would be estimated for all values of the independent variable. For that to be true, the regression line would have to have a slope of 0 (i.e., a horizontal line). If that is the case, we must ask ourselves, "How is testing the omnibus null hypothesis different from testing the null hypothesis that the slope is equal to zero?"

In bivariable analysis, testing the omnibus null hypothesis and testing the null hypothesis that the slope is equal to 0 are exactly the same thing. One way to prove that this is true is to take the square root of the F-ratio. This square root is exactly equal to Student's t-value used in testing the null hypothesis that the slope is equal to 0. In bivariable analysis, the omnibus null hypothesis adds no new information. When we get to multivariable regression analysis in Chapter 10, however, testing the omnibus null hypothesis will provide very useful information about the relationship between the dependent and independent variables.

7.1.2   Correlation Analysis

Another aspect of the relationship between a continuous dependent variable and a continuous independent variable is the strength of the association between the variables. What we imply by the "strength" of the association is the consistency with which changes in the value of the dependent variable are associated with changes of a given amount in the value of the independent variable. This strength of the association between two continuous variables can be examined graphically in a scatter plot.

---

[17] As an alternative to calculating P-values, hypothesis testing can be conducted by comparing the value in the table required to reject H_0 (the critical value) to the calculated value.

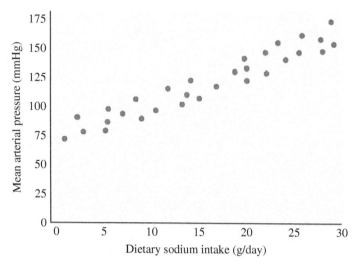

Figure 7.6 Scatter plot showing a strong association between dietary sodium intake and mean arterial blood pressure. There is a strong association when the dependent variable values change in a highly consistent manner as independent variable values increase.

In Figure 7.1, we saw a tendency for mean arterial blood pressure values to increase with increases in dietary sodium intake, but there were exceptions. There are quite a few of these exceptions in Figure 7.1, so the strength of that relationship can be considered to be of a moderate degree. For comparison, Figure 7.6 shows a relationship that is considered to be strong and Figure 7.7 shows a relationship that is considered to be weak. Notice that there are fewer and numerically smaller exceptions for the strong association and more and numerically larger exceptions for the weak association.

Examination of scatter plots is one way we might investigate the strength of the association between two continuous variables, but it is not the only way. We can look at the strength of the association numerically as well, by calculating a number that reflects the strength of the association. One number that does this is the covariance. We encountered the covariance in our discussion of regression analysis, where covariance was used in the numerator of the estimate slope of the regression line (Equation (7.4)).

As the name implies, covariance tells us how two continuous variables vary together. It is equal to a positive value when there is a direct association between the variables and a negative value when there is an inverse association between those variables.[18] Furthermore, the numeric magnitude of the covariance is an indication of how strong the association is.

---

[18] The concept of direct and inverse associations was introduced earlier in this chapter when we were discussing regression analysis. There, a direct association was identified by a positive slope and an inverse association was identified by a negative slope.

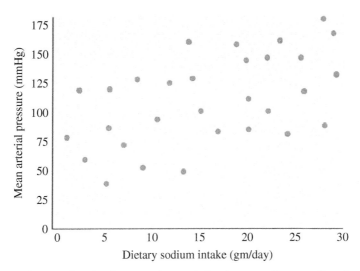

Figure 7.7   Scatter plot showing a weak association between dietary sodium intake and mean arterial blood pressure. There is a weak association when dependent variable values do not change in a consistent manner as independent variable values increase.

To see how this works, take a look at the scatter plot in Figure 7.8 to which a grid has been added to separate the scatter plot into four quadrants, based on the means of the dependent and independent variables. In the upper right quadrant, the values of the dependent and independent variables are larger than their means. Consequently, data values in this quadrant contribute positive values to the numerator of the covariance (when the mean of each variable is subtracted from each observed data

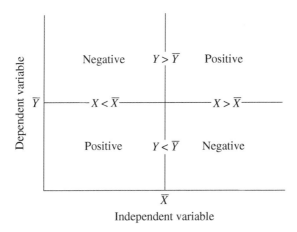

Figure 7.8   Contributions of data values in the four quadrants of a scatter plot to the numerator of the covariance.

value). In the lower left quadrant, both the dependent and independent variable values are less than their respective means. Since both the differences are negative and because these negative differences are multiplied together, they also contribute positive values to the numerator of the covariance. In the remaining two quadrants, one of the data values is greater than its mean and the other is less than its mean. Data in these quadrants contribute negative values to the numerator of covariance.

In a direct association, most of the data values fall in the upper right and lower left quadrants of the scatter plot. These are the quadrants in which data contribute positive values to the numerator of the covariance. Therefore, data in these quadrants will cause the covariance to have a positive numeric value. In an inverse association, most of the data fall in the upper left and lower right quadrants of the scatter plot, giving the covariance a negative value. This is why a direct association is indicated by a positive covariance and an inverse association is indicated by a negative covariance.

Covariance tells us more than just the direction of the association. It also tells us the strength of the association, with larger numeric values corresponding to stronger associations. To examine this, let us take a look at Figures 7.9–7.11.

All three scatter plots in Figures 7.9–7.11 show direct associations of different strengths. Notice that stronger the direct association, the more the data values are

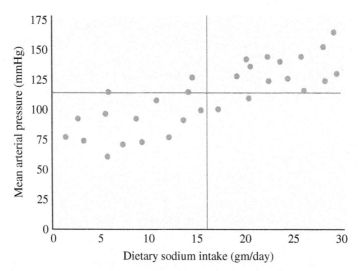

Figure 7.9   Scatter plot showing a moderate association between dietary sodium intake and mean arterial pressure. The means of the dependent and independent variables are used to separate the scatter plot into four quadrants. Data points in the upper right and lower left quadrants contribute positive values to the covariance. Data points in the upper left and lower right quadrants contribute negative values to the covariance. Most of the data points in this example are in the upper right and lower left quadrants, resulting in a covariance with a moderately high positive value.

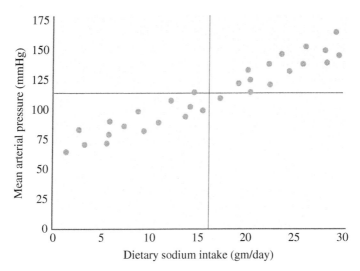

Figure 7.10 Scatter plot from Figure 7.6 showing a strong association between dietary sodium intake and mean arterial pressure. Almost all of the data points in this example are in the upper right and lower left quadrants, resulting in a covariance with a high positive value.

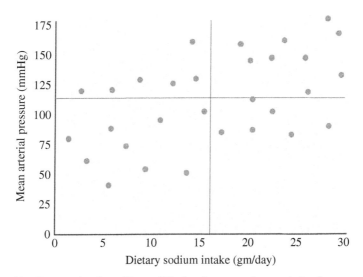

Figure 7.11 Scatter plot from Figure 7.7 showing a weak association between dietary sodium intake and mean arterial pressure. Although most of the data points in this example are in the upper right and lower left quadrants, quite a few are in the upper left and lower right quadrants. Thus, the covariance will have a small positive value.

confined to the lower left and upper right quadrants. For a weaker direct association, there are also data values in the upper left and lower right quadrants (see
Figure 7.11). Since these are the quadrants that contribute negative values to
the numerator of the covariance, they decrease the numeric magnitude of the
covariance in a direct association.

For inverse associations, just the opposite is true: most of the data values are in
the upper left-hand and lower right-hand quadrants. These are the quadrants that
contribute negative values to the covariance. For weaker inverse associations, data
will also fall in the other two quadrants, which contribute positive values to the
covariance.

So, covariance can tell us about both the direction and the strength of the association between a continuous dependent variable and a continuous independent
variable. The strength of the association is reflected by the numeric magnitude of the
covariance. Unfortunately, the numeric value of the covariance also reflects the scale
on which the dependent and independent variables were measured. Consequently,
interpretation of the numeric magnitude of the covariance varies for different data
and for the same data measured on different scales (e.g., weight measured in pounds
as opposed to weight measured in kilograms). This feature substantially reduces the
utility of covariance as a measure of the strength of the association between two
continuous variables.

What we need is a dimensionless index that reflects only the strength of the association and not the scale of measurement. Fortunately, we can calculate such an
index by dividing the covariance by its maximum possible value. That maximum
value is equal to the square root of the product of the variances of the two variables. The index of the strength of the association calculated in this way is called
the **correlation coefficient**. Equation (7.18) shows how the population's correlation
coefficient (ρ) is estimated from the sample's observations.

$$\rho \triangleq r = \frac{\frac{\sum (Y_i - \overline{Y}) \cdot (X - \overline{X})}{n-1}}{\sqrt{s_Y^2 \cdot s_X^2}} \tag{7.18}$$

where

ρ = population's correlation coefficient (rho)

r = sample's estimate of the correlation coefficient

s_Y^2 = sample's estimate of the variance of dependent variable values

s_X^2 = sample's estimate of the variance of independent variable values

Since the square root of the product of the variance estimates is the maximum
numeric magnitude for the covariance, the correlation coefficient will be equal to
+1 when the covariance is at its maximum positive value. The minimum numeric
magnitude of the covariance is equal to the negative square root of the product of

the variances. Thus, the maximum negative value of the correlation coefficient is -1 when the covariance is at its maximum negative value.

A perfect direct association is represented by a correlation coefficient of $+1$ and a perfect inverse association is represented by a correlation coefficient of -1. Also, no association between the variables results in a correlation coefficient equal to 0. Interpretation of a correlation coefficient for those three values is fairly straightforward. Unfortunately, interpretation of other numeric values of the correlation coefficient (i.e., between 0 and $+1$ and between 0 and -1) is a little more complicated.

For instance, what does a correlation coefficient of 0.5 tell us about the strength of the association between two continuous variables? Since 0.5 is halfway between 0 and $+1$, we might expect the strength of that association to be half as strong as a perfect direct association. But this is not the case, since the correlation coefficient does not have a linear (i.e., straight line) relationship with the strength of association between two continuous variables.[19] Fortunately, we can change the correlation coefficient into a value that does have a linear relationship with the strength of the association between two continuous variables. This is done by squaring the correlation coefficient. This square of the correlation coefficient is called the **coefficient of determination** or, more commonly, **R-squared (R^2)**. Equation (7.19) illustrates the calculation of the coefficient of determination.

$$R^2 = r^2 \tag{7.19}$$

where

$R^2 =$ sample's estimate of the coefficient of determination

$r =$ sample's estimate of the correlation coefficient

R^2 tells us the proportion of variation of the dependent variable that is associated with the independent variable. Although it is part of correlation analysis, R^2 can be calculated from the results of regression analysis.[20] Equation (7.20) shows how this calculation can be performed:

$$R^2 = \frac{\text{Regression sum of squares}}{\text{Total sum of squares}} \tag{7.20}$$

Equation (7.20) adequately illustrates what we mean when we say that R^2 tells us about the proportion of variation in the dependent variable that is associated with the

---

[19] Actually, 0.5 is one-quarter of the way between no association and a perfect direct association! We will soon see why this is true.

[20] This is one reason why most computer programs for regression analysis include the coefficient of determination in the output. If we look back at Example 7.4, we can see that the coefficient of determination is part of the information in the first table of the output from that we ignored when we were concentrating on information relevant to regression analysis. It is the value labeled "R-square." It is also in the output from R in Example 7.4. There, it is in the second to last line and is labeled "Multiple R-squared."

independent variable. The total variation in the dependent variable is represented by the total sum of squares. The total sum of squares consists of the regression sum of squares (the variation of dependent variable values "explained" by the independent variable in the regression equation) and the residual sum of squares (the variation of dependent variable values not "explained" by the independent variable in the regression equation). R^2 tells us what proportion of the total variation is the "explained" variation.

The next example illustrates calculation and interpretation of a correlation coefficient.

■ **EXAMPLE 7.6**

Let us calculate a correlation coefficient to examine the strength of the association between dietary sodium intake and mean arterial blood pressure using the data described in Example 7.1.

To calculate a correlation coefficient, we need an estimate of the covariance and estimates of the univariable variances of the dependent and independent variables. The covariance can be estimated from the sum of cross products calculated in Example 7.1.

$$\frac{\sum(Y_i - \overline{Y}) \cdot (X_i - \overline{X})}{n-1} = \frac{5,574.2}{30-1} = 192.2 \, \text{mmHg/g/day}$$

Also, from information in Example 7.1, we can estimate the variance of the independent variable:

$$s_X^2 = \frac{\sum(X_i - \overline{X})^2}{n-1} = \frac{2,234.24}{30-1} = 77.04 \, \text{g/day}^2$$

We also need to estimate the univariable variance estimate for the dependent variable. The following table summarizes the calculations we perform in preparation to estimate this variance:

Patient	X_i	Y_i	$\sum(Y_i - \overline{Y})$	$\sum(Y_i - \overline{Y})^2$
TH	1.0	78	−34	1,156
ER	2.3	93	−19	361
EI	2.9	75	−37	1,369
SN	5.2	97	−15	225
OT	5.4	62	−50	2,500
HI	5.5	115	3	9
NG	7.0	72	−40	1,600
ON	8.4	93	−19	361
EA	9.0	74	−38	1,444
RT	10.5	108	−4	16

Patient	X_i	Y_i	$\sum(Y_i - \overline{Y})$	$\sum(Y_i - \overline{Y})^2$
HL	11.8	78	−34	1,156
IK	13.3	92	−20	400
EA	13.8	115	3	9
NI	14.2	127	15	225
CE	15.1	100	−12	144
RE	16.9	101	−11	121
GR	18.8	128	16	256
ES	19.8	142	30	900
SI	20.0	110	−2	4
ON	20.2	136	24	576
TO	22.0	144	32	1,024
CH	22.1	124	12	144
EE	23.3	140	28	784
RS	24.1	126	14	196
TA	25.5	144	32	1,024
TI	25.8	116	4	16
ST	27.8	152	40	1,600
IC	28.0	124	12	144
IC	28.0	124	12	144
IA	28.9	164	52	2,704
NS	29.2	130	18	324
Total	477.8	3,360	0	20,792

The sample's estimate of the univariable variance is

$$\sigma_Y^2 \triangleq s_Y^2 = \frac{\sum(Y_i - \overline{Y})^2}{n-1} = \frac{20{,}792}{30-1} = 717.0 \, \text{mmHg}^2$$

Now, we are ready to use Equation (7.18) to calculate the sample's estimate of the population's correlation coefficient.

$$\rho \triangleq r = \frac{\frac{\sum(Y_i - \overline{Y}) \cdot (X_i - \overline{X})}{n-1}}{\sqrt{s_Y^2 \cdot s_X^2}} = \frac{\frac{5{,}574.2}{30-1}}{\sqrt{717.0 \cdot 77.04}} = 0.818$$

Thus, the sample's estimate of the correlation coefficient is equal to 0.818. To interpret that correlation coefficient, we use Equation (7.19) to calculate the coefficient of determination (i.e., R^2).

$$R^2 = r^2 = 0.818^2 = 0.669$$

That coefficient of determination tells us that 0.669 (or 66.9%) of the variation in mean arterial pressure is associated with variation in dietary sodium intake.   ∎

There are two ways to estimate correlation coefficients in Excel. One is to examine the first table in the "Regression" output. Go back to Example 7.4 and look at the first table. The correlation coefficient is called the "Multiple R," and "R Square" is just below the correlation coefficient.[21] The other way is to use the "Correlation" procedure in "Data Analysis." That procedure is useful if you want to estimate correlation coefficients for several variables. It produces a matrix of correlation coefficients for all possible pairs of variables.

In R, the "cor(data)" command produces a matrix of correlation coefficients similar to the output from the Correlation procedure in Excel. Another way to estimate a correlation coefficient for a pair of variables is by using the "cor.test(IV,DV)" command. This is illustrated in Example 7.7.

7.1.2.1 *Taking Chance into Account.*

Under certain conditions, we can take chance into account for the sample's estimate of the population's correlation coefficient using the same kind of Gaussian approach we have used for means, slopes, and intercepts. This can be done when the population's correlation coefficient is equal to 0.[22]

At first, this might seem to be an unrealistic restriction, but the most commonly used null hypothesis for the correlation coefficient is that the population's value is equal to 0. Since we always assume the null hypothesis is true when taking chance into account using hypothesis testing, we can use the Gaussian approach to test the null hypothesis.

When we assume the population's correlation coefficient is equal to 0, the sampling distribution has a mean equal to 0 and a standard error equal to Equation (7.21):

$$\sigma_r \triangleq s_r = \sqrt{\frac{1-r^2}{n-2}} \qquad (7.21)$$

where

s_r = standard error for the sample's estimate of the correlation coefficient

r = sample's estimate of the correlation coefficient

To test the null hypothesis that the population's correlation coefficient is equal to 0, we can apply the usual Gaussian approach in which we convert the sample's estimate to a value from a distribution with a mean equal to 0 and a standard deviation of 1. Since we are also estimating the variances of the dependent and independent variables, we need to use Student's t-distribution to take into account

---

[21] The third value ("Adjusted R Square") has no interpretation here.

[22] The reason for this is that the correlation coefficient has a restricted range of possible values (from 1 to +1), but means, slopes, and intercepts vary (theoretically) from $-\infty$ to $+\infty$. The effect of this restricted range of possible values is to make the sampling distribution for the correlation coefficient symmetric only when the mean of that sampling distribution is equal to the midpoint of its range of possible values (when the correlation coefficient is equal to 0).

the independent role of chance in making these estimates.[23] Equation (7.22) shows this calculation.

$$t = \frac{r - \rho_0}{s_r} \tag{7.22}$$

where

t = Student's t-value with $n - 2$ degrees of freedom

r = sample's estimate of the correlation coefficient

ρ_0 = population's correlation coefficient, according to the null hypothesis (i.e., equal to 0)

s_r = standard error for the sample's estimate of the correlation coefficient (from Equation (7.21))

Now, let us take a look at an example in which we take chance into account for the sample's estimate of the population's correlation coefficient.

■ EXAMPLE 7.7

In Example 7.6 we found that the sample's estimate of the population's correlation coefficient representing the strength of the association between dietary sodium intake and mean arterial blood pressure is equal to 0.818. Now, let us take chance into account by testing the null hypothesis that the population's correlation coefficient is equal to 0 versus the alternative hypothesis that is not equal to 0. Let us allow a 5% chance of making a type 1 error.

First, we use Equation (7.21) to calculate the standard error for estimates of the correlation coefficient.

$$s_r = \sqrt{\frac{1 - r^2}{n - 2}} = \sqrt{\frac{1 - 0.818^2}{30 - 2}} = 0.1087$$

Next, we convert the sample's estimate to a Student's t-value using Equation (7.22),

$$t = \frac{r - \rho_0}{s_r} = \frac{0.818 - 0}{0.1087} = 7.53$$

To interpret that value, we compare it with a value from Table B.2 that corresponds to 28 degrees of freedom and a two-sided α of 0.05 (i.e., the critical value). That t-value is 2.048. Since 7.52 is larger than 2.048, we reject the null hypothesis and, through the process of elimination, accept the alternative hypothesis (i.e., that the population's correlation coefficient is not equal to 0).

This example illustrates how we can take chance into account in correlation analysis by hand. In practice, we use a computer to perform these calculations for us.

---

[23] At first, it may seem as if we are not estimating either variance in Equation (7.21), but those variance estimates are included in $1 - r^2$ in the numerator of the standard error. There, r^2 is an algebraic simplification of including the covariance and the two variances in calculation of the standard error.

In Excel, correlation analysis is usually done using the "Regression" analysis tool. The P-value associated with the F-ratio testing the omnibus null hypothesis in the regression output is the same as the P-value testing the null hypothesis that the population's correlation coefficient is equal to 0.[24] In R, we can use the "cor.test(IV,DV)" command to perform the t-test for the correlation coefficient. This is illustrated below while specifying that the data are in a data set named "Example7_1":

```
>with(Example7_1,cor.test(SODIUM,ARTPRESS))

Pearson's product-moment correlation

data: SODIUM and ARTPRESS
t = 7.5205, df = 28, p-value = 3.427e-08
alternative hypothesis: true correlation is not equal to 0
95 percent confidence interval:
 0.6487119 0.9099893
sample estimates:
 cor
0.8178424
```

That output also contains a confidence interval for the correlation coefficient. Calculation of a confidence interval for a correlation coefficient is a little more complicated than calculation of other confidence intervals we have seen. How this is done is beyond the scope of this text. ∎

7.1.2.2 *Naturalistic Versus Purposive Samples.*

In Flowchart 5, the choice between performing regression analysis and correlation analysis appears to be determined by the purpose of the analysis. If dependent variable values are to be estimated, regression analysis is the right choice. If the strength of the association between the dependent and independent variables is our interest, we should choose correlation analysis. In the latter case, however, there is an additional criterion that must be met if the strength of the association between the two variables in the population is being estimated. This is because the sample's estimate of the population's correlation coefficient is influenced by how independent variable values are sampled.

There are two ways we can sample independent variable values from the population. One possibility is to select a sample that contains a random subset of the independent variable values in the population.[25] When independent variable values are selected randomly, the distribution of independent variable values in the sample represents the distribution of independent variable values in the population, at least

---

[24] In fact, the F-ratio in regression analysis is equal to the square of the Student's t-value in correlation analysis.

[25] This is distinct from a random sample of dependent variable values. As discussed in Chapter 2, all statistical procedures assume that the dependent variable has been sampled randomly. Now, we are referring to how the independent variable has been sampled. Few statistical procedures assume that the independent variable has been sampled randomly as well.

on the average. We call a sample that is the result of randomly sampling independent variable values a **naturalistic sample**.[26]

In contrast to sampling independent variable values randomly, these values can be selected so that they have a distribution in the sample that is different from their distribution in the population. Such a sample is called a **purposive sample**.[27] There are a number of reasons a researcher might choose to take a purposive sample. A common reason is to "oversample" values of the independent variable that do not occur very often in the population. For example, the National Hospital Discharge Survey (NHDS) planned to include all of the very largest hospitals in the United States, although lower percentages of smaller hospitals were also included. One reason for this is that there are very few of these larger hospitals in the population. To be able to describe the discharges at the larger hospitals and smaller hospitals with the same precision, a greater proportion of the larger hospitals had to be included in the sample. As a result, the distribution of hospital sizes in the sample was not representative of their distribution in the population. Thus, the NHDS uses a purposive sample of hospital size in its sample.

The following example illustrates the distinction between a naturalistic sample and a purposive sample.

■ EXAMPLE 7.8

Suppose that we are interested in the relationship between age and renal clearance rates. Further, suppose that the relationship in the population is represented in the following scatter plot:

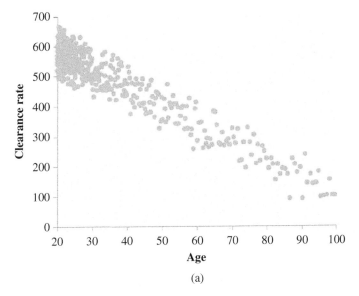

(a)

---

[26] A naturalistic sample results from taking a simple random sample mentioned in Chapter 2.
[27] A purposive sample results from taking a stratified random sample mentioned in Chapter 2.

The scatter plot shows the renal clearance rate (measured as plasma/min/1.73 m^2) decreasing with increasing age. It also demonstrates that there are fewer persons in the population in older age groups. This is evident from the fact that there are fewer points in the scatter plot for each higher decade of life.

Now, let us consider how to sample this population and the implications of our choice on interpretation of the estimate of the correlation coefficient.

One choice is to take a naturalistic sample. To take a naturalistic sample, members of the population are selected regardless of their age. When the value of the independent variable does not influence the probability of being included in the sample, chance will create a distribution of independent variable values in the sample that, on the average, reflects the population's distribution. The following scatter plot illustrates a naturalistic sample of 50 persons taken from that population. The points in darker shade represent the individuals in the population who are selected for the sample.

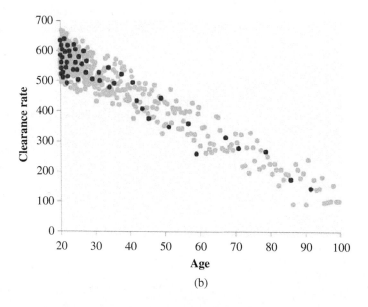

(b)

This naturalistic sample shows the same age distribution as the population's age distribution; namely, there are fewer persons in each older age group. With this naturalistic sample, renal clearance rates can be estimated with fair precision for younger persons, but they cannot be estimated with much precision for older persons, since there are few older persons in the sample.

If we are interested in more precisely estimating clearance rates for older persons, we need to determine each person's age before we can decide whether or not they should be included in the sample. Then, we need to select persons for the sample according to their age (i.e., take a stratified sample), making the probability of being selected higher for older persons than for younger persons. The following scatter plot illustrates a sample of 50 persons who would be selected from the population in this way:

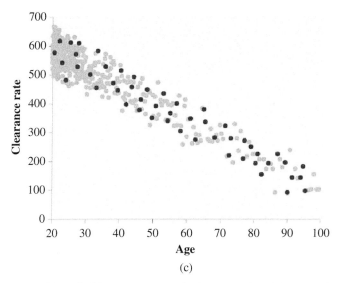

(c)

This oversampling of older persons results in a sample with approximately the same number of persons throughout the range of ages studied. Consequently, estimates for older persons will have the same precision as estimates for younger persons. This sample, however, is a purposive sample. This fact limits the kind of analysis that would be appropriate for these data (i.e., correlation analysis would not be appropriate).

Another approach to sampling a population such as this is to limit the range of independent variable values to those values that are well represented in the population (i.e., take a **restricted** sample). For this population, suppose we decided to eliminate persons 60 years old or older from the sampling process, and then take a naturalistic sample of persons between the ages of 20 and 50 years. The following scatter plot illustrates a restricted sample:

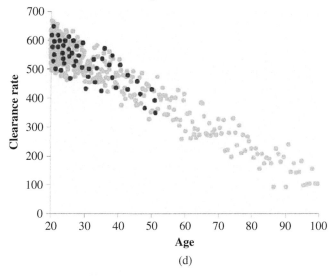

(d)

This sampling method confines the ages in the sample to those that are well represented in the population. It does not allow estimates for older persons; instead it focuses on the younger persons for whom precise estimates can be made without oversampling. Between the ages of 20 and 59 years, the distribution of ages in the sample represents the distribution of ages in the population in that age range. Thus, relative to persons between 20 and 59 years of age in the population, this is a naturalistic sample. Relative to the initial population, however, this is a purposive sample. ■

When we have a purposive sample, we can perform a regression analysis that can be interpreted relative to the population. That is to say, such analyses provide unbiased estimates of the slope in the population. The only effect of purposive sampling on the estimate of the slope is to change the precision of this estimate.[28] It will not have an effect on the value of the estimate itself (i.e., on the average, samples' estimates will be equal to the population's parameters).

This is not the case for the sample's estimate of the population's correlation coefficient. Estimates of the correlation coefficient will change in value as the distribution of independent variable values in the sample changes. Only naturalistic samples produce estimates of the correlation coefficient that are equal, on the average, to the population's correlation coefficient. With purposive samples, the estimate of the correlation coefficient will be higher than the population's value (even on the average) when the ages of persons in the sample are more dispersed than the ages of persons in the population (as in the first purposive sample in Example 7.8 in which older persons were oversampled). Similarly, the estimate of the correlation coefficient will be lower than the population's value when the ages of persons in the sample are less dispersed (as in the second purposive sample in Example 7.8, in which older persons were excluded from the sample). The ways in which methods of sampling independent variable values affect estimates of the slope, intercept, and correlation coefficient are illustrated in the next example.

■ EXAMPLE 7.9

In Example 7.8, we considered a naturalistic and two purposive samples from a population with fewer persons of older ages. We were interested in the relationship between age and renal clearance rates. This population was generated in a computer simulation that assumed that the population's regression equation had an intercept equal to 700 cc of plasma/min/1.73 m^2 and a slope equal to 6 cc of plasma/min/ 1.73 m^2/year. The coefficient of determination (R^2) in this simulated population was equal to 0.9 (which corresponds to a correlation coefficient of approximately 0.95). Now, let us see what the estimates for the slope, intercept, and correlation coefficient are for each of the three samples taken from that population.

---

[28] The precision of the estimates of the slope and intercept increase as the variability of independent variable values in the sample increases. This is illustrated mathematically (for the slope) in Equation (7.15), where the sum of squares for the independent variable values in the sample is included in the denominator of the standard error calculation.

To begin with, let us take a look at the first sample in Example 7.8. That was a naturalistic sample, so we expect all of the estimates to be close to the population's values. The following Excel output came from analyzing these data using the "Regression" analysis tool.

SUMMARY OUTPUT

Regression statistics	
Multiple R	0.9577
R square	0.9171
Adjusted R square	0.9154
Standard error	35.95523
Observations	50

ANOVA

	df	SS	MS	F	Significance F
Regression	1	686,677	686,677	531.1	1.32E-27
Residual	48	62,055	1,292.77584		
Total	49	748,731			

	Coefficients	Standard error	t Stat	P-value	Lower 95%
Intercept	706.99334	10.70865	66.02	8.96494E-49	685.4621561
X variable 1	−6.26329	0.27176	−23.05	1.31E-27	−6.809700102

At the bottom of this output, we can see that the naturalistic sample's estimate of the intercept and slope are 706.99334 cc of plasma/min/1.73 m^2 and 6.26329 cc of plasma/min/1.73 m^2/year. These are close to the actual values (700 and 6). In addition, if we were to continue taking naturalistic samples from this population, we would find that the means of the slope and intercept from these samples would be, in the long run, exactly equal to the population's values. Thus, the estimates of the slope and intercept from a naturalistic sample are unbiased estimates[29] of the slope and intercept in the population.

The sample's estimate of the correlation coefficient is equal to the square root of the estimate of R^2 that is included in the output from the "Regression" analysis tool. In this sample, the estimate of R^2 is 0.9171, which is very close to the actual value in the population (0.9).

Similar to the estimates of the slope and intercept, the mean of estimates of the correlation coefficient from repeated naturalistic samples would be exactly equal to the population's value. Thus, naturalistic samples provide unbiased estimates of the slope, intercept, and correlation coefficient.

Next, let us take a look at the first purposive sample in Example 7.8, which resulted from oversampling persons of older ages. The following is the result of using the "Regression" analysis tool to analyze these data.

[29] Recall from Chapter 2 that an unbiased estimate is equal to the population's value on the average.

SUMMARY OUTPUT

Regression statistics	
Multiple R	0.9685
R square	0.938
Adjusted R square	0.9368
Standard error	37.60455
Observations	50

ANOVA

	df	SS	MS	F	Significance F
Regression	1	1027,536	1027,659	726.72	1.21E-30
Residual	48	67,877	1,414.10189		
Total	49	1095,536			

	Coefficients	Standard error	t Stat	P-value	Lower 95%	Upper 95%
Intercept	725.58134	10.70865	66.02	8.96494E-49	704.0501561	747.1125239
X variable 1	–6.29827	0.27176	–23.05	1.31E-27	–6.844680102	–5.7518599

As in the naturalistic sample, this purposive sample gives us an estimate of the slope (6.29827) that is close in value to the actual slope (6). The intercept (725.58134) is not as close to the actual intercept (700) as that from the naturalistic sample, but this is due to the role of chance in selecting this sample from the simulated population.[30] Even so, if we were to take all possible samples of this kind from the population, the mean of the estimates of the slope and the intercept from these samples would be exactly equal to the actual slope and the intercept. Taking a purposive sample does not bias the point estimates of the slope and intercept.

The estimate of R^2 (0.9380), however, is larger than the actual value in the population (0.9).[31] This would be true even if we were to take all possible samples of this same size and calculate the mean of the estimates of the correlation coefficient from each sample. In that case, the mean would be larger than the actual value. This purposive sample has increased the variation in ages by oversampling older persons and, as a result, overestimates the population's correlation coefficient.

Finally, let us take a look at the second purposive sample in Example 7.8. This sample resulted from restricting the sample to persons 50 years old or younger. The following is the result of using the "Regression" analysis tool to analyze these data:

[30] In a simulation, chance is used to select a particular sample. Thus, we can see the effect of this role of chance in a simulation by occasionally obtaining estimates that are not very close to the value of the population's parameter. On the average, however, those estimates would be exactly equal to the parameter.

[31] At first, 0.9380 does not seem to be very much larger than 0.9, but we need to keep in mind that R^2 has an upper limit of +1. 0.9380 represents an increase that is more than 1/3 (0.0380/0.1000) of the maximum possible increase.

SUMMARY OUTPUT

Regression statistics	
Multiple R	0.833966
R square	0.6955
Adjusted R square	0.6892
Standard error	35.85928
Observations	50

ANOVA

	df	SS	MS	F	Significance F
Regression	1	140,985	140,958	109.6209	5.51E-14
Residual	48	61,732	1,285.88764		
Total	49	202,708			

	Coefficients	Standard error	t Stat	P-value	Lower 95%	Upper 95%
Intercept	713.0502	17.97786	39.66	2.40359E-38	704.0501561	747.1125239
X variable 1	-6.62744	0.63294	-10.47	5.51E-14*	7.900051163	-5.35482884

As in the previous two samples, this purposive sample gives us estimates of the slope (6.62744) and the intercept (713.05020) that are close in value to the actual slope (6) and intercept (700). Also, as in the previous two samples, the mean of the estimates of the slope and the intercept from all possible samples of this same type would be exactly equal to the actual slope and the intercept. The estimate of R^2 (0.6955), however, is smaller than the actual value of R^2 (0.9). This would be true even if we were to take all possible samples like this one and calculate the mean of the estimates of the correlation coefficient from each sample. This purposive sample has decreased the variation in ages by excluding older persons and as a result, underestimates the population's R^2 (and correlation coefficient). ∎

7.2   ORDINAL INDEPENDENT VARIABLE

When a bivariable sample contains a continuous dependent variable, we can choose among a variety of statistical procedures for continuous or nominal independent variables. There are not, however, any well-accepted procedures used in health research for a sample consisting of a continuous dependent variable and an ordinal independent variable. Such a sample is analyzed either by converting the continuous dependent variable to an ordinal scale and using techniques discussed in Chapter 8 or by creating a collection of nominal variables from the ordinal independent variable and using statistical procedures described in Chapter 10.

7.3   NOMINAL INDEPENDENT VARIABLE

When the independent variable represents nominal data, the effect is to separate dependent variable values into two groups.[32] Suppose, for instance, that we conduct

[32] Remember that a nominal variable can represent only two possible values. Therefore, a single nominal independent variable divides a sample into two, and only two, groups. If the sample contains more than

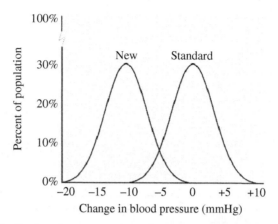

Figure 7.12   Distribution of continuous dependent variable values divided into two groups by a nominal independent variable.

a clinical trial of an antihypertensive medication to compare a new treatment with standard therapy. The independent variable, in this case, is a nominal variable indicating group membership (new or standard therapy) and dependent variable is the change in blood pressure. Figure 7.12 illustrates the way we think about the distribution of continuous dependent variable values when the independent variable represents nominal data.

7.3.1   Estimating the Difference between the Groups

The most common method of comparing two groups of continuous dependent variable values is by comparing the means of the groups. We compare means by examining their difference. For example, when comparing changes in blood pressure measurements between persons who received a new drug versus those who received standard therapy, we would make the comparison by examining the difference between the means of the change in blood pressure values in the two treatment groups.[33]

To estimate the difference between the means of the groups in the population, we take the difference between the sample's estimates of those means (Equation (7.23))). This is an unbiased estimate of the difference between the means in the population.

$$\mu_1 - \mu_2 \triangleq \overline{Y}_1 - \overline{Y}_2 = \frac{\sum Y_{1,i}}{n_1} - \frac{\sum Y_{2,i}}{n_2} \tag{7.23}$$

two groups, those groups must be represented by more than one nominal independent variable. Then, we would have a multivariable dataset.

[33]One reason we compare means as a difference is that a linear combination (such as a sum or difference) of measures of location of a distribution (like means) will have a Gaussian distribution if the components of the linear combination have Gaussian distributions. In other words, we can apply the central limit theorem to linear combinations of measures of location just as we can apply it to these measures of location themselves.

where

μ_1 = population's mean in group 1
μ_2 = population's mean in group 2
$\overline{Y}_1$ = sample's estimate of the mean in group 1
$\overline{Y}_2$ = sample's estimate of the mean in group 2

7.3.2 Taking Chance into Account

We can take chance into account for the estimate of the difference between means either by testing a null hypothesis or calculating a confidence interval for that difference. In either case, we need to consider the sampling distribution for differences between the means (i.e., the distribution of differences between the means from all possible samples of the same size). This sampling distribution tends to be a Gaussian distribution, so we can use the same approach to conducting hypothesis testing and interval estimation we have used for other Gaussian sampling distributions.

If the sampling distribution for the differences between the means is a Gaussian distribution, its parameters must be a mean and a standard error. The mean of this sampling distribution is equal to the difference between the population's means.[34] The standard error of the sampling distribution of the difference between two means is calculated from the standard errors of the univariable sampling distributions for each of the means[35] as illustrated in Equation (7.24).

$$\sigma_{\overline{Y}_1 - \overline{Y}_2} \triangleq s_{\overline{Y}_1 - \overline{Y}_2} = \sqrt{s_{\overline{Y}_1}^2 + s_{\overline{Y}_2}^2} = \sqrt{\frac{s_1^2}{n_1} + \frac{s_2^2}{n_2}} \qquad (7.24)$$

where

$s_{\overline{Y}_1 - \overline{Y}_2}$ = standard error for the difference between the means in two groups of continuous dependent variable values

$s_{\overline{Y}_1}^2, s_{\overline{Y}_2}^2$ = sample's estimate of the squared univariable standard errors for the means in groups 1 and 2

s_1^2, s_2^2 = sample's estimates of the variances of dependent variable values in groups 1 and 2

n_1, n_2 = numbers of observations in groups 1 and 2

We will take a look at an example in which we calculate this standard error shortly, but first we need to consider how we will go about estimating the variance of dependent variable values when there are two groups of these values. In Figure 7.12, the dispersions of the two distributions of dependent variable values are identical.

---

[34]For any unbiased estimate, the mean of the sampling distribution is equal to the population's value being estimated. This is what we imply when we say that an unbiased estimate is equal to the population's value, "on the average."

[35]Another aspect of a linear combination that makes it attractive as a way to compare measures of location is that the standard error of the combination can easily be calculated from the standard errors of its components.

This is done for simplicity. Having the dispersions of these two distributions equal to the same value implies that we can use all of the data in our sample to estimate that single, common variance. The alternative is to use the sample's observations in each group by themselves to estimate the population's variance of values in that group.[36]

If we can assume that the variances are equal in the two groups of dependent variable values, then we can use all of the observations in the sample (i.e., dependent variable values associated with both groups) to estimate a single variance in the population that applies to both groups, rather than having to estimate separate variances for each of the two groups. As a result, we can have greater confidence in that estimate and greater statistical power (i.e., greater ability to avoid a type II error in statistical hypothesis testing). Assuming that the variances are the same in the population for different groups of dependent variable values is known as the assumption of **homoscedasticity**.[37]

When we assume homoscedasticity, we can use information from both groups to estimate the population's variance. It is important to keep in mind that assuming homoscedasticity does not require that the sample's estimates of the variance observed in each of the two groups have the same value. Rather, we expect that the sample's observations in each of these groups will give us different variance estimates by chance alone, even if they are estimating the same variance in the population. The issue here is whether or not the observed variances (i.e., the sample's estimates) are different enough for us to suspect that they are estimating different values in the population. We will consider how to decide about this assumption shortly. For now, let us say that we are willing to assume homoscedasticity. In that case, we want to arrive at a single estimate of the variance.

To understand how we derive a single estimate of the population's variance from the sample's two estimates, we need to learn about an important statistical concept. That is the concept of a **weighted average**.

In everyday language, the terms "average" and "mean" are considered to be synonyms. In statistics, we draw a distinction between the two. An average (more often called a weighted average) is the sum of the products of each observation or estimate times a particular number (called a weight) divided by the sum of those weights. This is easier to appreciate if we look at Equation (7.25).

$$\text{Weighted average} = \frac{\sum w_i \cdot Y_i}{\sum w_i} \tag{7.25}$$

where

w_i = weight for the ith observation or estimate

Y_i = value of the ith observation or estimate

---

[36] This implies that there are three ways chance can influence the sample. The first is in the estimates of the difference between the means of the two distributions. The second and third ways are in the variance estimates for each of the two groups of dependent variable values.

[37] We will discuss the assumption of homoscedasticity in more detail in Chapter 13.

In contrast, a mean is a special type of weighted average in which each observation is given a weight equal to 1.[38] The use of a weighted average with weights equal to 1 implies that we are unable to say that one observation is closer to the population's mean than is any other observation. Thus, each observation is given the same weight as every other observation when estimating the mean.

Now, let us apply this principle of weighted averages to estimation of the population's variance of the distribution of data when we have estimates of that variance from two groups of dependent variable values.

We know from Chapter 4 that the number of degrees of freedom in a sample is used as a parameter of Student's t-distribution to reflect the degree of precision with which we can estimate the population's variance of the distribution of data. The greater the number of degrees of freedom, the less the penalty that must be paid for estimating the population's variance from the sample's observations.[39] Since degrees of freedom can be used in that context to reflect how precisely we can estimate the population's variance, it makes sense for us to use degrees of freedom as the weights for the variance estimates from each of the two groups in the sample. The weighted average of these two variance estimates using degrees of freedom as the weights is called the **pooled estimate** of the variance. Equation (7.26) shows how to calculate the pooled estimate of the variance of the distribution of data in the population from the sample's observations.

$$\sigma_Y^2 \triangleq s_{pooled}^2 = \frac{\sum(n_i - 1) \cdot s_i^2}{\sum(n_i - 1)} = \frac{((n_1 - 1) \cdot s_1^2) + ((n_2 - 1) \cdot s_2^2)}{(n_1 - 1) + (n_2 - 1)} \qquad (7.26)$$

where

σ_Y^2 = variance of the distribution of dependent variable values in the population

s_{pooled}^2 = pooled estimate of the variance of dependent variable values

$(n_i - 1)$ = degrees of freedom in the ith group of dependent variable values

s_i^2 = variance estimate in the ith group of dependent variable values

When we assume homoscedasticity, we should use the pooled estimate of the variance to calculate the standard error of the difference between the means rather than using the separate variance estimates. Equation (7.27) shows how Equation (7.24) is modified to use the pooled estimate in calculating the standard error for the differences between the means.

$$\sigma_{\bar{Y}_1 - \bar{Y}_2} \triangleq s_{\bar{Y}_1 - \bar{Y}_2} = \sqrt{s_{\bar{Y}_1}^2 + s_{\bar{Y}_2}^2} = \sqrt{\frac{s_{pooled}^2}{n_1} + \frac{s_{pooled}^2}{n_2}} \qquad (7.27)$$

[38] Mathematically, the mean can be presented as a weighted average as follows: $\bar{Y} = \frac{\sum 1 \cdot Y_i}{\sum 1} = \frac{\sum Y_i}{n}$

[39] Recall from Chapter 4 that the "penalty" applied by Student's t-distribution is to make it harder to reject the null hypothesis (by making the P-value larger) and to make confidence intervals wider.

where

$s_{\overline{Y}_1-\overline{Y}_2}$ = standard error for the difference between the means in two groups of continuous dependent variable values

s^2_{pooled} = pooled estimate of the variance of dependent variable values from Equation (7.26)

n_1, n_2 = number of observations in groups 1 and 2

So, there are two ways to calculate the standard error for the differences between the means of two groups of continuous dependent variable values. Equation (7.27) is the way we calculate the standard error if we are willing to assume that the population's variances of the distributions of data are equal in the two groups (i.e., when we assume homoscedasticity). In that case, we use the pooled estimate of the population's variance in calculating the standard error. If we are unwilling to assume homoscedasticity, however, we use the separate, group-specific estimates of the population's variance in each group of dependent variable values. That calculation is shown in Equation (7.24).

Now that we understand the choices for the standard error of the difference between two means, we are ready to take chance into account for the sample's estimate of that difference. To do this, we can either test a null hypothesis[40] or calculate a confidence interval for the difference between the means in the population. In either case, we use Student's t-distribution so that we can have degrees of freedom to take into account the independent role(s) of chance in estimating the population's variance(s) of the distributions of data in each group. Equations (7.28) (for hypothesis testing) and (7.29) (for interval estimation) illustrate these calculations.

$$t = \frac{(\overline{Y}_1 - \overline{Y}_2) - (\mu_1 - \mu_2)}{s_{\overline{Y}_1-\overline{Y}_2}} \qquad (7.28)$$

$$\mu_1 - \mu_2 \triangleq (\overline{Y}_1 - \overline{Y}_2) \pm (t_{\alpha/2} \cdot s_{\overline{Y}_1-\overline{Y}_2}) \qquad (7.29)$$

where

t = Student's t-value representing the observed difference between the means

$t_{\alpha/2}$ = Student's t-value representing $1 - \alpha$ confidence split between the tails of Student's t-distribution

$\overline{Y}_1, \overline{Y}_2$ = sample's estimate of the means in group 1 and 2

μ_1, μ_2 = population's means in groups 1 and 2

---

[40]The most commonly addressed null hypothesis for a difference between means is that the difference in the population is equal to 0. This is tantamount to hypothesizing that the means for the two groups are equal to each other.

$s_{\overline{Y}_1 - \overline{Y}_2}$ = standard error for the difference between the means calculated from Equation (7.24) when we cannot assume homoscedasticity or from Equation (7.27) when we can assume homoscedasticity

When we assume homoscedasticity, the degrees of freedom for Student's t-value are equal to $n_1 + n_2 - 2$. This is the same as the value that is used in the denominator when we calculated the pooled estimate of the variance (Equation (7.26))). It is equal to the sum of the univariable degrees of freedom (i.e., $n_i - 1$) in each group.

When we are unwilling to assume that the variances are equal in the two groups, we have an additional role of chance. In that case, chance can have an independent influence on the estimates of both variances. This additional role of chance is reflected in the degrees of freedom we use to identify a t-value.[41] The degrees of freedom will be fewer than $n_1 + n_2 - 2$ when we are unwilling to assume homoscedasticity.[42] The effect of having fewer degrees of freedom, with all else being equal, is to make rejecting the null hypothesis harder and to make confidence intervals wider.[43]

In the next example, we see how we can take chance into account in examining the difference between the means of dependent variable values in two groups specified by a nominal independent variable.

■ EXAMPLE 7.10

Suppose we are interested in comparing mean arterial blood pressure values between two groups of persons: first a group of 30 persons who follow a low-sodium diet and a second group of 50 persons who do not try to control their dietary sodium intake. Imagine that we observed the following results:

Group	n	Arterial blood pressure $\overline{Y}$	s^2
Diet	30	105.9	109.86
Control	50	126.7	585.32

While assuming the variances are equal to the same value in the population, let us test the null hypothesis that the difference between the mean arterial blood pressure is equal to 0 (versus the alternative hypothesis that the difference between the means is not equal to 0) while allowing a 5% chance of making a type I error.

Since we are told to assume the variances are equal to the same value in the population, we will calculate a standard error based on the pooled estimate of the variance of dependent variable values. In preparation, we use Equation (7.26) to

---

[41] This is often called Welch's approximate t

[42] The calculation of the degrees of freedom when we are not willing to assume homoscedasticity is a bit complicated. In practice, the computer does this calculation for us.

[43] When calculating a confidence interval with unequal variances, first perform a t-test on the computer to get the degrees of freedom.

calculate the pooled estimate of that variance:

$$\sigma_Y^2 \triangleq s_{\text{pooled}}^2 = \frac{\sum(n_i - 1) \cdot s_i^2}{\sum(n_i - 1)} = \frac{((n_1 - 1) \cdot s_1^2) + ((n_2 - 1) \cdot s_2^2)}{(n_1 - 1) + (n_2 - 1)}$$

$$= \frac{((30 - 1) \cdot 109.86) + ((50 - 1) \cdot 585.32)}{(30 - 1) + (50 - 1)} = 408.55 \text{ mmHg}^2$$

So, our best estimate of the variance of dependent variable values is equal to 408.55 mmHg^2. This value is closer to the variance estimate among controls than it is to the estimate among persons on the diet. This is so because the estimate of the variance is more precise (i.e., more individuals and thus, more degrees of freedom) among controls.

Next, we use Equation (7.27) to calculate the standard error for the difference between two means:

$$\sigma_{\overline{Y}_1 - \overline{Y}_2} \triangleq s_{\overline{Y}_1 - \overline{Y}_2} = \sqrt{\frac{s_{\text{pooled}}^2}{n_1} + \frac{s_{\text{pooled}}^2}{n_2}} = \sqrt{\frac{408.55}{30} + \frac{408.55}{50}} = 4.67 \text{ mmHg}$$

Now, we are ready to convert the observed difference between the means to a t-value. To do that, we use Equation (7.28).

$$t = \frac{(\overline{Y}_1 - \overline{Y}_2) - (\mu_1 - \mu_2)}{s_{\overline{Y}_1 - \overline{Y}_2}} = \frac{(105.9 - 126.7) - 0}{4.67} = -4.46$$

To interpret this value, we can compare it with the value in Table B.2 (Student's t-distribution), which corresponds to a two-sided $\alpha = 0.05$ and 78 degrees of freedom. There is no listing for that number of degrees of freedom in Table B.2. Instead, we find a t-value of 1.992 for 75 degrees of freedom and of 1.990 for 80 degrees of freedom. Our calculated value (-4.46) is larger (for a two-sided test, we ignore the sign of the calculated t-value) than either of these values. Thus, we can reject the null hypothesis and accept, through the process of elimination, the alternative hypothesis that the difference between the two means is not equal to 0. ∎

In Example 7.10, we assumed that the variances for the groups are equal in the population. When we looked at the estimates of that variance, we might have been concerned that they were not similar enough to assume homoscedasticity. Deciding how similar estimates of the population's variance have to be to make it sensible to use a pooled estimate is a bit tricky. What most people do is test the null hypothesis that the population's variances are equal to each other. This may not be the best method, since it is affected by statistical power.[44] Its use, however, is

---

[44] Statistical power will determine how different the sample's estimates of the variance need to be before the null hypothesis, stating that they are equal can be rejected. The problem with this is that the sample's estimates of the variance can be quite different in a small sample without rejecting the null hypothesis. On the other hand, estimates that are numerically similar can lead to rejection of the null hypothesis if the sample is large. Thus, this criterion for assuming homoscedasticity has different results for samples of different sizes.

encouraged by computer programs that provide the results of this hypothesis test any time Student's t-test is performed. For now, we will use that criterion for assuming homoscedasticity.

To have Excel conduct this test of homogeneity, we use the analysis tool in "Data Analysis" called "F-test: Two-Sample for Variances." In R, we use the "var.test" command. In both of these, it is important to list the group with the larger variance first to give us an F-ratio greater than 1. Then the alternative hypothesis is one-sided stating that the F-ratio is greater than 1. Excel uses the alternative by default, but it must be stated as part of the "var.test" command.

Depending on the result of the F-test, we either conduct Student's t-test assuming homoscedasticity or not assuming homoscedasticity. In Excel, this means we use either "t-test: Two Sample Assuming Equal Variances" or "t-test: Two Sample Assuming Unequal Variances" in "Data Analysis."[45] In R, we need to specify "TRUE" or "FALSE" for "equal.variances =" in the "t.test" command.[46] These processes are illustrated in the next example.

■ **EXAMPLE 7.11**

Let us begin by using "F-test: Two-Sample for Variances" in Excel to test for homoscedasticity in the data described in Example 7.10. Since the control group has the greater variance, we select it as "Variable 1."[47] Selecting "F-test: Two-Sample for Variances" gives us the following dialog box:

(a)

---

[45] We can also use Excel's "t.test" function.
[46] The default is "FALSE," so when not assuming homoscedasticity we can leave this information out of the "t.test" command.
[47] Despite the labels in Excel, These are not different variables, but rather different groups of the dependent variable.

This results in the following output:

F-Test two-sample for variances

	Control	Diet
Mean	126.7	105.9333333
Variance	585.3163265	109.8574713
Observations	50	30
df	49	29
F	5.327961037	
P(F<=f) one-tail	3.93744E–06	
F critical one-tail	1.777387217	

(b)

The "bottom line" in this output is the P-value ("P(F<=f) one-tail") for test of the hypothesis that the variances are equal in the population. Here, that value is equal to 3.93744×10^{-6}. Since the P-value is less than 0.05, we reject the null hypothesis. Thus, we need to use the analysis tool that does not assume homoscedasticity ("t-test: Two-Sample Assuming Unequal Variances" to perform a t-test testing the null hypothesis that the means are equal).

In R, we use the "var.test" command. These data are contained in a data set called "Example7_10," so we begin that command telling R where the data are listed. Also, as part of that command, we need to specify the one-sided alternative hypothesis.

>with (Example7_10,var.test(Control,Diet,alternative=c("greater")))

```
 F test to compare two variances

data: Control and Diet
F = 5.328, num df = 49, denom df = 29, p-value = 3.937e-06
alternative hypothesis: true ratio of variances is
 greater than 1
95 percent confidence interval:
 2.997637 Inf
sample estimates:
ratio of variances
 5.327961
```

The P-value in that output is the same as the one in the Excel output. This means that when using the "t.test" command in R, we will have to specify "var.equal=FALSE."

Now, we are ready to perform Student's t-test. In Excel, the "t-test: Two Sample Assuming Unequal Variances" procedure gives us the following dialog box:

(c)

From that procedure, we get the following output:

t-Test: Two-Sample Assuming Unequal variances		
	Control	Diet
Mean	126.7	105.9333333
Variance	585.3163265	109.8574713
Observations	50	30
Hypothesized mean difference	0	
df	72	
t Stat	5.297301517	
P(T<=t) one-tail	6.12668E-07	
t Critical one-tail	1.666293696	
P(T<=t) two-tail	1.22534E-06	
t Critical two-tail	1.993463567	

(d)

Here, the bottomline is the "two-tailed" P-value (1.22534×10^{-6}). Since this P-value is less than 0.05, we can reject the null hypothesis that the two means are equal in the population.

In R, we use the "t.test" command. As before, we need to specify the data are contained in the data set "Example7_10." Since we are unable to assume homoscedasticity, we also need to specify "var.equal=FALSE" in that command.[48]

>with (Example7_10,t.test(Control,Diet,var.equal=FALSE))

---

[48] Strictly speaking, we do not need to specify this, since it is the default.

```
Welch Two Sample t-test

data: Control and Diet
t = 5.2973, df = 72.469, p-value = 1.21e-06
alternative hypothesis: true difference in means is
not equal to 0
95 percent confidence interval:
 12.95268 28.58065
sample estimates:
mean of x mean of y
 126.7000 105.9333
```

The P-value from R is very close but not equal to the P-value from Excel. The reason they are not identical is that Excel and R use slightly different algorithms to calculate the degrees of freedom when we cannot assume homoscedasticity.   ■

In the next chapter, we will take a look at bivariable analysis of an ordinal dependent variable. These analyses are the nonparametric methods that correspond to the analyses presented in this chapter.

CHAPTER SUMMARY

In this chapter, we encountered bivariable data sets that contain a continuous dependent variable and an independent variable. In previous chapters, we discussed univariable data sets containing only a dependent variable. In those univariable data sets, our interest was in the dependent variable under all conditions. The independent variable in bivariable data sets, in contrast, specifies special conditions that focus our interest on values of the dependent variable. Continuous independent variables allow us to examine how values of the dependent variable are related to each value of the independent variable along a continuum. Nominal independent variables define two groups of values of the dependent variable between which we can compare estimates of parameters.

The first type of independent variable we examined in this chapter was a continuous independent variable. When we have a continuous dependent variable and a continuous independent variable, we might be interested in estimating dependent variable values that correspond to particular values of the independent variable. When this is our interest, we use linear regression analysis. Alternatively, (or in addition), we might be interested in determining the strength of the association between the variables. With this interest, we use correlation analysis.

Regression analysis can be used to estimate parameters of a straight line that mathematically describe how values of the dependent variable change corresponding to changes in the values of the independent variable. The equation for that straight line includes the intercept (the value of the dependent variable when the independent variable is equal to 0) and the slope (the amount the dependent variable changes for each unit change in the independent variable). The population's intercept is symbolized by α and its estimate from the sample by a. The population's slope is symbolized by β and the sample's estimate by b.

To understand hypothesis testing in regression analysis, it is helpful to understand sources of variation of data represented by the dependent variable. There are three sources of variation, each referred to as a sum of squares or, when divided by its degrees of freedom, as a mean square. The total mean square is the same as the univariable variance of data. The total variation has two components. One component is the variation in values of the dependent variable that is unexplained by the regression line. When this sum of squares is divided by its degrees of freedom, it is called the residual mean square. The other component is the variation in values of the dependent variable that is explained by the regression line. This source of variation is called the regression sum of squares or, when divided by its degrees of freedom (always equal to 1 for bivariable data sets), it is known as the regression mean square.

The residual mean square is used in estimation of the standard errors used in regression analysis. For hypothesis testing about the population's slope, the standard error is calculated from the residual mean square and the sum of squares of the independent variable.

Hypothesis testing for the slope or intercept uses Student's t-distribution. The number of degrees of freedom for that distribution is the number of degrees of freedom used in calculation of the residual mean square ($n - 2$).

In addition to testing specific hypotheses about the slope and intercept in regression analysis, we can test the omnibus hypothesis. The omnibus hypothesis is a statement that knowing values of the independent variable does nothing to improve estimation of values of the dependent variable. It is tested by examining the ratio of the regression mean square and the residual mean square. This ratio is known as the F-ratio.

The F-ratio has a special distribution known as the F-distribution. This distribution is related to Student's t-distribution, but it has two, instead of one, parameters for degrees of freedom. One parameter for degrees of freedom is associated with the numerator of the F-ratio (always equal to 1 when we have 1 independent variable), and the other is associated with the denominator of that ratio (equal to $n - 2$ when we have one independent variable). Table B.4 provides values from the F-distribution.

When the null hypothesis that knowing values of the independent variable does nothing to improve estimation of values of the dependent variable is true, we expect the F-ratio to be equal to 1, on the average. When that null hypothesis is false, the explained variation in values of the dependent variable (i.e., the regression mean square) will be greater than the unexplained variation (i.e., the residual mean square) in those values. Then, the F-ratio will be greater than 1. Thus, tests of hypotheses using the F-ratio are all one-tailed.

When we have only one independent variable, the F-ratio also tests the null hypothesis that the slope of the population's regression line is equal to 0. In fact, the square root of the F-ratio, in this case, is equal to Student's t-value that we would obtain if we tested the null hypothesis that the population's slope is equal to 0.

Alternatively, we might be interested in the way values of the dependent variable vary relative to variation in values of the independent variable. A measure of how two continuous variables vary together is the covariance. The covariance is the sum of the products of the differences between each value of a variable and its mean. Covariance has the desirable property of having a positive value when there is a direct relationship between the variables (as values of the independent variable increase, so do values of the dependent variable) and a negative value when there is an inverse relationship between the variables (as values of the independent variable increase, the values of dependent variables decrease). The magnitude of the covariance reflects the strength of the association between the independent and dependent variables.

The covariance, on the other hand, has a distinct disadvantage in that its magnitude is not only a reflection of the strength of the association between the independent and dependent variables, but is also affected by the scale of measurement. This disadvantage can be overcome by dividing the covariance by the square root of the product of the variances of the data represented by the two variables. The resulting value has a range from -1 to $+1$, with -1 indicating a perfect inverse relationship, $+1$ indicating a perfect direct relationship, and 0 indicating no relationship between the independent and dependent variables. This value is called the correlation coefficient. We symbolize the population's correlation coefficient with ρ (rho) and the sample's estimate of the correlation coefficient with r.

To evaluate the strength of the association between the independent and dependent variables, we square the correlation coefficient. The square of the correlation coefficient (symbolized by R^2) is known as the coefficient of determination. The coefficient of determination (or that coefficient times 100%) indicates the proportion (or percentage) of variation in the dependent variable that is associated with the independent variable.

Interval estimation of the correlation coefficient is not very commonly used in health statistics. More often, we encounter tests of the null hypothesis that the population's correlation coefficient is equal to 0 (indicating no association between the variables).

Since estimation of the standard error of the correlation coefficient requires estimation of the variances of the data represented by the independent and dependent variables, hypothesis testing involves conversion of the sample's observations to Student's t scale to take into account the influence of chance on those estimates. The number of degrees of freedom for that conversion is equal to the sample's size minus two. Two is subtracted from the sample's size because two variances of data in the population are estimated from the sample's observations.[49]

---

[49] Another way to think about this is that it take a minimum of three points to consider variation from a straight line.

For the correlation coefficient to have relevance, values of both the dependent and independent variables must be randomly sampled from the population of interest. The assumption that the dependent variable is randomly sampled from the population is universal to all statistical procedures. Few procedures assume that the independent variable is also randomly sampled (this is referred to as a naturalistic sample). The value of the correlation coefficient, however, can change dramatically as the distribution of the independent variable in the sample changes (such as can occur when a purposive sample is taken in which the distribution of values of the independent variable in the sample is under the control of the investigator).

A nominal independent variable separates values of the dependent variable into two groups. Comparison of values of the dependent variable between those two groups is accomplished by examining the difference between the means in the groups. The standard error for the difference between means is equal to the square root of the sum of the squares of the standard errors of the means in the groups.

In calculating the standard error for the difference between two means, we often assume that the variance of the data in the two groups is the same. This allows us to use all the observations in our sample to estimate a single variance. That estimate of the variance of data is a weighted average of the separate estimates in each group with their degrees of freedom as the weights. The resulting single estimate of the variance of data represented by the dependent variable is known as the pooled variance estimate.

Under the assumption that the variances of data are equal in the two groups, the pooled estimate of the variance is used in place of individual variances when calculating the standard error for the difference between means.

Hypothesis testing for the difference between means uses Student's t-distribution. The number of degrees of freedom is equal to the sum of the degrees of freedom in each of the two groups $(n - 2)$.

EXERCISES

7.1. Suppose we are interested in the relationship between nerve diameter and nerve conduction velocity. To investigate this relationship, we test nine nerves of various diameters. These data are in the Excel file EXR7_1.xls on the website accompanying this textbook. Analyze these data as a regression. Based on the results of this analysis, which of the following is the nerve conduction velocity you would expect for a nerve with a diameter of 10 μm?

A. 6
B. 8
C. 15
D. 32
E. 48

7.2. Suppose we are interested in the changes in diastolic blood pressure (DBP) related to age and make the observations in the Excel file called EXR7_2.xls on the website accompanying this textbook. Based on those data, perform a regression analysis. From those results what DBP would we expect, on the average, for persons who are 50 years old?

  A. 76
  B. 80
  C. 83
  D. 86
  E. 89

7.3. Suppose we are interested in the relationship between nerve diameter and nerve conduction velocity. To investigate this relationship, we test nine nerves of various diameters. These data are in the Excel file EXR7_1.xls on the website accompanying this textbook. Analyze these data as a regression. Based on the results of this analysis, test the null hypothesis that the intercept is equal to 0 in the population versus the alternative hypothesis that it is not equal to 0. If you allow a 5% chance of making a type I error, which of the following is the best conclusion to draw?

  A. Reject both the null and alternative hypotheses
  B. Accept both the null and alternative hypotheses
  C. Reject the null hypothesis and accept the alternative hypothesis
  D. Accept the null hypothesis and reject the alternative hypothesis
  E. It is best not to draw a conclusion about the null and alternative hypotheses from these observations

7.4. Suppose we are interested in the changes in diastolic blood pressure related to age and make the observations in the Excel file EXR7_2.xls on the website accompanying this textbook. Based on those data, perform a regression analysis. Test the null hypothesis that the slope is equal to 0 in the population versus the alternative hypothesis that it is not equal to 0. If we allow a 5% chance of making a type I error, which of the following is the best conclusion to draw?

  A. Reject both the null and alternative hypotheses
  B. Accept both the null and alternative hypotheses
  C. Reject the null hypothesis and accept the alternative hypothesis
  D. Accept the null hypothesis and reject the alternative hypothesis
  E. It is best not to draw a conclusion about the null and alternative hypotheses based on these observations

7.5. Suppose we are interested in the relationship between nerve diameter and nerve conduction velocity. To investigate this relationship, we test nine nerves of various diameters. These data are in the Excel file EXR7_1.xls on the website accompanying this textbook. Analyze these data as a regression. Based on the results of this analysis, test the null hypothesis that knowing nerve diameter does not help estimate nerve conduction velocity versus the alternative hypothesis that it does help. If you allow a 5% chance of making a type I error, which of the following is the best conclusion to draw?

A. Reject both the null and alternative hypotheses

B. Accept both the null and alternative hypotheses

C. Reject the null hypothesis and accept the alternative hypothesis

D. Accept the null hypothesis and reject the alternative hypothesis

E. It is best not to draw a conclusion about the null and alternative hypotheses based on these observations

7.6. Suppose we are interested in the changes in DBP related to age and make the observations in the Excel file EXR7_2.xls on the website accompanying this textbook. Based on those data, perform a regression analysis. From the results of the analysis, test the null hypothesis that knowing age does not help estimate DBP versus the alternative hypothesis that it does help. If you allow a 5% chance of making a type I error, which of the following is the best conclusion to draw?

A. Reject both the null and alternative hypotheses

B. Accept both the null and alternative hypotheses

C. Reject the null hypothesis and accept the alternative hypothesis

D. Accept the null hypothesis and reject the alternative hypothesis

E. It is best not to draw a conclusion about the null and alternative hypotheses based on these observations

7.7. Suppose we are interested in the relationship between nerve diameter and nerve conduction velocity. To investigate this relationship, we test nine nerves of various diameters. These data are in the Excel file EXR7_1.xls on the website accompanying this textbook. Analyze these data as a regression. Based on the results of that analysis, which of the following is an interval of values within which we are 95% confident that the slope in the population occurs?

A. −22.0 to 18.8

B. −2.9 to 6.9

C. 0.0 to 4.9

D. 2.9 to 6.9

E. 22.0 to 18.8

7.8. Suppose we are interested in the changes in DBP related to age and make the observations in the Excel file EXR7_2.xls on the website accompanying this textbook. Based on those data, perform a regression analysis. From the results of the analysis, which of the following is an interval of values within which we are 95% confident that the slope in the population occurs?

A. 0.42–0.57

B. 1.18–9.42

C. 2.59–21.52

D. 26.35–39.2

E. 50.60–60.86

7.9. Suppose we are interested in the relationship between nerve diameter and nerve conduction velocity. To investigate this relationship, we test eight nerves of various diameters. These data are in the Excel file EXR7_1.xls on the website accompanying this textbook. Analyze these data as a regression. Based on the results of that analysis, which of the following is the proportion of variation in nerve conduction velocity that is associated with differences in nerve diameter?

A. 0.756

B. 0.826

C. 0.890

D. 0.923

E. 0.991

7.10. Suppose we are interested in the changes in DBP related to age and make the observations in the Excel file EXR7_2.xls on the website accompanying this textbook. Based on those data, perform a regression analysis. Based on the results of that analysis, which of the following is the proportion of variation in DBP that is associated with differences in age?

A. 0.26

B. 0.44

C. 0.53

D. 0.61

E. 0.78

7.11. Suppose we are interested a diet designed to lower serum cholesterol. When we compare the amount of change in serum cholesterol between men and women, we make the observations in the Excel file EXR7_3 on the website accompanying this textbook. Use Excel or R to test the null hypothesis that the difference of the means of the changes in cholesterol is equal to 0 when comparing men and women in the population versus the alternative that it is not equal to 0. If we allow a 5% chance of making a type I error, which of the following is the best conclusion to draw?

A. Reject both the null and alternative hypotheses

B. Accept both the null and alternative hypotheses

C. Reject the null hypothesis and accept the alternative hypothesis

   D. Accept the null hypothesis and reject the alternative hypothesis

   E. It is best not to draw a conclusion about the null and alternative hypotheses based on these observations

7.12. Suppose we are interested in cholesterol levels among patients who had a myocardial infarction (cases) 14 days ago compared with patients who did not have a myocardial infarction (controls). The Excel file containing those data is EXR7_4 on the website accompanying this textbook. Use those data to compare the means between cases and controls. Test the null hypothesis that the difference of the means of the changes in cholesterol is equal to 0 when comparing cases and controls in the population versus the alternative that it is not equal to 0. If we allow a 5% chance of making a type I error, which of the following is the best conclusion to draw?

   A. Reject both the null and alternative hypotheses

   B. Accept both the null and alternative hypotheses

   C. Reject the null hypothesis and accept the alternative hypothesis

   D. Accept the null hypothesis and reject the alternative hypothesis

   E. It is best not to draw a conclusion about the null and alternative hypotheses based on these observations

7.13. Suppose we are interested a diet designed to lower serum cholesterol. When we compare the amount of change in serum cholesterol between men and women, we make the observations in the Excel file EXR7_3 on the website accompanying this textbook. Use Excel or R to calculate a 95% confidence interval for the difference between the means (men–women). Which of the following is closest to that interval?

   A. −0.62 to 15.58

   B. −0.58 to 15.44

   C. −0.10 to 16.13

   D. 0.00 to 15.72

   E. 0.92 to 15.26

7.14. Suppose we are interested in cholesterol levels among patients who had a myocardial infarction (cases) 14 days ago compared to patients who did not have a myocardial infarction (controls). The Excel file containing those data is EXR7_4 on the website accompanying this textbook. Which of the following is closest to an interval of estimates of the differences of the mean serum cholesterol between cases and controls (cases–controls) within which we can be 95% confident that the population's difference occurs?

   A. −3.2 to 53.5

   B. −1.0 to 44.4

   C. 0.0 to 38.2

   D. 1.0 to 44.4

   E. 3.2 to 53.5

CHAPTER 8

BIVARIABLE ANALYSIS OF AN ORDINAL DEPENDENT VARIABLE

When we begin a chapter that addresses an ordinal dependent variable, we can expect to see methods that we could use as nonparametric analyses for a continuous dependent variable. With that expectation, we look for methods that are parallel to those we encountered in Chapter 7. In that chapter, we learned about regression and correlation analyses for a continuous dependent variable with a continuous independent variable and about Student's t-test for a continuous dependent variable with a nominal independent variable.

If we look at Flowchart 6 with the expectation of finding nonparametric methods for regression, correlation, and Student's t-test, we will be disappointed. The most obvious feature of this flowchart is that it describes two, rather than three

Introduction to Biostatistical Applications in Health Research with Microsoft Office Excel® and R,
Second Edition. Robert P. Hirsch.
© 2021 John Wiley & Sons, Inc. Published 2021 by John Wiley & Sons, Inc.
Companion website: www.wiley.com/go/hirsch/healthresearch2e

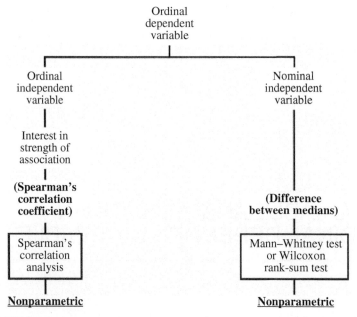

FLOWCHART 6 Flowchart showing bivariable analysis of an ordinal dependent variable. The point estimate that is most often used to describe the dependent variable is in bold. The common name of the statistical test is enclosed in a box. The general procedure that is used to test hypotheses and calculate confidence intervals is in bold and underlined.

types of statistical approaches. The missing method is a nonparametric approach that is parallel to regression analysis. There are no truly nonparametric methods for regression analysis. This is so because a slope cannot be defined for ordinal data.[1] Without a slope, we cannot have regression analysis, because regression analysis estimates values of the dependent variable corresponding to particular values of the independent variable.

8.1 ORDINAL INDEPENDENT VARIABLE

Even though we are unable to perform a regression analysis for an ordinal dependent variable, we still can consider the strength of the association between the dependent

[1]Recall from Chapter 7 that the slope tells us how much the value of the dependent variable changes for each unit change in the value of the independent variable. When the dependent variable is represented on an ordinal scale, we no longer consider how far apart dependent variable values are from each other; we only consider their rank order. Without considering how far apart dependent variable values are, we cannot think about how much the dependent variable values change. Thus, a slope has no meaning on an ordinal scale.

and independent variables. On an ordinal scale, however, the nature of the association is different from the association between two continuous variables.[2] On a continuous scale, an association has two properties. The first property of an association between two continuous variables is the consistency with which the values of the dependent variable change in a particular direction as the values of the independent variable increase.[3] The more consistent the direction of change in the values of the dependent variable, the stronger the association between the variables. The second property of an association between continuous variables is the consistency with which the numeric magnitude of the dependent variable values changes as the values of the independent variable increase. The more consistent the amount of the change in the values of the dependent variable as the values of the independent variable increase by a given amount, the stronger the association between the two variables.

Pearson's correlation coefficient is the correlation coefficient we use to assess the strength of the association between two continuous variables (see Equation (7.18)). A perfect association between two continuous variables is indicated by Pearson's correlation coefficient equal to 1 (+1 for a direct association or −1 for an inverse association). Figure 8.1 illustrates direct associations between two continuous variables and their corresponding values of Pearson's correlation coefficient.

In Figure 8.1, the only values that have a perfect association are those in which both the direction and the magnitude of the change in the values of the dependent variable are constant. When either the direction (▼s) or the magnitude (▲s) of the changes in the value of the dependent variable varies, the association is less than perfect. This is reflected by Pearson's correlation coefficient having a value closer to 0.

When we think about the association between two ordinal variables, the direction of the change in dependent variable values can be considered, but the magnitude of that change cannot. This is due to the fact that the magnitude of differences between data values is lost when continuous data are converted to an ordinal scale. This is illustrated in Figure 8.2.

So, a correlation coefficient for ordinal variables should take into account only in the direction of change in dependent variable values. There are several correlation coefficients that satisfy this criterion, but the one that is used most often in analysis of health research data is called **Spearman's correlation coefficient**. This correlation coefficient is the one that is most similar to Pearson's correlation coefficient, but is not influenced by the magnitude of changes in dependent variable values. In fact, Spearman's correlation coefficient can be calculated using the same equation that

---

[2]This difference will be true regardless of whether the independent variable is represented by a continuous or an ordinal variable. The convention, however, is to represent both variables on an ordinal scale.

[3]Recall from Chapter 7 that for a *direct* association, this would be the consistency with which the value of the dependent variable *increases* as the value of the independent variable increases. For an *inverse* association, this would be the consistency with which the value of the dependent variable *decreases* as the value of the independent variable increases.

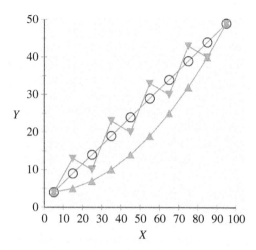

Figure 8.1   Scatter plot showing the aspects of an association between a continuous dependent variable (*Y*) and a continuous independent variable (*X*). The circles represent a perfect direct association between the variables: The value of the dependent variable increases by the same amount, as the value of the independent variable increases (*r* = 1.00). The ▲s represent an association in which the *magnitude* of the change in dependent variable values varies (*r* = 0.97). The ▼s represent an association in which the *direction* of change of the dependent variable values varies (*r* = 0.95).

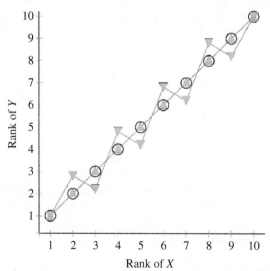

Figure 8.2   Scatter plot showing the continuous variables from Figure 8.1 when they are represented by their relative ranks. Now, both the circles (linear on the continuous scale) and the ▲s (changing magnitude on the continuous scale) represent perfect direct associations on an ordinal scale (r_s = 1.00). The ▼s (changing direction on the continuous scale), however, have an imperfect association on an ordinal scale (r_s = 0.95). This is because the ordinal scale has information about direction but not magnitude of an association.

is used to calculate Pearson's correlation coefficient (Equation (7.18)), substituting the ranks of the data values for the actual values of the data on the continuous scale. If there are no tied ranks,[4] Spearman's correlation coefficient is easier to calculate using the following shortcut equation[5]:

$$\rho_S \triangleq r_S = 1 - \frac{6 \cdot \sum d_i^2}{n \cdot (n^2 - 1)} \tag{8.1}$$

where

ρ_S = population's value of Spearman's correlation coefficient

r_S = sample's estimate of Spearman's correlation coefficient

d_i = difference between the rank of the dependent variable and the rank of the independent variable for the ith observation

n = sample's size

Later in the chapter we will discuss how Spearman's correlation coefficient can be estimated using this shortcut formula, but before we do that, let us consider how we can interpret its numeric value.

To begin with, let us recall from Chapter 7 how Pearson's correlation coefficient is interpreted. Pearson's correlation coefficient (r) is converted to a coefficient of variation (R^2) by squaring it. Then, the coefficient of variation is interpreted as the proportion of variation in the dependent variable that is associated with variation in the independent variable. Since Spearman's correlation coefficient is the same as Pearson's correlation coefficient, except that it is calculated from the ranks of the data, interpretation of Spearman's correlation coefficient is easier if we square it. Then, we can interpret the square of Spearman's correlation as the degree of association between the variables on an ordinal scale.[6]

Another aspect of the interpretation of Spearman's correlation coefficient is how it compares with the value of Pearson's correlation coefficient calculated on the same data. Usually, Spearman's correlation coefficient will be close to or larger (in absolute value) than Pearson's correlation coefficient. Keeping in mind that Pearson's correlation coefficient reflects the consistency in the change of magnitude of the dependent variable and Spearman's correlation coefficient is not affected by the magnitude of changes, we can interpret the relative values of these two correlation coefficients as a reflection of the consistency of the change in magnitude of the dependent variable. When the two correlation coefficients are close in value, this suggests that the magnitude of change of the dependent variable is consistent. This is illustrated by the ▾s in Figures 8.1 and 8.2. In other words, the relationship

---

[4] Recall from Chapter 5 that the term "tied ranks" refers to two (or more) data values that are equal to the same value on the continuous scale. Each of these observations is assigned the mean of the ranks they would be assigned if they had close, but not identical, values.

[5] If there are tied ranks, the "shortcut" is fairly complicated. In that circumstance, it is easier to use Equation (7.19), substituting the ranks for the data values.

[6] Strictly speaking, the square of Spearman's correlation indicates the proportion of variance in the ranks of the dependent variable that is associated with variation in the ranks of the independent variable.

between the dependent and independent variables is linear. If the value of Spearman's correlation coefficient is larger (in absolute magnitude) than the value of Pearson's correlation coefficient, it indicates that Pearson's correlation coefficient is affected by inconsistencies in the change in magnitude of the dependent variable.[7] That will be the case when the relationship between the variables is not linear. This is illustrated by the ▲s in Figures 8.1 and 8.2.

Now, let us take a look at an example of using the shortcut formula to estimate Spearman's correlation coefficient.

■ EXAMPLE 8.1

In Example 7.6, we calculated Pearson's correlation coefficient as a reflection of the strength of the association between dietary sodium intake and mean arterial blood pressure in a sample of 30 persons. That correlation coefficient was equal to 0.818. Now, let us use the shortcut formula (Equation (8.1)) to estimate Spearman's correlation coefficient for these data.

To begin with, we need to convert the data for both the independent and dependent variables to an ordinal scale. This is done by representing the data values with their relative ranks. This process is illustrated in the following table:

Patient	Dietary Sodium (X_i)	Rank of X_i	Arterial Pressure (Y_i)	Rank of Y_i	d_i	d_i^2
TH	1.0	1.0	78.0	5.5	−4.5	20.25
ER	2.3	2.0	93.0	8.5	−6.5	42.25
EI	2.9	3.0	75.0	4.0	−1.0	1.00
SN	5.2	4.0	97.0	10.0	−6.0	36.00
OT	5.4	5.0	62.0	1.0	4.0	16.00
HI	5.5	6.0	115.0	15.5	−9.5	90.25
NG	7.0	7.0	72.0	2.0	5.0	25.00
ON	8.4	8.0	93.0	8.5	−0.5	0.25
EA	9.0	9.0	74.0	3.0	6.0	36.00
RT	10.5	10.0	108.0	13.0	−3.0	9.00
HL	11.8	11.0	78.0	5.5	5.5	30.25
IK	13.3	12.0	92.0	7.0	5.0	25.00
EA	13.8	13.0	115.0	15.5	−2.5	6.25
NI	14.2	14.0	127.0	21.0	−7.0	49.00
CE	15.1	15.0	100.0	11.0	4.0	16.00
RE	16.9	16.0	101.0	12.0	4.0	16.00
GR	18.8	17.0	128.0	22.0	−5.0	25.00
ES	19.8	18.0	142.0	26.0	−8.0	64.00

---

[7]Sometimes, Pearson's correlation coefficient is larger (i.e., farther from 0) than Spearman's correlation coefficient. This happens when there is quite a bit of variation of independent variable values. For instance, this occurs when only extreme values of the independent variable are represented in the sample.

Patient	Dietary Sodium (X_i)	Rank of X_i	Arterial Pressure (Y_i)	Rank of Y_i	d_i	d_i^2
SI	20.0	19.0	110.0	14.0	16.0	256.00
ON	20.2	20.0	136.0	24.0	−5.0	25.00
TO	22.0	21.0	144.0	27.5	−7.5	56.25
CH	22.1	22.0	124.0	18.5	2.5	6.25
EE	23.3	23.0	140.0	25.0	−3.0	9.00
RS	24.1	24.0	126.0	20.0	3.0	9.00
TA	25.5	25.0	144.0	27.5	−3.5	12.25
TI	25.8	26.0	116.0	17.0	8.0	64.00
ST	27.8	27.0	152.0	29.0	−3.0	9.00
IC	28.0	28.0	124.0	18.5	8.5	72.25
IA	28.9	29.0	164.0	30.0	−2.0	4.00
NS	29.2	30.0	130.0	23.0	6.0	36.00
Total						1,068.50

Now, let us use Equation (8.1) to estimate Spearman's correlation coefficient.

$$\rho_S \triangleq r_S = 1 - \frac{6 \cdot \sum d_i^2}{n \cdot (n^2 - 1)} = \frac{6 \cdot 1,068.50}{30 \cdot (30^2 - 1)} = 0.762$$

In these data, there are five pairs of tied ranks. The presence of these tied ranks makes the estimate derived from the shortcut formula a biased estimate. Specifically, the estimate is closer to 0 than is the actual value of Spearman's correlation coefficient. If we were to use a method that corrects for these tied ranks, we would get 0.810; a value much closer to Pearson's correlation coefficient estimated for these data (0.818), but this formula is very complex. There is an easier way we will discuss next. ∎

We can use the method demonstrated in Example 8.1 if we need to estimate Spearman's correlation coefficient manually. In practice, however, we will be using a computer program to estimate Spearman's correlation coefficient. In Excel, we can calculate Spearman's correlation coefficient by converting the data to ranks using the "rank.avg" function (as we did in Example 5.2) and then using the "correl" function on the ranks. This results in Spearman's correlation coefficient regardless of the presence of tied ranks. In R, we can specify Spearman's correlation coefficient in the "cor" command. The next example demonstrates these processes.

■ **EXAMPLE 8.2**

In Example 8.1, we were interested in the strength of association between dietary sodium intake and mean arterial pressure. In Excel, these data are converted to a scale of ranks using the "rank.avg" function. The data set then appears as illustrated below:

Dietary Sodium (X_i)	Arterial Pressure (Y_i)	Rank of X	Rank of Y
1	78	1	5.5
2.3	93	2	8.5
2.9	75	3	4
5.2	97	4	10
5.4	62	5	1
5.5	115	6	15.5
7	72	7	2
8.4	93	8	8.5
9	74	9	3
10.5	108	10	13
11.8	78	11	5.5
13.3	92	12	7
13.8	115	13	15.5
14.2	127	14	21
15.1	100	15	11
16.9	101	16	12
18.8	128	17	22
19.8	142	18	26
20	110	19	14
20.2	136	20	24
22	144	21	27.5
22.1	124	22	18.5
23.3	140	23	25
24.1	126	24	20
25.5	144	25	27.5
25.8	116	26	17
27.8	152	27	29
28	124	28	18.5
28.9	164	29	30
29.2	130	30	23

If we were to use the "correl" function on the continuous variables, we would get 0.817842. This is Pearson's correlation coefficient. If we use that same function on the ranks, we get 0.809794. This is Spearman's correlation coefficient.

Determination of Spearman's correlation coefficient is more straightforward in R. We can use the "cor.test" command specifying "method=c("spearman")." This is illustrated below:

>with(Example7_1,cor.test(SODIUM,ARTPRES,method=c("spearman")))

```
Spearman's rank correlation rho

data: SODIUM and ARTPRESS
S = 854.97, p-value = 5.953e-08
alternative hypothesis: true rho is not equal to 0
sample estimates:
 rho
0.8097942
```

This gives us the same correlation coefficient we got using Excel.   ■

In Example 8.2, R provides us with a P-value testing the null hypothesis that Spearman's correlation coefficient in the population is equal to 0. If we estimate Spearman's correlation coefficient using a computer program that does not provide a P-value (e.g., Excel), we can test the null hypothesis that the correlation coefficient is equal to 0 in the population by using a statistical table. The next example shows how this is done.

■ EXAMPLE 8.3

In Example 8.2, we estimated Spearman's correlation coefficient to be 0.809794. Now, let us use a statistical table to test the null hypothesis that Spearman's correlation coefficient in the population is equal to 0.

We use Table B.5 to test this null hypothesis. Across the top of the table are one- and two-sided values of α. Sample sizes are listed down the left-most column. In the body of the table are the corresponding values of Spearman's correlation coefficient. The easiest way to use this table is to find the critical value for the correlation coefficient by identifying the row that corresponds to our sample's size ($n = 30$) and the column that corresponds to our selected value of α ($\alpha(2) = 0.05$). Where this row and column intersect, the critical value of Spearman's correlation coefficient is found.

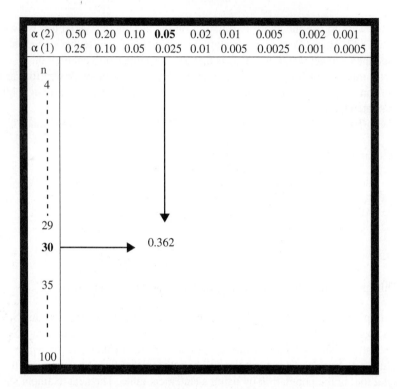

The critical value is equal to 0.362. Since our calculated value (0.809794) is greater than the critical value (0.362), we can reject the null hypothesis that there is no association between dietary sodium intake and mean arterial blood pressure in the population. ∎

In Chapter 7, we learned that the correlation coefficient in the sample can be assumed to estimate the correlation coefficient in the population only if the distribution of independent variable values in the sample represents their distribution in the population. A sample in which this is true is called a "naturalistic" sample. This principle applies to Spearman's correlation coefficient just as it does to Pearson's correlation coefficient. Thus, Spearman's correlation analysis should be used only when a naturalistic sample has been taken.

8.2   NOMINAL INDEPENDENT VARIABLE

When the independent variable represents nominal data, that independent variable divides dependent variable values into two groups. The purpose, then, is to compare those two groups. When we had a continuous dependent variable (i.e., in Chapter 7), we compared the means of the two groups by estimating their difference and by testing the null hypothesis that the difference between the means is equal to 0 in the population. Student's t-test was used to test this null hypothesis. The commonly used nonparametric tests that parallel Student's t-test are the **Mann–Whitney test** and the **Wilcoxon Rank-Sum test**.

Both the Mann–Whitney test and the Wilcoxon Rank-Sum test begin by converting the dependent variable values to an ordinal scale by ranking them. This ranking of dependent variable values is done regardless of the group to which the dependent variable values belong. We will see how this is done in the next example, but before we do so, we need to learn how to calculate and interpret statistics associated with each of those tests.

Calculations are easier for the Wilcoxon Rank-Sum test. All that is required is to add the ranks of the dependent variable values separately for each of the two groups of dependent variable values. An unusual feature of the Wilcoxon Rank-Sum test is that P-values get smaller for smaller values of the test statistic. Most statistics have just the opposite relationship with P-values: as those test statistics get larger, the P-values get smaller.[8]

The Mann–Whitney test gives us the same answer as the Wilcoxon Rank-Sum test, except that the Mann–Whitney test uses the sums of ranks in a calculation that produces a test statistic (U) that behaves as most test statistics do; namely, the P-value gets smaller as the test statistic gets larger. Equation (8.2) illustrates that calculation:

$$U = (n_1 \cdot n_2) + \frac{n_1 \cdot (n_1 + 1)}{2} - R_1 \qquad (8.2)$$

where

U = Mann–Whitney test statistic
n_1 = number of observations in group 1 (chosen arbitrarily)
n_2 = number of observations in group 2
R_1 = sum of the ranks of the dependent variable values in group 1

The choice of which group is considered to be group 1 in Equation (8.2) is arbitrary, but that choice affects the value of U. When we are performing a two-sided test, the Mann–Whitney test statistic is calculated both ways and then the larger of the two values is compared with the critical value in a table of Mann–Whitney test statistics.

---

[8] This is also true for the Wilcoxon Signed-Rank test that we encountered as the nonparametric parallel to the paired t-test in Chapter 4. There is no commonly used alternative to the Wilcoxon Signed-Rank test, but the Mann–Whitney test is a common alternative to the Wilcoxon Rank-Sum test.

To calculate the second value of U, Equation (8.2) can be used again, or the following shortcut formula can be used:

$$U' = (n_1 \cdot n_2) - U \qquad (8.3)$$

where

U' = Mann–Whitney test statistic value when the second group of dependent variable values is considered to be group 1

n_1 = number of observations in group 1

n_2 = number of observations in group 2

U = Mann–Whitney test statistic from Equation (8.2)

Now, let us take a look at an example of how to perform and interpret this non-parametric parallel to Student's t-test.

■ EXAMPLE 8.4

Suppose we were to compare blood pressure values between 12 persons who received a new medication intended to lower blood pressure and 8 persons who received standard therapy. Imagine that we observed the following results from that study:

New	Standard
130	137
114	130
121	143
127	146
115	134
124	150
113	142
110	138
126	
116	
125	
119	

Let us use these data to test the null hypothesis that blood pressure is the same in the two treatment groups.

To begin with, we need to convert the blood pressure values to an ordinal scale. We do that by ranking the dependent variable values from both groups. This is illustrated using Excel in the following table.

	A	B	C	D	E	F	G	H
1	New	Standard		IV	BP	Rank		
2	130	137		NEW	130	12.5		
3	114	130		NEW	114	3		
4	121	143		NEW	121	7		
5	127	146		NEW	127	11		
6	115	134		NEW	115	4		
7	124	150		NEW	124	8		
8	113	142		NEW	113	2		
9	110	138		NEW	110	1		
10	126			NEW	126	10		
11	116			NEW	116	5		
12	125			NEW	125	9		
13	119			NEW	119	6	78.5	=sum(F2:F13)
14				STD	137	15		
15				STD	130	12.5		
16				STD	143	18		
17				STD	146	19		
18				STD	134	14		
19				STD	150	20		
20				STD	142	17		
21				STD	138	16	131.5	=sum(F14:F21)

The sums of the ranks are equal to 78.5 in the new treatment group and 131.5 for the standard treatment group. If we were performing the Wilcoxon Rank-Sum test, we would compare the smaller of those sums (i.e., 78.5) to values in a table of Wilcoxon Rank-Sum test statistics. Alternatively, we can use those sums in Equation (8.2) to calculate the Mann–Whitney test statistic. Choosing the new treatment group as group 1, we get

$$U = (n_1 \cdot n_2) + \frac{n_1 \cdot (n_1 + 1)}{2} - R_1 = (12 \cdot 8) + \frac{12 \cdot 13}{2} - 78.5 = 95.5$$

The value of 95.5 is obtained if we arbitrarily assign the new treatment group to be group 1. If we had assigned the standard treatment group as group 1, we would have gotten the following test statistic (using Equation (8.3)):

$$U' = (n_1 \cdot n_2) - U = (12 \cdot 8) - 95.5 = 0.5$$

For a two-sided test, we select the larger of those two test statistics (95.5). Then, we compare that calculated value to the corresponding value in a table of Mann–Whitney U statistics (e.g., Table B.6).

Table B.6 has in its left-most column the number of observations in each of the two groups of dependent variable values. These are listed under the headings "n_S"

and "n_L." "n_S" corresponds to the group with the fewer observations and "n_L" corresponds to the group with the greater number of observations. In this example, the standard treatment group has eight observations and the new treatment group has 12 observations. Thus, we need to find the row that has eight in the "n_S" column and 12 in the "n_L" column. The critical value of the U statistic is in that row and in the column corresponding to a two-sided α of 0.05. This value is equal to 74.

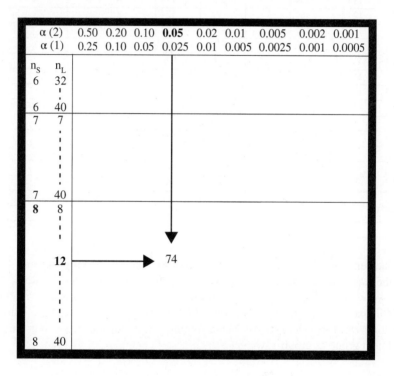

Since the calculated value of U (95.5) is greater than the critical value from the table (74), we can reject the null hypothesis and accept, through the process of elimination, the alternative hypothesis that the blood pressure is not the same in the two groups.

This can also be done in Excel or R. In Excel, the BAHR program "Nonparametric" can perform the Mann–Whitney test. The following is output analyzing the data in this example.

		Mann–Whitney Test			
Statistic =	95.5	z =	3.664705	P-value =	0.000248

That *P*-value is less than 0.05, so we can reject the null hypothesis and accept the alternative hypothesis. This is consistent with the result we got from performing the Mann–Whitney test by hand.

R performs the Wilcoxon Rank-Sum test using the "wilcox.test(group1,group2)" command. Specifying that these data are in a data set called "Example8_4," we get the following result:

>with(Example8_4,wilcox.test(New,Standard))

```
Wilcoxon rank sum test with continuity correction

data: New and Standard
W = 0.5, p-value = 0.0002862
alternative hypothesis: true location shift is not equal to 0
```

That *P*-value is less than 0.05, so we can reject the null hypothesis and accept the alternative hypothesis. This is consistent with the result we got from performing the Mann–Whitney test by hand and using Excel. ■

If the number of observations exceeds those in Table B.6, we can use a normal approximation to interpret Mann–Whitney statistics. The population's mean under the null hypothesis is:

$$\mu_U = \frac{n_1 \cdot n_2}{2} \tag{8.4}$$

Its standard error is:

$$\sigma_U = \sqrt{\frac{n_1 \cdot n_2 \cdot (n_1 + n_2 + 1)}{12}} \tag{8.5}$$

The test is:

$$z = \frac{U - \mu_U}{\sigma_U} \tag{8.6}$$

The next chapter is the last one on bivariable analysis. It discusses bivariable analysis of a nominal dependent variable.

CHAPTER SUMMARY

In Chapter 8, we discover a method of correlation analysis designed for an ordinal dependent variable and an ordinal independent variable. That procedure involves estimation and hypothesis testing for Spearman's correlation coefficient. We learned that there is no method of regression analysis for an ordinal dependent variable.

Spearman's correlation coefficient is calculated from data converted to ranks. Those data can be ordinal or continuous in their natural scale. When a Spearman's correlation coefficient is used to describe the strength of the association between two continuous variables, some of the assumptions of the continuous variable correlation coefficient (Pearson's correlation coefficient) are circumvented. Those assumptions concern the nature of the distributions of the variables. Another assumption of Pearson's correlation coefficient, that the relationship between the variables is linear, is also changed. Rather than assume a linear relationship between the variables on their natural (continuous) scale, we assume a linear relationship on an ordinal scale. This is much easier to achieve since it involves only a consistency in direction, not magnitude of dependent variable values.

Preparing to calculate Spearman's correlation coefficient, values of the dependent and independent variables are ranked separately. The easiest way to determine the value of Spearman's correlation coefficient is to use Excel to perform Pearson's correlation analysis on the ranked data or use R to perform Spearman's correlation analysis. If we wish to test the null hypothesis that the population's Spearman's correlation coefficient is equal to 0, hypothesis testing involves comparison of the sample's estimate of Spearman's correlation coefficient with a value in Table B.5 or use the P-value supplied by R.

When we have an ordinal dependent variable and a nominal independent variable, our interest is in comparing the two groups of dependent variable values defined by the two values of the nominal independent variable. When we considered a continuous dependent variable and a nominal independent variable in Chapter 7, we estimated the difference between means. In contrast, we make no estimates of the difference between the groups when we have an ordinal dependent variable. Therefore, point and interval estimation are not often used when the dependent variable is ordinal.

The method of statistical hypothesis testing we discussed in this chapter for an ordinal dependent variable and a nominal independent variable was the Mann–Whitney U test. We use this procedure to test the null hypothesis that the distribution of the dependent variable is the same in the two groups. The Mann–Whitney U statistic is calculated from the number of observations in each of the two groups and the sum of the ranks in one group (referred to as "group1"). The choice of group1 is arbitrary, but that choice will affect the value of the Mann–Whitney U statistic. So, we need to find out what the value of U would have been if we had selected the other group.

When we are considering a two-tailed alternative hypothesis, the appropriate value of the Mann–Whitney U statistic is the larger of U and U'. For a one-tailed hypothesis, the appropriate Mann–Whitney U statistic is calculated by choosing group 1 to be the group that is hypothesized to have the lower sum of ranks. The appropriate Mann–Whitney U value calculated from the observations in the sample is compared with a value in Table B.6 to complete statistical hypothesis testing.

An alternative to calculating the Mann–Whitney test statistic by hand is to use Excel. There you will find a program in the BAHR collection of programs provided with the textbook. Yet another alternative is to use R to perform the Wilcoxon Rank-Sum test. This gives us the same answer as the Mann–Whitney test.

EXERCISES

8.1. Suppose we are interested in a diet designed to lower serum cholesterol. When we compare the amount of change in serum cholesterol between men and women, we make the observations in the Excel file EXR7_3 on the website accompanying this textbook. Use the Mann–Whitney test to test the null hypothesis that the distribution of the changes in cholesterol is the same for men and women in the population versus the alternative that it is not the same. If we allow a 5% chance of making a type I error, which of the following is the best conclusion to draw?

A. Reject both the null and alternative hypotheses

B. Accept both the null and alternative hypotheses

C. Reject the null hypothesis and accept the alternative hypothesis

D. Accept the null hypothesis and reject the alternative hypothesis

E. It is best not to draw a conclusion about the null and alternative hypotheses based on these observations

8.2. Suppose we are interested in birth weights among mothers who have been exposed to second-hand smoke. The observations are in the Excel file EXR8_3 on the website accompanying this textbook. Test the null hypothesis that the distribution of birth weights is the same for exposed and unexposed mothers in the population versus the alternative that it is not the same using the Mann–Whitney test. If we allow a 5% chance of making a type I error, which of the following is the best conclusion to draw?

A. Reject both the null and alternative hypotheses

B. Accept both the null and alternative hypotheses

C. Reject the null hypothesis and accept the alternative hypothesis

D. Accept the null hypothesis and reject the alternative hypothesis

E. It is best not to draw a conclusion about the null and alternative hypotheses based on these observations

8.3. Suppose that we are interested in the association between the level of exercise each week and the amount of weight change over a four-week period. The Excel file containing these data is EXR8_1 on the website accompanying this textbook. Use Excel or R to perform a correlation analysis on the ranks of the variables. Which of the following is the estimate of Spearman's correlation coefficient?

A. −0.427

B. 0.000

C. 0.257

D. 0.427

E. 1.000

8.4. In a study of serum cholesterol levels among patients who had a myocardial infarction 14 days ago compared with those same patients who had a myocardial infarction 2 days ago. We find the data in the Excel file EXR8_2 on the website accompanying this textbook. Which of the following is Spearman's correlation coefficient comparing those measurements?

A. 0.12

B. 0.25

C. 0.39

D. 0.51

E. 0.69

8.5. Suppose that we are interested in the association between the level of exercise each week and the amount of weight change over a four-week period. The Excel file containing these data is EXR8_1 on the website accompanying this textbook. Test the null hypothesis that Spearman's correlation coefficient comparing variables is equal to 0 in the population versus the alternative hypothesis that it is not equal to 0. Which of the following is the best conclusion to draw?

A. Reject both the null and alternative hypotheses

B. Accept both the null and alternative hypotheses

C. Reject the null hypothesis and accept the alternative hypothesis

D. Accept the null hypothesis and reject the alternative hypothesis

E. It is best not to draw a conclusion about the null and alternative hypotheses based on these observations

8.6. In a study of serum cholesterol levels among patients who had a myocardial infarction 14 days ago compared with those same patients who had a myocardial infarction 2 days ago we find the data in the Excel file EXR8_2. Use Excel or R to test the null hypothesis that there is no association between the ranks of the measurements at 14 days compared to 2 days versus the alternative that there is an association. If we allow a 5% chance of making a type I error, which of the following is the best conclusion to draw?

A. Reject both the null and alternative hypotheses

B. Accept both the null and alternative hypotheses

C. Reject the null hypothesis and accept the alternative hypothesis

D. Accept the null hypothesis and reject the alternative hypothesis

E. It is best not to draw a conclusion about the null and alternative hypotheses based on these observations

CHAPTER 9

BIVARIABLE ANALYSIS OF A NOMINAL DEPENDENT VARIABLE

Nominal data, which can only be equal to either of two possible values, are the simplest type of data we encounter in health research. Even so, Flowchart 7 reveals a greater diversity of bivariable statistical methods for nominal dependent variables than we have seen for either continuous or ordinal dependent variables. The reason for this diversity is the simplicity of nominal data. Because nominal data are

Introduction to Biostatistical Applications in Health Research with Microsoft Office Excel® and R,
Second Edition. Robert P. Hirsch.
© 2021 John Wiley & Sons, Inc. Published 2021 by John Wiley & Sons, Inc.
Companion website: www.wiley.com/go/hirsch/healthresearch2e

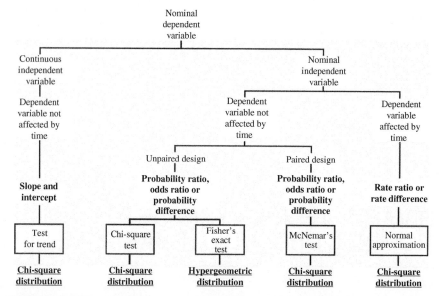

FLOWCHART 7   Flowchart showing bivariable analysis of a nominal dependent variable. The point estimate that is most often used to describe the dependent variable is in bold. The common name of the statistical test is enclosed in a box. The standard distributions that are used to test hypotheses and calculate confidence intervals are in bold and underlined.

comparatively simple, we understand these data better than other types of data. This better understanding allows us to interpret nominal dependent variables in a variety of ways. We will find this to be true especially when the independent variable also represents nominal data.

9.1   CONTINUOUS INDEPENDENT VARIABLE

When we are analyzing a set of data that has a nominal dependent variable and a continuous independent variable, our interest most often is in estimating the probability of the event addressed by the dependent variable (e.g., probability of cure) along the continuum of independent variable values (e.g., dose of medication). Figure 9.1 illustrates this sort of relationship graphically.

The implication in Figure 9.1 is that the relationship between the nominal dependent variable and the continuous independent variable is a linear (i.e., straight line) one. This is not the only possible relationship, but it is the one that is assumed by the **test for trend**, a statistical method that is often used to describe how the probability of the event represented by a nominal dependent variable changes as the value of a

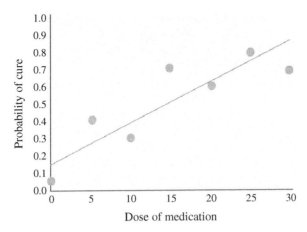

Figure 9.1   Scatter plot showing the relationship between a nominal dependent variable and a continuous independent variable.

continuous independent variable changes. Mathematically, this relationship can be described for the population as shown in Equation (9.1):

$$\theta = \alpha + (\beta \cdot X) \tag{9.1}$$

where

θ = probability of the event in the population when the independent variable is equal to X

α = population's intercept of the line, indicating the probability of the event when the continuous independent is equal to 0 in the population

β = population's slope of the line, indicating how much the probability of the event changes as the value of the independent variable increases by one-unit

X = value of the independent variable

Other than the fact that the dependent variable is represented by θ instead of by μ, Equation (9.1) looks like the population's regression equation we considered for a continuous dependent variable and a continuous independent variable in Chapter 7 (Equation (7.1)). Namely, dependent variable values are equal to the intercept plus the slope times the value of the independent variable.

9.1.1 Estimation

Not only does Equation (9.1) look like a regression equation, but also the parameters of that equation are estimated from the sample's observations in the same way as we estimate the parameters of a linear regression line. Specifically, we use the method of least squares, which minimizes the squared differences between observed and estimated values of the dependent variable.

An important difference between a continuous dependent variable and a nominal dependent variable is that a continuous dependent variable represents quantitative information (i.e., numeric magnitude), while a nominal dependent variable represents qualitative information (i.e., categories). A regression equation estimates the numeric magnitude of the dependent variable. Thus, to have a regression equation that relates to a nominal dependent variable, that nominal dependent variable must be represented numerically.

There are two ways to satisfy this need for a numeric representation of a nominal variable. One is to make multiple observations of the nominal dependent variable for each distinct value of the independent variable. Then, the number of times the event is observed among those multiple observations can be expressed as the probability of the event occurring when the independent variable is equal to that specific value. This approach is illustrated in the following example.

■ EXAMPLE 9.1

Suppose the data in Figure 9.1 are from a study in which we are interested in the probability that an infection is cured for different doses of an antibiotic. In this study, we randomly assign 10 persons to each of 7 doses of the antibiotic (1, 5, 10, 15, 20, 25, 30 mg). Imagine we observed the following results:

Dose in mg (X)	Number of Persons Observed (n)	Number of Persons Cured (a)
1	10	1
5	10	4
10	10	3
15	10	7
20	10	6
25	10	8
30	10	9

From these results, let us calculate the probability of being cured for each of the seven groups of observations.

The probability of having the event represented by a nominal dependent variable is calculated in the same way that we calculated univariable probabilities in Chapter 6 (Equation (6.2)). These calculations are summarized in the following table:

Dose in mg (X)	Number of Persons Observed (n)	Number of Persons Cured (a)	Probability of Cure (p)
1	10	1	0.1
5	10	4	0.4
10	10	3	0.3
15	10	7	0.7
20	10	6	0.6
25	10	8	0.8
30	10	9	0.9

The probabilities of being cured in this table correspond to the •s in Figure 9.1. ■

When this approach is used to represent a nominal dependent variable quantitatively, the sample's estimates of the slope and the intercept of the equation describing the association between the nominal dependent variable and the continuous independent variable (i.e., Equation (9.1)) are calculated as shown in Equations (9.2) and (9.3), respectively:

$$\beta \triangleq b = \frac{\sum n_i \cdot (p_i - \bar{p}) \cdot (X_i - \bar{X})}{\sum n_i \cdot (X_i - \bar{X})^2} \tag{9.2}$$

where

β = population's slope
b = sample's estimate of the slope
n_i = number of observations in the ith group
p_i = probability of the event in the ith group
$\bar{p}$ = probability of the event in all groups combined
X_i = independent variable value in the ith group
$\bar{X}$ = mean of the independent variable values in all groups combined

$$\alpha \triangleq a = \bar{p} - (b \cdot \bar{X}) \tag{9.3}$$

where

α = (alpha) population's intercept
a = sample's estimate of the intercept

The next example shows how this method can be used to estimate the slope and the intercept of the straight-line equation that describes the relationship between a nominal dependent variable and a continuous independent variable.

■ EXAMPLE 9.2

Let us estimate the parameters of the equation that describes the relationship between the probability of an infection being cured and the dose of an antibiotic for the data in Example 9.1.

To begin with, we need to estimate the mean of the independent variable values and the overall probability of the event. In preparation, we need to add up the number of events, the number of observations, and the product of the number of observations and the values of the independent variable (we need this product to calculate the mean of the independent variable values because each group has n_i observations of its independent variable value). The following table summarizes these calculations.

Dose in mg (X_i)	Number of Persons Observed (n_i)	Number of Persons Cured (a_i)	Probability of Cure (p_i)	$X_i \cdot n_i$
1	10	1	0.1	10
5	10	4	0.4	50
10	10	3	0.3	100
15	10	7	0.7	150
20	10	6	0.6	200
25	10	8	0.8	250
30	10	9	0.9	300
Total	70	38		1,060

Now, we can estimate the mean of the independent variable values as a weighted average (Equation (7.25)) with the number of observations as the weights.

$$\overline{X} = \frac{\sum n_i \cdot X_i}{\sum n_i} = \frac{1,060}{70} = 15.14 \text{ mg}$$

The overall probability of the event is:

$$\overline{p} = \frac{\sum a_i}{\sum n_i} = \frac{38}{70} = 0.54$$

Next, we use these two estimates to calculate the values we will need to estimate the slope and the intercept. The following table summarizes these calculations:

X_i	n_i	a_i	$X_i - \overline{X}$	$p_i - \overline{p}$	$n_i \cdot (X_i - \overline{X}) \cdot (p_i - \overline{p})$	$n_i \cdot (X_i - \overline{X})^2$
1	10	1	−14.14	−0.44	62.63	2,000.20
5	10	4	−10.14	−0.14	14.49	1,028.78
10	10	3	−5.14	−0.24	12.49	264.49
15	10	7	−0.14	0.16	−0.22	0.20
20	10	6	4.86	0.06	2.78	235.92
25	10	8	9.86	0.26	25.35	971.63
30	10	9	14.86	0.36	53.06	2,207.35
Total	70	38			170.57	6,708.57

Now, we are ready to use Equations (9.2) and (9.3) to estimate the slope and the intercept.

$$\beta \triangleq b = \frac{\sum n_i \cdot (p_i - \overline{p}) \cdot (X_i - \overline{X})}{\sum n_i \cdot (X_i - \overline{X})^2} = \frac{170.57}{6,708.57} = 0.025$$

$$\alpha \triangleq a = \overline{p} - (b \cdot \overline{X}) = 0.54 - (0.025 \cdot 15.14) = 0.158$$

These estimates of the slope and intercept can be used to estimate the probability of being cured for a particular dose. To make an estimate, the dose is substituted for X in the following equation (this is the sample's estimate of Equation (9.1)).

$$\theta = \alpha + (\beta \cdot X) \triangleq \hat{p} = a + (b \cdot X) = 0.158 + (0.025 \cdot X)$$

Thus, for a dose of 7.5 mg, we would expect to see the following proportion of the people treated with that dose to be cured.

$$\hat{p} = a + (b \cdot X) = 0.158 + (0.025 \cdot 7.5) = 0.35$$

In other words, we estimate that 35% of the people receiving a dose of 7.5 mg will be cured. ∎

We have taken a look at one way we can estimate the slope and intercept of the straight-line equation that we use in the test for trend to describe the relationship between a nominal dependent variable and a continuous independent variable. That was to represent the nominal dependent variable as the probability of the event occurring in a group of persons all of whom have the same, specific value of the continuous independent variable (e.g., they all have the same dose of medication).

Another way is to represent the nominal dependent variable numerically and, then use the same methods that were used in Chapter 7 to estimate the slope and the intercept for a continuous dependent variable.

The trick in this approach is to choose numeric values for the nominal dependent variable that are qualitative and not quantitative. We cannot represent the nominal dependent variable with numbers that convey any quantitative value, because nominal data are not quantitative. We cannot say, for instance, that having the event is twice the value used for not having the event. Instead, we need to select numeric values that separate those observations in which the event occurs from those observations in which the event does not occur without quantitative implication.

The key to solving this problem is to use zero to represent one value of the nominal dependent variable and the number one to represent the other value. When we do this, the numeric variable that represents the nominal variable is called an **indicator** (or **dummy**) **variable**. If we represent the nominal dependent variable with an indicator variable, then we can use linear regression calculations to estimate the slope and the intercept. This approach will give us exactly the same estimates as those obtained using the first method.[1]

If we are using a computer to estimate the slope and intercept for us, this second method becomes important. Neither Excel nor R, like most statistical packages, have a straightforward method for the test for trend. Instead, we can use the "Regression" analysis tool in Excel or the "lm(DV~IV)" command in R while representing the dependent variable with an indicator variable. The next example shows the result of using this approach for the data in Examples 9.1 and 9.2.

■ EXAMPLE 9.3

Let us use Excel to estimate the slope and intercept as part of a test for trend. To do this, we represent being cured with an indicator variable equal to 1 and not being cured with that indicator variable equal to 0. Then, we use Excel's "Regression" analysis tool with the indicator variable as the dependent variable. The data set then looks like the following:

---

[1]This second approach is the same as the first approach with each "group" containing only one observation. If the observation is an event, the probability of having the event in that "group" is equal to 1. If the observation is not an event, the probability of having the event in that "group" is equal to 0. Then, Equations (9.2) and (9.3) become identical to Equations (7.4) and (7.6), which were used to estimate the slope and the intercept for a continuous dependent variable.

	A	B	C
1	Dose	Result	Indicator
2	1	cure	1
3	1	not	0
4	1	not	0
5	1	not	0
6	1	not	0
7	1	not	0
8	1	not	0
9	1	not	0
10	1	not	0
11	1	not	0
12	5	cure	1
13	5	cure	1
14	5	cure	1
15	5	cure	1
16	5	not	0
17	5	not	0
18	5	not	0
19	5	not	0
20	5	not	0
21	5	not	0
22	10	cure	0
23	10	cure	0
24	10	cure	0
25	10	not	0
26	10	not	0
27	10	not	0
28	10	not	0
29	10	not	0
30	10	not	0
31	10	not	0
32	15	cure	1
33	15	cure	1
34	15	cure	1
35	15	cure	1
36	15	cure	1

	A	B	C
37	15	cure	1
38	15	cure	1
39	15	not	0
40	15	not	0
41	15	not	0
42	20	cure	1
43	20	cure	1
44	20	cure	1
45	20	cure	1
46	20	cure	1
47	20	cure	1
48	20	not	0
49	20	not	0
50	20	not	0
51	20	not	0
52	20	cure	1
53	25	cure	1
54	25	cure	1
55	25	cure	1
56	25	cure	1
57	25	cure	1
58	25	cure	1
59	25	cure	1
60	25	not	0
61	25	not	0
62	30	cure	1
63	30	cure	1
64	30	cure	1
65	30	cure	1
66	30	cure	1
67	30	cure	1
68	30	cure	1
69	30	cure	1
70	30	cure	1
71	30	not	0

Then, the "Regression" dialog box looks like the following:

And, the output looks like the following:

Summary output						
Regression statistics						
Multiple R	0.499658748					
R Square	0.249658864					
Adjusted R square	0.238624436					
Standard error	0.437817069					
Observations	70					
ANOVA						
	df	*SS*	*MS*	*F*	*Significance F*	
Regression	1	4.336931127	4.336931127	22.62544589	1.06463E–05	
Residual	68	13.03449744	0.191683786			
Total	69	17.37142857				
	Coefficients	*Standard error*	*t Stat*	*P-value*	*Lower 95%*	*Upper 95%*
Intercept	0.157836457	0.096386181	1.63754238	0.106136998	–0.034499173	0.350172087
Dose	0.025425894	0.005345369	4.756621268	1.06463E–05	0.014759377	0.036092412

Most of the information in this output is not applicable to analysis of a nominal dependent variable, but the estimates of the intercept and slope are the same as those calculated in the test for trend in Example 9.2.

In R, we can use the "lm(DV~IV)" command to estimate the slope and the intercept.

>with (Example9_3,lm(Indicator~Dose)

```
Call:
lm(formula = Indicator ~ Dose)

Coefficients:
(Intercept)          Dose
    0.15784       0.02543
```

These estimates are the same as those we obtained using Excel.   ∎

The t-values in the output in Example 9.3 that test the null hypotheses (that the slope or intercept are equal to 0 in the population) are not interpretable for a nominal dependent variable. Similarly, the F-ratio that tests the omnibus null hypothesis is not interpretable for a nominal dependent variable.[2] Instead, we need to use a special procedure to test these null hypotheses. This procedure is what we will consider next.

9.1.2   Hypothesis Testing

Although the methods for estimating the slope and the intercept in the test for trend are the same as the methods used for regression analysis of a continuous dependent variable, the method for testing hypotheses is not the same. When we discussed regression analysis in Chapter 7, one method of hypothesis testing we encountered used an F-ratio to compare the regression mean square (the average explained variation in the dependent variable) with the residual mean square (the average unexplained variation in the dependent variable) as shown in Equation (7.17). The F-ratio, however, cannot be applied to a nominal dependent variable.[3]

The null hypothesis of interest in the test for trend is that the independent variable does not help estimate the probability of the event. This is parallel to the omnibus

---

[2]The reason these tests are inappropriate for a nominal dependent variable is that both the t- and F-distributions take into account the role of chance in estimating the variance of dependent variable values in the population. With a nominal dependent variable, however, there is no independent role of chance in estimating the variance. This was addressed in Chapter 6 where the normal approximation to the binomial was discussed.

[3]Use of a single value for the unexplained variation in the dependent variable (i.e., a single error mean square) requires the assumption that the unexplained variation is the same regardless of the value of the independent variable. This is the assumption of homoscedasticity. When we learned about the normal approximation to the binomial in Chapter 6, however, we found that the variation of a nominal dependent variable changes as the probability of the event changes. Thus, it does not make sense to assume homoscedasticity in hypothesis testing for a nominal dependent variable.

null hypothesis in regression analysis.[4] We test this null hypothesis for a nominal dependent variable by comparing the amount of variation in the dependent variable values that is explained by the relationship with the independent variable (i.e., "regression") to the univariable (i.e., "total") variance of dependent variable values. These values are the same as the regression sum of squares and the total mean square in regression analysis. They are compared as a ratio, but it is not an F-ratio. Instead, it is a **chi-square** statistic. Equation (9.4) shows us how this chi-square statistic is calculated from the output of the "Regression" analysis tool or when groups of observations are made for each value of the independent variable:

$$\chi^2 = \frac{\sum n_i \cdot (\hat{p}_i - \bar{p})^2}{\bar{p} \cdot (1 - \bar{p})} = \frac{\text{regression sum of squares}}{\text{total mean square}} \tag{9.4}$$

where

χ^2 = chi-square statistic

n_i = number of observations in the ith group

$\hat{p}_i$ = estimated probability of the event in the ith group

p_i = observed probability of the event in the ith group

$\bar{p}$ = overall probability of the event (for all groups combined)

The chi-square distribution is a member of the Gaussian family of standard statistical distributions. This is the fourth member of that family we have encountered.[5] The first of these was the standard normal distribution, which is a Gaussian distribution with a mean equal to 0 and a standard deviation equal to 1 (Chapter 2). The chi-square distribution comes from the standard normal distribution, but is distinguished from it by two features. First, the chi-square values are the square of standard normal deviates.[6] This is to prevent the occurrence of negative values. Second, an additional parameter is added to the mean and standard deviation of the standard normal distribution. This parameter is called **degrees of freedom**. These degrees of freedom reflect how much information the sample contains for estimation of the probability of the event. That amount of information is equal to the number of independent variables. In bivariable analysis, we have only one independent variable. Thus, the number of degrees of freedom for chi-square statistics in bivariable analysis is equal to 1.[7]

---

[4]Recall from Chapter 7 that the test of the omnibus null hypothesis in bivariable regression analysis is the same as testing the null hypothesis that the slope is equal to 0 in the population. The same is true when the dependent variable represents nominal data. The test of this parallel hypothesis also tests the null hypothesis that the slope in Equation (9.1) is equal to 0.

[5]The other members of the Gaussian family we have encountered are the standard normal, Student's t-distribution, and the F-distribution.

[6]We encountered this feature in Chapter 6 when we tested the null hypothesis that the proportion of persons in the population preferring one thing over another is equal to 0.5.

[7]This is the same as the degrees of freedom in the numerator of the F-ratio used to test the omnibus hypothesis in regression analysis with a continuous dependent variable (Equation (7.17))

Now, we are ready to take a look at an example of how we can perform hypothesis testing in the test for trend.

■ EXAMPLE 9.4

Let us test the null hypothesis that knowing a patient's dose of antibiotic does not help to estimate the probability that the patient's infection will be cured. As an alternative hypothesis, let us consider that knowing the dose does help estimate the probability of cure. Also, suppose we are willing to take a 5% chance of making a type I error.

To calculate the chi-square statistic in Equation (9.4), we need the regression sum of squares and the total mean square. Excel gives us the regression sum of squares but not the total mean square. If we were to rely on output from Excel, we would have to calculate the total mean square by dividing the total sum of squares by the total degrees of freedom.

R also can give us the information we need to calculate the chi-square statistic in Equation (9.4). We can get that information using the "summary.aov" command as follows:

>with Example9_4,summary.aov(lm(Indicator~Dose)))

```
            Df Sum Sq Mean Sq F value   Pr(>F)
Dose         1  4.337   4.337   22.62 1.06e-05 ***
Residuals   68 13.034   0.192
---
Signif. codes:  0 '***' 0.001 '**' 0.01 '*' 0.05 '.' 0.1 ' ' 1
```

Here, the regression degrees of freedom, sum of squares, and mean square are labeled with the name of the independent variable. Also, the total degrees of freedom and sum of squares is missing. You can calculate those values by adding the regression and residual values. Then, the total mean square can be calculated by dividing the total sum of squares by the total degrees of freedom.

From the output in Example 9.3, we know that these values are 4.336931127 for the regression sum of squares, 17.37142857 for the total sum of squares, and 69 for the total degrees of freedom. Substituting these values in Equation (9.4), we get the following result:

$$\chi^2 = \frac{\text{regression sum of squares}}{\text{total mean square}} = \frac{4.336931127}{17.37142857/69} = 17.23$$

To evaluate a chi-square statistic, we compare our calculated value with a value in a table of the chi-square distribution that corresponds to $\alpha = 0.05$ and one degree of freedom. Table B.7 is such a table. From that table, we find that the critical value of chi-square is equal to 3.841.

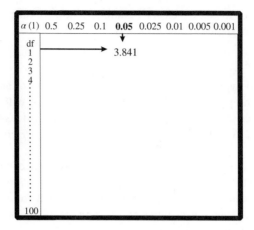

Since the calculated chi-square value (17.23) is greater than the critical value (3.841), we can reject the null hypothesis that knowing dose does not help us in estimating the probability of cure and accept, through the process of elimination, the alternative hypothesis that knowing the dose helps in estimating the probability of cure.

The test for trend can also be performed in R using the "prop.trend.test" command. In this test, Example9_1a contains the number of observations at each dose and Example9_1b contains the number cured at each dose. The values of the independent variable are given as scores.

>prop.test.trend(Example9_1b,Example9_1a,score=c(1,5,10,15,20,25,30))

```
Chi-squared Test for Trend in Proportions

data:  Example9_1b out of Example9_1a ,
 using scores: 1 5 10 15 20 25 30
X-squared = 17.476, df = 1, p-value = 2.909e-05
```

This chi-square is very close to the one we got using the results of a regression analysis. R uses a different method to approximate this chi-square. ∎

9.2 NOMINAL INDEPENDENT VARIABLE

A look at Flowchart 7 reveals that there are a variety of methods for estimation and hypothesis testing when both the dependent and independent variables represent nominal data. The choice of methods is determined in part by whether the nominal dependent variable is affected by time. What it means for a nominal dependent variable to be affected by time was discussed in Chapter 6, when we were thinking about univariable analysis of a nominal dependent variable. In essence, we use rates, rather than probabilities, to represent events when more events are observed the longer we look for them and if we have looked longer in some cases than in others. In the current chapter, we will begin by thinking about dependent variables that are not affected by time and, then we will see how these methods apply to nominal dependent variables affected by time.

9.2.1   Dependent Variable Not Affected by Time: Unpaired Design

When the independent variable represents nominal data and the nominal dependent variable is not affected by time, there is another distinction between the statistical methods we use—whether the data were collected in a paired or in an unpaired design. The choice of design affects hypothesis testing and some estimation processes. First, we will consider the unpaired design. Then, we will see how a paired design affects these statistical methods.

9.2.1.1   Estimation. A nominal independent variable has the effect of dividing dependent variable values into two groups; we want to compare estimates of the population's parameters between these groups. When the nominal dependent variable is not affected by time, the parameter estimates we compare are probabilities or related measures.

In Chapter 7, we compared means by looking at the difference between two means. The reason we took this approach is that differences between means are easier for the statistician to consider than are ratios of means. The same is true of probabilities: differences between probabilities are easier for the statistician to interpret than are ratios of probabilities. Even so, we often wish to compare two probabilities by looking at their ratio, especially when these probabilities are measures of disease frequency (i.e., prevalence or risk).

The reason for this interest in ratios is that probabilities that reflect disease frequency are usually small in numeric magnitude. When we take the difference between two small probabilities, the difference is also a small number. Ratios of small probabilities, on the other hand, can be large. For example, suppose that the risk of developing lung cancer during a certain period of time is 0.00001 if you smoke and 0.000001 if you do not smoke. The difference between those probabilities is 0.000009. This gives us a very different perspective on the risk of lung cancer among smokers compared to nonsmokers than if we examined the ratio of these two probabilities. That ratio is equal to 10. This implies that smokers are at 10 times the risk of developing lung cancer than are nonsmokers!

Neither of our choices (a difference or a ratio of probabilities or rates) is the better choice in all applications. Which measure we choose to reflect the relationship between two groups of nominal data depends on the question we are asking.

If we are interested in the *actual* distinction between two groups of nominal dependent variable values, we should estimate the difference between probabilities or rates. For example, if we wish to determine the practicality of treating two diseases, we would want estimates that reflected both the efficacy of the treatments and the underlying risks of the diseases. In this application, we would be more impressed with the treatment of a disease with a relatively large difference between the probabilities of recovery than we would be for a disease with a small difference, even if

TABLE 9.1. A General 2 × 2 Table for the Organization of Observations of a Nominal Dependent Variable and a Nominal Independent Variable

		Outcome		
		Event	No Event	
Group	Group 1	a	b	$a+b$
	Group 2	c	d	$c+d$
		$a+c$	$b+d$	n

the ratios of those probabilities were the same for the two diseases (e.g., probabilities of recovery of 0.000001 and 0.0000001 versus probabilities of recovery of 0.01 and 0.1).

If, on the other hand, we are interested in the *relative* distinction between two groups of nominal dependent variable values, we should estimate the ratio of probabilities or rates. For example, if we wish to determine how strongly a particular exposure is associated with a disease, we would not want estimates that reflect the underlying frequency of the disease. In this application, it does not matter if the event is rare or common in a particular population, the biologic relationship is the same.

When we have a nominal dependent variable and a nominal independent variable, we have a particular way in which we organize our observations in preparation for analysis. This organization is called a **contingency table** or, more commonly, a **2 × 2 table** (pronounced "2 by 2" table). A 2 × 2 table contains two rows and two columns. Although it is not a rule that is consistently followed in the medical literature, most persons expect columns to correspond to the event (e.g., disease) and the rows to correspond to the groups (e.g., exposure). Table 9.1 shows a general 2 × 2 table set up in that way.

The frequencies in each of the four boxes (called **cells**) in the 2 × 2 table are called the **cell frequencies**. a, b, c, and d represent these cell frequencies. The frequencies on the outside of the 2 × 2 table are called the **marginal frequencies**. Each of the marginal frequencies is equal to the sum of two cell frequencies, except the one in the lower right corner. There, we find the sample's size.

With our observations arranged in a 2 × 2 table, calculation of probabilities and their differences and ratios is rather straightforward. For example, the probability of the event in group 1 is $a/(a+b)$ and the probability of the event in group 2 is $c/(c+d)$. Thus, the difference between and the ratio of two probabilities can be expressed using the notation from a 2 × 2 table as shown in Equations (9.5) and (9.6), respectively[8]:

$$\text{Probability difference} = \theta_1 - \theta_2 \triangleq p_1 - p_2 = \frac{a}{a+b} - \frac{c}{c+d} \qquad (9.5)$$

[8] These equations assume that the 2 × 2 table is arranged as shown in Table 9.1.

where

$\theta_1 - \theta_2$ = difference between the probabilities of the event in the population

$p_1 - p_2$ = difference between the probabilities of the event in the sample

a = number of observations in group 1 with the event

b = number of observations in group 1 without the event

c = number of observations in group 2 with the event

d = number of observations in group 2 without the event

$$\text{Probability ratio} = \frac{\theta_1}{\theta_2} \triangleq \frac{p_1}{p_2} = \frac{a/(a+b)}{c/(c+d)} \tag{9.6}$$

where

$\dfrac{\theta_1}{\theta_2}$ = ratio of the probabilities of the event in the population

$\dfrac{p_1}{p_2}$ = ratio of the probabilities of the event in the sample

Now, let us take a look at an example in which we calculate and interpret a probability difference and a probability ratio.

■ EXAMPLE 9.5

In a clinical trial of a treatment for coronary artery disease, 100 persons were given the experimental treatment and 36 of them died within the study period. In addition, another 100 persons were given the standard treatment and, of those persons, 54 died within the same period of time. Let us compare the risk of dying with the experimental treatment to the risk of dying with the standard treatment.

First, let us organize these observations in a 2 × 2 table.

		Outcome		
		Died	Survived	
Treatment	Standard	54	46	100
	New	36	64	100
		90	110	200

The risks of death for those two treatment groups are:

$$p(\text{death}|\text{standard treatment}) = \frac{a}{a+b} = \frac{54}{100} = 0.54$$

$$p(\text{death}|\text{new treatment}) = \frac{c}{c+d} = \frac{36}{100} = 0.36$$

BIVARIABLE ANALYSIS OF A NOMINAL DEPENDENT VARIABLE

We can compare these risks either by examining their difference or by examining their ratio. If we were interested in the practicality of the new treatment (i.e., taking into account the number of lives saved), it would be better to examine the risk difference (Equation (9.5)) than the risk ratio, since the risk difference takes into account the underlying risk of death in coronary artery disease patients.

$$\theta_1 - \theta_2 \triangleq p_1 - p_2 = p(\text{death}|\text{standard treatment}) - p(\text{death}|\text{new treatment})$$
$$= 0.54 - 0.36 = 0.18$$

This risk difference tells us that for every 100 patients receiving the new treatment, 18 (or 18%) more persons will survive the period of time studied than would have survived that period of time if they had been given the standard treatment.

If, on the other hand, we are interested in the relative efficacy of the new treatment compared to the standard treatment (i.e., the biologic relationship), the risk ratio (Equation (9.6)) is the better choice, since it is not influenced by the underlying risk of death in coronary artery disease patients.

$$\frac{\theta_1}{\theta_2} \triangleq \frac{p_1}{p_2} = \frac{p(\text{death}|\text{standard treatment})}{p(\text{death}|\text{new treatment})} = \frac{0.54}{0.36} = 1.50$$

This risk ratio tells us that the risk of death (in the period of time studied) for persons given the standard treatment is 1.5 times the risk of death for persons given the new treatment.

As a further demonstration of the distinction between a probability difference and a probability ratio, let us change the underlying risk of death in the sample from 0.45 (90/200) to 0.225 (45/200); half of what it was. Then, the 2 × 2 table would be:

		Outcome		
		Died	Survived	
Treatment	Standard	27	73	100
	New	18	82	100
		45	155	200

Now, the risks of death for those two treatment groups are

$$p(\text{death}|\text{standard treatment}) = \frac{a}{a+b} = \frac{27}{100} = 0.27$$
$$p(\text{death}|\text{new treatment}) = \frac{c}{c+d} = \frac{18}{100} = 0.18$$

Finally, let us use Equation (9.5) to estimate the risk difference and Equation (9.6) to estimate the risk ratio from the data in this 2 × 2 table.

$$\theta_1 - \theta_2 \triangleq p_1 - p_2 = p(\text{death}|\text{standard treatment}) - p(\text{death}|\text{new treatment})$$
$$= 0.27 - 0.18 = 0.09$$

$$\frac{\theta_1}{\theta_2} \triangleq \frac{p_1}{p_2} = \frac{p(\text{death}|\text{standard treatment})}{p(\text{death}|\text{new treatment})} = \frac{0.27}{0.18} = 1.50$$

Reducing the overall risk of death reduced the risk difference to the same degree. Instead of preventing 18 out of 100 (18%) deaths by using the new treatment, now only 9 out of 100 (9%) deaths are prevented. This change is not because of a change in efficacy (the risk of death is still 1.5 times as likely using the standard treatment), but instead due to a reduction of the risk of death regardless of which treatment is used. The risk ratio is unchanged. ■

In addition to probabilities and rates, nominal dependent variables can be expressed as **odds**. Odds are the number of observations that had the event divided by the number of observations that did not have the event (Equation (9.7)):

$$\text{Odds of event in group } 1 = \frac{\text{events in group } 1}{\text{nonevents in group } 1} = \frac{a}{b} \qquad (9.7)$$

Odds are not rates, because they do not contain time in the denominator. Neither are odds probabilities, because the numerator is not contained in the denominator. When the probability of an event is small, however, odds have a value that is very close to the value of the probability of the event. For example, if the probability of an event is 0.5, this implies that, for every two observations, one observation will have the event and the other observation will not. The odds for that event would be equal to 1/1 or 1.0. If, on the other hand, the probability of an event is 0.05, then only 1 out of every 20 observations would have the event and the remaining 19 of those 20 observations would not. The odds of that event would be equal to 1/19 or 0.053, which is much closer to the corresponding probability.

We did not discuss odds in Chapter 6 when we were thinking about univariable samples with a nominal dependent variable because odds are used in health statistics only to compare nominal dependent variables between groups. Then, the odds of an event in the two groups are compared only as a ratio. This ratio is called an **odds ratio**. Equation (9.8) illustrates how the odds ratio is estimated from 2 × 2 table data:

$$\text{OR} \triangleq \widehat{\text{OR}} = \frac{\text{odds of event in group } 1}{\text{odds of event in group } 2} = \frac{a/b}{c/d} = \frac{a \cdot d}{b \cdot c} \qquad (9.8)$$

where

OR = ratio of the odds of the event in the population
$\widehat{\text{OR}}$ = ratio of the odds of the event in the sample
  a = number of observations in group 1 with the event
  b = number of observations in group 1 without the event
  c = number of observations in group 2 with the event
  d = number of observations in group 2 without the event

Now, let us take a look at an example of calculating and interpreting an odds ratio.

■ **EXAMPLE 9.6**

In Example 9.5, we looked at data from a clinical trial of a new treatment for coronary artery disease. Those data are summarized in the following table.

		Outcome		
		Died	Survived	
Treatment	Standard	54	46	100
	New	36	64	100
		90	110	200

Let us calculate an odds ratio to reflect the association between treatment group and outcome.

To calculate the odds ratio, we use Equation (9.8):

$$\text{OR} \triangleq \widehat{\text{OR}} = \frac{\text{odds of death in group 1}}{\text{odds of death in group 2}} = \frac{a/b}{c/d} = \frac{a \cdot d}{b \cdot c} = \frac{54 \cdot 64}{46 \cdot 36} = 2.09$$

The odds ratio tells us that the odds of dying if someone receives the standard treatment is about twice the odds of dying if someone receives the new treatment.   ■

The odds ratio is an important estimate of the relationship between two groups of nominal variables for several reasons. To the statistician, odds ratios are attractive because they have statistical properties that make analyses easier to develop. To the health researcher, odds ratios are attractive because they are less affected by certain types of bias[9] and because they are the only sensible way to compare nominal dependent variables in **case–control studies**.

A case–control study is a very useful approach to studying common characteristics (that we call risk factors) and their relationships with rare diseases. In this type of study, the researcher identifies a certain number of persons with the disease (the cases) and a certain number of persons without the disease (the controls). Since disease status defines the groups to be compared, the independent variable in a case–control study is an indicator of whether a person is a case or a control. In case–control studies, the researcher always determines the numbers of cases and

---

[9]For example, samples' odds ratios are unbiased estimates of the population's odds ratio under the condition of nondifferential (i.e., the same in both groups) sampling bias. If nondifferential sampling bias exists, however, sample estimates of differences and ratios of probabilities and rates are biased estimates of their corresponding population's values.

TABLE 9.2. A 2 × 2 Table for Observations from a Case–Control Study[a]

		Disease Group		
		Case	Control	
Risk Factor	Exposed	a	b	$a + b$
	Not Exposed	c	d	$c + d$
		$a + c$	$b + d$	n

[a] Here, disease status is the independent variable and the presence or absence of some characteristic (called a risk factor) is the dependent variable.

controls to be included.[10] Thus, case–control studies always use purposive sampling.

Once cases and controls have been identified, the researcher determines the frequency of some characteristic (or risk factor) believed to influence the occurrence of the disease of interest. Since the frequency of the risk factor is what is being determined here, the dependent variable in a case–control study is the presence or absence of this risk factor. At first, this might seem to be backward since, as health researchers, we are primarily interested in disease frequency, not presence or absence of some risk factor. It is important to recognize, however, that the dependent variable must be randomly sampled from the population. In a case–control study, only the presence or absence of the risk factor meets this criterion.

Table 9.2, shows observations from a case–control study arranged in a 2 × 2 table.

The next example shows the calculation and interpretation of an odds ratio in a case–control study.

■ EXAMPLE 9.7

Suppose we conducted a case–control study of the relationship between consumption of a particular food preservative and stomach cancer. In this study, we identified 100 persons with stomach cancer and 100 persons without stomach cancer and asked them about their consumption of food containing the preservative. Among those persons with stomach cancer, 25 ate foods containing the preservative. Among those persons without stomach cancer, 14 ate foods containing the preservative. Let us compare the odds of consumption of the preservative between cases and controls.

---

[10] Since case–control studies are applied to diseases that occur rarely, researchers usually include all persons who develop the disease over a specified period of time. Controls are selected so that there are usually between one and four controls per case in the sample. Thus, the researcher selects the proportion of persons in the sample who have the disease and that proportion is between 0.5 (one control per case) and 0.2 (four controls per case). This results in a purposive sample.

First, we organize this information in a 2×2 table

		Disease Group		
		Case	Control	
Food	Exposed	25	14	39
Preservative	Not Exposed	75	86	161
		100	100	200

To calculate the odds ratio, we use Equation (9.8).

$$\text{OR} \triangleq \widehat{\text{OR}} = \frac{\text{odds of exposure among cases}}{\text{odds of exposure among controls}} = \frac{a/b}{c/d} = \frac{a \cdot d}{b \cdot c} = \frac{25 \cdot 86}{14 \cdot 75} = 2.05$$

This odds ratio tells us that the odds of having been exposed to the food preservative is about twice as high among the cases as among the controls. ■

If we wanted to estimate probabilities from observations in a case–control study, we could only calculate the probability of having the risk factor for cases and controls since the frequency of the risk factor is the only variable that has been randomly sampled. The probability of having the risk factor, however, is not really of interest to us. Rather, we would like to compare the estimates of the probabilities of having the disease for persons who have the risk factor relative to persons who do not have the risk factor. Unfortunately, we cannot estimate probabilities of having the disease from case–control data since the researcher has determined how many cases and how many controls were included in the sample.

There is a similar limitation with odds in case–control studies. We would like to compare the odds of having the disease between persons with and without the risk factor, but we can only estimate the odds of having the risk factor for cases and controls for the same reason we are limited to estimating probabilities of having the risk factor. When we compare odds in an odds ratio, however, we find that the ratio of the odds for having the risk factor (i.e., from a case–control study) is identical to the odds for having the disease (i.e., from other types of studies). With the odds ratio, it does not matter which variable is the dependent variable and which is the independent variable; the odds ratio will have exactly the same value. In addition, when the disease we are studying is rare, the odds ratio is very close in value to the ratio of probabilities of having the disease.[11]

9.2.2 Hypothesis Testing

Regardless of which estimate is used to represent the association between the nominal dependent and independent variables, the null hypothesis usually tested is that

---

[11] Thus, we can think of an odds ratio in a case–control study as similar to a risk ratio in a cohort study.

those variables are statistically independent of each other. What is meant by statistical independence here is exactly the same thing that was meant when we first encountered the term in Chapter 1. Namely, statistical independence implies that the probability of one event is the same whether or not another event occurs. Generally, statistical independence can be described as shown in Equation (9.9) (same as Equation (1.8)):

$$p(B|A) = p(B|\overline{A}) = p(B) \tag{9.9}$$

where

$p(B\,|\,A)$ = probability of event B occurring given that event A occurs

$p(B|\overline{A})$ = probability of event B occurring given that event A does not occur

$p(B)$ = probability of event B occurring regardless of whether or not event A occurs (i.e., the unconditional probability of event B occurring)

Equation (9.10) shows how this description of statistical independence applies to 2×2 table data by using the terminology in Table 9.1:

$$p(\text{event}|\text{group } 1) = p(\text{event}|\text{group } 2) = p(\text{event}) \tag{9.10}$$

where

$p(\text{event}\,|\,\text{group } 1)$ = probability of the event represented by the dependent variable occurring for persons in group 1

$p(\text{event}\,|\,\text{group } 2)$ = probability of the event represented by the dependent variable occurring for persons in group 2

$p(\text{event})$ = probability of the event represented by the dependent variable occurring for persons in both groups combined

Since statistical independence is defined as having the probability of the event equal to the same value in each of the two groups, testing the null hypothesis of statistical independence is the same as testing the null hypothesis that the probability difference is equal to 0 or that the probability or odds ratios are equal to 1.

In Chapter 1, we were interested in statistical independence when we considered the multiplication rule of probability theory: the way in which the probability of the intersection of events is calculated. The importance of statistical independence in the multiplication rule is to permit the probability of the intersection to be calculated by multiplying unconditional probabilities. A general form of this calculation is shown in Equation (9.11):

$$p(A \text{ and } B) = p(A) \cdot p(B) \tag{9.11}$$

where

$p(A$ and $B) =$ probability that both events A and B will occur in the same observation (i.e., the intersection of events A and B)

$p(A) =$ probability that event A will occur regardless of whether or not event B occurs (i.e., the unconditional probability of event A)

$p(B) =$ probability that event B will occur regardless of whether or not event A occurs (i.e., the unconditional probability of event B)

Equation (9.12) shows this same relationship, but in terms of a 2×2 table:

$$p(\text{event and group } 1) = p(\text{event}) \cdot p(\text{group } 1) \tag{9.12}$$

where

$p(\text{event and group } 1) =$ probability that a person has the event represented by the dependent variable and is in group 1 (i.e., the intersection of having the event and being in group 1)

$p(\text{event}) =$ probability that the event represented by the dependent variable will occur regardless of in which group a person is in (i.e., the unconditional probability of the event occurring)

$p(\text{group } 1) =$ probability that a person is in group 1 regardless of whether or not the event represented by the dependent variable occurs (i.e., the unconditional probability of being in group 1)

In a 2×2 table, the probability of the intersection of being in a particular group and having the event is the same as the probability of an observation being in a particular cell of the table. The probability of having the event and being in group 1 to the left of the equal sign in Equation (9.12) equals the probability of an observation being in the upper left-hand cell of the table. The unconditional probabilities relate to the marginal frequencies of that table. Table 9.3 shows how those probabilities relate to the frequencies in a 2×2 table

TABLE 9.3. A 2×2 Table that Shows the Probabilities that, When Multiplied by the Sample's Size (n), Are Equal to the Cell and Marginal Frequencies in a 2×2 Table

		Outcome		
		Event	No Event	
Group	Group 1	$p(\text{event and group } 1)$	$p(\overline{\text{event}} \text{ and group } 1)$	$p(\text{group 1})$
	Group 2	$p(\text{event and group } 2)$	$p(\overline{\text{event}} \text{ and group } 2)$	$p(\text{group 2})$
		$p(\text{event})$	$p(\overline{\text{event}})$	1

In Table 9.3, we can see that the probabilities associated with each of the four cells of the 2 × 2 table are the probabilities of someone in the sample being in one of the groups specified by the independent variable and either having or not having the event represented by the dependent variable. If any of those four probabilities is multiplied by the total number of observations in the sample (i.e., n), the product would be equal to the corresponding cell frequency (a, b, c, or d). The probabilities on the margins of the 2 × 2 table represent the unconditional probabilities of either being in a particular group or having (or not having) the event.

We test the null hypothesis of statistical independence by using the unconditional probabilities on the margins of the 2 × 2 table to calculate the probabilities in the cells of that table. Then, these calculated probabilities for the cells of the 2 × 2 table are multiplied by the sample's size to obtain the cell frequencies we would expect to observe, on the average, if the variables are statistically independent (i.e., if the null hypothesis is true). Equations (9.13) through (9.16) illustrate how these expected values are calculated:

$$E(a) = p(\text{event}) \cdot p(\text{group 1}) \cdot n = \frac{a+c}{n} \cdot \frac{a+b}{\not{n}} \cdot \not{n} = \frac{(a+c) \cdot (a+b)}{n} \qquad (9.13)$$

$$E(b) = p(\overline{\text{event}}) \cdot p(\text{group 1}) \cdot n = \frac{b+d}{n} \cdot \frac{a+b}{\not{n}} \cdot \not{n} = \frac{(b+d) \cdot (a+b)}{n} \qquad (9.14)$$

$$E(c) = p(\text{event}) \cdot p(\text{group 2}) \cdot n = \frac{a+c}{n} \cdot \frac{c+d}{\not{n}} \cdot \not{n} = \frac{(a+c) \cdot (c+d)}{n} \qquad (9.15)$$

$$E(a) = p(\overline{\text{event}}) \cdot p(\text{group 2}) \cdot n = \frac{b+d}{n} \cdot \frac{c+d}{\not{n}} \cdot \not{n} = \frac{(b+d) \cdot (c+d)}{n} \qquad (9.16)$$

where

$E(a), E(b),$
$E(c), E(d)$ = cell frequencies that are expected in a 2 × 2 table, on the average, if the null hypothesis of statistical independence is true (i.e., the expected values)

$p(\text{group 1}),$
$p(\text{group 2})$ = unconditional probability that a person is in group 1 (or group 2 as specified by the independent variable

$p(\text{event}),$
$p(\overline{\text{event}})$ = unconditional probability that a person has (or does not have) the event represented by the dependent variable

$(a+b), (c+d),$
$(a+c), (b+d)$ = marginal frequencies from the 2 × 2 table

n = total number of observations (i.e., sample's size)
$= a+b+c+d$

Now, let us take a look at an example that illustrates how we can calculate these expected values for the cell frequencies in a 2 × 2 table.

■ **EXAMPLE 9.8**

In Examples 9.5 and 9.6, we looked at data from a clinical trial of a treatment for coronary artery disease. Those data are summarized in the following table:

		Outcome		
		Died	Survived	
Treatment	Standard	54	46	100
	New	36	64	100
		90	110	200

These are the observed frequencies for the 2 × 2 table. Now, let us calculate the cell frequencies that we would expect to observe (on the average) if the dependent and independent variables were statistically independent.

To calculate these expected frequencies, we use the marginal frequencies in the 2 × 2 table and Equations (9.13) through (9.16).

$$E(a) = \frac{(a+c) \cdot (a+b)}{n} = \frac{90 \cdot 100}{200} = 45$$

$$E(b) = \frac{(b+d) \cdot (a+b)}{n} = \frac{110 \cdot 100}{200} = 55$$

$$E(c) = \frac{(a+c) \cdot (c+d)}{n} = \frac{90 \cdot 100}{200} = 45$$

$$E(d) = \frac{(b+d) \cdot (c+d)}{n} = \frac{110 \cdot 100}{200} = 55$$

A convenient way to organize these expected frequencies is to include them in the cells of the 2 × 2 table along with the corresponding observed values. To distinguish the expected values from the observed values, the expected values appear in brackets.

		Outcome		
		Died	Survived	
Treatment	Standard	54 {45}	46 {55}	100
	New	36 {45}	64 {55}	100
		90	110	200

■

In Example 9.8, we can see there is a difference between the observed cell frequencies and those that we expect to see (on the average) if survival outcome is statistically independent of the treatment group. The question now is, "Are these differences large enough to lead us to reject the null hypothesis?" We answer this question by calculating a chi-square value. That chi-square value represents the difference between each observed cell frequency and its corresponding expected cell frequency, relative to the magnitude of the expected frequency for each cell. This calculation is illustrated in Equation (9.17):

$$\chi^2 = \frac{(a - E(a))^2}{E(a)} + \frac{(b - E(b))^2}{E(b)} + \frac{(c - E(c))^2}{E(c)} + \frac{(d - E(d))^2}{E(d)} \qquad (9.17)$$

where

$$\chi^2 = \text{chi-square statistic (with one degree of freedom)}$$
$$a, b, c, d = \text{cell frequencies observed in the sample}$$
$$E(a), E(b), E(c), E(d) = \text{cell frequencies expected, on the average, if the null}$$
$$\text{hypothesis of statistical independence is true}$$

To test the null hypothesis that the dependent and independent variables are statistically independent, the chi-square value calculated in Equation (9.17) is compared with the value from Table B.7 that corresponds to one degree of freedom and $\alpha = 0.05$. This chi-square is often called **Pearson's chi-square** to distinguish it from other chi-square tests. This test is illustrated in the next example.

■ **EXAMPLE 9.9**

In Example 9.8 we calculated the expected cell frequencies and organized them in a 2 × 2 table.

		Outcome		
		Died	Survived	
Treatment	Standard	54 {45}	46 {55}	100
	New	36 {45}	64 {55}	100 100
		90	110	200

Now, let us test the null hypothesis that the dependent and independent variables are statistically independent.

To test the null hypothesis of statistical independence, we use Equation (9.17) to calculate a chi-square statistic.

$$\chi^2 = \frac{(a - E(a))^2}{E(a)} + \frac{(b - E(b))^2}{E(b)} + \frac{(c - E(c))^2}{E(c)} + \frac{(d - E(d))^2}{E(d)}$$

$$= \frac{(54 - 45)^2}{45} + \frac{(46 - 55)^2}{55} + \frac{(36 - 45)^2}{45} + \frac{(64 - 55)^2}{55} = 6.545$$

Thus, the calculated value of chi-square is equal to 6.545. To test the null hypothesis that the dependent and independent variables are statistically independent, we compare this calculated value with a value from Table B.7 that corresponds to one degree of freedom and $\alpha = 0.05$. That value is equal to 3.841. Since the calculated value (6.545) is larger than the critical value from the table (3.841), we reject the null hypothesis and accept, through the process of elimination, the alternative hypothesis. The alternative hypothesis states that the dependent and independent variables in the population are not statistically independent. In other words, the risk of dying is different for the two treatments.   ∎

The chi-square test is a normal approximation. Although it is the test we encounter most often to test the null hypothesis of statistical independence for data in a 2×2 table, there are two other tests based on normal approximations that are used often enough in health research that they deserve mention. One of these is a normal approximation for the difference between the two probabilities. Equation (9.18) shows how a standard normal deviate is calculated to represent the observed difference between the probability estimates:

$$ z = \frac{(p_1 - p_2) - (\theta_1 - \theta_2)}{\sqrt{[\overline{\theta} \cdot (1 - \overline{\theta})/n_1] + [\overline{\theta} \cdot (1 - \overline{\theta})/n_2]}} \tag{9.18}$$

where

z = standard normal deviate representing the observed difference between the probabilities

p_1, p_2 = observed probabilities of the event represented by the dependent variable

θ_1, θ_2 = actual probabilities of the event represented by the dependent variable in the population

$\overline{\theta}$ = overall (univariable) probability of the event in the population

n_1, n_2 = number of observations in groups 1 and 2

Although Equations (9.17) and (9.18) look like different tests, they are not. Not only do they test the same null hypothesis,[12] but they are also numerically identical, except for the fact that the chi-square value is equal to the square of the standard normal deviate.

A third normal approximation test for 2×2 table data is the **Mantel–Haenszel test**.[13] It can be used to test the same null hypotheses that are tested by the chi-square

[12]These hypotheses are: H_0: $\theta_1 - \theta_2 = 0$, H_0: $\theta_1/\theta_2 = 1$, H_0: OR = 1, and H_0: the dependent and independent variables are statistically independent

[13]Sometimes the Mantel–Haenszel test statistic is presented as a standard normal deviate, rather than as a chi-square value. This standard normal deviate is simply the square root of the chi-square value.

test and the normal approximation for the difference between two probabilities. It is very similar (but not identical) to these tests.[14] Equation (9.19) illustrates the Mantel–Haenszel chi-square test:

$$\chi^2 = \frac{(a - E(a))^2}{[(a+b)\cdot(c+d)\cdot(a+c)\cdot(b+d)]/[n^2\cdot(n-1)]}$$ (9.19)

where

χ^2 = chi-square statistic representing the relationship between the observed and expected frequencies for any one of the cells in a 2 × 2 table

a = observed frequency in the upper left-hand cell in a 2 × 2 table

$E(a)$ = expected frequency for the upper left-hand cell, assuming that the dependent and independent variables are statistically independent (from Equation (9.13))

$(a+b), (c+d),$
$(a+c), (b+d)$ = marginal frequencies from the 2 × 2 table

n = total number of observations in the 2 × 2 table

The next example compares these three tests for a 2 × 2 table.

■ EXAMPLE 9.10

In Example 9.9, we used the chi-square test to test the null hypothesis that the dependent and independent variables are statistically independent for the data in the following 2 × 2 table:

		Outcome		
		Died	Survived	
Treatment	Standard	54 {45}	46 {55}	100
	New	36 {45}	64 {55}	100
		90	110	200

Now, let us test this same null hypothesis using the normal approximation for the difference between the probabilities and the Mantel–Haenszel test.

[14]The advantage of the Mantel–Haenszel test is that it can be applied to a collection of 2 × 2 tables as we will see in Chapter 12.

First, let us take a look at the normal approximation for the difference between the probabilities of death for the two treatment groups. This test uses Equation (9.18).

$$z = \frac{(p_1 - p_2) - (\theta_1 - \theta_2)}{\sqrt{[\bar{\theta} \cdot (1 - \bar{\theta})/n_1] + [\bar{\theta} \cdot (1 - \bar{\theta})/n_2]}}$$

$$= \frac{(0.54 - 0.36) - 0}{\sqrt{[0.45 \cdot (1 - 0.45)/100] + [0.45 \cdot (1 - 0.45)/100]}} = 2.56$$

This standard normal deviate is compared with a value from Table B.1 that corresponds to 0.05 split between the two tails of the standard normal distribution. That value from the table is equal to 1.96. Since the calculated value (2.56) is larger than the critical value (1.96), we can reject the null hypothesis and accept, through the process of elimination, the alternative hypothesis, which states that the dependent and independent variables are not statistically independent. This is the same conclusion we drew in Example 9.9 using the chi-square test. In fact, the square of this standard normal deviate (2.56^2) is exactly equal to the chi-square value calculated in Example 9.9.

Next, let us test this same null hypothesis using the Mantel–Haenszel test from Equation (9.19).

$$\chi^2 = \frac{(a - E(a))^2}{[(a+b) \cdot (c+d) \cdot (a+c) \cdot (b+d)]/[n^2 \cdot (n-1)]}$$

$$= \frac{(54 - 45)^2}{(90 \cdot 110 \cdot 100 \cdot 100)/(200^2 \cdot 199)} = 6.513$$

This result (6.513) is very close, but not identical, to the result from the chi-square test (6.454) and the square of the result from the normal approximation for the difference between the probabilities (also 6.454). This difference is due to a slightly different approximation used in the Mantel–Haenszel test.   ∎

The three hypothesis tests we have considered are all normal approximations applied to the **hypergeometric distribution**. The hypergeometric distribution is the actual sampling distribution for 2 × 2 tables. It is a discrete distribution (i.e., represented graphically using a bar graph), while the Gaussian distribution is a continuous distribution (i.e., represented graphically using a frequency polygon). Some statisticians think we can get a better approximation if we correct for the lack of continuity in the hypergeometric distribution. The most common **continuity correction** involves subtracting ½ from the absolute difference between observed and expected cell frequencies.[15] The corrected calculation for the chi-square test is illustrated in

---

[15]This is sometimes called **Yate's correction**.

Equation (9.20) and in the next example:

$$\chi^2 = \frac{\left(|a - E(a)| - \frac{1}{2}\right)^2}{E(a)} + \frac{\left(|b - E(b)| - \frac{1}{2}\right)^2}{E(b)}$$

$$+ \frac{\left(|c - E(c)| - \frac{1}{2}\right)^2}{E(c)} + \frac{\left(|d - E(d)| - \frac{1}{2}\right)^2}{E(d)} \tag{9.20}$$

■ EXAMPLE 9.11

In Example 9.9, we used the chi-square test to test the null hypothesis that the dependent and independent variables are statistically independent for the data in the following 2 × 2 table:

Now, let us perform that chi-square test using the correction for continuity. We use Equation (9.20) to obtain the corrected calculation of chi-square.

$$\chi^2 = \frac{\left(|a - E(a)| - \frac{1}{2}\right)^2}{E(a)} + \frac{\left(|b - E(b)| - \frac{1}{2}\right)^2}{E(b)} + \frac{\left(|c - E(c)| - \frac{1}{2}\right)^2}{E(c)}$$

$$+ \frac{\left(|d - E(d)| - \frac{1}{2}\right)^2}{E(d)}$$

$$= \frac{\left(|54 - 45| - \frac{1}{2}\right)^2}{45} + \frac{\left(|36 - 45| - \frac{1}{2}\right)^2}{45} + \frac{\left(|46 - 55| - \frac{1}{2}\right)^2}{55}$$

$$+ \frac{\left(|64 - 55| - \frac{1}{2}\right)^2}{55} = 5.838$$

This chi-square corrected for continuity (5.838) is less than the uncorrected chi-square (6.545), but it is still greater than the value from Table B.7 corresponding to one degree of freedom and $\alpha = 0.05$ (3.841). Thus, we draw the same conclusion: we reject the null hypothesis. ■

The chi-square using a continuity correction is always smaller than the chi-square without the correction. This means it is a little harder to reject the null hypothesis than without the correction. Usually, the P-value from the continuity-corrected chi-square is closer to the "true" P-value (which we will discuss shortly). So, it is probably the better choice.

The advantage of using normal approximations for a nominal dependent variable is that normal approximations are easier to calculate than using the actual sampling distribution (i.e., the **hypergeometric distribution** for a 2 × 2 table). However, with computers to perform these calculations for us, their difficulty should be moot. Given a choice, we should use the actual sampling distribution. We learned in Chapter 6 that using the actual sampling distribution for a nominal dependent variable is called an exact procedure. In the case of 2×2 tables, this exact procedure is called **Fisher's exact test**. We will see the result of Fisher's exact test in the next example.

We have performed these hypothesis tests by hand so that we can see how they work. In practice, however, we will us a computer to perform these tests. In the next example, we will see how we can use Excel and R to analyze 2×2 tables.

■ EXAMPLE 9.12

One of the Excel programs supplied with this text is a 2×2 table analyzer. If we were to use that program to analyze the 2×2 table first encountered in Example 9.5, we would get the following output:

Observed		Outcome			Expected		Outcome		
		Yes	No				Yes	No	
Group	A	54	46	100	Group	A	45	55	100
	B	36	64	100		B	45	55	100
		90	110	200			90	110	200

Parameter	PE	SE	95% IE		Test	Chi-sq	P-value
p(Yes|A)	0.54	0.04984	0.442314	0.637686	Pearson's (uncorrected)	6.545455	0.010515
p(Yes|B)	0.36	0.048	0.26592	0.45408	Pearson's (corrected)	5.838384	0.01568
Probability diff	0.18	0.069195	0.044377	0.315623	Mantel-Haenszel	6.51272/	0.010711
Probability ratio	1.5	0.162161	1.091583	12.523/4	Fisher's exact		0.015462
Odds ratio	2.086957	0.289241	1.183876	3.678921			

This program provides us with lots of information about the 2×2 table. First, it gives us the observed and expected frequencies in 2×2 tables. Then, it gives us point and interval estimates for the univariable probabilities, the probability difference, the probability ratio, and the odds ratio (on the left). Finally, it gives us the results of testing the null hypotheses that the probability difference is equal to 0, the probability ratio is equal to 1, and the odds ratio is equal to 1 (on the right). All of those null hypotheses are true when the dependent and independent variable are statistically independent of each other.

If we compare the results of using the 2×2 table analyzer to the results we obtained by hand, we see that they are identical.

The last hypothesis test on the right side of the output is Fisher's exact test. Note that P-value from Fisher's exact test is closest to the corrected chi-square. This is usually the case, making the corrected chi-square the best among the normal approximations. Even so, you commonly encounter uncorrected chi-square tests in the health research literature.

We can perform Pearson's chi-square in R using the "chisq.test" command. The input we will use is a matrix[16] that contains the 2×2 table data.

---

[16]See Appendix E.

>chisq.test(Example9_5)

```
Pearson's Chi-squared test with Yates' continuity correction

data:   Example9_5
X-squared = 5.8384, df = 1, p-value = 0.01568
```

By default, "chisq.test" gives us the continuity-corrected chi-square. If we want the uncorrected chi-square, we have to add "correct=FALSE" to the command.
>chisq.test(Example9_5,correct=FALSE)

```
Pearson's Chi-squared test

data:   Example9_5
X-squared = 6.5455, df = 1, p-value = 0.01052
```

To perform Fisher's exact test in R, we use the "fisher.test" command.
>fisher.test(Example9_5)

```
Fisher's Exact Test for Count Data

data:   Example9_5
p-value = 0.01546
alternative hypothesis: true odds ratio is not equal to 1
95 percent confidence interval:
 1.139707 3.829553
sample estimates:
odds ratio
  2.079135
```

For the most part, the results from R are the same as the results from the 2×2 table analyzer in Excel. One exception is the odds ratio given in the Fisher's exact test output. That odds ratio in the R output is not calculated in the usual way and is not very useful. ∎

9.2.3 Dependent Variable Not Affected by Time: Paired Design

When we make two measurements of the dependent variable on each individual or on two individuals who are essentially identical, we call it a **paired design**. The purpose of a paired design is to control for some of the person-to-person variability and, as a result, to provide more precise estimates of relationships between groups. For a continuous dependent variable, we did this by taking the difference between the two measurements for each pair (i.e., as in the paired t-test discussed in Chapter 4). For a nominal dependent variable, we have a different way to represent paired data. This is done by numerating different outcomes for each pair of observations.

TABLE 9.4. A Paired 2 × 2 Table[a]

		Group 1		
		Event	No Event	
Group 2	Event	A	B	b
	No Event	C	D	d
		a	c	n_p

[a] The letters A, B, C, and D in the cells of the paired 2 × 2 table represent the frequencies of each possible outcome for a pair. The letters a, b, c, and d represent the frequencies of each outcome for the individuals who make up the pairs as shown in Table 9.1. n_p is the number of pairs in the sample ($n_p = n/2$).

For each pair of observations, there are four possible outcomes. First, both members of a pair could have the event represented by the nominal dependent variable. Second, neither member of a pair could have that event. These first two types of pairs are called **concordant pairs**. The more concordant pairs we observe, the more effective the pairing. That is to say, the pairing resulted in the selection of two persons who had about the same likelihood of having the event.

The concordant pairs do not, however, reflect the difference between the groups being compared. This difference is reflected by the **discordant pairs**. These are the pairs in which one member of the pair had the event while the other member of that pair did not have the event. The discordant pairs are those pairs between which group membership is more likely to be reflected in the outcomes of the members of the pairs. This is because pairing intends to match individuals who are identical in all aspects related to the outcome, except for group membership.

Since this paired analysis tracks the outcomes by pairs, we organize the events in a different type of 2 × 2 table. This **paired 2 × 2 table** distinguishes between the two groups specified by the nominal independent variable by having one group represented by the columns and the other group represented by the rows. Then, each column for the first group and each row for the second group specify the outcome for that member of the pair. This format is illustrated in Table 9.4.

The next example illustrates data organized in a paired 2 × 2 table and how they relate to an unpaired 2 × 2 table.

■ EXAMPLE 9.13

In previous examples, we examined data from a clinical trial of a treatment for coronary artery disease in which 100 persons were given the experimental treatment (36 of whom died within the study period) and another 100 persons were given the standard treatment (54 of whom died within the same period of time). The following 2 × 2 table was used in Example 9.5 to organize these data:

		Outcome		
		Died	Survived	
Treatment	Standard	54	46	100
	New	36	64	100
		90	110	200

Now, let us suppose that these data come from a paired design in which each of the 100 persons in the new treatment group is matched to one of the 100 persons in the standard treatment group.

The unpaired and paired 2 × 2 tables are related in that the cell frequencies of the unpaired table are the marginal frequencies of the paired table. Therefore, the paired table contains all of the information in the unpaired table. That is to say, both tables tell us what happened to the 200 individuals in the study. In addition, the paired table tells us what happened to each pair. The following is an example of how the paired table could appear for these data:[17]

		Standard Treatment		
		Died	Survived	
New Treat-ment	Died	30	6	36
	Survived	24	40	64
		54	46	100

This table tells us that there were 30 pairs in which both members of the pair died and 40 pairs in which both members of the pair survived. These are the concordant pairs. The discordant pairs are those in which one member of the pair died and the other member of the pair survived. In 24 of these pairs, it was the member who received the standard treatment who died. In six of these pairs, it was the member who received the new treatment who died. ∎

9.2.3.1 *Estimation.*
Having a paired study does not affect the point estimates of the probability difference or of the probability ratio. We still use Equations (9.5, 9.6) and the cell frequencies from the unpaired 2 × 2 table (or marginal frequencies from the paired table). It does not matter whether the study is paired or not; these estimates will be identical. The point estimate of the odds ratio, on the other hand, is affected by the paired design. Thus, we must use the paired 2 × 2 table to estimate the odds ratio when the study has a paired design. Equation (9.21) illustrates how the point estimate of the odds ratio is calculated from a paired 2 × 2 table[18]:

$$\text{OR} \triangleq \widehat{\text{OR}} = \frac{C}{B} \qquad (9.21)$$

---

[17]This is just 1 of 37 possible paired tables that could result from this study. It was selected arbitrarily.
[18]Equation (9.21) assumes that the paired 2 × 2 table has the group in the numerator of the odds ratio specifying columns. If that group is specifying rows, take the inverse of this equation (B/C).

where

OR = population's value of the odds ratio

$\widehat{OR}$ = sample's estimate of the odds ratio

   C = number of discordant pairs in which the member in group 1 did not have the event and the member in group 2 had the event

   B = number of discordant pairs in which the member in group 1 had the event and the member in group 2 did not have the event

The next example shows how these point estimates are calculated from the paired 2×2 table.

■ EXAMPLE 9.14

In Example 9.13, we organized the data from a clinical trial of a treatment for coronary artery disease as if it had a paired design in which one member from each of 100 pairs of persons was given the experimental (i.e., new) treatment and the other member was given the standard treatment. The particular paired 2×2 table selected in Example 9.13 is as follows:

		Standard Treatment		
		Died	Survived	
New Treat-	Died	30	6	36
ment	Survived	24	40	64
		54	46	100

Now, let us calculate point estimates of the probability difference, probability ratio, and odds ratio comparing survival in the two treatment groups.

First, we use Equation (9.5) to estimate the probability difference. When the data appear in a paired 2×2 table, we can perform this calculation using the frequencies in the margins of the paired table (see Table 9.4). For this particular table we get

$$\theta_1 - \theta_2 \triangleq p_1 - p_2 = \frac{a}{a+c} - \frac{b}{b+d} = \frac{54}{54+46} - \frac{36}{36+64} = 0.18$$

Then, we use Equation (9.6) to estimate the probability ratio from the paired 2×2 table.

$$\frac{\theta_1}{\theta_2} \triangleq \frac{p_1}{p_2} = \frac{a/(a+c)}{b/(b+d)} = \frac{54/(54+46)}{36/(36+64)} = 1.5$$

These values are the same as the probability difference and the probability ratio point estimates obtained from the unpaired 2×2 table in Example 9.5.

Now, we calculate the point estimate for the odds ratio. When the study has a paired design, we cannot use Equation (9.8), since it applies only to the unpaired

2 × 2 table. Instead, we use Equation (9.21) to estimate the odds ratio from the paired table.

$$\text{OR} \triangleq \widehat{\text{OR}} = \frac{C}{B} = \frac{24}{6} = 4.0$$

This is not the same as the estimate of the odds ratio that we calculated from the unpaired 2 × 2 table in Example 9.6. That unpaired odds ratio was equal to 2.09. In general, odds ratios from paired studies will be further from one in numeric magnitude than the corresponding odds ratios from unpaired studies. This difference between paired and unpaired odds ratio estimates reflects the advantage of pairing. ∎

9.2.3.2 *Hypothesis Testing.*

The principal advantage of using a paired design is to increase statistical power (i.e., improve our chance of rejecting a false null hypothesis). This advantage applies equally to probability differences, probability ratios, and odds ratios. Equation (9.22) shows how we can test the null hypotheses that the probability difference is equal to 0, that the probability ratio is equal to 1, that the odds ratio is equal to 1, or that there is statistical independence between group membership and the outcome[19]:

$$\chi^2 = \frac{(C - B)^2}{C + B} \tag{9.22}$$

where

χ^2 = chi-square value with one degree of freedom

C = number of discordant pairs in which the member in group 1 did not have the event and the member in group 2 had the event

B = number of discordant pairs in which the member in group 1 had the event and the member in group 2 did not have the event

The statistical test that uses Equation (9.22) on data from a paired 2 × 2 table is called McNemar's test. The following example shows McNemar's test applied to the paired 2 × 2 table in Example 9.13.

∎ EXAMPLE 9.15

In Example 9.13, we organized the data from a clinical trial of a treatment for coronary artery disease as if it had a paired design in which one member from each of 100 pairs of persons was given the experimental (i.e., new) treatment and the other member was given the standard treatment. The particular paired 2 × 2 table selected in Example 9.13 is as follows

---

[19]Earlier in this chapter we learned, if any of these null hypotheses are rejected, then all four are rejected.

		Standard Treatment Group		
New Treatment Group	Died	30	6	36
	Survived	24	40	64
		54	46	100

Now, let us use these data to test the null hypothesis that the probability ratio is equal to 1 in the population.

Since these data are from a study with a paired design, we need to test this null hypothesis using McNemar's test. From Equation (9.22) we get

$$\chi^2 = \frac{(C - B)^2}{C + B} = \frac{(24 - 6)^2}{24 + 6} = 10.8$$

The chi-square value calculated by using McNemar's test has one degree of freedom, so we compare it with a value from Table B.7 for $\alpha = 0.05$ and one degree of freedom. This value is equal to 3.841. Since 10.80 is larger than 3.841, we reject the null hypothesis that the probability ratio in the population is equal to 1 and accept, through the process of elimination, that it is not equal to 1. The fact that this test has greater statistical power than the chi-square test for unpaired data (Equation (9.17)) is illustrated by the fact that McNemar's test yields a larger chi-square value (10.80) than does the unpaired chi-square test in Example 9.9 (6.55). A larger chi-square value implies that it is easier to reject the null hypothesis.

Even though McNemar's test is easy to calculate by hand, the paired 2×2 table analyzer program in the BAHR collection of programs in Excel will perform these calculations for you.

		Group A							
		Yes	No						
Group B	Yes	30	6	36					
	No	24	40	64					
		54	46	100					
Parameter	PE	SE	95%IE				Test	CHISQ	P-value
Probability diff	0.18	0.141421	−0.09719	0.457186			McNemar's		10.8	0.001015
Probability ratio	1.5	0.188746	1.036162	2.171476					
Odds ratio	4	0.456435	1.635062	9.78556					

R also performs McNemar's test with the "mcnemar.test(matrix)" command.
>mcnemar.test(Example9_13)

```
McNemar's Chi-squared test with continuity correction

data:  Example9_13
McNemar's chi-squared = 9.6333, df = 1, p-value = 0.001911
```

R gives us a smaller value of chi-square and, thus, a larger *P*-value. This is because, by default, R uses a continuity correction in its calculation of chi-square. ∎

9.2.4 Dependent Variable Affected by Time

In Chapter 6, we considered a nominal dependent variable to be affected by time if two criteria were met. The first criterion is that the event represented by the dependent variable is observed more often the longer we look for it. This is true of most events we encounter in health research and practice. The second criterion is that we look longer for the event in some cases than we do in others. If both of these criteria are met, we need to use special statistical methods that take time into account. In Chapter 6, we did that by using rates (i.e., incidence), rather than probabilities, as estimates of the frequency of events. We take that same approach in bivariable analysis.

When we have nominal dependent and independent variables and the dependent variable is not affected by time, we organize the observations in a 2 × 2 table. We do something similar when the dependent variable is affected by time, but we do not keep track of the number of observations in which the event does not occur. Table 9.5 illustrates the way we organize data from a bivariable sample when the nominal dependent variable is affected by time.

In bivariable analysis, when the independent variable represents nominal data, we can estimate the incidence of the event in each of the two groups specified by the nominal independent variable. The way we make those estimates is the same as the way we did in univariable analysis (Equation (6.5)). When we have two estimates of the incidence of an event, however, our interest is in comparing the estimates. We can make this comparison either by considering the difference between, or the ratio of, the estimates. These estimates are illustrated in Equations (9.23) and (9.24):

$$\text{ID} \triangleq \widehat{\text{ID}} = \frac{a}{\text{PT}_1} - \frac{b}{\text{PT}_2} \tag{9.23}$$

TABLE 9.5. A Table for Organizing Observations for a Nominal Dependent Variable and a Nominal Independent Variable When the Dependent Variable Is Affected by Time[a]

		Independent Variable		
		Group 1	Group 2	
Dependent Variable	Events	a	b	$a+b$
	Person-Time	PT_1	PT_2	

[a] The letters a and b represent the frequencies (i.e., counts) of the events in each of two groups. PT_1 and PT_2 represent the total amount of follow-up time (person-time) over which events were observed in each group.

where

ID = population's incidence difference
$\widehat{\text{ID}}$ = sample's estimate of the incidence difference
a, b = number of events observed in groups 1 and 2, respectively, in the sample
PT_1, PT_2 = amount of follow-up time spent looking for events in groups 1 and 2, respectively, in the sample

and

$$\text{IR} \triangleq \widehat{\text{IR}} = \frac{a/PT_1}{b/PT_2} \tag{9.24}$$

where

IR = population's incidence ratio
$\widehat{\text{IR}}$ = sample's estimate of the incidence ratio
a, b = number of events observed in groups 1 and 2, respectively, in the sample
PT_1, PT_2 = amount of follow-up time spent looking for events in groups 1 and 2, respectively, in the sample

When the nominal dependent variable is not affected by time, the choice between a probability difference and a probability ratio is based on whether or not we want the measure to reflect the underlying frequency of the event. The same is true in bivariable analysis when the nominal dependent is affected by time. The incidence difference is used to compare rates when we want to reflect the underlying rate of disease and the incidence ratio is used to compare rates when we do not want to reflect the underlying rate of disease. We will take a look at an example of how to calculate and interpret these estimates shortly, but first, let us see how we can take chance into account for two rates.

Regardless of whether we are interested in the difference between or the ratio of two rates, the method we use to take chance into account is the same, as long as the null hypothesis corresponds to the rates being equal to the same value in the population. For the difference between rates, the null hypothesis is that the difference is equal to 0. For the ratio of two rates, the corresponding null hypothesis is that the ratio is equal to 1. Equation (9.25) illustrates the method for testing these null hypotheses:

$$\chi^2 = \frac{(a - [(a+b) \cdot PT_1]/(PT_1 + PT_2))^2}{[(a+b) \cdot PT_1 \cdot PT_2]/(PT_1 + PT_2)^2} \tag{9.25}$$

where

χ^2 = chi-square value with one degree of freedom

a, b = number of events observed in groups 1 and 2, respectively

PT_1, PT_2 = amount of follow-up time spent looking for events in groups 1 and 2, respectively

Now, let us take a look at an example in which we compare two rates.

■ EXAMPLE 9.16

In Example 6.2, we followed 11 persons for up to 3 years looking for the development of retinopathy and found 7 new cases during a total of 21.8 person-years. This led to an estimate of the rate at which new cases of retinopathy appear in the population equal to 0.32 per year. Now, let us suppose that these 11 persons represent a group that has been diagnosed with diabetes and that we have another group of 11 persons without diabetes among whom 6 cases of retinopathy were observed over a total of 40 person-years of follow-up. Let us compare those rates between the two groups.

First, let us organize these data in a table like Table 9.5.

		Diabetes		
		Yes	No	
Retinopathy	Cases	7	6	13
	Person-Time	21.8	40.0	

Next, we need to decide whether we want to make this comparison in a way that reflects the underlying rate of disease. Most likely, we would be interested only in the strength of the association between retinopathy and diabetes (i.e., without reflecting the underlying incidence of retinopathy). If this is the case, we want to make the comparison by calculating a rate ratio using Equation (9.24).

$$\text{IR} \triangleq \widehat{\text{IR}} = \frac{a/PT_1}{b/PT_2} = \frac{7/21.8}{6/40.0} = 2.14$$

This implies that persons with diabetes develop retinopathy at more than twice the rate as do persons without diabetes. Now, let us take chance into account by testing the null hypothesis that the incidence of retinopathy is the same in these two groups. We do that by using Equation (9.25).

$$\chi^2 = \frac{(a - [(a+b) \cdot PT_1]/(PT_1 + PT_2))^2}{[(a+b) \cdot PT_1 \cdot PT_2]/(PT_1 + PT_2)^2}$$

$$= \frac{(7 - [13 \cdot 21.8]/(21.8 + 40.0))^2}{(13 \cdot 21.8 \cdot 40.0)/(21.8 + 40)^2} = 1.96$$

To test the null hypothesis that the rate ratio in the population is equal to 1, we compare the calculated chi-square value with one from Table B.7 that corresponds to $\alpha = 0.05$ and one degree of freedom. This chi-square value is 3.841. Since 1.96 is less than 3.841, we fail to reject the null hypothesis.   ■

We have finished discussing bivariable methods that are commonly used in the health research literature. Now, we are ready to take a look at multivariable methods.

CHAPTER SUMMARY

Some of the statistical procedures we have examined in this chapter for a nominal dependent variable and one independent variable are very similar to the procedures described in Chapter 7 for bivariable data sets containing a continuous dependent variable. An example is the test for trend which involves estimation of a straight line to describe probabilities as a function of a continuous independent variable.

Testing the omnibus null hypothesis in trend analysis for a nominal dependent variable and a continuous independent variable is similar to the F-test in regression analysis in that hypothesis testing in trend analysis involves examination of a ratio of two estimates of the variation of data represented by the dependent variable. In regression analysis, the F-ratio is calculated by dividing the explained variation (the regression mean square) by the unexplained variation (the residual mean square). In trend analysis, we divide the explained variation by the total variation. The reason for this difference between regression analysis and trend analysis is that the total variation of a nominal dependent variable is a function of the point estimates and, therefore, is not subject to separate effects of chance. The ratio in trend analysis has a distribution that is the square of the standard normal distribution. The square of the standard normal distribution is represented by the chi-square distribution with one degree of freedom.

Another parallel between bivariable data sets that contain a continuous dependent variable and those that contain a nominal dependent variable can be seen when the independent variable is nominal. In both cases, the nominal independent variable has the effect of dividing values of the dependent variable into two groups. Similar to comparing means of a continuous dependent variable between two groups, comparison of probabilities between two groups of nominal dependent variable values can be accomplished by examining the difference between those probabilities.

Means are always compared by examining their difference. Estimates of nominal dependent variable values (e.g., probabilities) can be compared by examining their difference or by examining their ratio. A ratio of nominal dependent variable estimates allows us to consider the relative, rather than absolute, distinction between two groups. Differences can be used to compare probabilities or rates. Probabilities and rates can also be compared as a ratio.

Another ratio that can be used to compare values of a nominal dependent variable is the odds ratio. The odds ratio is equal to the odds of the event represented by the dependent variable in one group divided by the odds of that event in the other group. Odds are equal to the number of observations in which the event occurred divided by the number of observations in which the event did not occur.

The difference and ratios we have examined thus far assume that two nominal variables are measured for each individual and that only the values of those variables indicate any relationship among the individuals in a set of observations. In another type of data set for a nominal dependent variable and a nominal independent variable, individuals are paired based on one or more characteristics thought to be associated with values of the dependent variable. In this paired sample, one member of the pair has one value of the nominal independent variable, and the other member of the pair has the other value of the independent variable.

Paired nominal data are arranged in a 2×2 table that is different from the type of 2×2 table used to organize unpaired nominal data. Ratios and differences between probabilities are calculated from a paired 2×2 table using different formulas from those used for an unpaired 2×2 table, but the point estimates are the same regardless of which formula is used. That is not true for odds ratios, which must be estimated using the formula for paired data if the data are paired.

Statistical hypothesis testing for nominal dependent and independent variables uses the same statistical procedures to test the most common null hypothesis about differences as is used to test the most common null hypothesis about ratios. Those null hypotheses are that the difference is equal to 0 and that the ratio is equal to 1. If one of those null hypotheses is true, then both are true, since they both imply that the nominal dependent variable estimates in the two groups are equal.

Thus, we need only one method of hypothesis testing for probabilities (and odds) and one test for rates. In this chapter, we encountered three alternative methods to test null hypotheses about probabilities. The reason for presenting three alternative methods is that all three are commonly found in health research literature. The first method involves conversion of the difference between probabilities to a standard normal deviate. The standard error for that difference is calculated using a weighted average of the point estimates of the probability of the event in the population.

Another method, known as the chi-square test, is based on the 2×2 table. In this approach, observed frequencies for the four combinations of dependent and independent variable values are compared with what we would expect if the probability of the event were the same for each of the two groups. Calculation of expected values is based on the simplified version of the multiplication rule of probability theory. Then, observed and expected frequencies are compared for each cell of the 2×2 table. Their sum is a chi-square value with one degree of freedom.

The results of those two methods of hypothesis testing are exactly the same with the chi-square value being the square of the standard normal deviate. The popularity of the chi-square test is due, in part, to its ability for expansion to consider more than one dependent and/or independent variable. The chi-square test uses redundant information since only one cell of a 2×2 table needs to be known to determine values in all four cells assuming the marginal frequencies are known.

The third procedure we examined for probabilities and odds uses only one cell of the 2×2 table. This procedure is a slightly different normal approximation, known as the Mantel–Haenszel test.

For statistical hypothesis testing on paired nominal data, we calculate a chi-square statistic using a special method known as McNemar's test.

To test the null hypothesis that the difference between rates is equal to 0 or that the ratio of rates is equal to 1, we use a method that is similar to the Mantel–Haenszel procedure.

EXERCISES

9.1. Suppose we are interested in the number of immunizations necessary to provide protection against hepatitis B infections. To investigate this, we identify a group of persons in a population in which hepatitis B is endemic who had 0, 1, 2, 3, 4, or 5 immunizations and follow them for a period of 10 years. Imagine we observe the data in the Excel file EXR9_1 on the website accompanying this textbook. These data use an indicator of hepatitis B as the dependent variable and the number of immunizations as the independent variable. From that information, estimate the 10-year risk of hepatitis B for a person who had three immunizations. Which of the following is closest to that estimate?

A. 0.09

B. 0.12

C. 0.15

D. 0.19

E. 0.24

9.2. In the Framingham Heart Study, 4,658 persons had their body mass index (BMI) calculated and were followed for 32 years to determine how many persons would develop heart disease (HD). Those data are in the Excel file EXR9_2 on the website accompanying this textbook. From those observations, estimate the probability that a person with a BMI of 30 would develop HD during a 32-year period. Which of the following is closest to that estimate?

A. 0.14

B. 0.21

C. 0.29

D. 0.33

E. 0.39

9.3. Suppose we are interested in the number of immunizations necessary to provide protection against hepatitis B infections. To investigate this, we identify a group of persons in a population in which hepatitis B is endemic who had 0, 1, 2, 3, 4, or 5 immunizations and follow them for a period of 10 years. Imagine we observe the data in the Excel file EXR9_1 on the website accompanying this textbook. These data use an indicator of hepatitis B as the dependent variable and the number of immunizations as the independent variable. From that information, test the null hypothesis that the number of immunizations does not help estimate risk versus the alternative hypothesis that it does help. If you allow a 5% chance of making a type I error, which of the following is the best conclusion to draw?

A. Reject both null and alternative hypotheses

B. Accept both null and alternative hypotheses

C. Reject the null hypothesis and accept the alternative hypothesis

D. Accept the null hypothesis and reject the alternative hypothesis

E. It is best not to draw a conclusion about the null and alternative hypotheses from these data

9.4. In the Framingham Heart Study, 4,658 persons had their BMI calculated and were followed for 32 years to determine how many persons would develop HD. Those data are in the Excel file EXR9_2 on the website accompanying this textbook. From those observations, test the null hypothesis that knowing BMI does not help estimate the probability of HD versus the alternative that it does help. If you allow a 5% chance of making a type I error, which of the following is the best conclusion to draw?

A. Reject both null and alternative hypotheses

B. Accept both null and alternative hypotheses

C. Reject the null hypothesis and accept the alternative hypothesis

D. Accept the null hypothesis and reject the alternative hypothesis

E. It is best not to draw a conclusion about the null and alternative hypotheses from these data

9.5. Suppose we are interested in the number of immunizations necessary to provide protection against hepatitis B infections. To investigate this, we identify a group of persons in a population in which hepatitis B is endemic who had 0, 1, 2, 3, 4, or 5 immunizations and follow them for a period of 10 years. Imagine we observe the data in the Excel file EXR9_1 on the website accompanying this textbook. These data use an indicator of hepatitis B as the dependent variable and the number of immunizations as the independent variable. From that information, determine the 10-year risk of hepatitis B for persons who had no immunizations. Which of the following is closest to that risk?

A. 0.119

B. 0.146

C. 0.161

D. 0.261

E. 0.322

9.6. Suppose that we were to conduct a cohort study in which we identified 31 patients who had been diagnosed as having systemic hypertension and another group of 30 patients who had not been diagnosed with hypertension. We followed each of the groups to determine how many developed diabetes. At the end of the follow-up period, there were 25 persons who developed diabetes, 7 of whom did not have hypertension. From that information, which of the following is closest to the estimate of the odds ratio comparing the two groups of patients?

A. 1.50

B. 2.49

C. 3.14

D. 4.55

E. 13.76

9.7. Suppose that we were to conduct a cohort study in which we identified 31 patients who had been diagnosed as having systemic hypertension and another group of 30 patients who had not been diagnosed with hypertension. We followed each of the groups to determine how many developed diabetes. At the end of the follow-up period, there were 25 persons who developed diabetes, 7 of whom did not have hypertension. From that information, which of the following is closest to the estimate of the risk ratio comparing the risk of diabetes among exposed persons and among unexposed persons?

A. 0.52

B. 0.61

C. 1.05

D. 2.49

E. 5.14

9.8. Suppose we are interested in the number of immunizations necessary to provide protection against hepatitis B infections. To investigate this, we identify a group of persons in a population in which hepatitis B is endemic who had 0, 1, 2, 3, 4, or 5 immunizations and follow them for a period of 10 years. Imagine we observe the data in the Excel file EXR9_1 on the website accompanying this textbook. From these data, estimate the 10-year risk ratio comparing persons who received no immunization to persons who received at least one immunization. Which of the following is closest to that risk ratio?

A. 0.22

B. 0.58

C. 1.08

D. 1.65

E. 1.80

9.9. Suppose that we were to conduct a cohort study in which we identified 31 patients who had been diagnosed as having systemic hypertension and another group of 30 patients who had not been diagnosed with hypertension. We followed each of the groups to determine how many developed diabetes. At the end of the follow-up period, there were 25 persons who developed diabetes, 7 of whom did not have hypertension. From that information, test the null hypothesis that the risk ratio is equal to 1 in the population versus the alternative hypothesis that it is not equal to 1. If you allow a 5% chance of making a type I error, which of the following is the best conclusion to draw?

A. Reject both null and alternative hypotheses

B. Accept both null and alternative hypotheses

C. Reject the null hypothesis and accept the alternative hypothesis

D. Accept the null hypothesis and reject the alternative hypothesis

E. It is best not to draw a conclusion about the null and alternative hypotheses from these data

9.10. Suppose we are interested in the number of immunizations necessary to provide protection against hepatitis B infections. To investigate this, we identify a group of persons in a population in which hepatitis B is endemic who had 0, 1, 2, 3, 4, or 5 immunizations and follow them for a period of 10 years. Imagine we observe the data in the Excel file EXR9_1 on the website accompanying this textbook. From these data, test the null hypothesis that the risk ratio comparing persons with no immunizations to persons with at least one immunization is equal to 1 in the population versus the alternative hypothesis that it is not equal to 1. If you allow a 5% chance of making a type I error, which of the following is the best conclusion to draw?

A. Reject both null and alternative hypotheses

B. Accept both null and alternative hypotheses

C. Reject the null hypothesis and accept the alternative hypothesis

D. Accept the null hypothesis and reject the alternative hypothesis

E. It is best not to draw a conclusion about the null and alternative hypotheses from these data

PART FOUR

MULTIVARIABLE ANALYSES

If there is one thing on which we can all agree, it is the fact that the science of health and disease is complex. There are few (if any) measurements that we can make on individuals that are not related to other characteristics of these individuals. To do justice to this complexity, our analyses of data from health research should take these interrelationships into account. This can be done by considering more than one independent variable. When we have a data set with more than one independent variable, we call it a **multivariable** data set.

Usually, we conduct statistical analyses with one independent variable of particular interest. We know that independent variables specify conditions under which we wish to examine the dependent variable. These conditions are defined for one of two reasons. The first reason is that we wish to examine the relationship between the dependent variable and independent variable. For example, in data from a clinical trial of a therapeutic intervention, we have a nominal independent variable that specifies to which treatment group someone has been assigned. Our interest in analyzing these data is to compare values of the dependent variable between the treatment groups. In bivariable analyses, every independent variable has served this purpose.

The second reason we might want to use independent variables to specify conditions is to examine the relationship between the dependent variable and one or more independent variables while taking into account or controlling for the effects of other characteristics. For example, if we were interested in the relationship between dose

Introduction to Biostatistical Applications in Health Research with Microsoft Office Excel® and R,
Second Edition. Robert P. Hirsch.
© 2021 John Wiley & Sons, Inc. Published 2021 by John Wiley & Sons, Inc.
Companion website: www.wiley.com/go/hirsch/healthresearch2e

of an antihypertensive medication and diastolic blood pressure, we would probably want to control for any differences in age among the persons at different doses. The reason for this is that diastolic blood pressure increases with age. If the persons who received the higher doses were younger than the persons who received the lower doses, we would see an apparent dose–response relationship, even if the dose of the medication does not change diastolic blood pressure. An apparent association that is caused by another characteristic like this is most often called **confounding**.

In health research, there are two approaches to decrease the impact of confounding on observed associations. First, we can design a study with features that reduce the impact of confounding. One such feature is **matching**. In matching, two (or more) measurements are made on the same individual or on individuals who are the same as far as characteristics that are potential confounders are concerned. If there is no difference in these characteristics, they cannot be confounders.

The second design feature that can be used to decrease the impact of confounding is **randomization**. In randomization, persons are randomly assigned to groups. This tends to make the groups similar in all characteristics, including those that are potential confounders. Unlike matching, however, randomization does not guarantee that potential confounders will have the same distribution in the groups. Just by chance, there could still be confounding.

The second approach to controlling confounding is to include potential confounders as independent variables in multivariable analyses. In the next three chapters, we will see how independent variables can serve this important function.

CHAPTER 10

MULTIVARIABLE ANALYSIS OF A CONTINUOUS DEPENDENT VARIABLE

In Chapter 7, we discussed bivariable analysis of a continuous dependent variable. In that chapter we considered, in turn, continuous and nominal independent variables. When the independent variable represents continuous data, the choices for bivariable analysis include regression analysis and correlation analysis. The same is true

Introduction to Biostatistical Applications in Health Research with Microsoft Office Excel® and R,
Second Edition. Robert P. Hirsch.
© 2021 John Wiley & Sons, Inc. Published 2021 by John Wiley & Sons, Inc.
Companion website: www.wiley.com/go/hirsch/healthresearch2e

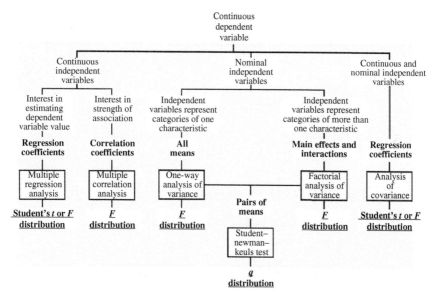

FLOWCHART 8 Flowchart showing multivariable analysis of a continuous dependent variable. The point estimate that is most often used to describe the dependent variable is in bold. The common name of the statistical test is enclosed in a box. The standard distribution used to test hypotheses and calculate confidence intervals is in bold and underlined.

in multivariable analysis, only they now include more than one continuous independent variable and are called **multiple regression analysis** and **multiple correlation analysis**.

When the independent variable represents nominal data, the bivariable analysis we use is Student's t-test. The purpose of this test is to compare dependent variable values between the two groups specified by the nominal independent variable. In a multivariable analysis, we can have more than one nominal independent variable and, as a result, more than two groups of dependent variable values. The multivariable methods that we use to compare these groups include **analysis of variance** and **posterior tests**.

Multivariable analysis of a continuous dependent variable includes statistical methods for which there is no bivariable parallel. These methods are used when a data set includes a mixture of continuous and nominal independent variables. The multivariable method used in this case is called **analysis of covariance (ANCOVA)**. These statistical methods are summarized in Flowchart 8.

10.1 CONTINUOUS INDEPENDENT VARIABLES

One thing statisticians like is a linear relationship. We saw this in bivariable regression and correlation analyses when the relationship between a continuous dependent variable and a continuous independent variable was considered to be a straight line. Even though there is more than one continuous independent variable in multiple regression and correlation analyses, the assumed relationship between the dependent variable and those continuous independent variables continues to be linear. However, with more than one independent variable, the relationship is more complicated than that can be described as a straight line. In this case, the linear relationship includes the effects of each of the independent variables added together. This is easiest to see in the context of multiple regression analysis.

10.1.1 Multiple Regression Analysis

In multiple regression analysis, we have a continuous dependent variable and more than one continuous independent variable. The way the independent variables are related to the dependent variable is by adding their effects. This is illustrated in Equation (10.1):

$$\mu_{Y|X_1,X_2,\dots,X_k} = \alpha + (\beta_1 \cdot X_1) + (\beta_2 \cdot X_2) + \cdots + (\beta_k \cdot X_k) \tag{10.1}$$

where

$\mu_{Y|X_1,X_2,\dots,X_k}$ = mean of the dependent variable in the population corresponding to a particular set of values for each of the k independent variables

α = intercept of the population's multiple regression equation

β_i = regression coefficient (i.e., slope) for the ith (out of k) independent variable in the population

X_i = value of the ith (out of k) independent variable

10.1.1.1 *Estimation of Regression Coefficients.* In multiple regression analysis, we tend to use the term "**regression coefficient**" instead of "slope" to refer to the number by which we multiply independent variable values. The reason for this is that "slope" implies a two-dimensional relationship. This fits a bivariable regression equation, but multivariable regression equations have more than two dimensions.

Equation (10.2) shows the multiple regression equation as it is estimated from the sample's observations:

$$\hat{Y} = a + (b_1 \cdot X_1) + (b_2 \cdot X_2) + \cdots + (b_k \cdot X_k) \tag{10.2}$$

Estimates of the intercept and regression coefficients in the multiple regression equation are based on the same least squares approach we used to estimate the slope and intercept of the bivariable regression equation in Chapter 7.[1] In that chapter, we took a look at the mathematical equation that is used in the method of least squares

[1] In Chapter 7, we found that the least squares method of estimation involves calculations that minimize the sum of the squared differences between observed and estimated values of the dependent variable.

to estimate the slope of the bivariable regression equation. It was done as an aid to understanding, rather than as a suggestion that we will, in practice, be determining the value of that estimate manually. We recognize that the computer will be doing the calculations for us when we are actually analyzing data. Now that we are considering multiple regression analysis, we need to rely on other methods to understand the logic behind estimation of the regression coefficients, since having more than one independent variable makes the math virtually useless for most of us as a method to understand the logic. So, we will leave these calculations to the computer.

10.1.1.2 *Control of Confounding.*

Since multiple regression analysis involves two or more independent variables, we must now confront an issue that does not exist when we have only one independent variable. This is how the relationship between the dependent variable and each of the independent variables is influenced by the inclusion of the other independent variables in the analysis. Multiple regression analysis (and all other multivariable analyses) does this by taking into account the relationship between the dependent variable and all of the other independent variables before considering the relationship between the dependent variable and a particular independent variable.

To see how this works, let us consider a multiple regression equation with only two independent variables. Suppose we are interested in examining the relationship between diastolic blood pressure (DBP, the dependent variable) and dietary sodium intake and age (NA and Age, the independent variables). Equation (10.3) shows the estimated regression equation for those three variables:

$$\widehat{\text{DBP}} = a + (b_1 \cdot \text{NA}) + (b_2 \cdot \text{Age}) \tag{10.3}$$

where
$\widehat{\text{DBP}}$ = estimated diastolic blood pressure (dependent variable)
a = sample's estimate of the intercept
NA = dietary sodium intake (independent variable)
b_1 = sample's estimate of the regression coefficient for dietary sodium intake
Age = age (independent variable)
b_2 = sample's estimate of the regression coefficient for age

Now suppose the research question for these data is, "How does dietary sodium intake affect diastolic blood pressure?" Then, the reason for age being included as an independent variable is to control for its effect on diastolic blood pressure. The concern is that both diastolic blood pressure and dietary sodium intake increase with age. If this is true, an observed association between diastolic blood pressure and dietary sodium intake might only be due to the relationship of both with age.

This can lead to a type of bias known as confounding.[2] By including age as an independent variable in the multiple regression equation, we can control for its effect as a confounder before considering the relationship between dietary sodium intake and diastolic blood pressure. Example 10.1 shows how this process affects estimates of regression coefficients.

■ EXAMPLE 10.1

Suppose we determine diastolic blood pressure (DBP) and average dietary sodium intake (NA) for 40 persons between 40 and 79 years of age. Imagine we make the following observations:

	A	B	C				
1	AGE	NA	DBP	21	59	2,498	106
2	40	2,019	92	22	60	2,663	99
3	41	2,628	79	23	61	2,736	114
4	42	2,404	71	24	62	2,500	111
5	43	2,382	81	25	63	2,890	84
6	44	2,581	71	26	64	2,541	129
7	45	2,332	84	27	65	2,618	96
8	46	2,231	85	28	66	2,841	118
9	47	2,385	87	29	67	2,712	120
10	48	2,275	63	30	68	2,481	100
11	49	2,607	92	31	69	2,707	101
12	50	2,496	87	32	70	2,765	119
13	51	2,583	75	33	71	2,541	98
14	52	2,391	85	34	72	2,721	117
15	53	2,403	81	35	73	2,494	110
16	54	2,321	71	36	74	3,034	113
17	55	2,457	97	37	75	3,068	99
18	56	2,478	104	38	76	2,887	123
19	57	2,640	111	39	77	2,567	106
20	58	2,440	93	40	78	2,805	123
				41	79	2,791	101

Now, let us perform a bivariable regression analysis with DBP as the dependent variable and NA as the only independent variable. We will do this just as we did in Chapter 7 using the "Regression" analysis tool in "Data Analysis" under the "Data" tab in Excel.

---

[2]Confounding occurs when there is a correlation between independent variables, but not all of the independent variables have biologic relationships with the dependent variable. In this circumstance, there can be a statistical association that does not reflect a biologic relationship.

SUMMARY OUTPUT					
Regression statistics					
Multiple R	0.531200628				
R square	0.282174107				
Adjusted R square	0.263283952				
Standard error	14.40685489				
Observations	40				
ANOVA					
	df	*SS*	*MS*	*F*	*Significance F*
Regression	1	3100.416218	3100.416218	14.93762787	0.000420689
Residual	38	7887.183782	207.5574679		
Total	39	10987.6			
	Coefficients	*Standard error*	*t Stat*	*P-value*	*Lower 95%*	*Upper 95%*
Intercept	−8.157165883	27.40641543	−0.297637095	0.767601353	−63.63855334	47.32422157
NA	0.041027729	0.010615407	3.864922751	0.000420689	0.01953796	0.062517497

We can also do this in R using the "summary(lm(DV~IV))" command[3]:

>summary(lm(DBP~SODIUM,data=Example10_1))

```
Call:
lm(formula = DBP ~ SODIUM, data = Example10_1)

Residuals:
 Min 1Q Median 3Q Max
-26.735 -7.579 -0.428 11.050 32.906

Coefficients:
 Estimate Std. Error t value Pr(>|t|)
(Intercept) -8.15717 27.40642 -0.298 0.767601
SODIUM 0.04103 0.01062 3.865 0.000421 ***
---
Signif. codes: 0 '***' 0.001 '**' 0.01 '*' 0.05 '.' 0.1 ' ' 1

Residual standard error: 14.41 on 38 degrees of freedom
Multiple R-squared: 0.2822, Adjusted R-squared: 0.2633
F-statistic: 14.94 on 1 and 38 DF, p-value: 0.0004207
```

From that output, it appears that dietary sodium is a predictor of diastolic blood pressure, since the *P*-value for the omnibus null hypothesis is 0.00042, which is less than 0.05, and the regression coefficient is 0.0410, which is significantly different from 0.

---

[3]We have to use "SODIUM" as the name for dietary sodium intake instead of "NA" because "NA" is a reserved term in R standing for missing data.

Now, let us add age as a second independent variable. Doing this will control for the relationship between age and DBP before examining the relationship between NA and DBP. In Excel, we get:

SUMMARY OUTPUT						
Regression statistics						
Multiple R	0.736695047					
R square	0.542719592					
Adjusted R square	0.518001732					
Standard error	11.65311026					
Observations	40					
ANOVA						
	df	*SS*	*MS*	*F*	*Significance F*	
Regression	2	5,963.185788	2981.592894	21.95657691	5.16866E-07	
Residual	37	5,024.414212	135.7949787			
Total	39	10,987.6				
	Coefficients	*Standard error*	*t Stat*	*P-value*	*Lower 95%*	*Upper 95%*
Intercept	30.94403234	23.74741838	1.303048266	0.200609557	–17.1728078	79.06087247
AGE	1.031600814	0.22467789	4.591465659	4.94534E-05	0.576360168	1.486841461
NA	0.001972819	0.012086246	0.163228477	0.871226852	–0.02251624	0.026461879

In R, we get the following:

>summary(lm(DBP~AGE+SODIUM,data=Example10_1))

```
Call:
lm(formula = DBP ~ AGE + SODIUM, data = Example10_1)

Residuals:
 Min 1Q Median 3Q Max
-21.949 -8.350 0.741 8.285 27.021

Coefficients:
 Estimate Std. Error t value Pr(>|t|)
(Intercept) 30.944032 23.747418 1.303 0.201
AGE 1.031601 0.224678 4.591 4.95e-05 ***
SODIUM 0.001973 0.012086 0.163 0.871
---
Signif. codes: 0 '***' 0.001 '**' 0.01 '*' 0.05 '.' 0.1 ' ' 1

Residual standard error: 11.65 on 37 degrees of freedom
Multiple R-squared: 0.5427, Adjusted R-squared: 0.518
F-statistic: 21.96 on 2 and 37 DF, p-value: 5.169e-07
```

Now, the relationship between DBP and NA is very different. Instead of 0.0410, the regression coefficient for NA is 0.002 and it is no longer significantly different from 0 (P-value $= 0.87123$). This tells us that the apparent relationship we observed between NA and DBP in the first regression analysis was almost entirely due to the confounding effect of age. ∎

From this example, we can see how controlling for age affects the regression coefficient for dietary sodium intake. Now, let us take a closer look at the regression coefficient for age.

Multiple regression analysis cannot discriminate between independent variables that are included in a multiple regression equation because they address the research question (like dietary sodium intake) and those that have been included to control their effect as a confounder (like age). Thus, the regression coefficient for age in the multiple regression equation reflects the relationship between age and diastolic blood pressure after controlling the potential confounding effect of dietary sodium intake just like the regression coefficient for dietary sodium intake reflects the relationship between dietary sodium intake and diastolic blood pressure after controlling the potential confounding effect of age. It works both ways. This is illustrated in the next example.

■ EXAMPLE 10.2

The following output is the result of using the "Regression" analysis tool in Excel to perform a bivariable regression analysis with age as the only independent variable:

SUMMARY OUTPUT						
Regression statistics						
Multiple R	0.736471524					
R square	0.542390306					
Adjusted R square	0.530347946					
Standard error	11.50289697					
Observations	40					
ANOVA						
	df	*SS*	*MS*	*F*	*Significance F*	
Regression	1	5,959.56773	5,959.56773	45.04019894	6.0632E-08	
Residual	38	5,028.03227	132.3166387			
Total	39	10,987.6				
	Coefficients	*Standard error*	*t Stat*	*P-value*	*Lower 95%*	*Upper 95%*
Intercept	34.48405253	9.549566282	3.611059551	0.000878398	15.15196628	53.81613878
AGE	1.057410882	0.157559149	6.711199516	6.0632E-08	0.738449061	1.376372703

The following is the same model in R:

```
Call:
lm(formula = DBP ~ AGE, data = Example10_1)

Residuals:
```

```
Min 1Q Median 3Q Max
-22.240 -8.303 1.059 8.397 26.842

Coefficients:
 Estimate Std. Error t value Pr(>|t|)
(Intercept) 34.4841 9.5496 3.611 0.000878 ***
AGE 1.0574 0.1576 6.711 6.06e-08 ***
---
Signif. codes: 0 '***' 0.001 '**' 0.01 '*' 0.05 '.' 0.1 ' ' 1

Residual standard error: 11.5 on 38 degrees of freedom
Multiple R-squared: 0.5424, Adjusted R-squared: 0.5303
F-statistic: 45.04 on 1 and 38 DF, p-value: 6.063e-08
```

Just as for NA, the relationship between age and DBP appears to have a stronger relationship with DBP when it is the only independent variable. This is evident by the increase in the value of the regression coefficient and the decrease of the P-value when age is the only independent variable compared to when NA is included as a second independent variable.

The regression coefficient for age is equal to 1.05741 mmHg/year when it is the only independent variable in a bivariable regression analysis. This is of higher numeric magnitude than when dietary sodium intake is also included in the multiple regression equation (1.03160 mmHg/year). The difference between the two regression coefficients for age is much smaller than the difference between the regression coefficients for dietary sodium intake. This implies that controlling for dietary sodium intake does affect the relationship between diastolic blood pressure and age, but it does not have a substantial impact on that relationship. ■

Estimates of the regression coefficients for independent variables in a multiple regression equation reflect the relationship between the corresponding independent variable and the dependent variable after taking into account all of the other independent variables. The fact that some independent variables are included in a multiple regression equation because they reflect the research question (like dietary sodium intake) and others are included to control for their effect as a confounder (like age) is reflected in the way in which the results are interpreted, not in the way calculations are performed. Estimation for all independent variables in a multiple regression equation is based on the same logical process.

10.1.1.3 *Variability of Dependent Variable Values.*
What we saw happen to the regression coefficients for age and dietary sodium intake when we compared bivariable and multivariable regression equations in Examples 10.1 and 10.2 is the result of a relationship between those independent variables that we call **multicollinearity**. Multicollinearity affects the results of multivariable analyses when independent variables have two characteristics. First, for multicollinearity to exist, the independent variables need to be correlated with each other. By being correlated, we mean that the independent variables share some of their variability. Second, some

of that shared variability needs to include variability that is used to "explain" (i.e., estimate) the dependent variable. When two or more independent variables have both of these characteristics, we say that they are **collinear**.

The usual result of multicollinearity on estimates of regression coefficients is to reduce the absolute numeric magnitude of the regression coefficients for the collinear independent variables. The magnitude of that reduction depends on how much of the variability used by a particular independent variable to estimate dependent variable values is correlated with the other independent variable(s) in the multiple regression equation. The key to understanding how to interpret the results of multiple regression analysis is to understand the relationships between the variability of the independent variables and how that variability contributes to estimation of dependent variable values.

As in bivariable regression analysis, we can think of the variability of dependent variable values in multiple regression analysis as being divided between variation that is explained by the relationship with the independent variables and variation that is not explained by that relationship. Also, as in bivariable regression analysis, the explained variation is called the **regression** variation and the unexplained variation is called the **residual** variation. Unlike bivariable regression analysis, however, a multiple regression equation contains two or more independent variables. Thus, we can consider how much of the variation in dependent variable values is explained by all of the independent variables taken together, or how much is explained by individual independent variables taking the other independent variables into account.[4] The latter is a feature of multivariable analyses that is referred to as the **independent contribution** of an independent variable.

In the example of age, dietary sodium intake, and diastolic blood pressure, most of the variability in dietary sodium intake that is used to estimate diastolic blood pressure values is associated with age. We know this is the case because the regression coefficient for dietary sodium intake is much closer to 0 in the multiple regression equation than in the bivariable regression equation. Because the regression coefficient is close to 0, the estimated value of diastolic blood pressure changes very little as dietary sodium intake increases in value. Thus, dietary sodium intake has little independent contribution to estimation of diastolic blood pressure values.

The same is not true for age. Since the regression coefficient for age is not much closer to 0 in the multiple regression equation than in the bivariable regression equation, we can conclude that little of the variability in diastolic blood pressure explained by age is the same as the variability associated with dietary sodium intake. Thus, age has a considerable independent contribution to estimation of diastolic blood pressure values.

To see how this works, let us take a look at the R^2 values in the Excel and R output in Examples 10.1 and 10.2. We learned in Chapter 7 that these values tell us the

---

[4]We could also consider the contribution of subsets of independent variables, but this would be useful only if these subsets represent interesting biologic relationships.

TABLE 10.1. R^2 Values for the Regression Equations in Examples 10.1 and 10.2*

Regression Equation	R^2	Difference
$\widehat{\text{DBP}} = a + b_1 \cdot \text{NA} + b_2 \cdot \text{Age}$	0.5427	–
$\widehat{\text{DBP}} = a + b \cdot \text{Age}$	0.5424	0.0003
$\widehat{\text{DBP}} = a + b \cdot \text{NA}$	0.2822	0.2605

[a] The column labeled "Difference" is the R^2 value for the corresponding equation subtracted from the R^2 value for the equation including both independent variable.

proportion of the variation in the dependent variable that is associated with the independent variable.[5] Table 10.1 summarizes the R^2 values from the three regression analyses in these two examples.

Notice that the R^2 value for the regression equation that includes both independent variables (called the "**full model**") is larger than the values for either of the regression equations excluding one of independent variables (called a "**reduced model**"). This will always be the case. Adding more independent variables, even if they are just random numbers, will cause the R^2 value to increase. This is because every independent variable will be associated to some degree with the dependent variable, if only by chance.

These relationships can also be represented graphically. In this graphic approach, the variability of a variable is represented as a rectangle and associations between variables are represented by overlap of their rectangles. The amount of overlap of the rectangles relative to the size of the rectangles reflects the strength of these associations. Figures 10.1 through 10.3 are graphic representations of the associations among diastolic blood pressure, dietary sodium intake, and age seen in Examples 10.1 and 10.2.

Table 10.1 also looks at how much larger the R^2 value is in the equation that includes both independent variables compared to those in equations including only one of the independent variables. Differences between these R^2 values are presented in the last column of this table. The difference is very small for age (0.0003) and not very small for dietary sodium intake (0.2605). At first, it might seem this indicates that dietary sodium intake is associated with the greater proportion of variation in diastolic blood pressure, but just the opposite is true. The difference of 0.0003 for the equation that includes only age tells us that dietary sodium intake contributes only 0.0003 over and above that contributed by age in the equation that includes both of the independent variables. Earlier, we learned that this is often referred to as the "independent contribution" of an independent variable. The independent contribution of dietary sodium intake is that it explains 0.0003 of the variation in diastolic

[5] The R^2 value is really a part of correlation analysis, rather than regression analysis. For R^2 to reflect the proportion of variation in the dependent variable explained by the independent variables in the population, the independent variables must all be from a naturalistic sample. Here, we are interested in the amount of explained variation in the sample, without extrapolating the results to the population.

$$\widehat{DBP} = a + b \cdot AGE$$

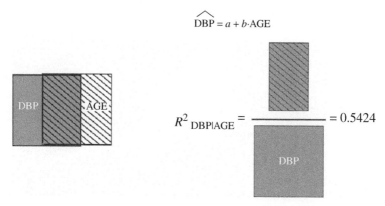

$$R^2_{\text{DBP|AGE}} = \frac{\qquad}{\qquad} = 0.5424$$

Figure 10.1 Graphic representation of the bivariable regression equation that estimates diastolic blood pressure from age. The area of overlap represents the association between the variables. The R^2 value for this regression equation corresponds to the area in which the rectangle for age overlaps the rectangle for diastolic blood pressure divided by the entire rectangle for diastolic blood pressure.

$$\widehat{DBP} = a + b \cdot NA$$

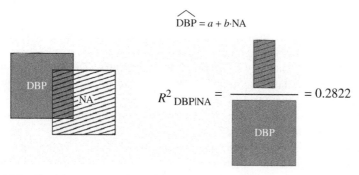

$$R^2_{\text{DBP|NA}} = \frac{\qquad}{\qquad} = 0.2822$$

Figure 10.2 Graphic representation of the bivariable regression equation that estimates diastolic blood pressure from dietary sodium intake. The area of overlap represents the association between the variables. The R^2 value for this regression equation corresponds to the area in which the rectangle for dietary sodium intake overlaps the rectangle for diastolic blood pressure divided by the entire rectangle for diastolic blood pressure.

blood pressure over and above the variation explained by age. Likewise, the independent contribution of age is that it explains 0.2605 of the variation in diastolic blood pressure over and above the variation explained by dietary sodium intake. Figures 10.4 and 10.5 show how these independent contributions of the independent variable relate to variation in diastolic blood pressure (the dependent variable).

This reduced overlap between diastolic blood pressure and dietary sodium intake in Figure 10.5 is consistent with the results of the multiple regression analysis in Example 10.1. Namely, when age was included as an independent variable in the

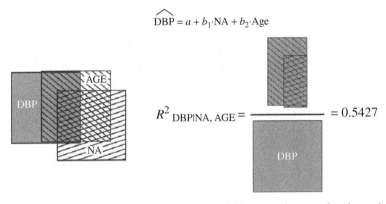

$$\widehat{\text{DBP}} = a + b_1 \cdot \text{NA} + b_2 \cdot \text{Age}$$

$$R^2_{\text{DBP|NA, AGE}} = \frac{}{} = 0.5427$$

Figure 10.3 Graphic representation of the multivariable regression equation that estimates diastolic blood pressure from the combination of dietary sodium intake and age. The areas of overlap represent the associations among the variables. The R^2 value for this regression equation corresponds to the area in which the rectangles for dietary sodium intake and/or age overlap the rectangle for diastolic blood pressure divided by the entire rectangle for diastolic blood pressure.

Independent contribution of age

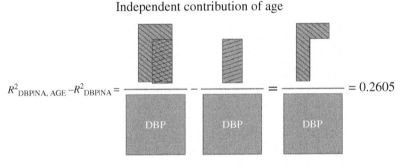

$$R^2_{\text{DBP|NA, AGE}} - R^2_{\text{DBP|NA}} = \frac{}{} - \frac{}{} = \frac{}{} = 0.2605$$

Figure 10.4 Graphic representation of the regression equation that estimates diastolic blood pressure from dietary sodium intake and age. The areas of overlap represent the association among the variables. The difference in R^2 values indicates the independent contribution of Age to the regression equation.

multiple regression equation, very little variability in diastolic blood pressure was explained by dietary sodium intake.

For more general applications, we can calculate the independent contribution of any particular independent variable in a multiple regression equation by subtracting the R^2 value for the reduced model that includes all but that particular independent variable from the R^2 value for the full model that includes all of the independent variables. This difference is called the **partial R^2** or the **coefficient of partial determination**. It is illustrated in Equation (10.4).

$$R^2_{\text{Partial}} = R^2_{\text{Full}} - R^2_{\text{Reduced}} \tag{10.4}$$

Independent contribution of NA

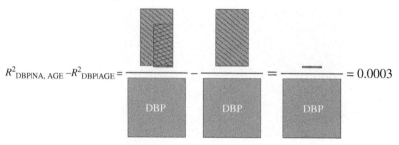

$$R^2_{\text{DBP|NA, AGE}} - R^2_{\text{DBP|AGE}} = \dfrac{\qquad}{\qquad} - \dfrac{\qquad}{\qquad} = \dfrac{\qquad}{\qquad} = 0.0003$$

Figure 10.5 Graphic representation of the regression equation that estimates diastolic blood pressure from dietary sodium intake and age. The areas of overlap represent the association among the variables. The difference in R^2 values indicates the independent contribution of dietary sodium intake to the regression equation.

where

R^2_{Partial} = coefficient of partial determination for independent variable X_i

$R^2_{\text{Full}} = R^2$ from the full model (i.e., including all of the independent variables)

$R^2_{\text{Reduced}} = R^2$ from the reduced model that includes all of the independent variables except the one for which the partial R^2 is calculated (X_i)

Earlier in this chapter, we recalled from Chapter 7 that the R^2 in bivariable regression analysis tells us the proportion of variation in dependent variable values explained by the independent variable. R^2 in multivariable regression analysis tells us the proportion of variation in dependent variable values explained by all of the independent variables taken together and the partial R^2 tells us the proportion of variation in dependent variable values explained by a particular independent variable over and above the variation explained by the other independent variables.

10.1.1.4 Hypothesis Testing. In bivariable regression analysis, we took chance into account by testing three null hypotheses:

$H_0 : \alpha = 0$ (i.e., the population's intercept is equal to 0)

$H_0 : \beta = 0$ (i.e., the population's slope is equal to 0)

H_0:The independent variable does not help estimate dependent variable values (i.e., the omnibus null hypothesis)

These same null hypotheses are tested in multiple regression analysis, but with some distinctions. The first of these is that there are separate null hypotheses to be tested for the regression coefficients for each of the independent variables. Also, the omnibus null hypothesis addresses all of the independent variables taken together instead of an individual independent variable.

In the bottom part of the "Regression" output in Excel and in the middle of the "summary(lm())" output in R, we find the sample's estimate of the intercept and the sample's estimates of the regression coefficients that correspond to each of the independent variables. Also, in that part of the output, we find the standard errors for each of the estimates, Student's t-values resulting from a test of the null hypothesis that the corresponding population's value is equal to 0, and its P-value. If the P-value is equal to or less than α, (which is usually equal to 0.05), we reject the null hypothesis and, through the process of elimination, accept the alternative hypothesis that the population's parameter is not equal to 0. This sounds like the way we interpret the P-values from bivariable regression analysis, but there is an important difference: these P-values in multiple regression analysis also reflect multicollinearity.

To see how this works, it helps to look at how a Student's t-value can be used to test the null hypothesis that a particular regression coefficient is equal to 0 in the population. One way to do this is by dividing the sample's estimate of the regression coefficient by its standard error just like in bivariable regression analysis (Equation (7.11)). This is illustrated for multiple regression analysis in Equation (10.5).

$$t = \frac{b_i - \beta_{0_i}}{s_{b_i}} \tag{10.5}$$

where

t = Student's t-value that corresponds to the sample's estimate of the regression coefficient for the ith independent variable

b_i = sample's estimate of the regression coefficient for the ith independent variable

β_{0_i} = value of the regression coefficient for the ith independent variable in the population according to the null hypothesis (equal to 0)

s_{b_i} = sample's estimate of the standard error for the estimate of the regression coefficient for the ith independent variable

For better understanding of how to interpret the results of these tests, it is helpful to consider another way by which those t-values could be calculated. This way uses the independent variable's unique contribution to estimation of dependent variable values as expressed by the partial R^2 (Equation (10.4)). The partial R^2 is multiplied by the total sum of squares to determine the amount of variation in the dependent variable explained by the independent variable and then compared (by division) with the unexplained variation (error mean square). The square root of that value is exactly equal to Student's t-value testing the null hypothesis that the corresponding regression coefficient is equal to 0 in the population as shown in Equation (10.5). This relationship is illustrated in Equation (10.6).

$$t = \frac{b_i - \beta_{0_i}}{s_{b_i}} = \sqrt{\frac{R^2_{\text{Partial}} \cdot \text{total SS}}{\text{residual MS}}} \tag{10.6}$$

where

t = Student's t-value used to test the null hypothesis that the regression coefficient for the ith independent variable is equal to 0 in the population

R^2_{Partial} = coefficient of partial determination for independent variable X_i (from Equation (10.4))

total SS = total sum of squares from the multiple regression equation that includes all of the independent variables (i.e., the full model)

residual MS = residual mean square from the multiple regression equation that includes all of the independent variables (i.e., the full model)

The numerator of Equation (10.6) reflects the unique contribution of that independent variable to estimation of dependent variable values. If that independent variable is collinear with one (or more) other independent variable(s) in the multiple regression equation, the numeric magnitude of the numerator will be reduced. The greater the degree of multicollinearity, the greater the reduction in numeric magnitude and, as a result, the smaller Student's t-value. A smaller value of Student's t makes it harder to reject the null hypothesis. Thus, multicollinearity affects hypothesis testing in multiple regression analysis by making it harder to reject the null hypothesis that a particular regression coefficient is equal to 0 in the population. This effect is illustrated in the next example.

■ EXAMPLE 10.3

Let us compare hypothesis testing for the regression coefficient of dietary sodium intake with and without age in the model to see how multicollinearity affects hypothesis testing.

To begin with, we will look again at the result of testing the null hypothesis that the regression coefficient for dietary sodium intake is equal to 0 when dietary sodium intake is the only independent variable (i.e., from bivariable regression analysis). The "Regression" output from Excel for that bivariable regression analysis is (as seen in Example 10.1):

SUMMARY OUTPUT						
Regression statistics						
Multiple R	0.531200628					
R square	0.282174107					
Adjusted R square	0.263283952					
Standard error	14.40685489					
Observations	40					
ANOVA						
	df	*SS*	*MS*	*F*	*Significance F*	
Regression	1	3,100.416218	3,100.416218	14.93762787	0.000420689	
Residual	38	7,887.183782	207.5574679			
Total	39	10,987.6				
	Coefficients	*Standard error*	*t stat*	*P-value*	*Lower 95%*	*Upper 95%*
Intercept	–8.157165883	27.40641543	–0.297637095	0.767601353	–63.63855334	47.32422157
NA	0.041027729	0.010615407	3.864922751	0.000420689	0.01953796	0.062517497

To get the same information from R, we need to use two commands. The command "summary(lm())" gives us the R^2, the F-test, and the regression coefficients and the results of testing the null hypothesis that they are equal to 0 in the population. It does not give us the information in the "ANOVA" table. To get that information in R, we have to use the "summary.aov(lm())" command. The following shows the results of using both commands in R to analyze these data.

>summary(lm(DBP~SODIUM,data=Example10_1))

```
Call:
lm(formula = DBP ~ SODIUM, data = Example10_1)

Residuals:
 Min 1Q Median 3Q Max
-26.735 -7.579 -0.428 11.050 32.906

Coefficients:
 Estimate Std. Error t value Pr(>|t|)
(Intercept) -8.15717 27.40642 -0.298 0.767601
SODIUM 0.04103 0.01062 3.865 0.000421 ***
---
Signif. codes: 0 '***' 0.001 '**' 0.01 '*' 0.05 '.' 0.1 ' ' 1

Residual standard error: 14.41 on 38 degrees of freedom
Multiple R-squared: 0.2822, Adjusted R-squared: 0.2633
F-statistic: 14.94 on 1 and 38 DF, p-value: 0.0004207
```

>summary.aov(lm(DBP~SODIUM,data=Example10_1))

```
 Df Sum Sq Mean Sq F value Pr(>F)
SODIUM 1 3100 3100.4 14.94 0.000421 ***
Residuals 38 7887 207.6
---
Signif. codes: 0 '***' 0.001 '**' 0.01 '*' 0.05 '.' 0.1 ' ' 1
```

Note that the "Total" variation is not given in the output from R. If these are needed, the total degrees of freedom and the total sum of squares can be found by adding the other values given.

As we learned in Chapter 7, the P-value from the test of the null hypothesis that the regression coefficient (i.e., the slope) is equal to 0 in the population appears in the fourth column of the bottom table in output from the "Regression" analysis tool and in the middle of the first R output. Here, the P-value is 0.0004, which is less than 0.05. Thus, we are able to reject the null hypothesis that the regression coefficient is equal to 0 in the population.

Now, let us look at the same hypothesis test, but from multivariable regression analysis that includes age as another independent variable. The "Regression" output from Excel for this multivariable regression analysis is (as seen in Example 10.1):

SUMMARY OUTPUT						
Regression statistics						
Multiple R	0.736695047					
R square	0.542719592					
Adjusted R square	0.518001732					
Standard error	11.65311026					
Observations	40					
ANOVA						
	df	*SS*	*MS*	*F*	*Significance F*	
Regression	2	5,963.185788	2,981.592894	21.95657691	5.16866E-07	
Residual	37	5,024.414212	135.7949787			
Total	39	10,987.6				
	Coefficients	*Standard error*	*t Stat*	*P-value*	*Lower 95%*	*Upper 95%*
Intercept	30.94403234	23.74741838	1.303048266	0.200609557	–17.1728078	79.06087247
AGE	1.031600814	0.22467789	4.591465659	4.94534E-05	0.576360168	1.486841461
NA	0.001972819	0.012086246	0.163228477	0.871226852	–0.02251624	0.026461879

The corresponding results from R are as follows:

>summary(lm(DBP~AGE+SODIUM,data=Example10_1))

```
Call:
lm(formula = DBP ~ AGE + SODIUM, data = Example10_1)

Residuals:
 Min 1Q Median 3Q Max
-21.949 -8.350 0.741 8.285 27.021

Coefficients:
 Estimate Std. Error t value Pr(>|t|)
(Intercept) 30.944032 23.747418 1.303 0.201
AGE 1.031601 0.224678 4.591 4.95e-05 ***
SODIUM 0.001973 0.012086 0.163 0.871
---
Signif. codes: 0 '***' 0.001 '**' 0.01 '*' 0.05 '.' 0.1 ' ' 1

Residual standard error: 11.65 on 37 degrees of freedom
Multiple R-squared: 0.5427, Adjusted R-squared: 0.518
F-statistic: 21.96 on 2 and 37 DF, p-value: 5.169e-07
```

>summary.aov(lm(DBP~AGE+SODIUM,data=Example10_1))

```
 Df Sum Sq Mean Sq F value Pr(>F)
AGE 1 5960 5960 43.887 9.01e-08 ***
SODIUM 1 4 4 0.027 0.871
Residuals 37 5024 136
---
Signif. codes: 0 '***' 0.001 '**' 0.01 '*' 0.05 '.' 0.1 ' ' 1
```

Note that in the R, output from the "summary.aov(lm())" command has the "Regression" variation divided into parts according to the independent variables. To get the regression degrees of freedom and the regression sum of squares, we add those values for each independent variable.

In this output, the P-value testing the null hypothesis that the regression coefficient for dietary sodium intake is equal to 0 in the population is equal to 0.871. This is much larger than the P-value from the bivariable regression analysis. When the P-value in multivariable analysis is larger than the P-value from bivariable analysis, this is an indication that multicollinearity exists between that independent variable and at least one other independent variable in the multivariable regression equation.

Now, let us use Equation (10.6) to calculate Student's t-value for the test of this null hypothesis. For the numerator of this equation, we need the partial R^2 for dietary sodium intake. We could calculate this by subtracting the R^2 from the model that includes only AGE from the R^2 from the full model. We found that this is equal to 0.0003 in Table 10.1.

$$t = \sqrt{\frac{R^2_{\text{Partial}} \cdot \text{total SS}}{\text{residual MS}}} = \sqrt{\frac{0.0003 \cdot 10,987.6}{135.7949787}} = 0.1632$$

This result is the same as Student's t-value corresponding to the regression coefficient for dietary sodium intake at the bottom of the Excel output for the multiple regression analysis (when it is rounded to four decimals). Thus, testing the null hypothesis that a particular regression coefficient is equal to 0 in the population using the partial R^2 is equivalent to using the point estimate of the regression coefficient and its standard error.   ∎

So, one way that hypothesis testing in multiple regression analysis differs from hypothesis testing in bivariable regression analysis concerns the test that a particular regression coefficient is equal to 0 in the population. The difference is that the ability to reject this null hypothesis in multiple regression analysis can be reduced by multicollinearity. In essence, it is a test of the null hypothesis that the independent variable does not have a unique (i.e., independent) contribution to estimation of dependent variable values. It only considers the relationship between the dependent and an independent variable after taking all of the other independent variables into account.

Another null hypothesis we tested in bivariable regression analysis was the omnibus null hypothesis. The omnibus null hypothesis in bivariable regression analysis is that the independent variable does not help estimate dependent variable values. In multiple regression analysis, the omnibus null hypothesis states that *all of* the independent variables *taken together* do not help estimate dependent variable values. The F-ratio and its corresponding P-value used to test the omnibus null hypothesis in multiple regression analysis appear in the second part of the output from the "Regression" analysis tool and the bottom of the R output just like they do in bivariable regression analysis.

In Chapter 7, we found that the test of the omnibus null hypothesis in bivariable regression analysis yields exactly the same result as the test of the null hypothesis that the slope is equal to 0 in the population. Thus, the test of the omnibus null hypothesis in bivariable regression provides no new information. This is not the case in multiple regression analysis.

The omnibus null hypothesis in multivariable analysis tests the null hypothesis that all of the independent variables in a regression equation, taken together, do not help estimate dependent variable values. In bivariable regression analysis, only the single independent variable was considered. This made the test of the omnibus null hypothesis in bivariable regression analysis the same as the test that the slope is equal to 0. In multiple regression analysis, however, "all of the independent variables" refer to the entire collection of independent variables. Thus, the test of the omnibus null hypothesis in multiple regression analysis is no longer redundant. Instead, it addresses a unique aspect of the relationship between the dependent variable and the independent variables.

The F-ratio used to test the omnibus null hypothesis in multiple regression analysis is equal to the regression mean square divided by the residual mean square. This calculation appears in Equation (10.7).

$$F = \frac{\text{Regression mean square}}{\text{Residual mean square}} \tag{10.7}$$

Equation (10.7) is the same as the equation for the F-ratio in Chapter 7 (Equation (7.17)). A difference between these two F-ratios is in the degrees of freedom. In bivariable regression analysis, the degrees of freedom in the numerator of the F-ratio (i.e., the regression degrees of freedom) are equal to 1. In multivariable regression analysis, the degrees of freedom in the numerator of the F-ratio are greater than 1. In the example of diastolic blood pressure being estimated from dietary sodium intake and age, the regression degrees of freedom are equal to 2 (see, the second output in Example 10.1 or 10.3). In general, the regression degrees of freedom are equal to the number of independent variables in the regression equation. In bivariable regression analysis, there is one independent variable and, thus, one model degree of freedom. In multivariable regression analysis, there is more than one independent variable, corresponding to more than one model degree of freedom.

The F-ratio in multiple regression analysis considers all of the independent variables as a unit when the omnibus null hypothesis is tested. Since all of the independent variables are considered, the degree to which these independent variables share information used to estimate dependent variable values does not detract from the ability to reject the omnibus null hypothesis as it does when testing the null hypothesis for an individual regression coefficient. The test of the omnibus null hypothesis in multiple regression analysis is not influenced by multicollinearity in the way that a test of the null hypotheses for a particular regression coefficient is affected. This is because the influence of one independent variable is not "subtracted" from the influence of another independent variable when considering the omnibus null hypothesis. This can lead to apparent contradictions in the conclusions drawn from multiple regression analyses, as illustrated in the next example.

■ EXAMPLE 10.4

To take a closer look at how multicollinearity affects hypothesis testing in multiple regression analysis, let us add another independent variable to the multiple regression equation. To make this new independent variable collinear with age and dietary sodium intake, we will create it by squaring each person's age.[6] Then, the output from the "Regression" analysis tool in Excel is as follows:

SUMMARY OUTPUT						
Regression statistics						
Multiple R	0.746018211					
R square	0.556543172					
Adjusted R square	0.519588436					
Standard error	11.63391384					
Observations	40					
ANOVA						
	df	*SS*	*MS*	*F*	*Significance F*	
Regression	3	6,115.073755	2,038.357918	15.06013131	1.63641E-06	
Residual	36	4,872.526245	135.3479512			
Total	39	10,987.6				
	Coefficients	*Standard error*	*t stat*	*P-value*	*Lower 95%*	*Upper 95%*
Intercept	−25.17085877	58.03501872	−0.433718457	0.667081014	−142.8713321	92.52961455
AGE	2.976753096	1.84984053	1.60919444	0.116309432	−0.774897386	6.728403578
AGE^2	−0.016367344	0.015450494	−1.059341147	0.296500651	−0.047702398	0.01496771
NA	0.002168623	0.012067751	0.179704009	0.858392642	−0.022305911	0.026643157

When analyze these data using R, we get the following results:

>summary(lm(DBP~AGE+AGESQ+SODIUM,data=Example10_4))

---

[6]This creates what is called a **polynomial** regression equation. Polynomial regression analysis is used to allow the relationship between the independent and dependent variables to be curvilinear.

```
Call:
lm(formula = DBP ~ AGE + AGESQ + SODIUM, data = Example 10_4)

Residuals:
 Min 1Q Median 3Q Max
-21.936 -7.557 1.786 8.597 25.189

Coefficients:
 Estimate Std. Error t value Pr(>|t|)
(Intercept) -25.170859 58.035019 -0.434 0.667
AGE 2.976753 1.849841 1.609 0.116
AGESQ -0.016367 0.015450 -1.059 0.297
SODIUM 0.002169 0.012068 0.180 0.858

Residual standard error: 11.63 on 36 degrees of freedom
Multiple R-squared: 0.5565, Adjusted R-squared: 0.5196
F-statistic: 15.06 on 3 and 36 DF, p-value: 1.636e-06
```

Let us take a look at the results of hypothesis testing from this output.

If we look at the bottom of the Excel output or the middle of the R output, we see that we are not able to reject any of the null hypotheses that a particular regression coefficient is equal to 0 in the population. To conclude from this observation that the independent variables do not contribute to estimating diastolic blood pressure would be a mistake. This is evident when we consider the F-ratio and P-value for the omnibus null hypothesis in the middle of the Excel output or the bottom of the R output. This P-value is then 1.63641E-06. This tells us we can reject the omnibus null hypothesis that the entire collection of independent variables does not help estimate dependent variable values. The reason for this apparent discrepancy is the fact that, with the addition of the square of age, the independent variables share practically all of the information they use to estimate dependent variable values. So, none of the independent variables provides sufficient independent information to allow rejection of the null hypothesis that its regression coefficient is equal to 0. When taken as a group, however, the independent variables are able to estimate dependent variable values. We draw this conclusion because of our ability to reject the omnibus null hypothesis. This implies that, although there is substantial overlap between the independent variables, the entire collection of independent variables accounts for a significant degree of variability of the dependent variable in the sample. ■

The apparent contradiction in the conclusions drawn in Example 10.4 leads some to suggest that correlated independent variables should not be included in the same regression equation. This is poor advice, since it ignores the fact that multicollinearity is an intentional feature built into multiple regression analysis, and all other multivariable analyses. It is multicollinearity that allows us to control for the confounding effects of some measurements by including them as independent variables. There is a danger in multicollinearity, but that danger is not the inclusion of collinear variables in the multivariable analysis. Instead, the danger is we might try to interpret the results of multivariable analyses in the same way that we interpret the results of bivariable analyses. In multiple regression analysis, we can avoid this mistake by examining the test of the omnibus null hypothesis as well as tests of null hypotheses about individual regression coefficients. When these seem to disagree (as they do in Example 10.4), we know that the independent variables are collinear.

Even though we do not want to eliminate all collinear independent variables from multivariable analyses, we should be aware that inclusion of an independent variable may make it harder to see relationships between other independent variables and the dependent variable. If we are including independent variables in the regression equation for which we do not intend to control, the multicollinearity should be reduced by removing those independent variables from the multiple regression equation. The square of age in Example 10.5 is such an independent variable. Since it seems to play no independent role in estimation of diastolic blood pressure, it should be excluded from the regression equation.[7]

10.1.2   Multiple Correlation Analysis

The purpose of correlation analysis is to estimate the strength of the association between independent and dependent variables. In multiple correlation analysis, the association between the dependent variable and the entire collection of independent variables is analyzed. The way these independent variables are organized into a collection is through the multiple regression equation. In essence, the **multiple correlation coefficient** reflects the strength of the association between the observed values of the dependent variable and the estimated values of the dependent variable that result when all of the independent variable values are used in the multiple regression equation. Since the regression equation is necessary to calculate the multiple correlation coefficient, multiple correlation analysis is conducted using the "Regression" analysis tool, which reports the multiple correlation coefficient.[8] To test the null hypothesis that the multiple correlation coefficient is equal to 0 in the population, we use the P-value from the test of the omnibus null hypothesis. This is illustrated in the next example:

■ EXAMPLE 10.5

Let us use the output from Example 10.1 to perform multiple correlation analysis.

The following is the Excel output from Example 10.1 in which diastolic blood pressure is the dependent variable and dietary sodium intake and age are the independent variables:

---

[7]This process of removing independent variables that seem to have little independent contribution to estimation of dependent variable values is called "**modeling**."
[8]Or we can use R and take the square root of the R^2.

SUMMARY OUTPUT						
Regression statistics						
Multiple R	0.736695047					
R square	0.542719592					
Adjusted R square	0.518001732					
Standard error	11.65311026					
Observations	40					
ANOVA						
	df	*SS*	*MS*	*F*	*Significance F*	
Regression	2	5,963.185788	2,981.592894	21.95657691	5.16866E-07	
Residual	37	5,024.414212	135.7949787			
Total	39	10,987.6				
	Coefficients	*Standard error*	*t stat*	*P-value*	*Lower 95%*	*Upper 95%*
Intercept	30.94403234	23.74741838	1.303048266	0.200609557	–17.1728078	79.06087247
AGE	1.031600814	0.22467789	4.591465659	4.94534E-05	0.576360168	1.486841461
NA	0.001972819	0.012086246	0.163228477	0.871226852	–0.02251624	0.026461879

The following is the result of analyzing these data in R:
>summary(lm(DBP~AGE+SODIUM,data=Example10_1))

```
Call:
lm(formula = DBP ~ AGE + SODIUM, data = Example10_1)

Residuals:
 Min 1Q Median 3Q Max
-21.949 -8.350 0.741 8.285 27.021

Coefficients:
 Estimate Std. Error t value Pr(>|t|)
(Intercept) 30.944032 23.747418 1.303 0.201
AGE 1.031601 0.224678 4.591 4.95e-05 ***
SODIUM 0.001973 0.012086 0.163 0.871
---
Signif. codes: 0 '***' 0.001 '**' 0.01 '*' 0.05 '.' 0.1 ' ' 1

Residual standard error: 11.65 on 37 degrees of freedom
Multiple R-squared: 0.5427, Adjusted R-squared: 0.518
F-statistic: 21.96 on 2 and 37 DF, p-value: 5.169e-07
```

We can obtain the multiple correlation coefficient directly from the Regression procedure in Excel or by taking the square root of the R^2 in the output from R. Thus, the multiple correlation coefficient is equal to 0.7367. We can test the null hypothesis that this correlation coefficient is equal to 0 in the population by testing the omnibus null hypothesis. The *P*-value for this hypothesis test is 5.16866E-07. Since it is less than 0.05, we can reject the null hypothesis that the multiple correlation coefficient is equal to 0 in the population. ■

The multiple correlation coefficient is part of the regression output because the regression equation is required to calculate it. This does not imply, however, that it is appropriate to interpret the correlation coefficient as a reflection of the strength of the association between the dependent and independent variables in the population. As with the bivariable correlation coefficient, the multiple correlation coefficient requires a naturalistic sample before it can be considered an estimate of the population's value. In the case of multivariable analysis, all of the independent variables in the sample need to be representative of their distributions in the population for the sample to be naturalistic.

10.2   NOMINAL INDEPENDENT VARIABLES

When we had a nominal independent variable in bivariable analysis, the independent variable had the effect of dividing the dependent variable values into two groups. In multivariable analysis, we have more than one nominal independent variable and, thus more than two groups of dependent variable values. In general, $k - 1$ nominal independent variables identify k groups of dependent variable values. The next example describes such a set of data.

■ EXAMPLE 10.6

Suppose we are interested in comparing the serum cholesterol levels (the dependent variable) among persons in four geographic regions of the United States: Northeast (NE), Northwest (NW), Southeast (SE), and Southwest (SW). To do this, we select 10 persons from each region and measure their serum cholesterol levels. Imagine we make the following observations:

	NE	NW	SE	SW
	197	194	220	206
	183	185	202	196
	190	186	212	195
	212	212	221	222
	223	209	227	228
	202	194	224	205
	201	186	197	197
	202	196	201	203
	197	190	198	199
	213	218	218	219
Mean	202	197	212	207

This data set consists of four groups of dependent variable values. This is a multivariable data set, since it takes three nominal independent variables to specify these four groups of dependent variable values. For example, suppose we have the following three nominal independent variables: NE, NW, and SE. Furthermore, suppose NE is equal to "yes" if the person is from the Northeast and equal to "no" if the person is not from the Northeast. Likewise, NW and SE identify persons from the Northwest and Southeast. People from the Southwest are identified when NE, NW, and SE are all equal to "no." Thus, three nominal independent variables are required to specify four groups of dependent variable values. ∎

When we had only two groups of continuous dependent variable values (in Chapter 7), we were interested in comparing the means of these groups. Now that we have more than two groups of dependent variable values, we are still interested in the means of these groups. The difference is that in multivariable analysis we have more than two means to compare.

10.2.1   Analysis of Variance

As far as point estimation is concerned, the mean for each group of dependent variable values is estimated in the same way we estimated the mean for a single group of continuous dependent variable values (Equation (3.1)). To test the null hypothesis that the population's means are equal to the same value, however, we need to use a new method. The name of the method we use to compare the means in multivariable analysis is **analysis of variance**, which is often called **ANOVA**.

This might seem to be a strange name for a method used to compare means, but it refers to the fact that the variation of the means between the groups of dependent variable values is compared with the variation of dependent variable values within these groups. These two sources of variation of dependent variable values are illustrated graphically in Figure 10.6.

The variation of dependent variable values between groups reflects the differences between the means of the groups. If the means of the groups in the population are all equal to the same value (i.e., the null hypothesis is true), we would still expect to see some variation of the sample's estimates of those means just by chance. To test the null hypothesis that the population's means are all equal to the same value, we need to consider whether the observed differences between the groups' means in the sample are greater than what we would expect to see simply due to chance.

The amount of variation we would expect to see among the sample's means simply due to chance depends on how different the data values are from each other. In other words, it depends on the variance of the dependent variable values. The greater the variation in the data, the greater the variation we can expect to see between the

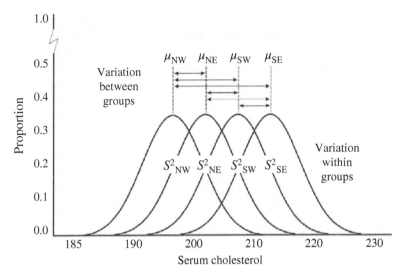

Figure 10.6 Illustration of the variation of dependent variable values between groups and the variation of dependent variable values within groups.

sample's means by chance alone. As a matter of fact, the chance variation in the estimates of the means will be equal, on the average, to the variance of the dependent variable values. Thus, we can test the null hypothesis that the means of the groups in the population are all equal to the same value by seeing how close the observed variation between the means in the sample is to the sample's estimate of the variance of dependent variable values. This is where we get the name, "analysis of variance."

When we had just two groups of continuous dependent variable values (in Chapter 7), we estimated the variance of dependent variable values by assuming that the variances in the two groups were equal in the population. This is the assumption of homoscedasticity. We make that same assumption here as well. The only difference is that we now have more than two estimates of the variance. The method of estimating the variance is, however, the same. That is, we use a weighted average of the group-specific variance estimates to represent our best estimate of the variance in the population (Equation (7.26)). The following equation illustrates how this is applied to more than two groups of dependent variable values:

$$\sigma_Y^2 \triangleq s_{Y|Xs}^2 = \frac{\sum [(n_i - 1) \cdot s_{Y|X_i}^2]}{\sum (n_i - 1)} \tag{10.8}$$

where

σ_Y^2 = variance of the distribution of dependent variable values in the population

$s_{Y|Xs}^2$ = estimate of the variance of dependent variable values pooling estimates for each set of values of the independent variables

$(n_i - 1)$ = degrees of freedom in the ith group of dependent variable values

$s_{Y|X_i}^2$ = variance estimate in the ith group of dependent variable values

So, in ANOVA, we have two measures of the variation in dependent variable values. The one that reflects the variation between the means in the sample is called the **between mean square**. The one that is a pooled estimate of the variance in dependent variable values (Equation (10.8)) is called the **within mean square**. We test the null hypothesis that the population's means are all equal to the same value by comparing the between mean square to the within mean square. The comparison is done by calculating an F-ratio. Equation (10.9) illustrates this calculation in terms of the between mean square and the within mean square:

$$F = \frac{\text{Between mean square}}{\text{Within mean square}} \qquad (10.9)$$

If the null hypothesis that all of the means are equal to the same value in the population is true, we expect to observe, on the average, an F-ratio equal to 1. This implies that the observed difference among the means is the same as we would expect to occur just by chance. If the null hypothesis is not true (i.e., that some of the means are not equal to the same value), we expect that, on the average, the between mean square will be greater than the within mean square. This is because the variation between groups due to differences between means in the population is added onto the differences between groups that is attributable to the variation in the dependent variable values themselves. So, the F-ratio will be greater than 1 (on the average) when the means of the groups in the population are not all equal to the same value.[9]

In Excel, we can use the "Anova: Single Factor" analysis tool to test the null hypothesis that the means are all equal to the same value in the population. The "Anova: Single Factor" analysis tool tests this null hypothesis using the F-ratio in Equation (10.9). In R, we can use the "aov(DV~factor)" command to do the same thing. In the next example, we will take a look at the output from the "Anova: Single Factor" analysis tool and the "aov(DV~factor)" command and see how to interpret them.

■ **EXAMPLE 10.7**

In Example 10.6 we looked at the serum cholesterol levels among persons from four geographic regions of the United States: Northeast (NE), Northwest (NW), Southeast (SE), and Southwest (SW). To do that, we selected 10 persons from each region and measured their serum cholesterol levels. Now, suppose we use the "Anova: Single Factor" analysis tool to analyze these data and we observe the following results:

---

[9]Occasionally, the calculated F-ratio can fall below 1. When this happens, we interpret it to be a random variation from an F-ratio of 1.

Anova: Single factor								
SUMMARY								
Groups	*Count*	*Sum*	*Average*	*Variance*				
NE	10	2,020	202	135.3333333				
NW	10	1,970	197	140.4444444				
SE	10	2,120	212	132.4444444				
SW	10	2,070	207	140				
ANOVA								
Source of variation	*SS*	*df*	*MS*	*F*	*P-value*	*F crit*		
Between groups	1,250	3	416.6666667	3.040129712	0.041324944	2.866265551		
Within groups	4,934	36	137.0555556					
Total	6,184	39						

In R, we can get the ANOVA table using the "aov(DV~factor)" command. In that output, the between variation is labeled with the name of the factor and the within variation is labeled "Residuals." The following is the result of analyzing these data using R:

>aov(CHOL~REGION,data=Example10_6)

```
 Df Sum Sq Mean Sq F value Pr(>F)
REGION 3 1250 416.7 3.04 0.0413 *
Residuals 36 4934 137.1
---
Signif. codes: 0 '***' 0.001 '**' 0.01 '*' 0.05 '.' 0.1 ' ' 1
```

Notice that the between degrees of freedom are equal to three. This reflects the fact that three nominal independent variables are needed to specify the four groups of dependent variable values (see, Example 10.6).

The F-ratio following the between mean square is the same as the F-ratio in Equation (10.9). It tests the null hypothesis that the means of serum cholesterol values in the four regions are equal to the same value in the population. Since the associated P-value is less than 0.05, we can reject that null hypothesis. ◼

10.2.1.1 *Factorial ANOVA.* The type of ANOVA we have been considering is called **one-way** ANOVA. This type of ANOVA is distinguished by the fact that the groups of dependent variables correspond to categories of a single characteristic. In the example of serum cholesterol values, the four groups were considered to be categories of a single characteristic: geographic location.

Sometimes, the groups of dependent variable values are specified by categories of more than one characteristic. For example, the four groups of serum cholesterol values in Example 10.6 that we thought of as representing four categories of a single characteristic (region) could also be thought of as representing two categories of each of two characteristics: North versus South and East versus West. The next example illustrates this way of thinking about the groups of dependent variable values.

■ EXAMPLE 10.8

The following table displays the data from Example 10.6 using two categories of two characteristics instead of four categories of one characteristic.

	North	South
East	197	220
	183	202
	190	212
	212	221
	223	227
	202	224
	201	197
	202	201
	197	198
	213	218
West	194	206
	185	196
	186	195
	212	222
	209	228
	194	205
	186	197
	196	203
	190	199
	218	219

The difference between this table and the table in Example 10.6 is in the way in which we label the means. Now, identifying a mean is a two-step process. First, we specify whether the mean is for persons in the North or in the South (specified by two columns). Once we make that determination, we further specify whether the mean is for persons from the East or the West (specified by two sets of rows).   ■

In statistical terminology, the characteristics that are used to identify groups of dependent variable values are called **factors**. Example 10.6 shows a one-way ANOVA. When we think about dependent variable values as categories of more than one factor, as in Example 10.8, the analysis is called **factorial** ANOVA.

When we have dependent variable values divided according to two (or more) factors, we have additional null hypotheses about the means that can be examined. These additional null hypotheses concern either **main effects** or **interactions**.

The main effect of a factor compares the means of the categories of that factor, ignoring the categories of the other factor(s). For instance, the main effect of the North/South factor in Example 10.8 compares the mean serum cholesterol among the 20 persons from the North, combining persons from the Northeast and Northwest ($[202 + 197]/2 = 199.5$ mg/dL), with the mean among the 20 persons from the South, combining persons from the Southeast and Southwest ($[212 + 207]/2 = 209.5$ mg/dL). The corresponding null hypothesis for the North/South main effect is that the mean serum cholesterol levels in the North are equal to the mean serum cholesterol levels in the South. Likewise, we can compare the mean serum cholesterol levels among persons in the East with the mean serum cholesterol levels among persons in the West combining persons from the North and South. This is the East/West main effect. The next example illustrates testing these main effects using Excel and R.

■ EXAMPLE 10.9

The following Excel output is the result of analyzing the data in Example 10.8 as a factorial ANOVA using the "Anova: Two-Factor with Replication" analysis tool in "Data Analysis" under the "Data" tab.

Anova: Two-factor with replication

SUMMARY		N	S	Total			
	E						
Count		10	10	20			
Sum		2,020	2,120	4,140			
Average		202	212	207			
Variance		135.3333333	132.4444444	153.1578947			
	W						
Count		10	10	20			
Sum		1,970	2,070	4,040			
Average		197	207	202			
Variance		140.4444444	140	159.1578947			
	Total						
Count		20	20				
Sum		3,990	4,190				
Average		199.5	209.5				
Variance		137.2105263	135.6315789				
ANOVA							
Source of variation		SS	df	MS	F	P-value	F crit
Sample		250	1	250	1.824077827	0.185257897	4.113165277
Columns		1,000	1	1,000	7.296311309	0.010467574	4.113165277
Interaction		0	1	0	0	1	4.113165277
Within		4,934	36	137.0555556			
Total		6,184	39				

The first part of that output is a summary of the data in Example 10.8. For each of the four groups of observations, the number, the sum, the mean, and the variance of each of the four groups are listed. In addition, the same values for the rows ignoring columns and for columns ignoring rows are provided (labeled as totals). These are the East/West and North/South main effects, respectively.

The last part of the output gives the results of the factorial ANOVA analysis. The row headed by "Sample" is the East/West main effect and the row headed by "Columns" is the North/South main effect. The P-values in each of these rows test the null hypothesis that there is no main effect. In other words, the null hypotheses that the means for East and West (ignoring North and South) and the means for North and South (ignoring East and West) are equal to the same value in the population. In this example, we are able to reject the null hypothesis that there is no main effect of North and South ($P = 0.0105$), but we cannot reject the null hypothesis that there is no main effect of East and West ($P = 0.1853$).

In R, we perform a factorial ANOVA using the "summary(aov(DV~Factor1* Factor2))" command. When we analyze these data, we get the following:

>summary(aov(CHOL~N_S*E_W,data=Example10_8))

```
 Df Sum Sq Mean Sq F value Pr(>F)
N_S 1 1000 1000.0 7.296 0.0105 *
E_W 1 250 250.0 1.824 0.1853
N_S:E_W 1 0 0.0 0.000 1.0000
Residuals 36 4934 137.1
---
Signif. codes: 0 '***' 0.001 '**' 0.01 '*' 0.05 '.' 0.1 ' ' 1
```

These results are the same as those obtained using Excel. ∎

In Example 10.9, consider the row headed by "Interaction" in the Excel output and the row headed "N_S:E_W" in the R output. This is the **interaction** between the North/South effect and the East/West effect. The interaction tells us whether or not it makes sense to look at the means of the categories for one factor (i.e., the main effect) while ignoring categories of the other factor(s). This makes sense only if the relationships among categories of the factor are the same regardless of the category of the other factor(s). If there is an interaction, the implication is that these relationships are different. In the case of an interaction, observation of the main effect of each factor is not helpful in understanding how the categories are related. This is illustrated in the next example.

■ **EXAMPLE 10.10**

The following figure illustrates mean serum cholesterol levels in the population from which the sample in Example 10.8 might have come. The main effects in this figure are represented by the differences between the means on the outside of the figure. The North/South main effect is that the serum cholesterol levels in the South is in average 10 mg/dL more than the serum cholesterol levels in the North. The East/West main effect is that the serum cholesterol levels in the West is in average 5 mg/dL less than the serum cholesterol levels in the East.

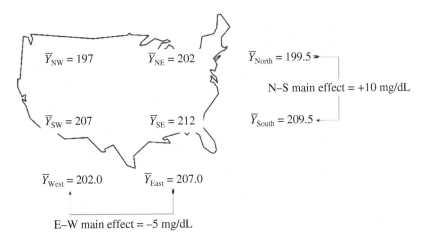

In this population, the main effects are enough to explain the differences between the means in the four geographic regions. For instance, if we know that the mean serum cholesterol level in the Northwest is equal to 197 mg/dL, we can add 5 mg/dL to get the mean cholesterol level in the Northeast or we can add 10 mg/dL to get the mean serum cholesterol level in the Southwest. To get the mean in the Southeast, we add both 5 and 10 mg/dL to the mean in the Northwest.

When we use the main effects in the sample to reflect the population's means in each group, we assume that there is no interaction between the factors. By this, we imply that it does not matter in which category of one factor the categories of another factor occur, the relationships among the means in the categories of that other factor will be the same.

In the case of this population, no interaction suggests that the difference between the mean in the North and the mean in the South will be 10 mg/dL, regardless of whether these means are from the East ($212 - 202 = 10$) or from the West ($207 - 197 = 10$). Likewise, it does not matter whether we compare the East with the West in the North or in the South, the difference between the means will be equal to 5 mg/dL.

Now, let us take a look at another possibility for mean serum cholesterol levels in the four geographic regions in the population: one that illustrates an interaction.

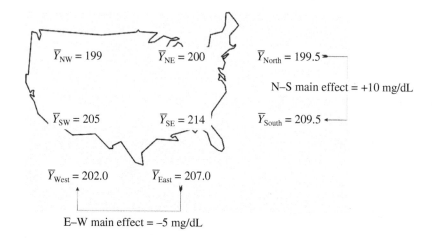

In this possibility, the main effects are the same as in the previous figure. Namely, there is a difference of 10 mg/dL between the serum cholesterol values in the North and the South and a difference of −5 mg/dL between the serum cholesterol values in the East and the West.

Although the main effects are the same as the previous population, they can no longer be interpreted in the same way. Now, the main effects are not enough to explain the differences between the mean levels of serum cholesterol in the geographic regions. For instance, if we add the East/West main effect to the mean in the Northwest, we get (199 + 5) = 204 mg/dL. When we did this for the previous population, we got the mean for the Northeast. This does not work when there is an interaction. Instead of the actual mean in the Northeast (200 mg/dL), we get 204 mg/dL for the Northeast by using the East/West main effect. Likewise, adding the North/South main effect to the mean in the Northwest yields the mean for the Southwest when there is no interaction, but not when there is an interaction. Instead of the actual mean in the Southwest (205 mg/dL), we get (199 + 10) = 209 mg/dL by adding the North/South main effect to the mean serum cholesterol level in the Northwest. When there is an interaction, the main effects do not describe the differences between the means. ∎

In Example 10.10, we saw that an interaction implies that main effects are not sufficient to describe the means in all the groups of dependent variable values. In that example, an interaction was assumed to exist as long as there were any differences not accounted for by the main effects. In practice, we expect to see, just by chance, some variation between the means not attributable to the main effects, even if the main effects are sufficient to describe the differences between the means in the population. To decide whether the apparent interaction in the sample is indicative of interaction in the population, we can test the null hypothesis of no interaction in a factorial ANOVA. The next example shows the test of the null hypothesis of no interaction for the data introduced in Example 10.10.

■ EXAMPLE 10.11

In Example 10.10, we looked at two possibilities for mean serum cholesterol levels in the four geographic regions in a population in which the main effects are an increase of 10 mg/dL between the North and South and a decrease of 5 mg/dL between the East and the West. Now, let us take a look at a set of data that might have come from the second population (i.e., the one with an interaction).

	North	South
East	220	222
	199	199
	193	198
	191	211
	205	217
	199	223
	212	202
	183	226
	203	215
	195	227
West	198	223
	199	205
	193	224
	215	202
	181	187
	189	213
	196	192
	194	203
	221	203
	204	198

The following Excel output is what we get when we analyze this new set of data using Excel's "Anova: Two-Factor with Replication" analysis tool to perform a factorial ANOVA.

Anova: Two-factor with replication

SUMMARY	North	South	Total			
East						
Count	10	10	20			
Sum	2,000	2,140	4,140			
Average	200	214	207			
Variance	113.7777778	122.4444444	163.4736842			
West						
Count	10	10	20			
Sum	1,990	2,050	4,040			
Average	199	205	202			
Variance	140	145.3333333	144.6315789			
Total						
Count	20	20				
Sum	3,990	4,190				
Average	199.5	209.5				
Variance	120.4736842	148.1578947				

ANOVA

Source of Variation	SS	df	MS	F	P-value	F crit
Sample	250	1	250	1.917341287	0.174672677	4.113165277
Columns	1,000	1	1,000	7.669365147	0.008823181	4.113165277
Interaction	160	1	160	1.227098424	0.275318642	4.113165277
Within	4,694	36	130.3888889			
Total	6104	39				

The test of the null hypothesis that there is no interaction in the population is presented at the end of the output in the row headed "Interaction." The next to last number in that row (0.2753) is the P-value for that null hypothesis. Since the P-value is greater than 0.05, we fail to reject the null hypothesis of no interaction. In this case, we assume that there is no interaction in the population and, thus, we can interpret the main effects as indicators of the differences between means. Here, we are able to reject the null hypothesis that the mean for the North is equal to the mean for the South ($P = 0.0088$), but we are unable to reject the null hypothesis that the mean for the East is the same as the mean for the West ($P = 0.1747$).

We draw the same conclusions using R.

>summary(aov(CHOL~N_S*E_W,data=Example10_11))

```
  Df Sum Sq Mean Sq F value Pr(>F)
N_S  1 1000 1000.0  7.669 0.00882 **
E_W  1  250  250.0  1.917 0.17467
N_S:E_W 1 160 160.0 1.227 0.27532
Residuals 36 4694 130.4
---
Signif. codes: 0 `***' 0.001 `**' 0.01 `*' 0.05 `.' 0.1 ` ' 1
```

So, the way we interpret the results of a factorial ANOVA depends on the result of the test of the null hypothesis that there is no interaction between the factors in the population. If we fail to reject this null hypothesis, we can interpret the main effects as explanations for differences between means. This makes interpretation of the data easier, since each main effect can be examined without having to consider the other factor(s). If, on the other hand, we reject the null hypothesis of no interaction between the factors, the main effects cannot be interpreted as an explanation of the differences between means. In this case, we must consider differences between all of the means, as we do in one-way ANOVA, testing the omnibus null hypothesis.

10.2.2 Posterior Testing

When the P-value for the test of the omnibus null hypothesis (i.e., all of the means in the population are equal to the same value) in one-way ANOVA is less than our usual α of 0.05, we reject that null hypothesis and, through the process of elimination, accept the alternative hypothesis. That alternative hypothesis must include all possible relationships among the means, except for the relationship specified in the null hypothesis.[10] Thus, the alternative hypothesis is that at least two of the means are different in the population. Exactly how many means are different and which means are different are not specified by this alternative hypothesis. To determine where the differences are, we need to use an additional type of analysis; one that reveals which means are different from each other. Such a test is called a **posterior test** because it is performed after the ANOVA has indicated that there are differences between the means.

The way we discover which means are different is to test null hypotheses that the difference between a pair of means is equal to 0. This could be done by performing several bivariable analyses. For example, if we have 4 means to compare, we could use Student's t-test to compare each pair of means. For 4 means, there are 10 pairs of means and, thus, 10 t-tests.

Although this appears to be a viable solution, it is not our best choice. The problem with doing 10 t-tests is that each one is associated with its own risks of making a type I or type II error (i.e., of rejecting a true null hypothesis or accepting a false null hypothesis). When we consider the entire collection of bivariable tests, the chance that we have made at least one error in the process performing those tests is higher than the chance of making an error on any single test.[11] If there are many bivariable tests required to examine each pair of means, the chance of making at least one error

---

[10]This is the principle we first encountered in Chapter 3. Since the alternative hypothesis is accepted through the process of eliminating the null hypothesis, the null and alternative hypotheses must be a collectively exhaustive set of possible relationships among the means.

[11]This is not unique to posterior testing. Any time we consider performing more than one statistical test, the chance of drawing an incorrect conclusion on at least one of the tests will be greater than the chance of drawing an incorrect conclusion on a single test. More generally, this simply says that the more times we do something with a chance of making a mistake, the greater the probability that on one (or more) of those times a mistake will occur.

can be very high indeed. For instance, 10 t-tests, each with a 5% chance of making a type I error, can have as much as a 40% chance that at least one type I error has occurred.[12] This is known as the **experiment-wise type I error**.

If the chance of drawing an incorrect conclusion in a series of statistical tests (i.e., the "experiment") can be reduced, we should consider reducing it, but we need to be careful in selecting a method to do that. One of the methods that is sometimes used to reduce the experiment-wise type I error is to make the value of α smaller for each of the statistical tests, so that the experiment-wise α is equal to 0.05. The greater the number of statistical tests, the smaller the value of α for each test. For 10 tests and an experiment-wise α of 0.05, the **test-wise type I error** rate would be 0.005. This approach is called the **Bonferroni** method. This method is not a good choice as a way to reduce the overall chance of making a type I error. The reason for this is the fact that lowering α makes it harder to reject null hypotheses that should be rejected. In other words, it increases the chance of making type II errors (i.e., it reduces the statistical power). So, the Bonferroni method simply trades one kind of error for another. This is not much of a bargain, especially since there are other posterior tests that can accomplish the same reduction in the experiment-wise chance of making at least one type I error with only a small reduction in statistical power.

One commonly used posterior test that controls the overall chance of making a type I error without much of a reduction in statistical power is the **Student–Newman–Keuls test**. This test is quite a bit like performing Student's t-tests to compare each pair of means. Equation (10.10) shows the calculation for comparing two means in the Student–Newman–Keuls test[13]:

$$q = \frac{(\overline{Y}_1 - \overline{Y}_2) - (\mu_1 - \mu_2)}{\sqrt{\frac{s^2_{Y|Xs}}{2} \cdot \left(\frac{1}{n_1} + \frac{1}{n_2}\right)}} \tag{10.10}$$

where
  q = Student–Newman–Keuls test statistic
  $\overline{Y}_i$ = observed mean in group i
  μ_i = population's mean in group i
  $s^2_{Y|Xs}$ = within mean square
  n_i = number of observations in group i

There are two important features that make the Student–Newman–Keuls test different from performing Student's t-tests. The first is that there is a specific order in which the comparisons are made in the Student–Newman–Keuls test. To begin with,

---

[12] This calculation assumes that the null hypothesis is true for all 10 t-tests and that the chance of making a type I error on each test is statistically independent of the chance of making a type I error on another test.

[13] Compare this with the calculation for Student's t-test (Equation (7.28)).

the means are arranged according to their numeric magnitudes. Then, the two most extreme means are compared. If the null hypothesis that these two means are the same in the population is rejected, then the next most extreme means are tested. If it is not rejected, then null hypotheses for the corresponding less-extreme means are automatically not rejected as well. It is following this protocol for comparing means that accounts for much of the reduction in the experiment-wise chance of making a type I error.

The second feature is that the Student–Newman–Keuls test uses a new standard distribution to determine statistical significance. This is the **q-distribution**. The q-distribution is like Student's t-distribution, but it has an additional parameter k that specifies the number of means involved in the comparison. Although, in practice, we will use a computer to do the calculations, it is easier to understand the Student–Newman–Keuls test by seeing it calculated at least once manually. The next example does that.

■ EXAMPLE 10.12

Let us use the Student–Newman–Keuls test to find out which means are significantly different for the data in Example 10.9.

The first step in the Student–Newman–Keuls test is to arrange the means according to their numeric magnitudes.

Region	NW	NE	SW	SE
Mean	197	202	207	212

Next, we test the null hypothesis that the two most extreme means are equal to the same value (i.e., their difference is equal to 0). These means are 197 mg/dL for persons from the NW and 212 mg/dL for persons from the SE.

$$H_0 : \mu_{NW} = \mu_{SE}$$

To make that comparison, we use Equation (10.10). This equation includes the within mean square. We can find the within mean square (137.055556) in the output from Example 10.7.

$$q = \frac{(\overline{Y}_1 - \overline{Y}_2) - (\mu_1 - \mu_2)}{\sqrt{\frac{s^2_{Y|Xs}}{2} \cdot \left(\frac{1}{n_1} + \frac{1}{n_2}\right)}} = \frac{(197 - 212) - 0}{\sqrt{\frac{137.06}{2} \cdot \left(\frac{1}{10} + \frac{1}{10}\right)}} = -4.05$$

To interpret that result, we compare it with the q-value in Table B.8 that corresponds to $\alpha = 0.05$. The way Table B.8 is set up, there are separate pages for specific values of α, with the value of α specified in the top row. The second page of the table corresponds to $\alpha = 0.05$.

To find the critical value with which we need to compare the absolute value of our calculated value of q, we need to know the degrees of freedom and the value of k. The degrees of freedom are the within degrees of freedom. In Example 10.7, we see that there are 36 degrees of freedom for the within variation. Thirty-six does not appear in Table B.8, so we use the next lower number of degrees of freedom (30).

The parameter k specifies the number of means involved in the comparison. We determine this value by counting the number of means being compared (always equal to 2) and the number of means between the 2 being compared (here, equal to 2). So, the value of k for the comparison of the means from the NW and SE is equal to 4.

Now, we go to Table B.8 and find that the critical value corresponding to α of 0.05, 30 degrees of freedom, and k equal to 4 is equal to 3.845.

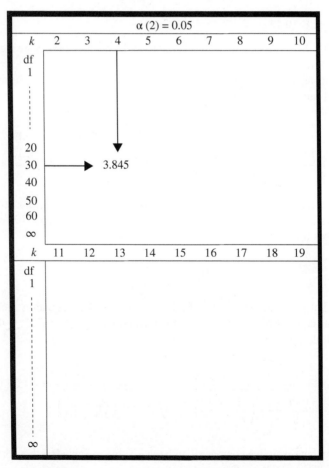

Then, we compare the calculated value (4.05) with the critical value (3.845). Since the calculated value is greater than the critical value, we can reject the null hypothesis that the mean serum cholesterol levels in the NW are equal to the mean serum cholesterol levels in the SE.

The fact that we reject this null hypothesis allows us to test null hypotheses for the next most extreme means. These are the null hypothesis that the mean for persons from the NW is equal to the mean for persons from the SW:

$$H_0 : \mu_{NW} = \mu_{SW}$$

and the null hypothesis that the mean for persons from the NE is equal to the mean for persons from the SE:

$$H_0 : \mu_{NE} = \mu_{SE}$$

It does not matter which of these two null hypotheses we test first. To test each of them, we use Equation (10.10) to calculate the q-value.

$$q = \frac{(\overline{Y}_1 - \overline{Y}_2) - (\mu_1 - \mu_2)}{\sqrt{\dfrac{s^2_{Y|Xs}}{2} \cdot \left(\dfrac{1}{n_1} + \dfrac{1}{n_2}\right)}} = \frac{(197 - 207) - 0}{\sqrt{\dfrac{137.06}{2} \cdot \left(\dfrac{1}{10} + \dfrac{1}{10}\right)}} = -2.70$$

$$q = \frac{(\overline{Y}_1 - \overline{Y}_2) - (\mu_1 - \mu_2)}{\sqrt{\dfrac{s^2_{Y|Xs}}{2} \cdot \left(\dfrac{1}{n_1} + \dfrac{1}{n_2}\right)}} = \frac{(202 - 212) - 0}{\sqrt{\dfrac{137.06}{2} \cdot \left(\dfrac{1}{10} + \dfrac{1}{10}\right)}} = -2.70$$

To interpret these results, we compare the absolute value of the calculated q-value with the q-value in Table B.8 that corresponds to $\alpha = 0.05$, 30 degrees of freedom, and $k = 3$ (we now have the two means being compared with one mean between them). This critical value is equal to 3.486.

For the null hypothesis that the mean for the NW is equal to the mean for the SW, the calculated q-value (-2.70) in absolute value is less than the critical value (3.486), so we fail to reject the null hypothesis. When we fail to reject a null hypothesis in the Student–Newman–Keuls test, we also fail to reject any null hypotheses for any two means that are both in between the means in the null hypothesis that we failed to reject. Thus, we fail to reject the following three null hypotheses even though only the first was actually tested.

$$H_0 : \mu_{NW} = \mu_{SW}$$

$$H_0 : \mu_{NW} = \mu_{NE}$$

$$H_0 : \mu_{NE} = \mu_{SW}$$

To keep track of the results of using the Student–Newman–Keuls test, it is useful to draw a line connecting the means for which we fail to reject the null hypothesis that the means are equal as follows:

Region	NW	NE	SW	SE
Mean	197	202	207	212

Then, we know that any pair of means also connected by that line has their null hypothesis not rejected, even though they were not directly tested.

For the null hypothesis that the mean for the NE is equal to the mean for the SE, the calculated q-value (-2.70) in absolute value is less than the critical value (3.486), so we fail to reject this null hypothesis and any null hypotheses for any two means that are both in between the means in that null hypothesis. Thus, we fail to reject the following three null hypotheses:

$$H_0 : \mu_{NE} = \mu_{SE}$$

$$H_0 : \mu_{NE} = \mu_{SW}$$

$$H_0 : \mu_{SW} = \mu_{SE}$$

As before, we can keep track of these results by drawing a line connecting the means for which we fail to reject the null hypothesis that the means are equal:

REGION	NW	NE	SW	SE
MEAN	197	202	207	212

From this table, we know that the difference between any two means is not statistically significant if they are connected by a line. In this example, only the means for the NW and SE are significantly different. ∎

Hopefully, Example 10.12 helps you understand how the Student–Newman–Keuls test works. Now, let us take a look at an example that shows the result of using Excel to carry out the Student–Newman–Keuls test to look for pairwise differences between means. Since Excel does not have a built-in procedure for the Student–Newman–Keuls test, we will use the "SNK" BAHR program.

■ EXAMPLE 10.13

Posterior testing can be performed in Excel by using the SNK BAHR program. The following is the dialog box we use in preparation to analyze the data in the one-way ANOVA shown in Example 10.7.

Student–Newman–Keuls Test

Group	n	Mean
NW	10	197
NE	10	202
SW	10	207
SE	10	212

Within mean square 137.06

Go   End

The following are the results obtained using that program to compare the means of the four geographic regions as part of the one-way ANOVA shown in Example 10.7.

		Student–Newman–Keuls Test	
NW	NE	SW	SE
197	202	207	212
2	1	4	3
$k = 4$			
NE	vs	SW	−4.05169
$k = 3$			
NE	vs	SE	−2.70112
NW	vs	SW	−2.70112
$k = 2$			
NE	vs	NW	−1.35056
NW	vs	SE	−1.35056
SE	vs	SW	−1.35056

This program sequentially tests hypotheses for means that are progressively less extreme. To interpret this output, the user needs to compare the q-values with critical values in Table B.8. For the comparison of the two most extreme means, the q-value is 4.052. We need to compare this calculated value with the critical value that represents an α of 0.05, 30 degrees of freedom (36 degrees of freedom is not listed), and k equal to 4. This critical value is equal to 3.845.[14]

Thus, there is a statistically significant difference between the means for the Northwest and Southeast. This significance permits us to consider the next most extreme means. These comparisons are associated with q-values that are both equal to 2.7011. The critical value for a k equal to 3 is 3.486. Since the absolute value of the calculated q-statistic (2.7011) is less than the critical value (3.486), we fail to reject the null hypotheses that the mean for the Northwest is the same as the mean for the Southeast and that the mean for the Northeast is the same as the mean for the Southeast. We also fail to reject any pairs of means that are less extreme than these means. Thus, the only statistically significant difference is between the means for the Northwest and Southeast.

R does not perform a Student–Newman–Keuls test, but it does perform another posterior test called Tukey's HSD test.[15] In this test, confidence intervals and P-values are adjusted for multiple comparisons. To perform Tukey's HSD test, we first save the results of an ANOVA then refer to those results in the "TukeyHSD(results)" command.

>temp<-aov(CHOL~REGION,data=Example10_9)
>TukeyHSD(temp)

```
Tukey multiple comparisons of means
95% family-wise confidence level

Fit: aov(formula = CHOL ~ REGION, data = Example10_9)

$REGION
 diff lwr upr p adj
NW-NE -5 -19.1005582 9.100558 0.7754596
SE-NE 10 -4.1005582 24.100558 0.2419179
SW-NE 5 -9.1005582 19.100558 0.7754596
SE-NW 15 0.8994418 29.100558 0.0334257
SW-NW 10 -4.1005582 24.100558 0.2419179
SW-SE -5 -19.1005582 9.100558 0.7754596
```

The only significant difference is between SE and NW. This result agrees with the result of using the Student–Newman–Keuls test.[16] ∎

---

[14] See, Example 10.12 for a more detailed explanation of how this critical value is selected.

[15] HSD stands for "Honest Significant Difference."

[16] These two tests will not always agree. Tukey's HSD has less statistical power than does the Student–Newman–Keuls test. The result is that some means that are significantly different according to the Student–Newman–Keuls test might not be significantly different according to Tukey's HSD test. This makes the Student–Newman–Keuls test the better choice.

The output in Example 10.13 is what we could expect if we were performing a one-way ANOVA or a factorial ANOVA with a statistically significant interaction. If we are using a factorial ANOVA design in which there is not a statistically significant interaction, means for each of the factors can be compared in their own separate analyses. The next example shows the result of the Student–Newman–Keuls test for the factorial ANOVA in Example 10.9.

■ EXAMPLE 10.14

The following is the result of using the "SNK" BAHR program to perform Student–Newman–Keuls tests on the main effects from the factorial ANOVA in Example 10.9:

Student–Newman–Keuls Test		Student–Newman–Keuls Test	
North	South	West	East
199.5	209.5	202	207
1	2	1	2
$k=2$		$k=2$	
North vs South −3.82003		West vs East −1.91001	

The critical value from Table B.8 is 2.888. The q-value for the comparison of the means in the North and South is greater than the critical value, so we are able to reject the null hypothesis that means for North and South are equal to the same value. The q-value for the comparison of the means in the East and West is less than the critical value, so we are unable to reject the null hypothesis that these means are equal in the population.

The following is the result of using R to analyze these data with the factorial model.

```
>temp<-aov(CHOL~NORTH+EAST,data=Example10_9)
>TukeyHSD(temp)
```

```
Tukey multiple comparisons of means
95% family-wise confidence level

Fit: aov(formula = CHOL ~ NORTH + EAST, data = Example 10_9)

$NORTH
 diff lwr upr p adj
YES-NO -10 -17.39911 -2.600891 0.0094377

$EAST
 diff lwr upr p adj
YES-NO 5 -2.399109 12.39911 0.179187
```

There, the only significant difference is between north and south. This agrees with the Excel output.

In this particular example, there are only two categories of each factor and, thus, only two means for each main effect. When there are only two categories, we do not need to perform a posterior test to determine which means are different. Instead, we know about these differences from the factorial ANOVA test for the main effects. In Example 10.9, we were able to reject the null hypothesis of no North/South main effect, but we were unable to reject the null hypothesis of no East/West main effect. These results are consistent with the Student–Newman–Keuls test results. Namely, the means for the North and South are statistically different, but the means for the East and West are not statistically different. ∎

10.3   BOTH CONTINUOUS AND NOMINAL INDEPENDENT VARIABLES

When a set of data consists of a mixture of continuous and nominal indepen-dent variables, we analyze these data using analysis of covariance (ANCOVA). ANCOVA can be thought of in two ways. One way to think about it is as an ANOVA in which the nominal independent variables specify the groups to be compared and the continuous independent variables are included to control for their effect on the dependent variable.[17] Another way to think about it is as a multiple regression analysis in which nominal independent variables are included in the regression equation. Although both ways are correct, it is the latter way that is more frequent in modern statistical thinking. Thus, we will discuss ANCOVA in terms of a parallel to multiple regression.

As an illustration of the type of study we would use for ANCOVA to analyze the data, let us suppose we are interested in looking at the relationship between two antihypertensive medications and diastolic blood pressure while controlling for the effect of time since diagnosis of hypertension. In this study, diastolic blood pres-sure is the continuous dependent variable, treatment (new treatment versus standard treatment) is a nominal independent variable, and time since diagnosis is a contin-uous independent variable. Then, we can think of the following multiple regression equation as representing the relationship among these variables in the population:

$$\mu_{\text{DBP}|\text{Time,Treatment}} = \alpha + (\beta_1 \cdot \text{Time}) + (\beta_2 \cdot \text{Treatment}) \tag{10.11}$$

where

$\mu_{\text{DBP}|\text{Time, Treatment}}$ = mean diastolic blood pressure value in the population that corresponds to persons with a certain time since diagnosis and assignment to a par-ticular treatment group

---

[17]It is this way of thinking about the ANCOVA that gives it its name. Continuous independent variables are called "covariates" in (older) statistical terminology.

Time = time since diagnosis of hypertension

Treatment = treatment group to which a person was assignedAs in regression analysis, we would like to use the regression equation to estimate the mean of the dependent variable values that correspond to specific values of the independent variables. This is accomplished by substituting values for the independent variables in the regression equation. This will not work for Equation (10.11), since Treatment is a nominal independent variable having values of "yes" or "no" (i.e., new treatment or standard treatment). Multiplying these values by a regression coefficient has no meaning as far as the regression equation is concerned. To have meaning, all of the independent variables in a regression equation must have a numeric value. So, to include it in a regression equation, we need to represent the nominal independent variable numerically.

10.3.1 Indicator (Dummy) Variables

The trick here is to represent the nominal independent variable numerically without assigning quantitative meaning to its inherent qualitative nature. We faced this same task in Chapter 9 when we wanted to use the "Regression" analysis tool to perform a test for trend. In that instance, we created an **indicator** (or **dummy**) **variable** by making the number 1 represent an observation in which the event occurred and 0 represent an observation in which the event did not occur.[18] These two numbers (0 and 1) are numeric, but they differ qualitatively instead of quantitatively.[19]

In our example of two treatment groups, we could set the indicator variable equal to 1 if the person received the new treatment and equal to 0 if the person received the standard treatment. Equation (10.12) illustrates the multiple regression equation shown in Equation (10.11), but with an indicator variable (TX) representing the nominal independent variable (Treatment):

$$\mu_{\text{DBP|Time,TX}} = \alpha + (\beta_1 \cdot \text{Time}) + (\beta_2 \cdot \text{TX}) \tag{10.12}$$

where

TX = indicator variable equal to 1 if the person received the new treatment or equal to 0 if the person received the standard treatment

To see how we can interpret the regression coefficients in Equation (10.12), let us first think about persons who receive the standard treatment. For these persons, TX is equal to 0. Then, Equation (10.12) becomes the following:

$$\mu_{\text{DBP|Time,TX=0}} = \alpha + (\beta_1 \cdot \text{Time}) + (\beta_2 \cdot 0) = \alpha + (\beta_1 \cdot \text{Time}) \tag{10.13}$$

[18]We will take a look at another method of defining these variables later in this chapter.
[19]We had a numbering system without the concept of zero for millennia. It is believed that the Babylonians first introduced the concept in the Old World and the Mayans independently introduced it in the New World. In the Old World, however, it was not a well-accepted concept until much later. Around 450 BC, Zeno of Elea, a Greek philosopher and cohort of Socrates, struggled with the concept of zero as part of a numbering system. In essence, his argument was that "nothing" cannot be included with "something," thus drawing a distinction between qualitative and quantitative information.

Since TX is equal to 0 in Equation (10.13), the regression coefficient for the indicator variable (β_2) disappears from the regression equation. What are left are the intercept, one regression coefficient (β_1), and the independent variable Time. Since there is only one independent variable in that equation, it is really just a bivariable regression equation with an intercept equal to α and with a slope equal to β_1.

Next, let us think about persons who receive the new treatment. They have a value of one for the indicator variable, and the resulting regression equation is

$$\mu_{DBP|Time,TX=1} = \alpha + (\beta_1 \cdot Time) + (\beta_2 \cdot 1) = \alpha + (\beta_1 \cdot Time) + \beta_2 \qquad (10.14)$$

In Equation (10.14), the indicator variable is equal to 1, so its regression coefficient remains in the regression equation. In fact, this is the only difference between the regression equation for persons who received the standard treatment (Equation (10.13)) and persons who received the new treatment (Equation (10.14)): Their diastolic blood pressure values differ by the value of β_2. When the indicator variable is equal to 1, it is really a bivariable regression equation. In this case, the intercept is equal to $\alpha + \beta_2$ and the slope is equal to β_1. The relationship between these two bivariable regression equations is illustrated graphically in Figure 10.7.

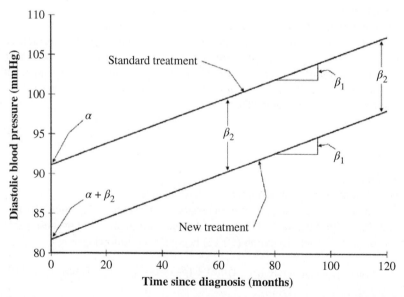

Figure 10.7   Illustration of how the regression coefficient for an indicator variable is interpreted. In this case, the indicator variable differentiates between two treatment groups. The regression coefficient for the indicator variable (β_2) specifies the difference between the means of the dependent variable for the two groups, regardless of the value of time since diagnosis. In this example, β_2 is a negative number, indicating that DBP is lower when the indicator variable is equal to 1.

10.3.2   Interaction Variables

If nominal independent variables are represented only by indicator variables, the regression coefficients for these indicator variables specify differences between mean values of the dependent variable regardless of the value of the continuous independent variable(s) or other indicator variable(s). In other words, the regression lines for the groups are parallel to each other (as seen in Figure 10.7). To allow the regression lines to have different slopes, we need to include another kind of variable in the regression equation. The variables that create differences in slopes are called **interaction variables**. An interaction variable is created by multiplying an indicator variable by another independent variable. This other independent variable can be either a continuous independent variable or another indicator variable. Equation (10.15) shows the regression equation describing the relationship between time since diagnosis, treatment group, and diastolic blood pressure with inclusion of an interaction variable:

$$\mu_{DBP|Time,TX} = \alpha + (\beta_1 \cdot Time) + (\beta_2 \cdot TX) + (\beta_3 \cdot Time \cdot TX) \qquad (10.15)$$

where

TX = indicator variable that is equal to 1 if the person received the new treatment or equal to 0 if the person received the standard treatment

$Time \cdot TX$ = interaction between time since diagnosis and treatment group, created by multiplying the continuous independent variable (Time) by the indicator variable (TX)

To see how to interpret the regression coefficient for the interaction, let us first take a look at how Equation (10.15) appears when the indicator variable is equal to 0. In the example of diastolic blood pressure and its relationship with time since diagnosis and treatment group, the indicator variable is equal to 0 for a person who receives the standard treatment. Equation (10.16) illustrates what happens to Equation (10.15) when the indicator variable is equal to 0:

$$\mu_{DBP|Time,TX=0} = \alpha + (\beta_1 \cdot Time) + (\beta_2 \cdot 0) + (\beta_3 \cdot Time \cdot 0) = \alpha + (\beta_1 \cdot Time)$$
$$(10.16)$$

When the indicator variable is equal to 0 (i.e., when a person receives the standard treatment), the interaction variable is also equal to 0. As a result, adding an interaction variable does not change the regression equation when the indicator is equal to 0. It is still a bivariable regression equation with an intercept equal to α and with a slope equal to β_1.

When the indicator variable is equal to 1, however, the interaction variable changes the regression equation. This is illustrated in Equation (10.17):

$$\mu_{DBP|Time,TX=1} = \alpha + (\beta_1 \cdot Time) + (\beta_2 \cdot 1) + (\beta_3 \cdot Time \cdot 1)$$
$$= \alpha + (\beta_1 \cdot Time) + \beta_2 + (\beta_3 \cdot Time) \qquad (10.17)$$

To see how the regression coefficient for the interaction variable is interpreted, let us do a little algebra and rearrange Equation (10.17):

$$\mu_{DBP|Time,TX=1} = \alpha + (\beta_1 \cdot Time) + \beta_2 + (\beta_3 \cdot Time)$$
$$= [\alpha + \beta_2] + ([\beta_1 + \beta_3] \cdot Time) \qquad (10.18)$$

Now, let us compare Equation (10.18) with Equation (10.16) to see how the equations differ between the treatment groups. In Equation (10.16), the slope of the regression line is equal to the regression coefficient for Time (β_1). In Equation (10.18), however, the slope of the regression line is equal to the sum of the regression coefficients for Time and for the interaction variable ($\beta_1 + \beta_3$). Thus, the regression coefficient for the interaction variable tells us about the difference between the slopes of the regression lines for persons in the two treatment groups.

Equation (10.18) also illustrates further how the regression coefficient for the indicator variable (β_2) is interpreted. Without an interaction variable in the regression equation (Equation (10.14)), the regression coefficient for the indicator variable revealed about the difference between the mean diastolic blood pressure values in the two treatment groups, regardless of a person's time since diagnosis. Since the regression lines were parallel before we included the interaction variable, it really did not matter at what time since diagnosis the means were compared; the difference between the means was equal to the same value.

When there is an interaction and, as a result, a difference between the slopes of the regression lines, the difference between the mean diastolic blood pressure values will change for persons with different times since diagnosis. Thus, the means of dependent variable values need to be compared for a specific value of the continuous independent variable (e.g., for persons with a particular time since diagnosis). Only if the continuous independent variable is equal to 0 does the regression coefficient for the indicator variable tell us the difference between the means. In other words, the regression coefficient for the indicator variable tells us the difference between the intercepts of the regression lines. This is illustrated graphically in Figure 10.8.

When interpreting the results of an ANCOVA, we must first consider the interaction variable(s). The reason for this is that, in the presence of an interaction, we cannot interpret the regression coefficient for the continuous independent variable (β_1) as the slope of the regression line without specifying which group is being considered. By definition, the presence of an interaction indicates that the slopes differ between the groups. Also, the presence of an interaction affects the way we interpret the regression coefficient for the indicator variable (β_2) as the difference in the means of the dependent variable values between the two groups. When there is an interaction, the difference between these means varies according to the value of the continuous independent variable. In this case, the regression coefficient for the indicator variable tells us the difference between means when the indicator variable is equal to 0. The next example illustrates how we can apply these principles when we use the "Regression" analysis tool in Excel to perform an ANCOVA.

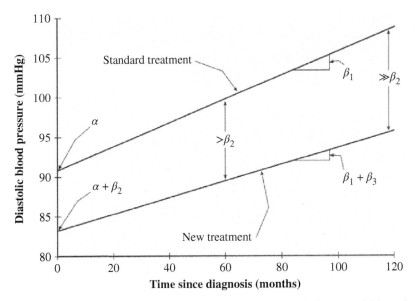

Figure 10.8 Illustration of how regression coefficients for an indicator variable and an interaction variable are interpreted. The regression coefficient for the indicator variable (β_2) differentiates between the intercepts of the two groups. The regression coefficient for the interaction variable (β_3) specifies the difference between the slopes of the regression lines for the two groups. In this example, β_2 and β_3 are negative numbers, indicating that the intercept and slope are lower when the indicator variable is equal to 1.

■ **EXAMPLE 10.15**

In our discussion of ANCOVA, we have been thinking about a study in which diastolic blood pressure (the dependent variable) is compared between persons who received a new antihypertensive medication and persons who received a standard treatment. These two groups are represented by a nominal independent variable. Also, the comparison between diastolic blood pressure and treatment group is performed while controlling for time since diagnosis (a continuous independent variable).

Now, let us suppose we have made these observations on 42 persons, 21 of whom were randomly assigned to receive the new treatment and 21 of whom were assigned to receive the standard treatment. To represent these treatment groups in the regression equation, we created an indicator variable (TX) that is equal to 1 if the person received the new treatment and equal to 0 if the person received the standard treatment. Also, we created an interaction variable (Time*TX) by multiplying time since diagnosis by the indicator variable. Now, suppose that we were to obtain the following output from the "Regression" analysis tool when we analyze these data.

SUMMARY OUTPUT

Regression statistics	
Multiple R	0.901390019
R square	0.812503966
Adjusted R square	0.797701647
Standard error	5.720031715
Observations	42

ANOVA

	df	SS	MS	F	Significance F
Regression	3	5,387.82987	1,795.94329	54.89031783	6.99042E-14
Residual	38	1,243.312987	32.71876282		
Total	41	6,631.142857			

	Coefficients	Standard error	t Stat	P-value	Lower 95%	Upper 95%
Intercept	60.81428571	8.543238252	7.118411535	1.7016E-08	43.51940406	78.10916737
TIME	0.757142857	0.206135634	3.673032367	0.000735131	0.339843082	1.174442632
TX	−10.98311688	9.567743519	−1.147931784	0.25817232	−30.35200103	8.385767259
TIME*TX	0.372727273	0.29151981	1.278565848	0.208803967	−0.217423729	0.962878274

As we learned previously, the first things we consider in ANCOVAs are the interactions. In this case, there is only one: the interaction between time since diagnosis and treatment group. The last row in the Excel output tells us about that interaction. The P-value for the test of the null hypothesis that the regression coefficient for the interaction is equal to 0 in the population is 0.2088. Since this P-value is greater than 0.05, we cannot reject the null hypothesis. In this circumstance, we can conclude that there is no significant interaction between time since diagnosis and treatment group. ■

In Example 10.15, we considered an ANCOVA in which the interaction term is not statistically significant. This implies that we cannot rule out the possibility that the regression coefficient in the population is equal to 0. Even so, the regression coefficient for the interaction term in the sample is *not* equal to zero. This means that the point estimates for the slopes of the regression lines are different. From Example 10.15, the slope for the regression line for persons who receive the standard treatment is equal to 0.7571 (the regression coefficient for the continuous independent variable Time). The slope for persons who receive the new treatment is equal to 0.7571 + 0.3727 = 1.1298 (0.3727 is the regression coefficient for the interaction). These two estimates of slopes are not significantly different, but they *are* numerically different.

If the interaction term is not significantly different from 0, it is often removed from the regression equation and the analysis repeated without it. Then, there is only one estimate of the slope that can be applied to both groups. This makes the interpretation of the results of the analysis more straightforward. This is illustrated in the next example.

■ EXAMPLE 10.16

In Example 10.15, we found that the regression coefficient for the interaction term was not significantly different from 0. This suggests that the slopes of the regression equations for the two groups were not significantly different from each other. If we want to have a single estimate of the slope that can be applied to both regression equations, we need to redo the analysis, leaving out the interaction term. When we do that, we get the following output from the "Regression" analysis tool:

SUMMARY OUTPUT

Regression statistics	
Multiple R	0.896904695
R square	0.804438031
Adjusted R square	0.794409213
Standard error	5.76639102
Observations	42

ANOVA

	df	SS	MS	F	Significance F
Regression	2	5,334.343506	2,667.171753	80.21263916	1.51372E-14
Residual	39	1,296.799351	33.2512654		
Total	41	6,631.142857			

	Coefficients	Standard error	t Stat	P-value	Lower 95%	Upper 95%
Intercept	53.17337662	6.15459934	8.639616275	1.35583E-10	40.72452442	65.62222882
TIME	0.943506494	0.146941249	6.420977753	1.34886E-07	0.646289763	1.240723224
TX	0.385064935	3.562125834	0.108099756	0.914470803	-6.820014645	7.590144515

Now, the two regression equations have the same slope (0.9435).[20] This makes interpretation of the results more straightforward. Now, the only difference between persons who received the new treatment and persons who received the standard treatment is that the mean diastolic blood pressure for those who received the new treatment is 0.3851 more than the diastolic blood pressure for those who received the standard treatment. Because the interaction term has been removed, this difference is applied to persons regardless of time since diagnosis (as in Figure 10.7). ■

Removing the interaction term(s) from an ANCOVA model has the effect of simplifying the relationship(s) between variables, but it also has an effect on the independent contributions of the independent variables that were involved in the

---

[20]This is the mean of the separate slopes from the model in which the interaction was included (Example 10.15).

interaction. Since an interaction is created by multiplying the independent variables together, it is not surprising that the interaction is correlated with those independent variables. If the correlated variation is used to estimate dependent variable values, there is multicollinearity among the independent variables and the interaction. When the interaction is removed from the regression equation, the multicollinearity is also removed. We can see this effect by comparing the results in Example 10.16 with the results in Example 10.15.[21]

10.3.3 General Linear Model

Thinking about ANCOVA as a regression analysis leads to the use of indicator variables to represent nominal independent variables in a regression equation. Strictly speaking, an ANCOVA includes at least one nominal independent variable and at least one continuous independent variable. In general, however, it is not necessary that the regression equation includes any continuous independent variables. For instance, consider the following regression equation:

$$\mu_{chol} = \alpha + (\beta_1 \cdot NS) + (\beta_2 \cdot EW) + (\beta_3 \cdot NS \cdot EW) \qquad (10.19)$$

where

μ_{chol} = mean serum cholesterol level in the population
NS = indicator variable that is equal to 1 if the person is from the North or equal to 0 if the person is from the South
EW = indicator variable that is equal to 1 if the person is from the East or equal to 0 if the person is from the West

Equation (10.19) consists of two indicator variables (NS and EW) representing two nominal independent variables. These nominal independent variables specify the geographic region in which a person lives. The dependent variable is a person's serum cholesterol level. This is the same as the example we used earlier in this chapter when we were discussing factorial ANOVA. The next example compares that factorial ANOVA with Equation (10.19) using Excel's "Regression" analysis tool.

■ EXAMPLE 10.17

In Example 10.9, we examined the following Excel output as a result of analyzing the data in Example 10.6 as a factorial ANOVA using the "Anova: Two-Factor with Replication" analysis tool.

---

[21] The same thing will happen if an interaction is removed from a factorial ANOVA.

Anova: Two-factor with replication				
SUMMARY	N	S	Total	
E				
Count	10	10	20	
Sum	2,020	2,120	4,140	
Average	202	212	207	
Variance	135.3333333	132.4444444	153.1578947	
W				
Count	10	10	20	
Sum	1,970	2,070	4,040	
Average	197	207	202	
Variance	140.4444444	140	159.1578947	
Total				
Count	20	20		
Sum	3,990	4,190		
Average	199.5	209.5		
Variance	137.2105263	135.6315789		

ANOVA						
Source of variation	SS	df	MS	F	P-value	F crit
Sample	250	1	250	1.824077827	0.185257897	4.113165277
Columns	1,000	1	1,000	7.296311309	0.010467574	4.113165277
Interaction	0	1	0	0	1	4.113165277
Within	4,934	36	137.0555556			
Total	6,184	39				

Now, let us reanalyze those same data using the "Regression" analysis tool and the regression equation as it appears in Equation (10.19). The following is the output we get from this analysis.

SUMMARY OUTPUT

Regression statistics	
Multiple R	0.449593751
R square	0.202134541
Adjusted R square	0.135645752
Standard error	11.70707289
Observations	40

ANOVA					
	df	SS	MS	F	Significance F
Regression	3	1,250	416.6666667	3.040129712	0.041324944
Residual	36	4,934	137.0555556		
Total	39	6,184			

	Coefficients	Standard error	t Stat	P-value	Lower 95%	Upper 95%
Intercept	207	3.702101505	55.91418812	1.36861E-36	199.4917901	214.5082099
NS	−10	5.235562158	−1.910014569	0.064123648	−20.6182122	0.618212205
EW	5	5.235562158	0.955007285	0.345943258	−5.618212205	15.6182122
NS_EW	5.61733E-15	7.404203011	7.58668E-16	1	−15.01641971	15.01641971

At first, there do not appear to be similarities between the factorial ANOVA and the regression analysis. If we examine the middle table, however, we see that the residual sum of squares is equal to 4,934, which is identical to the within sum of squares in the ANOVA. If we add up the main effects and interaction sums of squares the sum (1,250), the sum is equal to the regression sum of squares.

The similarities end here. There are no similarities between the main effects and the interaction between the ANOVA analysis and the regression analysis. This is because of the interpretation of the indicator values in the regression analysis. Next, we will take a closer look at the interpretation of these indicator variables.   ■

In Equation (10.19), we represented the relationship between geographic region and serum cholesterol with a regression equation that included two indicator variables: NS and EW. These indicator variables were given values of 0 and 1. This is a common choice for the values of indicator variables, but it is not the only choice. Let us take a closer look at what these regression coefficients imply and, then, we will consider another way in which to represent nominal independent variables in a regression equation.

Table 10.2 shows how the regression coefficients for zero/one indicator variables relate to the estimated mean of the dependent variable for each group of dependent variable values. The intercept (a) estimates the mean in the group that corresponds to all of the indicator variables being equal to 0. For serum cholesterol levels, this group includes persons from the Southwest. Thus, the estimate of the intercept in the regression output in Example 10.17 (207 mg/dL) is the estimate of the mean serum cholesterol level in the Southwest.

Now, let us consider the regression coefficients for the two indicator variables. Table 10.2 shows us that we add the regression coefficient for the North/South indicator variable ($b_1 = 10$ mg/dL) to the intercept ($a = 207$ mg/dL) to get the mean serum cholesterol level in the Northwest (197 mg/dL). Thus, the regression coefficient for the North/South indicator variable tells us how much serum cholesterol levels change, on the average, as we go from the Southwest to the Northwest. Likewise, Table 10.2 shows us that we add the regression coefficient for the East/West indicator variable ($b_2 = 5$ mg/dL) to the intercept ($a = 207$ mg/dL) to get the mean

TABLE 10.2. Interpretation of the Estimated Regression Coefficients When Two Nominal Independent Variables Are Represented by Indicator Variables That Have the Values of Either Zero or One

Region	$b_1 \cdot$ NS	$b_2 \cdot$ EW	$b_3 \cdot$ NS $\cdot$ EW	$\widehat{chol}$*	Mean
Southwest	$b_1 \cdot 0$	$b_2 \cdot 0$	$b_3 \cdot 0 \cdot 0$	a	207
Northwest	$b_1 \cdot 1$	$b_2 \cdot 0$	$b_3 \cdot 1 \cdot 0$	$a + b_1$	$207 - 10 = 197$
Southeast	$b_1 \cdot 0$	$b_2 \cdot 1$	$b_3 \cdot 0 \cdot 1$	$a + b_2$	$207 + 5 = 212$
Northeast	$b_1 \cdot 1$	$b_2 \cdot 1$	$b_3 \cdot 1 \cdot 1$	$a + b_1 + b_2 + b_3$	$207 - 10 + 5 + 0 = 202$

[a] Estimated value of the dependent variable.

serum cholesterol levels in the Southeast (212 mg/dL). So, the regression coefficient for the East/West indicator variable tells us how serum cholesterol levels change, on the average, as we go from the Southwest to the Southeast.

If we know the intercept and the regression coefficients for the indicator variables, we can calculate estimates of the mean serum cholesterol levels among persons in the Southwest, Northwest, and Southeast. This leaves only the mean in the Northeast. To estimate this mean, we add both of the regression coefficients for the indicator variables (10 and 5 mg/dL) to the intercept and, then, we add to that sum the regression coefficient for the interaction ($b_3 = 0$ mg/dL).

In this instance, the regression coefficient for the interaction is equal to 0. If the regression coefficient for the interaction is equal to 0 in the population, this implies that the difference between the means in the North and South is the same in the East as it is in the West. That is to say, the regression coefficient for the North/ South main effect is equal to the difference between the means in the Northeast and Southeast as well as to the difference between the means in the Northwest and Southwest.

When testing null hypotheses in this regression model, we are testing null hypotheses about mean serum cholesterol levels. For instance, testing the null hypothesis that the intercept is equal to 0 in the population is the same as testing the null hypothesis that the mean serum cholesterol in the Southwest is equal to 0 in the population. Testing the null hypothesis that one of the regression coefficients for an indicator is equal to 0 in the population is the same as testing the null hypothesis that each of those means is equal to the mean for the Southwest. When testing the null hypothesis that the interaction's regression coefficient is equal to 0, we are testing the hypothesis that the difference between the Southwest and the Northeast is equal to the difference between the Southwest and Northwest added to the difference between the Southwest and the Southeast. These null hypotheses are summarized in Table 10.3.

Now, let us compare these null hypotheses with the null hypotheses tested in factorial ANOVA. In factorial ANOVA, we test null hypotheses that address the

TABLE 10.3. Null Hypotheses Tested When Two Nominal Independent Variables Are Represented by Indicator Variables That Are Equal to Either Zero or One*

Null Hypothesis in Terms of	
Regression Parameters	Means
$H_0 : \alpha = 0$	$H_0 : \mu_{SW} = 0$
$H_0 : \beta_1 = 0$	$H_0 : \mu_{SW} = \mu_{NW}$
$H_0 : \beta_2 = 0$	$H_0 : \mu_{SW} = \mu_{SE}$
$H_0 : \beta_3 = 0$	$H_0 : \mu_{NE} = (3 \cdot \mu_{SW}) - \mu_{NW} - \mu_{SE}$ [24]

[a] These null hypotheses are stated first in terms of the parameters of the regression equation and, then, in terms of the means for each group of dependent variable values.

Another way to state this null hypothesis is to say $\mu_{SW} - \mu_{NW} = \mu_{SE} - \mu_{NE}$ (i.e., the difference between North and South is the same in the East as it is in the West) and $\mu_{SW} - \mu_{SE} = \mu_{NW} - \mu_{NE}$ (i.e., the difference between the West and the East is the same in the North as it is in the South).

main effects of each of the factors and their interaction(s). One of these main effects in this example is the difference between serum cholesterol values in the North and the South. These means differ from the ones in the null hypotheses in Table 10.3 in that the comparison between the North and the South in factorial ANOVA (i.e., the North/South main effect) is made regardless of whether it makes that comparison in the East or in the West. In Table 10.3, however, the comparison between North and South is restricted to persons from the West ($H_0 : \mu_{SW} = \mu_{NW}$). Likewise, the comparison between the East and the West in factorial ANOVA is made regardless of whether it makes that comparison in the East or in the West. In Table 10.3, however, the comparison between the East and the West is restricted to persons from the South ($H_0 : \mu_{SW} = \mu_{SE}$). So, when we make the indicator variables in Equation (10.19) equal to 0 and 1, the regression coefficients tell us how the group represented by a value of 1 for a particular indicator variable differs from the group represented by the intercept (i.e., the group for which there is no indicator variable). This is not the way comparisons are made in factorial ANOVA.

To make Equation (10.19) more like factorial ANOVA, we need to make another choice for the values of indicator variables. Another choice is to use the values of positive one and negative one. Like 0 and 1, the values of positive and negative one do not imply a quantitative difference between groups; thus, they are appropriate to represent the qualitative nature of nominal variables numerically. Equation (10.20) shows a regression equation with positive one/negative one indicator variables:

$$\mu_{chol} = \alpha + (\beta_1 \cdot NS') + (\beta_2 \cdot EW') + (\beta_3 \cdot NS' \cdot EW') \tag{10.20}$$

where

μ_{chol} = mean serum cholesterol level in the population
NS' = indicator variable that is equal to positive one if the person is from the North or equal to negative one if the person is from the South
EW' = indicator variable that is equal to positive one if the person is from the East or equal to negative one if the person is from the West

The next example illustrates the use of positive one/negative one indicator variables and how the regression coefficients relate to a factorial ANOVA.

■ EXAMPLE 10.18

The following Excel output is result of analyzing the data in Example 10.6 using the "Regression" analysis tool and representing the nominal independent variables in the regression equation with positive one/negative one indicator variables.

SUMMARY OUTPUT							
Regression statistics							
Multiple R	0.449593751						
R square	0.202134541						
Adjusted R square	0.135645752						
Standard error	11.70707289						
Observations	40						
ANOVA							
	df	*SS*	*MS*	*F*	*Significance F*		
Regression	3	1250	416.6666667	3.040129712	0.041324944		
Residual	36	4934	137.0555556				
Total	39	6184					
	Coefficients	*Standard error*	*t Stat*	*P-value*	*Lower 95%*	*Upper 95%*	
Intercept	204.5	1.851050753	110.477792	3.58015E-47	200.7458951	208.2541049	
NS	-5	1.851050753	-2.701168508	0.010467574	-8.754104927	-1.245895073	
EW	2.5	1.851050753	1.350584254	0.185257897	-1.254104927	6.254104927	
NS_EW	1.14102E-15	1.851050753	6.16418E-16	1	-3.754104927	3.754104927	

The F-ratio and the corresponding P-value in the table at the middle of this output are the same as those in the table at the middle of the "Regression" analysis tool output in Example 10.17. In both instances, these test the omnibus null hypothesis that all of the independent variables taken together do not help to estimate dependent variable values. Since all of the independent variables are nominal, this is the same as the ANOVA omnibus null hypothesis that the means in all of the groups of dependent variable values are equal to the same value in the population. The way we have defined the indicator variables does not change the fact that there are four groups of dependent variable values corresponding to four geographic regions. The only thing we have changed is the way these four groups of dependent variable values are represented in the regression equation.

The t-values and their corresponding P-values in the table at the bottom of this output are somewhat different from those values in the table at the bottom of the "Regression" analysis tool output in Example 10.17. This difference is due to the way the four groups of dependent variable values are represented by the indicator variables in those analyses. If we compare the P-values in the table at the bottom of this output with those in the table at the bottom of the "Anova: Two Factor with Replication" analysis tool output in Example 10.17, however, we see that they match. Specifically, the P-value for the NS indicator variable in this example is the same as the one testing the North/South main effect in Example 10.17 (0.0105) and the

TABLE 10.4. Interpretation of the Estimated Regression Coefficients When Two Nominal Independent Variables Are Represented by Indicator Variables That Have the Values of Either Positive One or Negative One

Region	$b_1 \cdot NS'$	$b_2 \cdot EW'$	$b_3 \cdot NS' \cdot EW'$	$\widehat{chol}$	Mean
Southwest	$b_1 \cdot -1$	$b_2 \cdot -1$	$b_3 \cdot -1 \cdot -1$	$a - b_1 - b_2 + b_3$	$204.5 - (-5) - 2.5 + 0 = 207$
Northwest	$b_1 \cdot +1$	$b_2 \cdot -1$	$b_3 \cdot +1 \cdot -1$	$a + b_1 - b_2 + b_3$	$204.5 + (-5) - 2.5 - 0 = 197$
Southeast	$b_1 \cdot -1$	$b_2 \cdot +1$	$b_3 \cdot -1 \cdot +1$	$a - b_1 + b_2 + b_3$	$204.5 - (-5) + 2.5 - 0 = 212$
Northeast	$b_1 \cdot +1$	$b_2 \cdot +1$	$b_3 \cdot +1 \cdot +1$	$a + b_1 + b_2 + b_3$	$204.5 + (-5) + 2.5 + 0 = 202$

P-value for the EW indicator variable in this example is the same as the one testing the East/West main effect in Example 10.17 (0.1853). Next, we will discover why this is the case. ■

The interpretation of regression coefficients for positive one/negative one indicator variables is different from the interpretation of the regression coefficients for zero/one indicator variables. To help understand their interpretation, let us take a look at Table 10.4 in which the mean serum cholesterol values for the four geographic regions are represented by the positive one/negative one indicator variables in Equation (10.20).

When positive one/negative one indicator variables are used, the intercept no longer represents the mean of one of the groups of dependent variable values, as it does when zero/one indicator variables are used. Instead, the intercept represents the overall mean[22] of the dependent variable values (i.e., the mean of the groups' means).[23] Then, the regression coefficients represent differences from that overall mean. The tests of the null hypotheses that these regression coefficients are equal to 0 in the population are described in relationship with the differences in means in Table 10.5.

So, zero/one indicator variables specify differences from the mean of the dependent variable values in one of the groups (when both indicator variables are equal to zero) and positive one/negative one indicator variables specify differences from the overall mean.

Thus, testing the null hypothesis that a regression coefficient for a positive one/negative one indicator variable is equal to 0 is the same as testing a main effect in factorial ANOVA. Likewise, testing the null hypothesis that a regression coefficient for an interaction between two positive one/negative one indicator variables is equal to 0 is the same as testing for an interaction in the factorial ANOVA. From these observations, we can conclude that regression analysis and ANOVA are really just different forms of the same type of analysis. In fact, this is true of all of the methods

---

[22] The overall mean is sometimes called the **grand mean**.
[23] That this is the case can be verified by adding the coefficients that correspond to all of the means and dividing by the number of means.

TABLE 10.5. Null Hypotheses Tested When Two Nominal Independent Variables Are Represented by Indicator Variables That Are Equal to Either Positive One or Negative One*

Null Hypothesis in Terms of	
Regression Parameters	Means
$H_0 : \alpha = 0$	$H_0 : \mu_{\text{means}} = 0$
$H_0 : \beta_1 = 0$	$H_0 : \mu_S = \mu_N$
$H_0 : \beta_2 = 0$	$H_0 : \mu_W = \mu_E$
$H_0 : \beta_3 = 0$	$H_0 : \mu_{SW} = (3 \cdot \mu_{\text{means}}) - \mu_N - \mu_E$

[a] These null hypotheses are stated first in terms of the parameters of the regression equation and, then, in terms of the means for each group of dependent variable values. μ_{means} refers to the mean of all of the means.

of analysis we have discussed for a continuous dependent variable; they can all be expressed as a regression equation.

This unity of methods used to analyze a continuous dependent variable is called the **general linear model**. This principle allows a regression equation to include nominal and/or continuous dependent variables.

The purpose of learning about the general linear model is twofold. First, it helps us understand the unifying principles behind all analyses for a continuous dependent variable. Second, it allows us to create analyses that are tailored to the research questions that are most relevant to us. In other words, understanding the general linear model means we are not restricted to a few study designs for which there are analyses in Excel or R. Instead, we can use indicator and interaction variables that best reflect our interest.

In the next chapter, we will look at nonparametric methods for multivariable data sets.

CHAPTER SUMMARY

When we have a continuous dependent variable and more than one continuous independent variable, we can perform statistical procedures that are extensions of correlation analysis and regression analysis discussed in Chapter 7 for a single independent variable. For more than one independent variable the procedures are called multiple correlation analysis and multiple regression analysis. Both of those procedures examine a linear combination of the independent variables multiplied by their corresponding regression coefficients (slopes).

In analysis of multivariable data sets, we can think about the relationship of the dependent variable to each of the independent variables or about its relationship to the entire collection of independent variables. In multiple regression analysis, both are considered. In multiple correlation analysis, however, only the association between the dependent variable and the entire collection of independent variables is considered.

To interpret the multiple correlation coefficient (or, more appropriately, its square, the coefficient of multiple determination) as an estimate of the strength of association in the population from which the sample was drawn, all the independent variables must be from a naturalistic sample. That is to say, their distributions in the sample must be the result of random selection from their distributions in the population.

In multiple regression analysis, we can examine the relationship between the dependent variable and the entire collection of independent variables. The way we do this is by testing the omnibus null hypothesis.

We can also examine each individual independent variable in multiple regression analysis. The relationship between the dependent variable and an individual independent variable in multiple regression analysis, however, is not necessarily the same as the relationship between those variables in bivariable regression analysis (i.e., when we have only one independent variable). The difference is that, in multiple regression analysis, we examine the relationship between an independent variable and the variability in data represented by the dependent variable that is not associated with the other independent variables.

If two or more independent variables share information (i.e., if they are correlated) and, in addition, that shared information is the same as the information they use to estimate values of the dependent variable, we say we have collinearity (for two independent variables) or multicollinearity (for more than two independent variables). Multicollinearity (or collinearity) can make estimation and hypothesis testing for individual regression coefficients difficult. On the other hand, it makes it possible to take into account the confounding effects of one or more independent variables, while examining the relationship between another independent variable and the dependent variable. Multicollinearity is a feature, not only of multiple regression analysis, but of all multivariable procedures.

When we have more than one nominal independent variable, we are able to specify more than two groups of dependent variable values. The means of the dependent variable values for those groups are compared using ANOVA procedures. ANOVA involves estimating three sources of variation of data represented by the dependent variable. The variation of the dependent variable without regard to independent variable values is called the total sum of squares. The total mean square is equal to the total sum of squares divided by the total degrees of freedom.

The best estimate of the population's variance of data represented by the dependent variable is found by taking a weighted average (with degrees of freedom as the weights) of the estimates of the variance of data within each group of values of the dependent variable. This estimate is called the within mean square. The within sum of squares is one of two portions of the total sum of squares. The remaining portion describes the variation among the group means. This is called the between sum of squares. The between sum of squares divided by its degrees of freedom (the number of groups minus one) gives us the average variation among group means called the between mean square.

We can test the omnibus null hypothesis that the means of the dependent variable in all the groups specified by independent variable values are equal in the population from which the sample was drawn by comparing the between mean square and the within mean square. This is done by calculating an F-ratio. If the omnibus null hypothesis is true, that ratio should be equal to 0, on the average.

In addition to testing the omnibus null hypothesis, it is often of interest to make pairwise comparisons of means of the dependent variable. To do this, we use a posterior test designed to keep the experiment-wise α error rate equal to a specific value (usually 0.05) regardless of how many pairwise comparisons are made. The best procedure to make all possible pairwise comparisons among the means is the Student–Newman–Keuls procedure. The test statistic for this procedure is similar to Student's t statistic in that it is equal to the difference between two means minus the hypothesized difference divided by the standard error for the difference.

It is also similar to Student's t statistic in that the standard error for the difference between two means includes a pooled estimate of the variance of data represented by the dependent variable. In ANOVA, the pooled estimate of the variance of data is the within mean square.

The important difference between Student's t procedure and the Student–Newman–Keuls procedure is that the latter requires a specific order in which pairwise comparisons are made. The first comparison must be between the largest and the smallest means. If and only if we can reject the null hypothesis that those two means are equal in the population can we compare the next less-extreme means.

If all the nominal independent variables identify different categories of a single characteristic (e.g., different races), we say we have a one-way ANOVA. If, on the other hand, some of the nominal independent variables specify categories of one characteristic (e.g., race), and other nominal independent variables specify categories of another characteristic (e.g., gender), we say we have a factorial ANOVA.

Factorial ANOVA involves estimation of total, within, and between variations of data represented by the dependent variable just like one-way ANOVA. The difference between factorial and one-way ANOVAs is that, in factorial ANOVA, we consider components (or partitions) of the between variation. Some of these components estimate the variation among the means of the dependent variable corresponding to categories of a particular factor and are called main effects. Other components reflect the consistency of the relationship among categories of one factor for different categories of another factor. This source of variation is called an interaction. Only if there does not seem to be a statistically significant interaction can the main effects be interpreted easily.

It is very common that a data set contains both continuous and nominal independent variables. The procedure we use to analyze such a data set is called ANCOVA. An ANCOVA can be thought of as a multiple regression in which the nominal independent variables are represented numerically, often with the values 0 and 1.

The numeric representation of a nominal independent variable is called a dummy or an indicator variable. An additional independent variable is created by multiplying an indicator variable by another independent variable. This is called an interaction.

In its simplest form, ANCOVA can be thought of as a method to compare regression equations for the categories specified by values of the nominal independent variables. In that interpretation, the regression coefficient for the indicator variable gives the difference between the intercepts of the regression equations, and the regression coefficient for the interaction gives the difference between the slopes for those regression equations.

Another way to think about ANCOVA is that it is a method used to compare group means while controlling for the confounding effects of a continuous independent variable. This is not really different than the regression interpretation. In fact, all the procedures we have examined for continuous dependent variables can be thought of as regression analyses. This is the principle of the general linear model.

EXERCISES

10.1. Suppose we are interested in the relationship between dietary sodium intake (NA) and diastolic blood pressure (DBP). To investigate this relationship, we measure both for a sample of 40 persons. Because DBP and NA both increase with age, we decide to control for age in our analysis. The data for this question are in the Excel file: EXR10_1 on the website accompanying this textbook. Based on those observations, which of the following is closest to the percent variation in DBP that is explained by the combination of NA and age?

A. 14.4%
B. 24.3%
C. 30.7%
D. 38.0%
E. 55.4%

10.2. Suppose we are interested in which blood chemistry measurements are predictive of urine creatinine. To investigate this, we identify 100 persons and measure their urine creatinine levels. We also measure serum creatinine, blood urea nitrogen (BUN), and serum potassium. These data are in the Excel file called EXR10_2 on the website accompanying this textbook. Use Excel or R to determine the percent of the variation in urine creatinine that is explained by the combination of serum creatinine, BUN, and serum potassium. Which of the following is closest to that value?

A. 73.3%
B. 69.3%
C. 53.7%

D. 48.0%

E. 43.0%

10.3. Suppose we are interested in the relationship between dietary sodium intake (NA) and diastolic blood pressure (DBP). To investigate this relationship, we measure both for a sample of 40 persons. Because DBP and NA both increase with age, we decide to control for age in our analysis. The data for this question is in the Excel file: EXR10_1 on the website accompanying this textbook. Based on those observations, test the null hypothesis that the combination of NA and age does not help estimate DBP, versus the alternative hypothesis that it does. If you allow a 5% chance of making a type I error, which of the following is the best conclusion to draw?

A. Reject both the null and alternative hypotheses

B. Accept both the null and alternative hypotheses

C. Reject the null hypothesis and accept the alternative hypothesis

D. Accept the null hypothesis and reject the alternative hypothesis

E. It is best not to draw a conclusion about the null and alternative hypotheses from these observations

10.4. Suppose we are interested in which blood chemistry measurements are predictive of urine creatinine. To investigate this, we identify 100 persons and measure their urine creatinine levels. We also measure serum creatinine, blood urea nitrogen (BUN), and serum potassium. These data are in the Excel file called EXR10_2 on the website accompanying this textbook. Use Excel or R to test the null hypothesis that the combination of serum creatinine, BUN, and serum potassium do not help estimate urine creatinine versus the alternative hypothesis that they do help. If you allow a 5% chance of making a type I error, what is the best conclusion to draw?

A. Reject both the null and alternative hypotheses

B. Accept both the null and alternative hypotheses

C. Reject the null hypothesis and accept the alternative hypothesis

D. Accept the null hypothesis and reject the alternative hypothesis

E. It is best not to draw a conclusion about the null and alternative hypotheses from these observations

10.5. Suppose we are interested in the relationship between dietary sodium intake (NA) and diastolic blood pressure (DBP). To investigate this relationship, we measure both for a sample of 40 persons. Because DBP and NA both increase with age, we decide to control for age in our analysis. The data for this question is in the Excel file: EXR10_1 on the website accompanying this textbook. Based on those observations, test the null hypothesis that the regression coefficient for NA, controlling for AGE, is equal to 0 in the population versus the alternative hypothesis that it is not equal to 0. If you allow a 5% chance of making a type I error, which of the following is the best conclusion to draw?

A. Reject both the null and alternative hypotheses

B. Accept both the null and alternative hypotheses

C. Reject the null hypothesis and accept the alternative hypothesis

D. Accept the null hypothesis and reject the alternative hypothesis

E. It is best not to draw a conclusion about the null and alternative hypotheses from these observations

10.6. Suppose we are interested in which blood chemistry measurements are predictive of urine creatinine. To investigate this, we identify 100 persons and measure their urine creatinine levels. We also measure serum creatinine, blood urea nitrogen (BUN), and serum potassium. These data are in the Excel file called EXR10_2 on the website accompanying this textbook. Use Excel or R to test the null hypothesis that the regression coefficient for serum creatinine, when controlling for BUN and serum potassium, is equal to 0 versus the alternative hypothesis that it is not equal to 0. If you allow a 5% chance of making a type I error, what is the best conclusion to draw?

A. Reject both the null and alternative hypotheses

B. Accept both the null and alternative hypotheses

C. Reject the null hypothesis and accept the alternative hypothesis

D. Accept the null hypothesis and reject the alternative hypothesis

E. It is best not to draw a conclusion about the null and alternative hypotheses from these observations

10.7. Suppose we are interested in the relationship between dietary sodium intake (NA) and diastolic blood pressure (DBP). To investigate this relationship, we measure both for a sample of 40 persons. Because DBP and NA both increase with age, we decide to control for age in our analysis. The data for this question are in the Excel file: EXR10_1 on the website accompanying this textbook. Based on those observations, which of the following independent variables contributes the most to the estimate of DBP, controlling for the other independent variables?

A. AGE

B. NA

C. They both contribute about the same to estimation of DBP

10.8. Suppose we are interested in which blood chemistry measurements are predictive of urine creatinine. To investigate this, we identify 100 persons and measure their urine creatinine levels. We also measure serum creatinine, blood urea nitrogen (BUN), and serum potassium. These data are in the Excel file called EXR10_2 on the website accompanying this textbook. Use Excel or R to determine which of the independent variables contributes the most to estimation of urine creatinine, while controlling for the other independent variables?

A. Serum creatinine

B. BUN

C. Serum potassium

D. They all contribute about the same to estimation of urine creatinine

10.9. Suppose we are interested in the survival time for persons with cancer of various organs. To investigate this, we identify 64 persons who died with cancer as the primary cause of death and record the period of time from their initial diagnosis to their death (in days). Those data are in the Excel file EXR10_3 on the website accompanying this textbook. Based on those data, test the null hypothesis that all five means are equal to the same value in the population versus the alternative that they are not all equal. If you allow a 5% chance of making a type I error, which of the following is the best conclusion to draw?

A. Reject both the null and alternative hypotheses

B. Accept both the null and alternative hypotheses

C. Reject the null hypothesis and accept the alternative hypothesis

D. Accept the null hypothesis and reject the alternative hypothesis

E. It is best not to draw a conclusion about the null and alternative hypotheses from these observations

10.10. Suppose we are interested in force of head impact for crash dummies in vehicles with different driver safety equipment. To study this relationship, we examine the results for 175 tests. Those data are in the Excel file: EXR10_4 on the website accompanying this textbook. Based on those data, test the null hypothesis that all four means are equal to the same value in the population versus the alternative that they are not all equal. If you allow a 5% chance of making a type I error, which of the following is the best conclusion to draw?

A. Reject both the null and alternative hypotheses

B. Accept both the null and alternative hypotheses

C. Reject the null hypothesis and accept the alternative hypothesis

D. Accept the null hypothesis and reject the alternative hypothesis

E. It is best not to draw a conclusion about the null and alternative hypotheses from these observations

10.11. Suppose we are interested in survival times for persons with cancer of various organs. To investigate this, we identify 64 persons who died with cancer as the primary cause of death and record the period of time from their initial diagnosis to their death (in days). Those data are in the Excel file: EXR10_3 on the website accompanying this textbook. Based on those data, perform tests comparing two means at a time in a way that avoids problems with multiple comparisons. If you allow a 5% chance of making a type I error, which of the following is the best conclusion to draw?

A. All five means are significantly different from each other

B. The mean for Bronchus is significantly different from all of the other means

C. The mean for Bronchus is significantly different from all of the other means except the mean for Stomach

D. The mean for Breast is significantly different from all of the other means

E. The mean for Breast is significantly different from all of the other means except the mean for Ovary

10.12. Suppose we are interested in force of head impact for crash dummies in vehicles with different driver safety equipment. To study this relationship, we examine the results for 175 tests. Those data are in the Excel file: EXR10_4 on the website accompanying this textbook. Based on those data, perform tests comparing two means at a time in a way that avoids problems with multiple comparisons. If you allow a 5% chance of making a type I error, which of the following is the best conclusion to draw?

A. All four means are significantly different from each other

B. Manual Belt is significantly different from the other three means, but the other three means are not significantly different from each other

C. All four means are significantly different from each other except Airbag and Motorized belt

D. All four means are significantly different from each other except Motorized Belt and Passive Belt

E. All four means are significantly different from each other except Passive Belt and Manual Belt

10.13. In a study of clinical depression, patients were randomly assigned to one of four drug groups (three active drugs and a placebo) and to a cognitive therapy group (active versus placebo). The dependent variable is a difference between scores on a depression questionnaire. The results are in the Excel file: EXR10_5 on the website accompanying this textbook. Based on those data, test the null hypothesis of no interaction between drug and therapy versus the alternative hypothesis that there is interaction allowing a 5% chance of making a type I error. Which of the following is the best conclusion to draw?

A. Reject both the null and alternative hypotheses

B. Accept both the null and alternative hypotheses

C. Reject the null hypothesis and accept the alternative hypothesis

D. Accept the null hypothesis and reject the alternative hypothesis

E. It is best not to draw a conclusion about the null and alternative hypotheses from these observations

10.14. In a multicenter study of a new treatment for hypertension, patients at nine centers were randomly assigned to a new treatment or standard treatment. The dependent variable is a difference in diastolic blood pressure from a pretreatment value. The results are in the Excel file: EXR10_6 on the website accompanying this textbook. Based on those data, test the null hypothesis of no interaction between drug and center versus the alternative hypothesis that there is interaction allowing a 5% chance of making a type I error. Which of the following is the best conclusion to draw?

A. Reject both the null and alternative hypotheses

B. Accept both the null and alternative hypotheses

C. Reject the null hypothesis and accept the alternative hypothesis

D. Accept the null hypothesis and reject the alternative hypothesis

E. It is best not to draw a conclusion about the null and alternative hypotheses from these observations

10.15. In a study of clinical depression, patients were randomly assigned to one of four drug groups (three active drugs and a placebo) and to a cognitive therapy group (active versus no therapy). The dependent variable is a difference between scores on a depression questionnaire. The results are in the Excel file: EXR10_5 on the website accompanying this textbook. Based on those data, test the null hypothesis of no differences between drug groups versus the alternative hypothesis that there is a difference, ignoring the possibility of an interaction. Allowing a 5% chance of making a type I error, which of the following is the best conclusion to draw?

A. Reject both the null and alternative hypotheses

B. Accept both the null and alternative hypotheses

C. Reject the null hypothesis and accept the alternative hypothesis

D. Accept the null hypothesis and reject the alternative hypothesis

E. It is best not to draw a conclusion about the null and alternative hypotheses from these observations

10.16. In a multicenter study of a new treatment for hypertension, patients at nine centers were randomly assigned to a new treatment or standard treatment. The dependent variable is a difference in diastolic blood pressure from a pretreatment value. The results are in the Excel file: EXR10_6 on the website accompanying this textbook. Based on those data, test the null hypothesis of no difference between drugs versus the alternative hypothesis that there is a difference, ignoring the possibility of an interaction. If you allow a 5%

chance of making a type I error, which of the following is the best conclusion to draw?

A. Reject both the null and alternative hypotheses
B. Accept both the null and alternative hypotheses
C. Reject the null hypothesis and accept the alternative hypothesis
D. Accept the null hypothesis and reject the alternative hypothesis
E. It is best not to draw a conclusion about the null and alternative hypotheses from these observations

10.17. In a study of clinical depression, patients were randomly assigned to one of four drug groups (three active drugs and a placebo) and to a cognitive therapy group (active versus no therapy). The dependent variable is a difference between scores on a depression questionnaire. The results are in the Excel file: EXR10_5 on the website accompanying this textbook. Based on those data, test the null hypothesis of no difference between therapy groups versus the alternative hypothesis that there is a difference, ignoring the possibility of an interaction. Allowing a 5% chance of making a type I error, which of the following is the best conclusion to draw?

A. Reject both the null and alternative hypotheses
B. Accept both the null and alternative hypotheses
C. Reject the null hypothesis and accept the alternative hypothesis
D. Accept the null hypothesis and reject the alternative hypothesis
E. It is best not to draw a conclusion about the null and alternative hypotheses from these observations

10.18. In a multicenter study of a new treatment for hypertension, patients at nine centers were randomly assigned to a new treatment or standard treatment. The dependent variable is a difference in diastolic blood pressure from a pre-treatment value. The results are in the Excel file: EXR10_6 on the website accompanying this textbook. Based on those data, test the null hypothesis of no difference among centers in the population versus the alternative hypothesis that there is a difference, ignoring the possibility of an interaction. If you allow a 5% chance of making a type I error, which of the following is the best conclusion to draw?

A. Reject both the null and alternative hypotheses
B. Accept both the null and alternative hypotheses
C. Reject the null hypothesis and accept the alternative hypothesis
D. Accept the null hypothesis and reject the alternative hypothesis
E. It is best not to draw a conclusion about the null and alternative hypotheses from these observations

10.19. Suppose we are interested in the relationship between body mass index (BMI) and serum cholesterol (the dependent variable) controlling for gender (SEX = 1 for women and SEX = 0 for men). To study this relationship, we analyze data from 300 persons who participated in the Framingham Heart Study. Those data are in Excel file: EXR10_7 on the website accompanying this textbook. Analyze those data as an ANCOVA. From that output, do you think the slopes of the regression lines for men and women are different?

  A. No, the slopes are the same

  B. Yes, the slopes are different, but not significantly different

  C. Yes, the slopes are different and they are significantly different

10.20. Suppose we are interested in the relationship between time since diagnosis of HIV and CD4 count. To investigate this relationship, we examine 1,151 HIV-positive patients. In making this comparison, we control for gender (SEX = 1 for women and SEX = 0 for men). These data are in the Excel file: EXR10_8 on the website accompanying this textbook. Which of the following is the best description of the relationship between time since diagnosis and CD4 in the sample?

  A. CD4 decreases with longer time since diagnosis for both men and women

  B. CD4 decreases with longer time since diagnosis for women only

  C. CD4 decreases with longer time since diagnosis for men only

  D. CD4 decreases with longer time since diagnosis for men and increases for women

  E. CD4 decreases with longer time since diagnosis for women and increases for men

CHAPTER 11

MULTIVARIABLE ANALYSIS OF AN ORDINAL DEPENDENT VARIABLE

As in previous chapters about ordinal dependent variables, we expect to find methods in this chapter that we could use as nonparametric analyses in the circumstance in which we are concerned about some of the assumptions made by a method in Chapter 10 (i.e., a method designed for a continuous dependent variable). With that expectation, we look in this chapter for methods that are parallel to those discussed in the previous chapter. In Chapter 10, we learned about multiple regression and correlation analyses for continuous independent variables, analysis of variance (ANOVA) for nominal independent variables, and analysis of covariance for a mixture of continuous and nominal independent variables. A look at Flowchart 11.1 quickly reveals that few of those analyses have nonparametric parallels.

When we discussed bivariable analysis of an ordinal dependent variable (Chapter 8), we found that there is no nonparametric parallel to regression analysis. The reason for this is that a slope cannot be estimated for an ordinal dependent

Introduction to Biostatistical Applications in Health Research with Microsoft Office Excel® and R,
Second Edition. Robert P. Hirsch.
© 2021 John Wiley & Sons, Inc. Published 2021 by John Wiley & Sons, Inc.
Companion website: www.wiley.com/go/hirsch/healthresearch2e

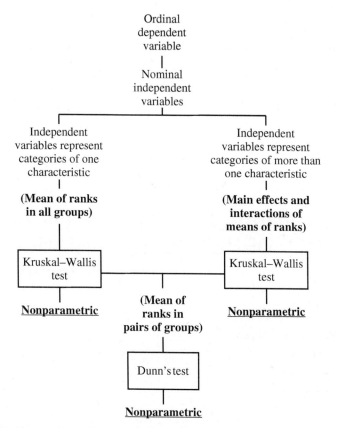

FLOWCHART 9   Flowchart showing multivariable analysis of an ordinal dependent variable. The point estimate that is most often used to describe the dependent variable is in bold. The common name of the statistical test is enclosed in a box. The method that is used to test hypotheses and calculate confidence intervals is in bold and underlined.

variable.[1] In multivariable analysis, this inability implies that we cannot have nonparametric parallels to multiple regression, multiple correlation,[2] or analysis of covariance. That leaves nonparametric parallels only to ANOVA and posterior testing: statistical methods in which all of the independent variables represent nominal data.

---

[1] A slope (or regression coefficient) tells us how much the numeric magnitude of the dependent variable changes for each one-unit change in the independent variable. On an ordinal scale, we cannot tell how far apart values are. Thus, an ordinal dependent variable precludes us from determining how much the dependent variable changes and, as a result, makes estimation of the slope (or regression coefficient) impossible.

[2] In multivariable analysis, the correlation coefficient tells us about the strength of the association between the dependent variable and all of the independent variables taken together. The way in which all the independent variables are represented is through the multiple regression equation. If regression coefficients cannot be estimated, the independent variables cannot be combined for multiple correlation analysis. Thus, we have bivariable correlation analysis on an ordinal scale, but we do not have multivariable correlation analysis on an ordinal scale.

11.1   NONPARAMETRIC ANOVA

The **Kruskal–Wallis test** is the nonparametric method used to perform one-way and factorial analyses of variance without assuming that the sampling distribution is a Gaussian distribution. To perform this test by hand, we begin by assigning relative ranks to the dependent variable values. This is done in the same way we assigned ranks to dependent variable values in preparation for a bivariable nonparametric parallel to Student's t-test: the Mann–Whitney test or the Wilcoxon Rank-Sum test (illustrated in Example 8.4). Specifically, all of the dependent variable values are ranked in order of their numeric magnitude without regard to which group those values belong.

Calculating the Kruskal–Wallis test statistic (usually symbolized by H) by hand can be tedious, especially if there are tied ranks.[3] Instead, it is much easier to make this calculation with the aid of a computer. This can be done even if the computer program you use does not have a procedure specifically for the Kruskal–Wallis test. In that case, the computer program's procedure for ANOVA for continuous dependent variable values can be used to help calculate the Kruskal–Wallis test statistic. This is done by changing the dependent variable values to ranks and using the computer to perform an ANOVA as we would for dependent variable values on a continuous scale. Then, we test the null hypothesis that the mean of the ranks[4] are the same for all the groups in the population (i.e., the nonparametric parallel to the omnibus null hypothesis that the means for all of the groups are equal to the same value) by calculating the Kruskal–Wallis test statistic from the results of the ANOVA. The Kruskal–Wallis test statistic is calculated from those results as illustrated in Equation (11.1).[5]

$$H = \frac{\text{Between sum of squares}}{\text{Total mean square}} \tag{11.1}$$

where

H = Kruskal–Wallis test statistic

To test the null hypothesis that the mean rank for each of the groups of dependent variable values is the same in the population, we can compare the value calculated in Equation (11.1) with a value in a table of Kruskal–Wallis test statistics (such as Table B.9) or, if the data set consists of more dependent variable values than found in such a table, the Kruskal–Wallis test statistic can be interpreted as a chi-square value with the same number of degrees of freedom as the between degrees of freedom in ANOVA.[6] This is illustrated in the next example.

---

[3]Recall from Chapter 5 that "tied ranks" refers to the average rank given to all dependent variable values that are equal to each other on the continuous scale.
[4]The mean of the ranks corresponds to the median on the continuous scale.
[5]This is also the way we calculated the test statistic for the chi-square test for trend procedure.
[6]Recall from Chapter 10 that the within degrees of freedom are equal to the number of nominal independent variables that are needed to specify the groups of continuous dependent variable values in an analysis of variance.

■ EXAMPLE 11.1

In Example 10.7, we compared serum cholesterol levels among persons in four geographic regions of the United States: Northeast (NE), Northwest (NW), Southeast (SE), and Southwest (SW). In that example, one-way ANOVA was used to test the null hypothesis that the means for all four groups of dependent variable values are equal to the same value in the population. Now, let us perform a Kruskal–Wallis test to test the nonparametric equivalent to that null hypothesis.

First, we need to convert those data to an ordinal scale. We do that by ranking the dependent variable values from lowest to highest regardless of the group they belong to. The data are from Example 10.6 and appear in the following table, along with their ranks.

NE	Rank	NW	Rank	SE	Rank	SW	Rank
197	13.5	194	7.5	220	34	206	25
183	1	185	2	202	21	196	10.5
190	5.5	186	3.5	212	28	195	9
212	28	212	28	221	35	222	36
223	37	209	26	227	39	228	40
202	21	194	7.5	224	38	205	24
201	18.5	186	3.5	197	13.5	197	13.5
202	21	196	10.5	201	18.5	203	23
197	13.5	190	5.5	198	16	199	17
213	30	218	31.5	218	31.5	219	33

Next, we use those ranks as the dependent variable values in Excel's "Anova: Single Factor" analysis tool.

Anova: single factor						
Summary						
Groups	Count	Sum	Average	Variance		
NE	10	189	18.9	122.3222222		
NW	10	125.5	12.55	128.7472222		
SE	10	274.5	27.45	89.85833333		
SW	10	231	23.1	115.7111111		
ANOVA						
Source of variation	SS	df	MS	F	P-value	F crit
Between groups	1208.25	3	402.75	3.527951822	0.024384921	2.866265551
Within groups	4109.75	36	114.1597222			
Total	5318	39				

We cannot use the *P*-values in this output. Instead, we use the between sum of squares and the total mean square in Equation (11.1) to calculate the Kruskal–Wallis test statistic. Since Excel does not provide the total mean square, we need to calculate it by dividing the total sum of squares by the total degrees of freedom.

$$H = \frac{\text{Between sum of squares}}{\text{Total mean square}} = \frac{1,208.25}{5,318/39} = 8.861$$

To test the null hypothesis that the mean of the ranks of serum cholesterol levels is the same in the four geographic regions in the population, we compare the calculated test statistic (8.861) with the critical value in Table B.9.

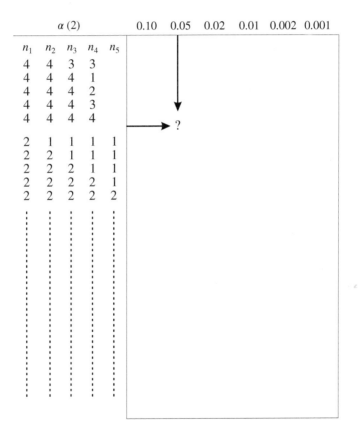

To find a critical value in Table B.9, we look for the same number of groups and the same number of observations in each of the groups in the leftmost columns of the table. In this case, we have 4 groups of dependent variable values and 10 observations in each group. A sample of this size is not listed in Table B.9 (the largest sample with four groups has four observations in each group).

If the sample is larger than the samples' sizes considered in Table B.9, we compare the calculated statistic (8.861) with a chi-square value in Table B.7 with 3 degrees of freedom (equal to the number of groups minus one). That critical value is equal to 7.815. Since the calculated value (8.861) is greater than the critical value (7.815), we reject the null hypothesis.

Another way to do this is to analyze the data in Excel or R. There, we do not have to convert the data to ranks. Instead, we use the BAHR "Nonparametric Analyses" program in Excel or the "Kruskal.test(DV~factor)" command in R.

In Excel, we get the following output.

	Kruskal-Wallis test (one-way)				
Statistic =	8.860803	DF =	3	P-value =	0.0312

In R, we get the following output.
>kruskal.test(CHOL~REGION,data=Example10_9)

```
Kruskal-Wallis rank sum test

data:  CHOL by REGION
Kruskal-Wallis chi-squared = 8.8608, df = 3, p-value = 0.0312
```

This gives us exactly the same result we got using Excel and calculating by hand. ∎

If the nominal independent variables represent more than one characteristic, we should use a method of analysis that takes this factorial design into account. As suggested earlier, the Kruskal–Wallis test can be extended to factorial designs. To do this, we convert the data to ranks and use those ranks as the dependent variable in the "Anova: Two-Factor with Replication" analysis tool. In this case, we need to use Excel to determine the ranks and perform a factorial ANOVA or we can use the BAHR program, in which case we do not need to convert the data to ranks. We cannot use R, however, since the "kruskal.test(DV~factor)" command can only analyze a one-way design.

In factorial ANOVA, we can test hypotheses about main effects and interactions as well as the omnibus null hypothesis (that the means of the ranks of all the groups are equal to the same value in the population). The nonparametric equivalent to factorial ANOVA tests null hypotheses about main effects by calculating the Kruskal–Wallis test statistic as shown in Equation (11.2) and also tests the null hypothesis that there is no interaction by calculating the Kruskal–Wallis test statistic as shown in Equation (11.3).

$$H = \frac{\text{Main effect sum of squares}}{\text{Total mean square}} \tag{11.2}$$

$$H = \frac{\text{Interaction sum of squares}}{\text{Total mean square}} \tag{11.3}$$

The next example demonstrates how we can perform a factorial Kruskal–Wallis test using Excel.

■ EXAMPLE 11.2

For this example, let us use the same data set we considered in the previous example, but now thinking of geographic region as having two characteristics: north versus south and east versus west. With this factorial design in mind, let us use the Kruskal–Wallis test to test hypotheses about the two main effects and the interaction.

To begin with, we need to convert serum cholesterol levels to ranks. This is done regardless of the group in which we find the dependent variable value. Thus, the ranks are the same as those given in Example 11.1.

Next, we use those ranks as the dependent variable in the "Anova: Two-Factor with Replication" analysis tool and specify two factors represented by the nominal independent variables. The following Excel output shows results from that analysis:

Anova: Two factor with replication						
Anova: Two factor with replication						
Summary	North	South	Total			
East						
Count	10	10	20			
Sum	189	274.5	463.5			
Average	18.9	27.45	23.175			
Variance	122.3222222	89.85833333	119.7440789			
West						
Count	10	10	20			
Sum	125.5	231	356.5			
Average	12.55	23.1	17.825			
Variance	128.7472222	115.7111111	145.0861842			
Total						
Count	20	20				
Sum	314.5	505.5				
Average	15.725	25.275				
Variance	129.5388158	102.3546053				
Anova						
Source of variation	*SS*	*df*	*MS*	*F*	*P-value*	*F crit*
Sample	286.225	1	286.225	2.5072328	0.122071489	4.113165277
Columns	912.025	1	912.025	7.989026096	0.007634223	4.113165277
Interaction	10	1	10	0.087596569	0.768955753	4.113165277
Within	4109.75	36	114.1597222			
Total	5.318	39				

Now, let us begin testing hypotheses about interaction and main effects. We learned in Chapter 10 that we need to test the null hypothesis that there is no interaction before we can look at the main effects. Testing for no interaction uses Equation (11.3).

$$H = \frac{\text{Interaction sum of squares}}{\text{Total mean square}} = \frac{10}{5,318/39} = 0.073$$

To interpret this test statistic, we compare it with a chi-square with the same degrees of freedom we would use to interpret the F-ratio for the interaction. In this case, there is one degree of freedom and the corresponding chi-square value from Table B.7 is equal to 3.814. Since the calculated value (0.073) is less than the tabled value (3.814), we fail to reject the null hypothesis that there is no interaction. This allows us to go on to interpret the main effects.

Next, let us test the North versus South main effect (NS). We do this by using Equation (11.2):

$$H = \frac{\text{NS sum of squares}}{\text{Total mean square}} = \frac{912.025}{5,318/39} = 6.688$$

To interpret this test statistic, we compare it with a chi-square with the same degrees of freedom we would use to interpret the F-ratio for this main effect. In this case, there is one degree of freedom and the corresponding chi-square value from Table B.7 is equal to 3.814. Since the calculated value (6.688) is greater than the tabled value (3.814), we reject the null hypothesis that there is no difference in the distribution of serum cholesterol values between the North and South.

Finally, we test the East versus West main effect (EW). We do this by using Equation (11.2).

$$H = \frac{\text{EW sum of squares}}{\text{Total mean square}} = \frac{286.225}{5,318/39} = 2.099$$

To interpret this test statistic, we compare it with a chi-square with the same degrees of freedom we would use to interpret the F-ratio for this main effect. In this case, there is one degree of freedom and the corresponding chi-square value from Table B.7 is equal to 3.814. Since the calculated value (2.099) is less than the tabled value (3.814), we fail to reject the null hypothesis that there is no difference in the distribution of serum cholesterol values between the East and West.

If we use the BAHR program "Nonparametric Analyses" to analyze the data, we get the following output.

Kruskal-Wallis test (two-way)			
	Statistic	DF	P-value
Groups	2.099055096	1	0.147390199
Columns	6.688411997	1	0.009704161
Interaction	0.073335841	1	0.786540315

The results of that analysis are identical with what we calculated by hand. ■

11.2 POSTERIOR TESTING

After performing an ANOVA, we do not know which groups are different (unless there are only two groups). To determine which are different, we need to perform a posterior test. The most commonly used posterior test for ordinal dependent variables is called **Dunn's test**. It is similar to the Student–Newman–Keuls test, introduced in Chapter 10 as a posterior test for continuous dependent variables. An important property of both the Student–Newman–Keuls test and Dunn's test is that they decrease the chance of making at least one type I error[7] when making pairwise comparisons without greatly decreasing our ability to reject false null hypotheses (i.e., decreasing statistical power).[8]

The key to maintaining statistical power in both posterior tests is to follow a protocol in selecting the order in which groups are compared. The protocol is the same for both the Student–Newman–Keuls test and Dunn's test. To begin with, we arrange the groups according to the numeric magnitude of the means of their ranks.[9] Then, the two most extreme groups are compared by testing the hypothesis that the mean ranks are the same in the two groups. If we are unable to reject that null hypothesis, then we stop making comparisons and fail to reject *all* of the pairwise null hypotheses. If, on the other hand, we reject this null hypothesis, we can compare the lowest group with the next to the highest group and the highest group with the next to the lowest groups. This continues until we have either rejected or failed to reject all pairwise null hypotheses. This was illustrated for the Student–Newman–Keuls test in Example 10.12.

We will take a look at an example of how to perform Dunn's test shortly, but first we need to see how Dunn's test statistic is calculated. That calculation is given by Equation (11.4).

$$Q = \frac{(\overline{Y}_{\text{rank}_1} - \overline{Y}_{\text{rank}_2}) - (\mu_{\text{rank}_1} - \mu_{\text{rank}_2})}{\sqrt{\text{TMS}/n_1 + \text{TMS}/n_2}} \tag{11.4}$$

where

Q = Dunn's test statistic

$\overline{Y}_{\text{rank}_i}$ = observed mean of the ranks in group i

μ_{rank_i} = population's mean of the ranks in group i

TMS = total mean square from an ANOVA performed on the ranks of dependent variable values

n_i = number of observations in group i

---

[7] Recall from Chapter 3 that a type I error occurs when we reject a true null hypothesis.

[8] This is in contrast to poorer posterior tests, such as using Bonferroni's "correction" to control the chance of making a type I error. These tests control the chance of making at least one type I error, but they do that in a way that needlessly decreases statistical power.

[9] The mean of the ranks is the same as the median when there is not the same rank being shared by more than one observation. When there are shared ranks (i.e., "tied" ranks), there are different ways we can define the median. The mean of the ranks is one of them.

To interpret the result of using Equation (11.4), we compare the calculated value with a corresponding value in Table B.10. To find the tabled value, we need to specify k, the number of groups involved in the comparison. This number is equal to two plus the groups that are between those being compared. This is easier to see in an example.

■ EXAMPLE 11.3

In Example 11.1, we used the ANOVA procedure to perform the Kruskal–Wallis test on serum cholesterol levels in persons from four geographic regions. In that example, we were able to reject the null hypothesis that the distributions of serum cholesterol levels are the same for all four geographic regions. Now, let us make pairwise comparisons among the four groups using Dunn's test.

To begin with, we need to calculate the mean ranks for each of the groups. This calculation is summarized in the following table:

NE	Rank	NW	Rank	SE	Rank	SW	Rank
197	13.5	194	7.5	220	34	206	25
183	1	185	2	202	21	196	10.5
190	5.5	186	3.5	212	28	195	9
212	28	212	28	221	35	222	36
223	37	209	26	227	39	228	40
202	21	194	7.5	224	38	205	24
201	18.5	186	3.5	197	13.5	197	13.5
202	21	196	10.5	201	18.5	203	23
197	13.5	190	5.5	198	16	199	17
213	30	218	31.5	218	31.5	219	33
Mean	18.90		12.55		27.45		23.10

Then we organize these means of ranks in order of their numeric magnitude:

Region	NW	NE	SW	SE
Mean	12.55	18.90	23.10	27.45

Now, we begin by testing the null hypothesis that the distribution of serum cholesterol levels is the same in the Northwest (the lowest mean) as in the Southeast (the highest mean). Using Equation (11.4), we get

$$Q = \frac{(\overline{Y}_{\text{rank}_{\text{NW}}} - \overline{Y}_{\text{rank}_{\text{SE}}}) - (\mu_{\text{rank}_{\text{NW}}} - \mu_{\text{rank}_{\text{SE}}})}{\sqrt{\text{TMS}/n_{\text{NW}} + \text{TMS}/n_{\text{SE}}}}$$

$$= \frac{(12.55 - 27.45) - 0}{\sqrt{[(5{,}318/39)/10] + [(5{,}318/39)/10]}} = -2.853$$

Next, we compare this calculated value (its absolute value) with a value from Table B.10 that corresponds to an α of 0.05 and k equal to four since there are two groups (NE and SW) between the Northwest and the Southeast.

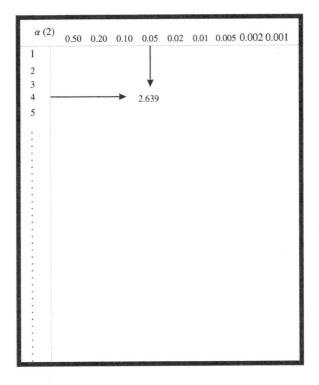

Our calculated value (-2.853) is larger (in absolute value) than the value from Table B.10 (2.639), which corresponds to an α of 0.05 and k equal to 4. Thus, we can reject the null hypothesis that the distribution of serum cholesterol levels among persons from the Northwest is the same as the distribution of serum cholesterol levels among persons from the Southeast.

Also, rejection of this null hypothesis permits us to make comparisons between groups in which the mean ranks are not as far apart as Northwest and Southeast. The groups that we can compare now are the Northwest with the Southwest and the Northeast with the Southeast. First, let us test the null hypothesis that the distribution of serum cholesterol levels in the Northwest is the same as the distribution in the Southwest.[10] Using Equation (11.4), we get

$$Q = \frac{(\overline{Y}_{\text{rank}_{NW}} - \overline{Y}_{\text{rank}_{SW}}) - (\mu_{\text{rank}_{NW}} - \mu_{\text{rank}_{SW}})}{\sqrt{\text{TMS}/n_{NW} + \text{TMS}/n_{SW}}}$$

$$= \frac{(12.55 - 23.10) - 0}{\sqrt{[(5,318/39)/10] + [(5,318/39)/10]}} = -2.020$$

We compare this calculated value with a value from Table B.10. In this case, k is equal to 3, since there is only one group between the two being compared. This tabled value is equal to 2.394. Since our calculated value (-2.020) is less (in absolute value) than the value from Table B.10 (2.394), we fail to reject the null hypothesis that the distribution of serum cholesterol levels among persons from the Northwest is the same as the distribution of serum cholesterol levels among persons from the Southwest. Following the protocol for comparing groups, this also implies that we fail to reject null hypotheses for any pairs of groups bracketed by the ones we just compared. Specifically, we fail to reject the null hypothesis that the distribution of serum cholesterol levels among persons from the Northwest is the same as the distribution of serum cholesterol levels among persons from the Northeast and we fail to reject the null hypothesis that the distribution of serum cholesterol levels among persons from the Northeast is the same as the distribution of serum cholesterol levels among persons from the Southwest. A convenient way to keep track of these results is to underline the groups that are not statistically different. Thus, the results so far are

Region	NW	NE	SW	SE
Mean	12.55	18.90	23.10	27.45

Even though we failed to reject the null hypothesis that the distribution of serum cholesterol levels among persons from the Northwest is the same as the distribution of serum cholesterol levels among persons from the Southwest, we are still able to compare the Northeast with the Southeast, since they are not connected by the line we just drew. Using Equation (11.4), we get

$$Q = \frac{(\overline{Y}_{\text{rank}_{NE}} - \overline{Y}_{\text{rank}_{SE}}) - (\mu_{\text{rank}_{NE}} - \mu_{\text{rank}_{SE}})}{\sqrt{\text{TMS}/n_{NE} + \text{TMS}/n_{SE}}}$$

$$= \frac{(18.90 - 27.45) - 0}{\sqrt{[(5,318/39)/10] + [(5,318/39)/10]}} = -1.637$$

[10]Which of the two pairs of means we compare first is arbitrary, since both comparisons can be made regardless of the result from either comparison.

Since there is one group between the two we just compared, we compare the absolute value of our calculated value (-1.637) with 2.639. This absolute value is less than the value from Table B.10, so we fail to reject the null hypothesis that the distribution of serum cholesterol levels among persons from the Northeast is the same as the distribution of serum cholesterol levels among persons from the Southeast. Following the protocol, this implies that we also fail to reject the null hypothesis that the distribution of serum cholesterol levels among persons from the Northeast is the same as the distribution of serum cholesterol levels among persons from the Southwest and the null hypothesis that the distribution of serum cholesterol levels among persons from the Southwest is the same as the distribution of serum cholesterol levels among persons from the Southeast. To illustrate this result, we add a second line to the list of mean ranks.

Region	NW	NE	SW	SE
Mean	12.55	18.90	23.10	27.45

We interpret this table by saying that any groups connected by a line are not statistically different from each other. In other words, the only statistical difference we observed is between the Northwest and the Southeast.

Dunn's test can also be performed in Excel using the BAHR program "Nonparametric Analyses." The following is the output we get when analyzing these data.

		Dunn's test				
	NW	NE	SW	SE		
	12.55	18.9	23.1	27.45		
$k = 4$		NW	vs	SE		$Q = -2.85318$
$k = 3$		NW	vs	SW		$Q = -2.02021$
		NE	vs	SE		$Q = -1.63723$
$k = 2$		NW	vs	NE		$Q = -1.21595$
		NE	vs	SW		$Q = -0.80425$
		SW	vs	SE		$Q = -0.83298$

Those results agree with what we calculated by hand.

In the next chapter, we will look at methods for a nominal dependent variable when there is more than one independent variable.

CHAPTER SUMMARY

When we have an ordinal dependent variable, we can examine that variable relative to more than one nominal independent variables. Statistical procedures for an ordinal dependent variable and more than one nominal independent variable are very similar in operation and interpretation to procedures for continuous dependent variables. A parallel procedure to a one-way ANOVA is the Kruskal–Wallis test. The test statistic for the Kruskal–Wallis test (H) is calculated from the between sum of squares and total mean square when ANOVA procedures are performed on ranks. Kruskal–Wallis test statistics calculated from a sample's observations can be compared to values in Table B.9 to test the omnibus null hypothesis. This is parallel to the F-ratio test in ANOVA. If the numbers of observations in each group are greater than the values in Table B.9, the Kruskal–Wallis test statistic can be considered to be a chi-square value with degrees of freedom equal to the number of groups minus one and compared to values in Table B.7.

When the dependent variable is continuous, we usually use a procedure such as the Student–Newman–Keuls test to compare two groups of values of the dependent variable. When the dependent variable is ordinal, we use a parallel procedure that we call Dunn's test. Dunn's test is very much like the Student–Newman–Keuls test except that the means of the ranks of the dependent variable values are compared rather than the means of the values of the dependent variable values themselves. The test statistic in Dunn's procedure is compared to values in Table B.10 to test the null hypothesis that the difference is equal to 0 in the population from which the sample was drawn.

To perform an analysis that is parallel to factorial ANOVA for continuous dependent variables on ordinal dependent variables, we take advantage of the fact that the Kruskal--Wallis test statistic can be calculated by dividing the between sum of squares for the ranks of values of the dependent variable by the total mean square for those ranks.

When we have more than one factor among the independent variables, we can partition the between sum of squares for the ranks in the same way that we partitioned the between sum of squares in factorial ANOVA. Null hypotheses that the means of the ranks of the categories within each factor are equal or that there is no interaction between factors in the population can be tested by dividing the appropriate partition of the between sum of squares by the total mean square and comparing the resulting test statistic to the values in Table B.9 or, for larger samples, Table B.7.

Following the Kruskal–Wallis test, we can use Dunn's test to discover which groups are significantly different from the others. Dunn's test compares the means of the ranks in each group by calculating Q statistics that are compared to values in Table B.10.

EXERCISES

11.1. In a study of clinical depression, patients were randomly assigned to one of four drug groups (three active drugs and a placebo) and to cognitive therapy (versus no therapy). The dependent variable is a difference between scores on a depression questionnaire. The results are in the Excel file: EXR10_5 on the website accompanying this textbook. Based on those data, test the null hypothesis of no interaction between drug and therapy versus the alternative hypothesis that there is interaction without assuming a Gaussian sampling distribution. Allowing a 5% chance of making a type I error, which of the following is the best conclusion to draw?

A. Reject both the null and alternative hypotheses

B. Accept both the null and alternative hypotheses

C. Reject the null hypothesis and accept the alternative hypothesis

D. Accept the null hypothesis and reject the alternative hypothesis

E. It is best not to draw a conclusion about the null and alternative hypotheses from these observations

11.2. In a multicenter study of a new treatment for hypertension, patients at nine centers were randomly assigned to a new treatment or standard treatment. The dependent variable is a difference in diastolic blood pressure from a pre-treatment value. The results are in the Excel file: EXR10_6 on the website accompanying this textbook. Based on those data, test the null hypothesis of no interaction between drug and center versus the alternative hypothesis that there is interaction without assuming a Gaussian sampling distribution. Allowing a 5% chance of making a type I error, which of the following is the best conclusion to draw?

A. Reject both the null and alternative hypotheses

B. Accept both the null and alternative hypotheses

C. Reject the null hypothesis and accept the alternative hypothesis

D. Accept the null hypothesis and reject the alternative hypothesis

E. It is best not to draw a conclusion about the null and alternative hypotheses from these observations

11.3. In a study of clinical depression, patients were randomly assigned to one of four drug groups (three active drugs and a placebo) and to cognitive therapy (versus no therapy). The dependent variable is a difference between scores on a depression questionnaire. The results are in the Excel file: EXR10_5 on the website accompanying this textbook. Based on those data, test the null hypothesis of no differences between drug groups versus the alternative hypothesis that there is a difference, ignoring the possibility of an interaction and not assuming a Gaussian sampling distribution. Allowing a 5% chance of making a type I error, which of the following is the best conclusion to draw?

A. Reject both the null and alternative hypotheses

B. Accept both the null and alternative hypotheses

C. Reject the null hypothesis and accept the alternative hypothesis

D. Accept the null hypothesis and reject the alternative hypothesis

E. It is best not to draw a conclusion about the null and alternative hypotheses from these observations

11.4. In a multicenter study of a new treatment for hypertension, patients at nine centers were randomly assigned to a new treatment or standard treatment. The dependent variable is a difference in diastolic blood pressure from a pre-treatment value. The results are in the Excel file: EXR10_6 on the website accompanying this textbook. Based on those data, test the null hypothesis of no difference between drugs versus the alternative hypothesis that there is a difference, ignoring the possibility of an interaction and not assuming a Gaussian sampling distribution. If you allow a 5% chance of making a type I error, which of the following is the best conclusion to draw?

A. Reject both the null and alternative hypotheses

B. Accept both the null and alternative hypotheses

C. Reject the null hypothesis and accept the alternative hypothesis

D. Accept the null hypothesis and reject the alternative hypothesis

E. It is best not to draw a conclusion about the null and alternative hypotheses from these observations

11.5. In a study of clinical depression, patients were randomly assigned to one of four drug groups (three active drugs and a placebo) and to cognitive therapy (versus no therapy). The dependent variable is a difference between scores on a depression questionnaire. The results are in the Excel file: EXR10_5 on the website accompanying this textbook. Based on those data, test the null hypothesis of no differences between therapy groups versus the alternative hypothesis that there is a difference, ignoring the possibility of an interaction and not assuming a Gaussian sampling distribution. Allowing a 5% chance of making a type I error, which of the following is the best conclusion to draw?

A. Reject both the null and alternative hypotheses

B. Accept both the null and alternative hypotheses

C. Reject the null hypothesis and accept the alternative hypothesis

D. Accept the null hypothesis and reject the alternative hypothesis

E. It is best not to draw a conclusion about the null and alternative hypotheses from these observations

11.6. In a multicenter study of a new treatment for hypertension, patients at nine centers were randomly assigned to a new treatment or standard treatment. The dependent variable is a difference in diastolic blood pressure from a pretreatment value. The results are in the Excel file: EXR10_6 on the website accompanying this textbook. Based on those data, test the null hypothesis of no difference among centers in the population versus the alternative hypothesis that there is a difference, ignoring the possibility of an interaction and not assuming a Gaussian sampling distribution. If you allow a 5% chance of making a type I error, which of the following is the best conclusion to draw?

   A. Reject both the null and alternative hypotheses
   B. Accept both the null and alternative hypotheses
   C. Reject the null hypothesis and accept the alternative hypothesis
   D. Accept the null hypothesis and reject the alternative hypothesis
   E. It is best not to draw a conclusion about the null and alternative hypotheses from these observations

CHAPTER 12

MULTIVARIABLE ANALYSIS OF A NOMINAL DEPENDENT VARIABLE

In clinical and epidemiologic research, nominal dependent variables are often used to represent the outcome of interest. Thus, chapters of this book that address nominal dependent variables are of particular interest to clinicians and epidemiologists. Also, research that involves human subjects, by necessity, entails control for extraneous characteristics as part of data analysis. Both of these requirements are addressed in this chapter, which discusses multivariable analysis of nominal dependent variables.

Introduction to Biostatistical Applications in Health Research with Microsoft Office Excel® and R,
Second Edition. Robert P. Hirsch.
© 2021 John Wiley & Sons, Inc. Published 2021 by John Wiley & Sons, Inc.
Companion website: www.wiley.com/go/hirsch/healthresearch2e

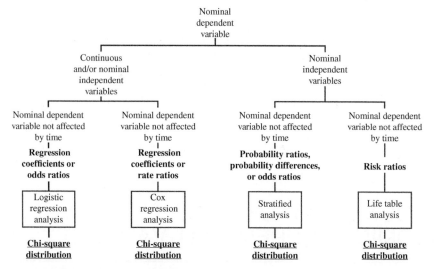

FLOWCHART 1   Flowchart showing multivariable analysis of a nominal dependent variable. The point estimate that is most often used to describe the dependent variable is in bold. The common name of the statistical test is enclosed in a box. The standard distribution that is used to test hypotheses and calculate confidence intervals is in bold and underlined.

Flowchart 10 outlines the methods that are most commonly used to analyze multivariable data sets with nominal dependent variables. They are divided into two groups. The first of these groups includes two types of regression analysis. They can be used regardless of the type of data (either continuous or nominal) represented by the independent variables.[1] Thus, these methods are broadly applicable. Their disadvantage is that they involve calculations so complex that it is virtually impossible to do them by hand. This is not an issue when we are using a computer to analyze these data, but it does make it a "black box" for which the process is difficult to visualize.

The methods in the second group are not as broadly applicable, since they are restricted to nominal independent variables (or continuous independent variables converted to a nominal scale). Their advantage, however, is that they can be done by hand, making it easier to understand how they work. As a result, they play an important role in analysis of health research data, even though the same data can be analyzed using regression analyses.

---

[1] In Chapter 10, we learned how to include nominal independent variables in regression equations by using indicator variables and interactions. This led us to the principle of the "general linear model," which asserts that all methods of analyzing continuous dependent variables can be represented as regression equations. The same is approximately true for nominal dependent variables, but since the methods for nominal dependent variables are not identical, we refer to them with the principle of the "generalized" linear model.

12.1 CONTINUOUS AND/OR NOMINAL INDEPENDENT VARIABLES

12.1.1 Maximum Likelihood Estimation

The reason why multivariable regression analysis for nominal dependent variables presents a challenge is that it uses a method of estimation that is substantially different from anything we have discussed so far. All other analyses that we have considered are based on what is called the method of "**least squares**." As described in Chapter 7, the goal of the method of least squares is to select estimates that minimize the squared differences between observed and estimated values of the dependent variable (Equation (7.3)). Thus, it is a mathematic representation of the method we would use to draw a line to fit a set of points in a scatter plot. Specifically, we draw the line to minimize the difference between the points (that represent the observed values) and the line (that represents the estimated values). The mathematical representation of this process results in formulae we can use to estimate means, slopes, regression coefficients, correlation coefficients, probabilities, rates, and all of the other estimates we have encountered so far.

The method of least squares could be used to estimate regression coefficients for multivariable analysis of nominal dependent variables as well, but, when there is a least one continuous independent variable, these estimates do not come as close to the true values (i.e., the values in the population) as do estimates based on the method of **maximum likelihood**. In maximum likelihood estimation, estimates are selected to maximize the likelihood (i.e., the conditional probability) of observing the sample's data if the population's regression coefficients were equal to the sample's estimates. This probability is illustrated in Equation (12.1):

$$p(\text{sample's data} \mid \beta = b) \tag{12.1}$$

where

β = population's regression coefficient(s)
b = sample's estimate(s) of regression coefficient(s)

So, the idea with the method of maximum likelihood is to select estimates that maximize the probability of getting a sample like the one we got, assuming that the sample's estimates are, in fact, equal to the population's parameters. This is an iterative process that involves making guesses about the value of the population's parameter and comparing the likelihood of each guess until the one with the highest likelihood is found. As a simple example, suppose that we have a sample of 10 persons, 2 of whom have a particular disease. From that sample, we want to estimate the prevalence of the disease in the population. The first step in the method of maximum likelihood is to make a guess about the prevalence. Some guesses for this sample are in the first column of Table 12.1. Then, the likelihood of obtaining

TABLE 12.1. Likelihood of Observing 2 out of 10 Persons with a Particular Disease if the Prevalence of the Disease is Equal to the Estimate

Guess	Likelihood
0.1	0.194
0.2	0.302
0.3	0.233
0.4	0.121
0.5	0.044
0.6	0.011
0.7	0.001
0.8	<0.001
0.9	<0.001

the sample for each guess is calculated. The likelihoods for this example are in the second column of Table 12.1.[2]

Finally, the maximum likelihood estimate of the prevalence is selected as the guess with the highest likelihood. Since the estimate of 0.2 has the highest likelihood (0.302) in Table 12.1, it is the maximum likelihood estimate of the prevalence.[3]

If you think this sounds like a lot of work, you are right! It is much easier to use Equation (12.2) as we did in Chapter 6 (Equation (6.3)).

$$\text{Prevalence} = \frac{\text{number of persons with the disease at time } t}{\text{total number of persons}} = \frac{2}{10} = 0.2 \quad (12.2)$$

Using a formula to calculate an estimate gives us the least squares estimate. In this example, the maximum likelihood estimate and the least squares estimate are equal to the same value. When we have a nominal dependent variable and there are no continuous independent variables, maximum likelihood estimates are equal to the same value as least squares estimates. In that case, using the formula makes sense. When the dependent variable is nominal and at least one independent variable is continuous, however, the two methods do not result in the same estimate. Further, the maximum likelihood estimate is the better estimate in that situation. Then, it makes sense to use the method of maximum likelihood, as long as we have a computer to make the guesses and search for the one with the highest likelihood of producing the sample's observations.

To interpret the results of analyses that use the method of maximum likelihood (like the regression analyses that appear in the Flowchart 10), understanding the difference between least squares and maximum likelihood estimation prepares us to encounter new types of information when interpreting the results of these analyses.

---

[2]These likelihoods were calculated using the binomial distribution.
[3]This is the maximum likelihood estimate to the nearest 10th. In practice, we would make more guesses with smaller differences between them, to see if a higher likelihood could be obtained.

In regression analyses that use least squares estimates (like those described in Chapters 7 and 10), we compare mean squares representing the explained and unexplained variation in dependent variable values in an F-ratio. In analyses that use maximum likelihood estimates, we compare likelihoods for full (including all of the independent variables) and reduced (excluding at least one of the independent variables) models in a **likelihood ratio** (Equation (12.3)):

$$\text{LR} = \frac{p(\text{sample's data} \mid \beta = b) \text{ for reduced model}}{p(\text{sample's data} \mid \beta = b) \text{ for full model}} \tag{12.3}$$

where

LR = likelihood ratio

Before we interpret a likelihood ratio, it is changed into a chi-square value with the number of degrees of freedom equal to the difference in the number of independent variables between the full and reduced models. Equation (12.4) shows that conversion.

$$\chi^2 = -2 \cdot \ln(\text{LR}) \tag{12.4}$$

We will see an example in which we interpret these chi-square values, but first let us take a closer look at one type of regression analysis for a nominal dependent variable.

12.1.2   Logistic Regression Analysis

In Chapter 9, we looked at a regression analysis for a nominal dependent variable called a test for trend (Equation (9.1)). This regression analysis uses a straight line to estimate the probability of an event based on a value of a continuous independent variable (Figure 9.1). One problem with using a straight line to

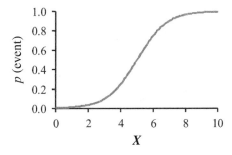

Figure 12.1   Sigmoid curve used to represent the relationship between a nominal dependent variable and a continuous independent variable. The sigmoid curve prevents estimates of the probability of an event from being less than 0 or greater than 1.

estimate probabilities is that a straight line continues forever, theoretically extending from $-\infty$ to $+\infty$. Probabilities, on the other hand, are restricted to the interval between 0 and 1. A solution to this problem is to use a curve, instead of a straight line, to estimate probabilities. One such curve is a **sigmoid curve** (Figure 12.1). This curve approaches, but never quite reaches 0 or 1.

A convenient way to create a sigmoid curve is by using a **transformation**. A transformation is a mathematical change in the dependent variable or an estimate.

In clinical and epidemiologic research, the most common transformation used to create a sigmoid curve is the **logit transformation**. A regression equation that uses the logit transformation is called a **logistic regression**.

In the logit transformation, we divide the probability of the event by its complement and take the natural logarithm of that fraction. Equation (12.5) illustrates a regression equation that uses the logit transformation:

$$\ln \frac{\theta}{1 - \theta} = \alpha + (\beta_1 \cdot X_1) + (\beta_2 \cdot X_2) + \cdots + (\beta_k \cdot X_k) \qquad (12.5)$$

where

$\ln$ = natural log scale (base e)

θ = probability of the event represented by the nominal dependent variable in the population

α = intercept of the regression equation in the population

β_i = regression coefficient for the ith (out of k) independent variable in the population

X_i = value of the ith (out of k) independent variable

When we use a transformation for the dependent variable, we perform all of the analyses on the transformed scale, and then we change the results of the analyses back to the original scale for interpretation. Equation (12.6) illustrates how we can change the logistic regression equation back to its original scale:

$$\theta \triangleq p = \frac{1}{1 + e^{-[a + (b_1 \cdot X_1) + (b_2 \cdot X_2 +) \cdots + (b_k \cdot X_k)]}} \qquad (12.6)$$

where

θ = probability of the event represented by the nominal dependent variable in the population

p = sample's estimate of the probability of the event represented by the nominal dependent variable

e = base of the natural log scale

a = sample's estimate of the intercept of the regression equation

b_i = sample's estimate of the regression coefficient for the ith (out of k) independent variable

X_i = value of the ith (out of k) independent variable

In logistic regression analysis, we usually change the log scale back to a linear scale, but we leave the probability of the event divided by its complement. This fraction is really the odds of the event, as shown algebraically in Equation (12.7)[4]:

$$\frac{\theta}{1-\theta} \triangleq \frac{p}{1-p} = \frac{\text{events}/\text{observations}}{1 - \text{events}/\text{observations}}$$

$$= \frac{\text{events}/\text{observations}}{\text{observations}/\text{observations} - \text{events}/\text{observations}}$$

$$= \frac{\text{events}}{\text{observations} - \text{events}} = \frac{\text{events}}{\text{nonevents}} = \text{odds} \qquad (12.7)$$

The advantage of leaving the dependent variable as the odds of the event is that the antilog[5] of each regression coefficient can be interpreted as an odds ratio comparing a one-unit difference in the value of that independent variable.[6] This is illustrated algebraically in Equation (12.8):

$$\text{OR} = \frac{e^{\ln\frac{\theta}{1-\theta}}}{e^{\ln\frac{\theta}{1-\theta}}} = \frac{e^{\alpha+(\beta_1 \cdot [X_1+1])+(\beta_2 \cdot X_2)+\cdots+(\beta_k \cdot X_k)}}{e^{\alpha+(\beta_1 \cdot X_1)+(\beta_2 \cdot X_2)+\cdots+(\beta_k \cdot X_k)}} = \frac{e^\alpha \cdot e^{\beta_1 \cdot [X_1+1]} \cdot e^{\beta_2 \cdot X_2} \cdot \ \cdots \ \cdot e^{\beta_k \cdot X_k}}{e^\alpha \cdot e^{\beta_1 \cdot X_1} \cdot e^{\beta_2 \cdot X_2} \cdot \ \cdots \ \cdot e^{\beta_k \cdot X_k}}$$

$$= \frac{e^{\beta_1 \cdot [X_1+1]}}{e^{\beta_1 \cdot X_1}} = e^{\beta_1} \triangleq \widehat{\text{OR}} = e^{b_1} \qquad (12.8)$$

In Excel, we can use the "Logistic Regression" BAHR program, provided with this book, to perform logistic regression analysis. In the next example, we will see output from this procedure and learn how to interpret it.[7] In R, we use the "glm()" command.[8] In that command, we get a logistic by specifying that the family of distributions to use is the binomial distribution. Logistic regression in Excel and R is illustrated in the next example.

---

[4] Compare with Equation (9.7).

[5] An antilog is found by taking the number as the power of the base of the logarithmic scale. For the natural log scale, that means taking the number as a power of e.

[6] We could also undo the odds part of the logit transformation to interpret regression coefficients as estimators of the probability ratio of the event, but these estimates require that a value be assigned to each independent variable, rather than to use only one independent variable at a time.

[7] To run the "Logistic Regression" program you must enable the "Solver" add-in. See the preface to the first edition to see how to do this.

[8] "glm" stands for generalized linear model.

■ EXAMPLE 12.1

In Examples 9.1 through 9.4, we considered data from a study in which we were interested in the probability that an infection is cured at different doses of an antibiotic. In this study, we randomly assigned 70 persons to 1 of 7 doses of the antibiotic. Suppose that we obtained the following data:

Dose (X)	Number Observed (n)	Number Cured (a)
1	10	1
5	10	4
10	10	3
15	10	7
20	10	6
25	10	8
30	10	9

This is a bivariable data set (since there is only one independent variable), but we can use it to see how to interpret the results of logistic regression analysis.

If we were to analyze these data using the "Logistic Regression"[9] BAHR program in Excel, we would obtain the following output:

Logistic Regression				
Omnibus H0	Log Lkhd	Chi Sq	DF	P-value
Intercept only	−48.2628			
Full model	−38.7552	19.01534	1	1.3E-05
Variable	Estimate	SE	Chi Sq	DF	P-value
Intercept	−1.61609	0.530615	10.99589	1	0.000913
Dose	0.1223	0.032039	19.01534	1	1.3E-05

As in linear and multiple regression analyses for a continuous dependent variable, logistic regression considers two kinds of hypotheses. One kind addresses all of the independent variables taken as a group. This is the test of the omnibus null hypothesis: that the entire collection of independent variables does not help estimate values of the dependent variable. The chi-square is based on the likelihood ratio that compares the full model (including all of the independent variables) with the reduced

---

[9]The BAHR collection of programs is on the companion website.

model (including none of the independent variables). Since this P-value is less than 0.05, we can reject the omnibus null hypothesis. The other kind of null hypothesis, in linear and multiple regression, considers the relationship between the dependent variable, and one independent variable while controlling for all of the other independent variables. Specifically, this null hypothesis states that the regression coefficient for the corresponding independent variable is equal to 0 in the population. P-values for these hypothesis tests are in the second table. In this case, there is only one independent variable and it has a P-value less than 0.05, so we reject this null hypothesis.

Estimates in logistic regression analysis include an intercept and a regression coefficient for each independent variable. They are listed in the same table as the P-values for the individual independent variables. Here, the estimate of the intercept is -1.61609 and the regression coefficient for Dose is 0.1223. Thus, the logistic regression equation is

$$\ln \frac{\theta}{1-\theta} \triangleq \ln \frac{p}{1-p} = a + (b \cdot \text{Dose}) = -1.61609 + (0.1223 \cdot \text{Dose})$$

Now, let us take look at the use of the "glm()" command in R to perform a logistic regression analysis of these data. These data exist in a data set called Example 9_3. We use "binomial" as the family of distributions to invoke the logistic regression.

>summary(glm(Indicator~Dose,data=Example9_3,family="binomial"))

```
Call:
glm(formula = Indicator ~ Dose, family = "binomial", data = Example9_3)

Deviance Residuals:
    Min       1Q   Median       3Q      Max
-2.0850  -0.7900   0.4914   0.8508   1.8419

Coefficients:
            Estimate Std. Error z value Pr(>|z|)
(Intercept) -1.61612    0.53062  -3.046 0.002321 **
Dose         0.12230    0.03204   3.817 0.000135 ***
---
Signif. codes:  0 '***' 0.001 '**' 0.01 '*' 0.05 '.' 0.1 ' ' 1

(Dispersion parameter for binomial family taken to be 1)

    Null deviance: 96.526  on 69  degrees of freedom
Residual deviance: 77.510  on 68  degrees of freedom
AIC: 81.51

Number of Fisher Scoring iterations: 4
```

Much of the information in that output we will not use. Instead, we focus on the table headed with "Coefficients." Here, we find the estimates of the intercept and slope as well as tests of the null hypotheses that these are equal to 0 in the population. The results are the same as those obtained from Excel. In R, the hypothesis tests use a z-value instead of a chi-square. These z-values are obtained using a different method from the method used by Excel to obtain the chi-square values[10].

One way to interpret the result of logistic regression analysis is to use the regression coefficient as an exponent of e (base of natural logarithms). As shown in Equation (12.8), this gives us an estimate of the odds ratio for a one-unit change in the independent variable. In this analysis, the odds ratio estimate is equal to 1.130.   ■

The odds ratio in Example 12.1 (1.130) is very close to one, suggesting that the odds of being cured does not change much as the dose changes. This odds ratio, however, is for a one-unit change in the independent variable. For continuous independent variables, odds ratios with intervals of change other than one separating the numerator and denominator make more sense. Equation (12.9) illustrates how odds ratios for other intervals of values of a continuous independent variable can be calculated[11]:

$$OR_\Delta = \frac{e^{\alpha+(\beta_1\cdot[X_1+\Delta])+(\beta_2\cdot X_2)+\cdots+(\beta_k\cdot X_k)}}{e^{\alpha+(\beta_1\cdot X_1)+(\beta_2\cdot X_2)+\cdots+(\beta_k\cdot X_k)}} = \frac{e^{\beta_1\cdot[X_1+\Delta]}}{e^{\beta_1\cdot X_1}} = e^{\beta_1\cdot\Delta} \triangleq e^{b_1\cdot\Delta} \qquad (12.9)$$

where

Δ = interval of independent variable values compared in an odds ratio

The choice of the interval can be somewhat arbitrary. When an interval is not suggested by the study's design or the nature of the event, an interval equal to about $\frac{1}{4}$ of the range[12] of values included in the sample is commonly used. In the next example, we will calculate an odds ratio for a larger interval of values for Dose.

■ EXAMPLE 12.2

In Example 12.1, we estimated an odds ratio of 1.130 for change in odds of cure for a one-unit (i.e., 1 mg) increase in the dose of a medication. Let us calculate an odds ratio for a larger change in dose.

In this study, doses were assigned in 5 mg increments, so it makes sense to calculate an odds ratio for that same 5 mg difference. To calculate this odds ratio, we use Equation (12.9):

$$OR_{\Delta=5} \triangleq e^{b_1\cdot\Delta} = e^{0.1223\cdot5} = e^{0.6115} = 1.843$$

[10]Excel calculates the chi-square values from the likelihood ratio. R calculates the z-values from the coefficients and the standard errors. Those two methods result in slightly different P-values.

[11]An equivalent way to do this is by taking the odds ratio for a one-unit change in a continuous independent variable to the Δth power (OR^Δ).

[12]In other words, the interval is equal to one quartile.

This odds ratio (1.843) gives us a different impression about how the odds of cure changes as dose is changed. It implies that the odds of cure almost doubles when the dose is increased by 5 mg.   ■

If the independent variable is a zero/one indicator variable, the antilog of its regression coefficient (i.e., e^b) is equal to the odds ratio comparing persons with the characteristic (i.e., when the indicator variable is equal to 1) with persons without the characteristic (i.e., when the indicator variable is equal to 0). Thus, we use Equation (12.8). For $-1/+1$ indicator variables (see Tables 10.4 and 10.5), this same odds ratio is calculated by taking the antilog of two times the regression coefficient (Equation (12.10)):

$$OR = \frac{e^{\alpha+(\beta_1\cdot+1)+(\beta_2\cdot X_2)+\cdots+(\beta_k\cdot X_k)}}{e^{\alpha+(\beta_1\cdot-1)+(\beta_2\cdot X_2)+\cdots+(\beta_k\cdot X_k)}} = \frac{e^{\beta_1\cdot+1}}{e^{\beta_1\cdot-1}} = e^{\beta_1\cdot2} \triangleq e^{b_1\cdot2} \qquad (12.10)$$

The next example illustrates the output from the "Logistic Regression" BAHR program when we add a nominal independent variable represented as a -1, $+1$ indicator variable.

■ EXAMPLE 12.3

In Example 12.1, we analyzed data from a study in which we randomly assigned 70 persons to 1 of 7 doses of an antibiotic. In that analysis, we were interested in the probability that an infection was cured for different doses of the antibiotic. Now, suppose that we are also interested in the relationship between the probability of cure and gender, so we randomize an equal number of men and women to each of the doses of the antibiotic. When we analyze these data using the "Logistic Regression" BAHR program, we obtain the following output:

Logistic Regression				
Omnibus HO	Log Lkhd	Chi Sq	DF	P-Value
Intercept only	−48.2628			
Full model	−33.6512	29.2232	1	4.51E-07
Variable	Estimate	SE	Chi Sq	DF	P-Value
Intercept	−1.88771	0.544086	12.03752	1	0.000521
Dose	0.141493	0.036973	20.7562	1	5.22E-06
Sex	0.957478	0.326296	10.20786	1	0.001398

This data set consists of a nominal dependent variable (CURE) and two independent variables: DOSE (a continuous independent variable) and GENDER (a nominal independent variable). The nominal independent is represented by an indicator variable (SEX) that has been assigned a value of +1 to women and −1 to men.

The results of testing the omnibus hypothesis (i.e., that the combination of dose and gender do not help estimate the probability of cure) appear in the first table. This omnibus null hypothesis is rejected, since the P-value is less than 0.05.

The relationships between each of the independent variables and the probability of cure (controlling for the other independent variable) are in the second table. This table lists the estimates of the intercept and each of the regression coefficients in the leftmost column. From that information, we know that the logistic regression equation is

$$\ln \frac{p}{1-p} = -1.88771 + (0.141493 \cdot \text{Dose}) + (0.957478 \cdot \text{Sex})$$

The same table lists (in the rightmost column) the P-values for tests of the null hypothesis that the corresponding parameter (listed in the leftmost column) is equal to 0 in the population. We are able to reject this null hypothesis for the regression coefficients for both gender ($P = 0.00000522$) and dose ($P = 0.001398$).

To interpret these regression coefficients, we usually calculate an odds ratio. Since the indicator variable is equal to −1 or +1, we need to use Equation (12.10) to calculate its corresponding odds ratio.

$$\text{OR} = \frac{e^{\alpha+(\beta_1\cdot+1)+(\beta_2\cdot X_2)+\ldots+(\beta_k\cdot X_k)}}{e^{\alpha+(\beta_1\cdot-1)+(\beta_2\cdot X_2)+\ldots+(\beta_k\cdot X_k)}} = \frac{e^{\beta_1\cdot+1}}{e^{\beta_1\cdot-1}} = e^{\beta_1\cdot 2} \triangleq e^{0.9574178\cdot 2} = 6.787$$

This odds ratio compares the odds of being cured for women with the odds of being cured for men.[13] The odds ratio of 6.787 tells us that women have more than six times the odds of being cured compared to men, when controlling for DOSE.   ■

In Example 12.3, we included an indicator variable in a logistic regression analysis. In the next example, we will include an interaction between dose and gender. By including an interaction, we imply that we are interested in determining if the relationship between dose and the odds of cure is different for the two genders.[14] If this is the case, we need to calculate separate odds ratios for men and women. Equation (12.11) shows how to calculate an odds ratio when the independent variable is included in an interaction:

---

[13] See Tables 10.4 and 10.5 to recall how we interpret a plus +1/−1 indicator variable.
[14] Equivalently, if there is an interaction, an odds ratio comparing the two genders will be different according to the dose of the antibiotic.

$$OR_\Delta = \frac{e^{\ln \frac{\theta}{1-\theta}}}{e^{\ln \frac{\theta}{1-\theta}}} = \frac{e^{\alpha+(\beta_1 \cdot [X_1+\Delta])+(\beta_2 \cdot X_2)+(\beta_3 \cdot [X_1+\Delta] \cdot X_2)}}{e^{\alpha+(\beta_1 \cdot X_1)+(\beta_2 \cdot X_2)+(\beta_3 \cdot X_1 \cdot X_2)}}$$

$$= \frac{\cancel{e^\alpha} \cdot e^{\beta_1 \cdot [X_1+\Delta]} \cdot \cancel{e^{\beta_2 \cdot X_2}} \cdot e^{\beta_3 \cdot [X_1+\Delta] \cdot X_2}}{\cancel{e^\alpha} \cdot e^{\beta_1 \cdot X_1} \cdot \cancel{e^{\beta_2 \cdot X_2}} \cdot e^{\beta_3 \cdot X_1 \cdot X_2}}$$

$$= e^{(\beta_1 \cdot \Delta)+(\beta_3 \cdot \Delta \cdot X_2)} \triangleq \widehat{OR}_\Delta = e^{(b_1 \cdot \Delta)+(b_3 \cdot \Delta \cdot X_2)} \qquad (12.11)$$

where

OR_Δ = population's odds ratio comparing two values of X_1 that differ by Δ

θ = probability of the event represented by the nominal dependent variable in the population

α = intercept of the logistic regression equation in the population

β_1, β_2 = regression coefficients for X_1 and X_2 in the population

β_3 = regression coefficient for the interaction between X_1 and X_2 in the population

Δ = difference in values of X_1 compared in the odds ratio

b_1 = sample's estimate of the regression coefficient for X_1

$\widehat{OR}_\Delta$ = sample's estimate of the odds ratio comparing two values of X_1

b_3 = sample's estimate of the regression coefficient for the interaction between X_1 and X_2

X_2 = value of X_2 for which the difference in values of X_1 are compared in the odds ratio

The next example demonstrates how we can calculate an estimate for an odds ratio when the logistic regression equation includes an interaction.

■ EXAMPLE 12.4

In Example 12.3, we created an indicator variable for gender. Now, we will add an interaction between gender and dose to obtain the following output:

Logistic regression				
Omnibus H0	Log Lkhd	Chi Sq	DF	P-value
Intercept only	−48.2628			
Full model	−31.2859	33.9538	1	5.64E-09
Variable	Estimate	SE	Chi Sq	DF	P-value
Intercept	−1.87637	0.60195	9.71569	1	0.001827
Dose	0.14449	0.03819	14.3187	1	0.000154
Sex	0.74495	0.60195	1.53264	1	0.215717
Dose*Sex	0.01566	0.03819	0.1681	1	0.681806

In the second table, we can see that the interaction between dose and gender occurs in the list of variables. Now, the logistic regression equation is

$$\ln \frac{p}{1-p} = -1.87637 + (0.14449 \cdot \text{Dose}) + (0.74495 \cdot \text{Sex})$$
$$+ (0.01566 \cdot \text{Dose} \cdot \text{Sex})$$

We interpret the interaction in this logistic regression equation just as we did in analysis of covariance (Chapter 10). Namely, the interaction tells us about the difference in slopes between the two genders. For men, the logistic regression equation is

$$\ln \frac{p}{1-p} = -1.87637 + (0.14449 \cdot \text{Dose}) + (0.74495 \cdot -1)$$
$$+ (0.01566 \cdot \text{Dose} \cdot -1) = -2.62132 + (0.12883 \cdot \text{Dose})$$

and for women it is

$$\ln \frac{p}{1-p} = -1.87637 + (0.14449 \cdot \text{Dose}) + (0.74495 \cdot +1)$$
$$+ (0.01566 \cdot \text{Dose} \cdot +1) = -1.13142 + (0.16015 \cdot \text{Dose})$$

Because we used a $-1/+1$ indicator variable, the numeric magnitude of the regression coefficient for the interaction tells us how the slopes of the two genders differ from the average of their slopes, rather than how different the slopes are from each other. Even so, the P-value testing the null hypothesis that the regression coefficient for the interaction is equal to 0 in the population also tests the null hypothesis that the slopes for men and women are equal to the same value in the population. The P-value is equal to 0.681806. Since it is greater than 0.05, we fail to reject this null hypothesis. In other words, there is not a statistically significant difference between the slopes for the two genders. Equation (12.11) shows us how to calculate an odds ratio for an independent variable that is involved in an interaction. Let us use that equation to calculate the odds ratio comparing men and women who receive a dose of 10 mg:

$$OR_{\text{Sex|Dose}=10} \triangleq \widehat{OR}_{\text{Sex|Dose}=10} = e^{(b_2 \cdot \Delta)+(b_3 \cdot \text{Dose} \cdot \Delta)} = e^{(0.74495 \cdot 2)+(0.01566 \cdot 10 \cdot 2)}$$
$$= e^{1.8031} = 6.068$$

Now, let us use that equation again to calculate the odds ratio comparing men and women who receive a dose of 20 mg:

$$OR_{\text{Sex|Dose}=20} \triangleq \widehat{OR}_{\text{Sex|Dose}=20} = e^{(b_2 \cdot \Delta)+(b_3 \cdot \text{Dose} \cdot \Delta)} = e^{(0.74495 \cdot 2)+(0.01566 \cdot 20 \cdot 2)}$$
$$= e^{2.1163} = 8.300$$

These two odds ratio estimates are different, but the difference is not statistically significant. We can see that this is true because the P-value for the null hypothesis that the coefficient for the interaction is equal to 0 in the population (0.681806) is greater than 0.05. In this case, the interaction might be removed from the logistic regression equation so that a single odds ratio can be estimated to compare men and women regardless of the dose. This odds ratio is the one estimated in Example 12.3 (6.787). ∎

12.1.3   Cox Regression Analysis

Logistic regression analysis is appropriate only when the nominal dependent variable is not affected by time.[15] If it is affected by time, we need to use a method of analysis that takes into account the different periods of time over which we looked for the event. **Cox regression**[16] analysis is the most commonly used regression analysis in this case.

The dependent variable in Cox regression is the rate (i.e., incidence) at which events occur.[17] Rates can have values from 0 to $+\infty$. To keep estimates of the rate from being less than 0, a logarithmic transformation is used. Equation (12.12) displays the Cox regression equation:

$$\ln(\text{rate}) = \alpha_t + (\beta_1 \cdot X_1) + (\beta_2 \cdot X_2) + \cdots + (\beta_k \cdot X_k) \tag{12.12}$$

where

$\ln(\text{rate})$ = natural log of the rate at which the event occurs in the population

α_t = function of time

β_i = regression coefficient for the ith (out of k) independent variable in the population

X_i = value of the ith (out of k) independent variable

For the most part, Equation (12.12) looks like other regression equations we have encountered. For instance, each of the independent variables is multiplied by a regression coefficient and, then, added together. However, there is one important difference. The intercept of other regression equations is a constant. In Cox regression analysis, what appears to be the intercept is really a function of time. This is how this analysis can take into account the different periods of time that persons were followed while looking for the event represented by the dependent variable.

When interpreting the result of Cox regression analysis, we usually take the regression coefficient as an exponent of e, the base of the natural logarithm scale.

---

[15] Recall from Chapter 6 that a nominal dependent variable is affected by time if (1) the longer we look for events, the more events we observe and (2) we look longer for events for some people than for others.

[16] Cox regression is also called "proportional hazards" regression.

[17] See Chapter 6 for a discussion of the difference between a rate and a probability.

The result is the ratio of the rates corresponding to a one-unit difference in the value of the independent variable as shown algebraically in Equation (12.13):

$$RR = \frac{e^{\ln(\text{rate})}}{e^{\ln(\text{rate})}} = \frac{e^{\alpha+(\beta_1\cdot[X_1+1])+(\beta_2\cdot X_2)+\cdots+(\beta_k\cdot X_k)}}{e^{\alpha+(\beta_1\cdot X_1)+(\beta_2\cdot X_2)+\cdots+(\beta_k\cdot X_k)}} = \frac{\cancel{e^\alpha}\cdot e^{\beta_1\cdot[X_1+1]}\cdot\cancel{e^{\beta_2\cdot X_2}}\cdot\ \cdots\ \cdot\cancel{e^{\beta_k\cdot X_k}}}{\cancel{e^\alpha}\cdot e^{\beta_1\cdot X_1}\cdot\cancel{e^{\beta_2\cdot X_2}}\cdot\ \cdots\ \cdot\cancel{e^{\beta_k\cdot X_k}}}$$

$$= \frac{e^{\beta_1\cdot[X_1+1]}}{e^{\beta_1\cdot X_1}} = e^{\beta_1} \triangleq \widehat{RR} = e^{b_1} \tag{12.13}$$

where

RR = population's rate ratio comparing a one-unit difference in the value of X_1

ln(rate) = natural log of the rate at which the event occurs in the population

α_t = function of time

β_i = regression coefficient for the ith (out of k) independent variable in the population

X_i = value of the ith (out of k) independent variable

$\widehat{RR}$ = sample's estimate of the rate ratio comparing a one-unit difference in the value of X_1

b_i = sample's estimate of the regression coefficient for the ith (out of k) independent variable

Excel does not have a program for Cox regression analysis, but this analysis can be performed in R. To access Cox regression analysis in R, it is necessary to load a package of programs called "Survival." To load this package, select the "Packages" tab in the lower righthand quadrant in RStudio then click on "Install." Type "Survival" in the blank for packages and click "Install." Now, "Survival" will appear in your list of packages. Click on the box to the left of "Survival" in the list to load it. You only need to install "Survival" once, but you will have to load it each time you start R if you want to use any of its programs.

Cox regression is performed with the "coxph(Surv(time,status)~IVs)" command where time is the variable that keeps track of the length of follow-up and status is the variable that indicates the condition under which a person left follow-up (e.g., 0 for withdrew without the event and 1 for withdrew with the event). The next example illustrates Cox regression analysis in R.

■ **EXAMPLE 12.5**

Suppose we were to conduct a study of an occupational exposure that we suspect is associated with liver toxicity. In this study, we identify 100 workers with the exposure and 100 workers without the exposure and follow them for up to five years to determine who develops liver disease. To control for the potential confounding effect of age, we include age as an independent variable. When we analyze those data with the "coxph()" command, we get the following result.

\>summary(coxph(Surv(Time,Death)~Exposure+Age,data=Example12_5))

```
Call:
coxph(formula = Surv(Time, Death) ~ Exposure + Age, data = Example12_5)

  n= 200, number of events= 52

            coef exp(coef) se(coef)     z Pr(>|z|)
Exposure 1.37413   3.95164  0.33097 4.152 3.3e-05 ***
Age      0.03258   1.03311  0.01908 1.707  0.0878 .
-
Signif. codes:  0 '***' 0.001 '**' 0.01 '*' 0.05 '.' 0.1 ' ' 1

         exp(coef) exp(-coef) lower .95 upper .95
Exposure     3.952     0.2531    2.0656     7.560
Age          1.033     0.9679    0.9952     1.072

Concordance= 0.734  (se = 0.041 )
Likelihood ratio test= 24.56  on 2 df,   p=5e-06
Wald test            = 21.06  on 2 df,   p=3e-05
Score (logrank) test = 24.14  on 2 df,   p=6e-06
```

The first table in that output gives the regression coefficient estimates, their standard errors and a z-value and corresponding P-value testing the null hypothesis that the coefficient in the population is equal to 0. There is an additional column in that table headed "exp(coef)." This is the regression coefficient taken as a power of e, the base of the natural log scale. As shown in Equation (12.13), this gives the rate ratio estimate for a one-unit change in the value of the independent variable. The second table also gives the rate ratios and their confidence intervals.

One thing you may have noticed about the first table is that there is no estimate of the intercept. This is because, unlike other regression equations, the intercept is not a constant, but rather a function of time. This is how Cox regression analysis controls for the fact that different people are followed for different periods of time.

The last part of the "coxph()" output gives tests of the omnibus null hypothesis that the entire collection of independent variables does not help estimate the dependent variable. The Wald test is the same as the method used by R to test null hypotheses about individual regression coefficients. The method I prefer to use is the likelihood ratio test. Usually, all three methods give very similar results. ∎

12.2 NOMINAL INDEPENDENT VARIABLES

When independent variables represent nominal data, they separate dependent variable values into groups. When this occurs in multivariable analysis of a nominal dependent variable, we select one of the independent variables to be compared directly with the dependent variable. Then, all of the remaining independent variables are assumed to represent characteristics for which we would like to control.

12.2.1 Stratified Analysis

If the nominal dependent variable is not affected by time and all of the independent variables are nominal, we can use **stratified analysis** to analyze our data. The idea in stratified analysis is to select one of the nominal independent variables to be compared with the nominal dependent variable in 2 × 2 tables. Then, the rest of the nominal independent variables are used to separate the data into groups (i.e., **strata**) within each of which we compare the dependent variable and the selected independent variable. This separation of the data into strata eliminates confounding by these variables. The next example demonstrates how this works.

■ EXAMPLE 12.6

Suppose we are interested in the relationship between exposure to a particular food additive and development of diabetes. Further, suppose we are concerned that gender might be a confounder because women are at higher risk for diabetes and are more likely to consume food with the additive than are men. In other words, we want to control for the potential confounding effect of gender. In stratified analysis, we can control for gender by separating the data into two gender strata. Imagine the following frequencies were observed:

Men		Diabetes		
		Yes	No	
Exposure	Yes	30	30	60
	No	30	30	60
		60	60	120

Women		Diabetes		
		Yes	No	
Exposure	Yes	100	10	110
	No	10	1	11
		110	11	121

There are a number of ways we could summarize the relationship between exposure and the risk of diabetes in each of these strata (i.e., **strata-specific estimates**), but with each we would see the same thing for these data. For example, the following are odds ratios comparing exposure to the occurrence of diabetes for each of the gender strata (using Equation (9.8)).

$$\widehat{OR}_{men} = \frac{a \cdot d}{b \cdot c} = \frac{30 \cdot 30}{30 \cdot 30} = 1.00$$

$$\widehat{OR}_{women} = \frac{a \cdot d}{b \cdot c} = \frac{100 \cdot 1}{10 \cdot 10} = 1.00$$

With odds ratios equal to 1, there is no apparent association between exposure and risk of diabetes in either of the two genders. If we had not divided the data into these two strata, however, we would have a different impression. Combining the data across the two strata, which is the wrong thing to do, we get the following[18]:

Both Genders		Diabetes		
		Yes	No	
Exposure	Yes	130	40	170
	No	40	31	71
		170	71	241

$$\widehat{OR} = \frac{a \cdot d}{b \cdot c} = \frac{130 \cdot 31}{40 \cdot 40} = 2.52$$

Now, it appears that there is a relatively strong relationship between exposure and diabetes.[19] This result, however, reflects the relationship between gender and diabetes (women are at higher risk of diabetes) and between gender and exposure (women are more often exposed), rather than a relationship between exposure and diabetes. By stratifying the data according to gender, we are able to control for its effect. ∎

When using stratified analysis, we sometimes see that the relationship between the dependent and independent variables used to construct the 2 × 2 tables is essentially the same regardless of which stratum is considered. This was true in Example 12.6. In that example, regardless of whether we are thinking about men or women, there is no association between exposure and risk of diabetes. When these strata-specific estimates are similar across strata, we do not need to report separate measures of association for each stratum. Instead, we would like to have a single measure of association that represents all strata. We call this single measure of association a **summary estimate**.

We might be tempted at this point to combine all the data into a single 2 × 2 table and calculate an estimate from this 2 × 2 table to serve as the summary estimate. Resist that temptation! To combine the data would be to remove control of confounding. Example 12.6 shows what can happen when control of confounders is removed; we can get a biased view of the association between the two variables. Instead of combining data across strata, we calculate a summary estimate by combining the strata-specific estimates.

There are two ways we commonly combine the strata-specific estimates to obtain a summary estimate. One way is to calculate a weighted average[20] of the

[18]We are doing this to illustrate what would happen if we combined the data over strata. In practice, combining the data is not an appropriate response to observation of similar strata-specific estimates.
[19]This observation of an association suggested by the combined data, even when there is no association in either of the strata, is sometimes called "Simpson's paradox."
[20]See Equation (7.25) for a description of a weighted average.

strata-specific estimates using the precision of each estimate as the weight. The result is called a **precision-based estimate**. The other way is to separately combine the numerators and the denominators of a ratio measure of association across strata, and then divide the sum of the numerators by the sum of the denominators. The result is called a **Mantel–Haenszel estimate**.

Of the two types of summary estimates, the Mantel–Haenszel estimate is the easier to calculate manually. Further, the two types of estimates are usually very close in value. So, if they are to be calculated by hand, use of the Mantel–Haenszel estimates is recommended. Equations (12.14) and (12.15) illustrate Mantel–Haenszel summary estimates of the odds ratio and risk ratio, respectively:

$$
OR \triangleq \overline{OR} = \frac{\sum_{i=1}^{k}(a_i \cdot d_i/n_i)}{\sum_{i=1}^{k}(b_i \cdot c_i/n_i)} \tag{12.14}
$$

$$
RR \triangleq \overline{RR} = \frac{\sum_{i=1}^{k}(a_i \cdot [c_i + d_i]/n_i)}{\sum_{i=1}^{k}(c_i \cdot [a_i + b_i]/n_i)} \tag{12.15}
$$

where

$\overline{OR}$ = summary estimate of the odds ratio

$\overline{RR}$ = summary estimate of the risk ratio

a_i, b_i, c_i, d_i = observed frequencies in the 2×2 table in the ith stratum of k strata[21]

n_i = number of observations in the ith stratum of k strata

In the next example, we will take a look at calculation of Mantel–Haenszel summary estimates of the odds ratio and risk ratio.

■ EXAMPLE 12.7

Suppose we are interested in the relationship between long-term steroid therapy and the risk of developing cataracts. To study this relationship, we identify 116 persons initiating this therapy and 100 persons initiating an alternative therapy. Then, we follow persons in both groups for five years to observe the development of cataracts. In analyzing these observations, we want to control for the effect of gender, since

---

[21] See Tables 9.1 and 9.2 to see how the cell frequencies are assigned to a 2×2 table for cohort and case–control studies, respectively.

women are more likely to be exposed to steroid therapy and are at greater risk of developing cataracts. Suppose we observe the following results[22]:

Women		Cataracts		
		Yes	No	
Therapy	Yes	31	49	80
	No	13	37	50
		44	86	130

Men		Diabetes		
		Yes	No	
Exposure	Yes	13	23	36
	No	9	41	50
		22	64	86

Let us use the "Stratified Analysis" BAHR program to help us calculate the Mantel–Haenszel summary estimates of the risk ratio and odds ratio from these data.

Women

Observed		Outcome		
		Yes	No	
Group	A	31	49	80
	B	13	37	50
		44	86	130

Expected		Outcome		
		Yes	No	
Group	A	27.07692	52.92308	80
	B	16.92308	33.07692	50
		44	86	130

Parameter	PE	SE	95% IE	
p(Yes|A)	0.3875	0.054468	0.280742	0.494258
p(Yes|B)	0.26	0.062032	0.138417	0.381583
Probability diff	0.1275	0.082552	−0.0343	0.289301
Probability ratio	1.490385	0.276914	0.866133	2.564555
Odds ratio	1.800628	0.395748	0.829004	3.911032

Test	Chi-Sq	P-value
Pearson's (uncorrected)	2.233946	0.135009
Pearson's (corrected)	1.700796	0.192184
Mantel–Haenszel	2.216761	0.136519
Fisher's exact		0.190707

Men

Observed		Outcome		
		Yes	No	
Group	A	13	23	36
	B	9	41	50
		22	64	86

Expected		Outcome		
		Yes	No	
Group	A	9.209302	26.7907	36
	B	12.7907	37.2093	50
		22	64	86

Parameter	PE	SE	95% IE	
p(Yes|A)	0.361111	0.080054	0.204206	0.518017
p(Yes|B)	0.18	0.054332	0.073509	0.286491
Probability diff	0.181111	0.09675	−0.00852	0.370742
Probability ratio	2.006173	0.374508	0.962898	4.179807
Odds ratio	2.574879	0.505868	0.955329	6.940018

Test	Chi-Sq	P-value
Pearson's (uncorrected)	3.606272	0.057562
Pearson's (corrected)	2.717667	0.099243
Mantel–Haenszel	3.564339	0.059033
Fisher's exact		0.100317

---

[22] Strata-specific estimates of the odds ratio and risk ratio are calculated using Equations (9.8) and (9.6), respectively.

In the analysis of these data, Excel has given us information about each stratum (i.e., for men and for women). This information includes a 2 × 2 table for each stratum as well as point and interval estimates for the odds ratio and the probability ratio. We interpret these results the same way we did in bivariable analysis (see Example 9.12). For women, the risk ratio estimate is equal to 1.4904 and the limits of the 95% confidence interval are 0.8661and 2.5645. Since this confidence interval includes 1, we cannot reject the null hypothesis that the risk ratio is equal to 1 for women in the population. For men, the risk ratio estimate is equal to 2.0062 and the limits of the 95% confidence interval are 0.9629 and 4.1798. As with women, this confidence interval includes 1, so we cannot reject the null hypothesis that the risk ratio is equal to 1 for men in the population.

This part of stratified analysis is like bivariable analysis, except that we are controlling for differences between genders by looking at one gender at a time. Now, we could use Equations (12.14) and (12.15) to calculate the summary estimates, but the program also provides us with those summary estimates.

Summary Estimates		
Parameter	Method	Estimate
Probability ratio	Mantel–Haenszel	1.655518
	Precision–based	1.709642
Odds ratio	Mantel–Haenszel	2.055673
	Precision–based	2.140471

Excel provides us with two types of summary estimates. One is the Mantel–Haenszel estimate we saw in Equations (12.14) and (12.15). The other is a precision-based estimate.[23] This is a weighted average of the strata-specific estimates with the weights being the inverse of the strata-specific variances (the square of the standard errors).

If we are willing to assume that the risk ratio comparing the risk of developing diabetes between exposed and unexposed persons is the same for women and men, then we do not have to provide separate estimates for the two genders. Instead, we estimate that the risk ratio is equal to 1.66 regardless of gender using the Mantel–Haenszel method. Likewise, if we are willing to assume that the odds ratio comparing the odds of developing diabetes between exposed and unexposed persons is the same for women and men, then we do not have to provide separate estimates for the two genders. Instead, we estimate that the odds ratio is equal to 2.06 regardless of gender using the Mantel–Haenszel method.   ∎

Next, we need to think about how to decide whether a summary estimate makes sense. If, in the population, there are different strengths of association in each of the

---

[23]Which type of estimate to use is somewhat arbitrary, but epidemiologists seem to prefer the Mantel–Haenszel estimates while statisticians seem to prefer the precision-based estimates.

strata, we do not want to provide a single estimate.[24] Instead, we want to provide strata-specific estimates if those values are different in the population.

In Example 12.6, the strata-specific estimates are both equal to 1. In that case, we would certainly use the same estimate (i.e., 1.00) for both genders. In practice, however, we cannot expect to see strata-specific estimates all exactly equal to each other when we take random samples, even if they are equal to the same value in the population. Instead, we expect to see some differences among those estimates due to the role of chance in selecting the sample. In Example 12.7, for instance, the strata-specific estimates are close, but not identical between men and women. The question is, "Are they close enough to assume they are estimating the same odds ratio and risk ratio in the population?"

To answer this question, we need a method to compare the strata-specific estimates that can take this role of chance into account. Most often, we make this decision by testing the null hypothesis that the strata-specific measures of association are equal to the same value in the population. This is called a **test of homogeneity**. If we are able to reject this null hypothesis, we conclude that there are different associations in each stratum in the population. In that case, we do not want to use a summary estimate. Instead, we report the strata-specific estimates. If, on the other hand, we fail to reject this null hypothesis, we conclude that a summary estimate makes sense. In that case, we report one estimate that applies to all of the strata.

A relatively straightforward approach involves calculation of a chi-square statistic with degrees of freedom equal to the number of strata (k) 1. That chi-square statistic is calculated as shown in Equation (12.16):

$$\chi^2_{k-1\text{df}} = \sum_{i=1}^{k} \frac{(Y_i - \overline{Y})^2}{1/w_i} = \sum_{i=1}^{k} \frac{(Y_i - \overline{Y})^2}{\text{SE}_i^2} \tag{12.16}$$

where

$\overline{Y}$ = any summary estimate, on a log scale for ratio estimates

Y_i = strata-specific estimate for the ith stratum, on a log scale for ratio estimates

w_i = weight corresponding to the ith stratum

SE_i = standard error of the estimate for the ith stratum

Now, let us take a look at an example that uses the "Stratified Analysis" BAHR program to perform a test of homogeneity for the odds ratio and the risk ratio.

■ EXAMPLE 12.8

In Example 12.7, we looked at the results of a study in which we examined the relationship between long-term steroid therapy and the risk of developing cataracts

---

[24]Epidemiologists refer to different strengths of association in different strata as **effect modification**. This is the same as what statisticians call an interaction.

while controlling for the potential confounding effects of gender. When we analyzed the data from Example 12.7 using the "Stratified Analysis" BAHR program, we observe the following output:

Homogeneity Tests		
Parameter	Chi-Sq	P-value
Probability ratio	0.136336	0.711951
Odds ratio	0.143023	0.705294

For both the odds ratio and the probability ratio (i.e., risk ratio) the P-values are greater than 0.05. Thus, we fail to reject the null hypothesis that the odds ratios for the two strata are equal to each other in the population and the null hypothesis that the risk ratios for the two strata are equal to each other in the population. This failure to reject those null hypotheses in a test of homogeneity implies that it is appropriate to report the summary estimates of the odds ratio and the risk ratio, rather than the strata-specific odds ratios and risk ratios.   ■

In this example, we were able to perform a test of homogeneity for the odds ratio and the risk ratio and conclude that it is appropriate to report the summary estimates. Now, let us test the null hypothesis that the summary estimates of the odds ratio and the risk ratio are equal to 1 in the population by using the **Mantel–Haenszel test**. We first encountered this test in Chapter 9, where it was an option for 2 × 2 table analysis (Equation (9.19)). This test can also be used to test two or more 2 × 2 tables. Equation (12.17) illustrates how this chi-square statistic can be used to test the null hypotheses that the probability ratio and odds ratio are equal to 1 and the hypothesis that the risk difference is equal to 0 in the population[25]:

$$\chi^2_{1df} = \frac{\left(\sum_{i=1}^{k} a_i - \sum_{i=1}^{k} E(a_i)\right)^2}{\sum_{i=1}^{k} [(a_i + b_i) \cdot (c_i + d_i) \cdot (a_i + c_i) \cdot (b_i + d_i)]/[n_i^2 \cdot (n_i - 1)]} \qquad (12.17)$$

where

χ^2_{1df} = chi-square statistic with one degree of freedom

a_i = observed frequency in the upper left-hand cell of the 2 × 2 table in the ith stratum of k strata

$E(a_i)$ = expected frequency for the upper left-hand cell of the 2 × 2 table in the ith stratum of k strata (from Equation (9.13))

---

[25] Recall from Chapter 9 that these three null hypotheses are always true together or false together. Thus, we do not need separate hypothesis tests for each estimate.

$(a_i + b_i), (c_i + d_i),$

$(a_i + c_i), (b_i + d_i)$ = marginal frequencies from the 2 × 2 table in the ith stratum of k strata

n_i = total number of observations in the 2 × 2 table in the ith stratum of k strata

In the next example, we see how the Mantel–Haenszel test is performed by the "Stratified Analysis" BAHR program in Excel and by the "mantelhaen()" command in R for stratified analysis.

■ EXAMPLE 12.9

In Example 12.7, we looked at the results of a study in which we examined the relationship between long-term steroid therapy and the risk of developing cataracts while controlling for the potential confounding effects of gender. In Example 12.8, we determined that it is appropriate to report the summary estimate of the risk ratio by performing a test of homogeneity. Now, let us test the null hypotheses that the summary estimate is equal to 1 in the population using the Mantel–Haenszel test.

The formula for calculation of the Mantel–Haenszel chi-square statistic is in Equation (12.17). We could use that formula to perform the Mantel–Haenszel test by hand or we could use a computer to perform the test for us. We will do the latter.

In Excel, this test is part of the output from the "Stratified Analysis" BAHR program. That output appears below:

Summary Chi-Square	
Chi-Sq	P-value
5.422003	0.019885

Since the P-value in that output is less than 0.05, we reject the null hypotheses that the odds ratio and the risk ratio are equal to 1 in the population.

This test is also performed by the "mantelhaen()" command in R. The only information required of that command is the name of a three-dimensional array that contains the data. These data are in an array called "Example12_6."

```
>mantelhaen(Example12_6)

Mantel-Haenszel chi-squared test with continuity correction

data:  Example12_6
Mantel-Haenszel X-squared = 4.7419, df = 1, p-value = 0.02944
alternative hypothesis: true common odds ratio is not equal to 1
95 percent confidence interval:
 1.115212 3.789224
sample estimates:
common odds ratio
        2.055673
```

Notice that this chi-square value is a little smaller and the *P*-value is a little larger than those obtained from Excel. The reason for this is that R uses a continuity correction. We discussed continuity corrections in Chapter 9. They tend to result in *P*-values that are closer to the *P*-value we get from an exact test.

This R output also provides us with the summary estimate of the odds ratio and its confidence interval. This summary estimate is the same as the Mantel–Haenszel estimate we obtained from Excel. ∎

12.2.2 Relationship Between Stratified Analysis and Logistic Regression

In Chapter 10, we learned about the principle of the general linear model. This principle unifies all of the analyses we have discussed for continuous dependent variables by allowing all of those analyses to be expressed as regression equations. We have a similar concept that applies to nominal dependent variables. It is called the principle of the **generalized linear model**. The reason for this new name is to reflect the fact that we can get very similar, rather than exact, results by expressing analyses for a nominal dependent variable as regression analyses. These are not exactly the same because most of the methods we use to analyze nominal dependent variables are normal approximations. Different approximations give slightly different results.

As an example of the generalized linear model, let us consider logistic regression and stratified analysis. Both methods are appropriate for a nominal dependent variable not affected by time. The distinction is that all of the independent variables in stratified analysis are nominal.[26] The next example demonstrates the effect of using logistic regression to perform a stratified analysis.

■ **EXAMPLE 12.10**

Suppose that we are interested in the relationship between a particular exposure and a disease, but we are concerned about the potential confounding effect of age. To analyze our data, we decide to use stratified analysis. To create age strata, we divide the data into three age groups: (1) less than 40 years, (2) 40–49 years, and (3) 50 or more years. Analyzing these data using the "Stratified Analysis" BAHR program for each stratum, suppose we get the following results:

---

[26]To continue this comparison, we can think of stratified analysis for a nominal dependent variable as being similar to factorial analysis of variance (ANOVA) for a continuous dependent variable. The categories of one "factor" in stratified analysis are used to separate dependent variable values into two groups within each stratum. Categories of the other "factor" are used to separate the data into strata. The "main effect" of the first factor in stratified analysis is represented by the summary estimate. This summary estimate makes sense only if there is homogeneity among strata. This is the same as having no interaction in factorial ANOVA.

<40

Observed		Outcome			Expected		Outcome		
		Yes	No				Yes	No	
Group	A	4	6	10	Group	A	1.904762	8.095238	10
	B	8	45	53		B	10.09524	42.90476	53
		12	51	63			12	51	63

Parameter	PE	SE	95% IE		Test	Chi-Sq	P-value
$p(Yes\|A)$	0.4	0.154919	0.096358	0.703642	Pearson's (uncorrected)	3.38424	0.065823
$p(Yes\|B)$	0.150943	0.049174	0.054562	0.247325	Pearson's (corrected)	1.961758	0.161325
Probability diff	0.249057	0.162536	−0.06951	0.567628	Mantel–Haenszel	3.330522	0.068005
Probability ratio	2.65	0.506095	0.982764	7.145664	Fisher's exact		0.172499
Odds ratio	3.75	0.750925	0.860658	16.33924			

40–49

Observed		Outcome			Expected		Outcome		
		Yes	No				Yes	No	
Group	A	8	24	32	Group	A	6.175439	25.82456	32
	B	3	22	25		B	4.824561	20.17544	25
		11	46	57			11	46	57

Parameter	PE	SE	95% IE		Test	Chi-Sq	P-value
$p(Yes\|A)$	0.25	0.076547	0.099969	0.400031	Pearson's (uncorrected)	1.523004	0.217165
$p(Yes\|B)$	0.12	0.064992	−0.00738	0.247385	Pearson's (corrected)	0.802654	0.370301
Probability diff	0.13	0.100416	−0.06682	0.326815	Mantel–Haenszel	1.496285	0.221244
Probability ratio	2.083333	0.62216	0.615411	7.052648	Fisher's exact		0.372323
Odds ratio	2.444444	0.738549	0.574797	10.39551			

>49

Observed		Outcome			Expected		Outcome		
		Yes	No				Yes	No	
Group	A	14	24	38	Group	A	10.31429	27.68571	38
	B	5	27	32		B	8.685714	23.31429	32
		19	51	70			19	51	70

Parameter	PE	SE	95% IE		Test	Chi-Sq	P-value
$p(Yes\|A)$	0.368421	0.078252	0.215048	0.521795	Pearson's (uncorrected)	3.954395	0.046749
$p(Yes\|B)$	0.15625	0.064186	0.030445	0.282055	Pearson's (corrected)	2.954272	0.085651
Probability diff	0.212171	0.101209	0.013802	0.41054	Mantel–Haenszel	3.897904	0.048346
Probability ratio	2.357895	0.462453	0.952525	5.836767	Fisher's exact		0.082832
Odds ratio	3.15	0.59172	0.987708	10.04599			

Summary Estimates		
Parameter	Method	Estimate
Probability ratio	Mantel–Haenszel	2.341754
	Precision–based	2.381543
Odds ratio	Mantel–Haenszel	3.033914
	Precision–based	3.114277

Homogeneity Tests		
Parameter	Chi-Sq	P-value
Probability ratio	0.051524	0.974567
Odds ratio	0.125585	0.939138

Summary Chi-Square	
Chi-Sq	P-value
8.23042	0.004119

From this output, we find a Mantel–Haenszel summary estimate of the odds ratio equal to 3.034.[27] From this output, we also find that the test of homogeneity is not significant. This implies that it makes sense to interpret a summary estimate. Finally, using this output, we find that we can reject the null hypothesis that the summary estimate of the odds ratio is equal to 1 in the population.

Now, let us use logistic regression analysis to represent this stratified analysis. To do this, we will create two indicator variables (0/1) to represent the three age strata. The following output shows the result of this analysis:

Logistic Regression				
Omnibus H0	Log Lkhd	Chi Sq	DF	P-value
Intercept only	−100.862			
Full model	−96.2089	9.305529	3	0.025493

Variable	Estimate	SE	Chi Sq	DF	P-value
Intercept	−1.73054	0.343438	34.02219	1	5.45E-09
Group	1.04583	0.389383	7.537363	1	0.006043
40–49	−0.36911	0.501035	0.546879	1	0.459596
GT49	0.112289	0.451425	0.061923	1	0.803482

Let us compare the results from stratified analysis with the results from logistic regression analysis.

In this example, we analyzed these data two ways. First, we used stratified analysis with strata defined by three age groups. In that analysis, the summary estimate of the odds ratio comparing the odds of disease between exposed and unexposed persons was 3.034 using the Mantel–Haenszel method.

Second, we used logistic regression analysis with indicator variables to represent the three age groups. From logistic regression, the estimate of the odds ratio comparing the odds of disease between exposed and unexposed persons is equal to 2.846 ($e^{1.04583}$). This is close, but not exactly equal to the summary estimates from stratified analysis.[28]

The same is true for the test of the null hypothesis that the odds ratio for exposure is equal to 1 in the population. In stratified analysis, the Mantel–Haenszel test is statistically significant. In logistic regression analysis, the chi-square test is statistically significant as well. ■

In Example 12.10, we controlled for age by defining age groups. When we do this, there is still variation in age among persons in each age group.[29] All we have

[27]We are focusing on the odds ratio because we want to compare stratified analysis with logistic regression analysis, which is usually interpreted using odds ratios.
[28]The fact that these are not exactly the same is why we refer to the "generalized" linear model for nominal dependent variables.
[29]Recall from Chapter 10 that multivariable analysis controls confounding by eliminating variation in the independent variable that is correlated with other independent variables before looking at the association between that independent variable and the dependent variable. When we represent a continuous

done is that we have reduced the variability of this continuous confounder, not eliminated it. The result is that we have not completely controlled for the confounding effect of age. The potential result of incomplete control of a confounder is illustrated in the next example.

■ **EXAMPLE 12.11**

In Example 12.10, we performed a logistic regression analysis in which age was represented by two indicator variables to separate the three age groups. Now, suppose we perform a different logistic regression analysis, including age as a continuous independent variable. Doing that produces the following output:

Logistic Regression				
Omnibus H0	Log Lkhd	Chi Sq	DF	P-value
Intercept only	−100.862			
Full model	−94.0754	13.57257	2	0.001129
Variable	Estimate	SE	Chi Sq	DF	P-value
Intercept	−0.00942	1.042321	17.41344	1	3.01E-05
Group	0.773144	0.373984	4.34663	1	0.037082
Age	0.051329	0.022313	5.53415	1	0.018649

Let us compare this output (including age as a continuous independent variable) with the logistic regression output in Example 12.10 (where age was represented as two indicator variables).

To check how well we have controlled for age as a confounder, we compare the apparent relationship between exposure (another independent variable) and disease (the dependent variable). If there is confounding, we will see an apparent relationship between exposure and disease, even though such a relationship does not exist.

In Example 12.10, the odds ratio comparing the odds of disease between exposed and unexposed persons was equal to 2.846 and was statistically significant. These are the results from controlling for age by defining three age groups. In the current example, however, the odds ratio comparing the odds of disease between exposed and unexposed persons is closer to 1 (2.167) and, although still significantly different from 1, its *P*-value is larger. The difference between the two analyses is that age is only partially controlled by defining age groups. In this circumstance, we say that there is **residual confounding** of the relationship between exposure and disease by age when age is represented by stratifying the data into age groups.   ■

---

independent variable as strata, there is still variation of the independent variable within strata. Thus, we cannot eliminate this variation on a nominal scale.

12.2.3 Life Table Analysis

When the nominal dependent variable is affected by time, we can take the differences in the length of follow-up into account by estimating rates. Another option is to consider time a confounder and stratify the data by time periods. Then, we are able to estimate risks instead of rates. The method we use to do this is called **life table analysis**.[30] Life table analysis shares an important property with stratified analysis. For both, we can perform the analyses by hand and, as a result, see what is happening in the analysis.

In Chapter 6, we saw how staggered admission can lead to a nominal dependent variable being affected by time (see Figure 6.2). In life table analysis, we measure time differently for each person followed. Time begins for each person when we begin following that person. This is called **study-relative time**. Figure 12.2 shows how study-relative time compares with calendar-relative time.

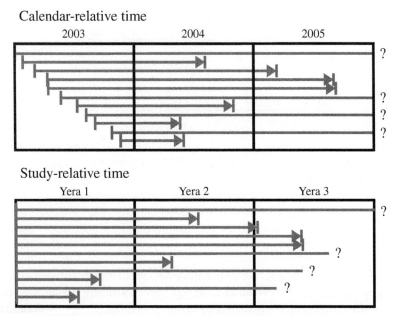

Figure 12.2 Staggered admission of 11 subjects during the first year of a three-year study. ⊢ Indicates the time at which the individual entered the study (and consequently, the time at which follow-up began), ▶| indicates follow-up ending because of occurrence of the event of interest, and? indicates end of follow-up without the event (because the study was concluded).[31] The upper figure shows follow-up according to calendar relative time. The lower figure shows follow-up according to study-relative time. Study-relative time starts at 0 for each subject when their follow-up begins, regardless of the date in calendar time.

---

[30]This comes from the fact that life tables were originally used with death as the event. These methods, however, can be used for any irreversible event for which a risk can be calculated.
[31]These are "censored" observations.

Life table analysis stratifies observations according to study-relative time. Since time is continuous, this is tantamount to representing time with one or more nominal independent variables. If we are doing the calculations manually, we customarily use only a few intervals for time. For the data in Figure 12.2, for instance, we would probably stratify time by year, creating three time strata. In each of these strata, we have two life tables, each specified by a particular value of the nominal independent variable that we want to compare with dependent variable values (e.g., exposure in a cohort study). Table 12.2 illustrates the usual format for each life table.

There are two probabilities that are calculated as part of life table analysis. The first is the probability of the event not occurring during that time period given that the person went through each of the previous time periods without the event occurring.[32] Equation (12.18) shows how this probability can be calculated:

$$p(\overline{\text{event}}_{t_i} \mid \overline{\text{event}}_{t_{<i}}) = 1 - \frac{a_{t_i}}{n_{t_i}} \tag{12.18}$$

where

$\overline{\text{event}}_{t_i}$ = not having the event during the ith time period

$\overline{\text{event}}_{t_{<i}}$ = not having the event prior to the ith time period

a_i = number of events during the ith time period

n_i = number of persons without the event at the beginning of the ith time period

The second probability in the life table is the probability of not having the event during the current time period and all previous time periods, thus it is called a **cumulative probability**. This probability is calculated by multiplying the probabilities in

TABLE 12.2. Format of a Life Table Applied to Data Observed in Figure 12.2[*]

Time Period	Persons	Events	Withdrawals	Probability of No Event	Cumulative Probability
1	11	2	0	0.82	0.82
2	9	3	0	0.67	0.55
3	6	2	4	0.67	0.36

[a] Each time period represents one year in study-relative time. In the "Persons" column is the number of persons without the event at the beginning of the time period. In the "Events" column is the number of persons who had the event during the time period. In the "Withdrawals" column is the number of persons for whom follow-up ended during the time period, but who did not have the event (i.e., censored observations). The probabilities are discussed in the last two columns.

[32]Notice that this is a conditional probability in which not having the event during the current time period is the conditional event and not having the event in previous time periods is the conditioning event. Conditional probabilities are discussed in Chapter 1.

Equation (12.18) for the current and all previous time periods.[33] This calculation is illustrated in Equation (12.19):

$$p(\overline{\text{event}}_{t_i} \text{ and } \overline{\text{event}}_{t_{<i}}) = \prod_{t=1}^{i} p(\overline{\text{event}}_{t_i} \mid \overline{\text{event}}_{t_{<i}}) \qquad (12.19)$$

where

$\overline{\text{event}}_{t_i}$ = not having the event during the ith (out of k) time period

$\overline{\text{event}}_{t_{<i}}$ = not having the event prior to the ith (out of k) time period

$\prod_{t=1}^{i}$ = product with t going from 1 (the first time period) to i (the time period $t - 1$ for which the probability is being calculated)

The next example illustrates use of the "Life Table" BAHR program to perform these calculations.

■ EXAMPLE 12.12

In Example 12.5, we supposed we conduct a cohort study of persons in a particular industry. In this study, we select 100 persons who are beginning to work in an area in which they will be exposed to a by-product of the manufacturing process and another 100 persons who are beginning to work in areas without this exposure. The event is developing liver toxicity. These persons are recruited over a five-year period (i.e., by staggered admission). At the end of each year of follow-up, we examine the cohort and determine who has developed liver toxicity. Imagine we make the following observations:

Year of Follow-up[*]	Exposed Persons	Events	Withdrawals	Unexposed Persons	Events	Withdrawals
1	100	0	20	100	0	20
2	80	4	16	80	2	18
3	60	11	9	60	1	19
4	40	10	10	40	3	17
5	20	15	5	20	6	14

[*]Study-relative time.

[33]This is the probability of the intersection of the probabilities of remaining event free in all of the time periods up to and including the current time period. We learned in Chapter 1 that we use the multiplication rule to find the intersection of events. Here we are assuming the probabilities of surviving each time period are statistically independent.

Let us use the "Life Table" BAHR program in Excel to create life tables for these two groups:

Life Table Analysis					

What is the name of this group?

Exposed

Time	Number	Events	Withdrawals	$p(t)$	$p(T)$
1	100	0	20	1.000	1.000
2	80	4	16	0.950	0.950
3	60	11	9	0.817	0.776
4	40	10	10	0.750	0.582
5	20	15	5	0.250	0.145

Life Table Analysis					

What is the name of this group?

Unexposed

Time	Number	Events	Withdrawals	$p(t)$	$p(T)$
1	100	0	20	1.000	1.000
2	80	2	18	0.975	0.975
3	60	1	19	0.983	0.959
4	40	3	17	0.925	0.889
5	20	6	14	0.700	0.621

Life tables are usually summarized by calculating risks. Risks are the complement of the cumulative probability of not experiencing the event. They can be calculated for each time period in the life table. Equation (12.20) illustrates that calculation:

$$\text{Risk}_i = 1 - p(\overline{\text{event}}_{t=i} \text{ and } \overline{\text{event}}_{t=i-1} \ \dots \ \text{and } \overline{\text{event}}_{t=1}) \qquad (12.20)$$

where

Risk_i = risk of having the event up to and including the ith time period

$\overline{\text{event}}_{t=i}$ = not having the event during the ith time period

The next example shows how these risks are calculated and compared in the Excel program.

■ EXAMPLE 12.13

In Example 12.12, we used Excel to construct life tables from data collected in a cohort study of the risk of liver damage related to exposure to a by-product of a manufacturing process. Let us use that same program to calculate risk estimates and compare them between exposed and unexposed persons.

	Risks			**95% Interval est.**	
Time	**Exposed**	**Unexposed**	**Risk Ratio**	**LL**	**UL**
1	0	0	0	0	0
2	0.05	0.025	2	0.388919978	10.28489209
3	0.224166667	0.04125	5.434343434	1.755603609	16.82161532
4	0.418125	0.11315625	3.695111848	1.816746146	7.51555279
5	0.85453125	0.379209375	2.253454968	1.587359374	3.19906089

Thus, the exposed group has twice the risk of liver disease after two years, 5.43 times the risk after three years, 3.70 times the risk after four years, and 2.25 times the risk after five years.   ■

Often, the results of life table analysis are summarized graphically in what is often called a **survival curve**. This name is a little misleading, since it suggests a curved line. Rather, survival "curves" are usually "staircase" plots in which the cumulative probability of avoiding the event is changed for each time period. Figure 12.3 shows the **survival plot** for the life tables in Example 12.12.

The survival plots in Figure 12.3 suggest that, as the length of follow-up increases, the differences in the risk of liver damage between the two exposure groups becomes greater. This is a common observation in survival plots. It is important to keep in mind, however, that the number of persons contributing to probability estimates decreases as the length of follow-up increases. This is because, as time goes on, fewer persons are followed, either because they have had the event or they have withdrawn from follow-up. Fewer persons are contributing to probability estimates. This results in less precise estimates. So, we need to be cautious about overinterpretation of differences seen during the later time periods.

So far, we have calculated probabilities by assuming that the persons who withdrew from the study[34] did so at the end of the time period. This assumption is reflected by the fact that all persons who withdrew are included in the denominator of Equation (12.18). When we make this assumption, the method of life table

---

[34] We learned in Chapter 6 that "withdrawals" include persons who are not followed any further for any reason, including termination of the study.

Survival plot

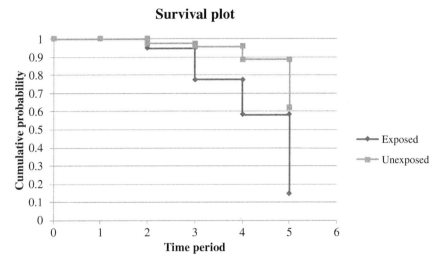

Figure 12.3 Survival plots for the cumulative probability of avoiding liver damage among persons who were exposed (lower line) or unexposed (upper line) to a manufacturing byproduct. These cumulative probabilities were determined in Example 12.12. Survival plots are part of the output from the "Life Table" BAHR program.

analysis we are using is called the **Kaplan–Meier** method.[35] This is the most commonly used type of life table analysis.

Another, more realistic, assumption we could make about the persons who withdrew is that their follow-up ended sometime during the time period. If we do not know when they withdrew, we can assume there was a uniform rate of withdrawal over the study period. For example, if 52 persons withdrew during a one-year time period, we could assume that, on the average, one person withdrew each week. This implies that the mean length of follow-up among withdrawals is equal to half the time period (e.g., 26 weeks). This is the same as saying that persons who withdrew were at risk for the event, on the average, for half the time of persons who did not withdraw.[36] To put this in a form that can be used in life table analysis, we assume this is the same as having half the number of persons who withdrew at risk for the entire time period. With this assumption about persons who withdraw from follow-up, we are using what is called the **Cutler–Ederer** or **actuarial** method of life table analysis. Equation (12.20) shows how this method affects calculation of the probability of avoiding the event (compare with Equation (12.18)):

$$p(\overline{\text{event}}_{t=i} \mid \overline{\text{event}}_{t<i}) = 1 - \frac{a_{t=i}}{n_{t=i} - (w_{t=i}/2)} \tag{12.21}$$

[35] This is also called the product-limit method, usually by statisticians rather than health researchers.
[36] In calculation of risks, we do not make an adjustment for the time that each person who had the event was followed. If we were calculating follow-up time (e.g., to estimate incidence), however, we would make the same adjustment. This is discussed in Chapter 6.

where

$\overline{event}_{t=i}$ = not having the event during the ith time period

$\overline{event}_{t<i}$ = not having the event prior to the ith time period

$a_{t=i}$ = number of events during the ith time period

$n_{t=i}$ = number of persons without the event at the beginning of the ith time

$w_{t=i}$ = number of withdrawals during the ith time period

The next example shows how the actuarial method affects risk estimates in life table analysis.

■ EXAMPLE 12.14

In Example 12.12, we constructed life tables using the Kaplan–Meier method. Now, let us reconstruct the life table for exposed and unexposed persons using the Cutler–Ederer method.

When we select the Cutler–Ederer method, the "Life Table" BAHR program uses Equation (12.21) to calculate the probabilities of not having evidence of liver damage in each period, given that there was no evidence of liver damage in previous periods as well as the cumulative probabilities. The Cutler–Ederer life table for exposed persons is

Life Table Analysis					
What is the name of this group?					
Exposed					
Time	Number	Events	Withdrawals	$p(t)$	$p(T)$
1	100	0	20	1.000	1.000
2	80	4	16	0.944	0.944
3	60	11	9	0.802	0.757
4	40	10	10	0.714	0.541
5	20	15	5	0.143	0.077

And for unexposed persons, the life table is

Life Table Analysis					
What is the name of this group?					
Unexposed					
Time	Number	Events	Withdrawals	$p(t)$	$p(T)$
1	100	0	20	1.000	1.000
2	80	2	18	0.972	0.972
3	60	1	19	0.980	0.953
4	40	3	17	0.905	0.862
5	20	6	14	0.538	0.464

To see the effect of using the actuarial method on risk estimates, let us use the "Life Table" BAHR program to perform Equation (12.20) to estimate the risks of liver damage.

	Risks			95% Interval est.	
Time	Exposed	Unexposed	Risk ratio	LL	UL
1	0	0	0	0	0
2	0.055555556	0.028169014	1.972222222	0.384243156	10.12291419
3	0.242742743	0.047413192	5.119730024	1.037886092	25.25482876
4	0.459101959	0.138135745	3.323556539	1.013467038	10.89924749
5	0.922728851	0.535919247	1.721768449	1.024639126	2.893200657

The Kaplan–Meier estimate of the five-year risk among the exposed was found in Example 12.12 to be 0.855. This is lower than the Cutler–Ederer estimate (0.923). This is true for all of the risks (except the risk of zero). The Cutler–Ederer estimates of risk will always be higher than the Kaplan–Meier estimate when there are withdrawals during the risk period. This is also evident in the survival plot. Compare the following survival plot with the one in Figure 12.3.

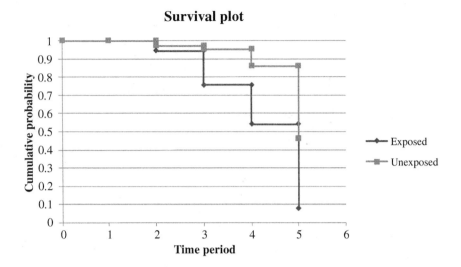

Survival plot

The difference between these two methods of calculating risk becomes less as the length of the time period between examinations becomes shorter. If examinations occurred so frequently that we know exactly when a person had the event or withdrew, both Kaplan–Meier and Cutler–Ederer methods would yield the same risk estimate. ∎

To take chance into account in life table analysis, we usually test the null hypothesis that the cumulative probabilities are the same in the groups being compared. The most common method we use to test this null hypothesis is a normal approximation called the **log-rank test**. Actually, this is not a new test, but just a new name. In Chapter 9, we learned about the Mantel–Haenszel test, which can be used for 2×2 table analyses (see Equation (9.19)). Earlier in this chapter, we learned that the Mantel–Haenszel test is also used in stratified analysis (see Equation (12.17)). The log-rank test is really just the Mantel–Haenszel test applied to data stratified by time period. The next example shows how we can conduct the log-rank test to test the null hypothesis that the risk ratio is equal to 1 in the population.

∎ EXAMPLE 12.15

In Example 12.12, we constructed life tables for a group of persons who were exposed to a by-product of a manufacturing process and another group of persons who were not exposed, comparing their risks of developing liver damage. In Example 12.13, we estimated the five-year risk ratio to be equal to 2.25. Now, let us test the null hypothesis that the risk ratio in the population is equal to 1.

First, we need to rearrange the data so that they are organized into strata that represent the four time periods:

Year 1		Liver Damage		
		Yes	No	
Exposure	Yes	0	100	100
	No	0	100	100
		0	200	200

Year 2		Liver Damage		
		Yes	No	
Exposure	Yes	4	76	80
	No	2	78	80
		6	154	160

Year 3		Liver Damage		
		Yes	No	
Exposure	Yes	11	49	60
	No	1	59	60
		12	108	120

Year 4		Liver Damage		
		Yes	No	
Exposure	Yes	10	30	40
	No	3	37	40
		13	67	80

Year 5		Liver Damage		
		Yes	No	
Exposure	Yes	15	5	20
	No	6	14	20
		21	19	40

To test this null hypothesis manually, we could use Equation (12.16) or the "Stratified Analysis" BAHR program in Excel. We will do the latter.

Summary Chi-Square		
Chi-Sq	P-value	
20.65432	5.5E-06	

The result of this analysis is a P-value of 0.0000055. Since this is less than 0.05, we reject the null hypothesis that the ratio of five-year risks is equal to 1 in the population. By the process of eliminating the null hypothesis, we accept the alternative hypothesis that the risk ratio is not equal to 1.

The log-rank test, *per se*, does not appear on the "Life Table" BAHR program output, but the confidence intervals of the risk ratios are **test-based confidence intervals**.[37] This means that the result of the log-rank test was used to calculate the confidence interval. Examination of the limits of the confidence interval will give us exactly the same conclusion as would the results of the log-rank test. ∎

This concludes our discussion of the most commonly used statistical methods in health research.

CHAPTER SUMMARY

We have two choices for our basic approach to multivariable analysis of a nominal dependent variable. One approach that is applicable to continuous and/or nominal independent variables is comparable to multiple regression analysis for a continuous dependent variable. The other approach is stratified analysis, which can be performed only with nominal independent variables or independent variables converted to a nominal scale.

In the regression approach to the analysis of nominal dependent variables, there are two techniques we encounter most often in health research. When the nominal dependent variable is expressed as a probability or as odds, we use logistic regression. Logistic regression uses a transformation of the nominal dependent variable known as the logit transformation. The logit transformation is equal to the natural logarithm of the ratio of the probabilities of an event and its complement. This is the same as the natural logarithm of the odds of the dependent variable (known as the log odds).

To estimate values of the logit-transformed dependent variable, logistic regression analysis uses a linear combination of the independent variables that is the same as in multiple regression analysis of continuous dependent variables.

---

[37] In a test-based confidence interval, the results of the hypothesis test are used to represent the standard error. For nominal dependent variables, the test-based interval is close to, but not exactly equal to, a conventional interval. Test-based intervals are used mostly when the standard error for the interval is difficult to estimate.

There are two ways in which the estimated values of the dependent variable in logistic regression can be expressed. One way is by estimating probabilities for specific values of all the independent variables.

The other way to interpret estimated values of the dependent variable in logistic regression is by estimating odds ratios for specific values of the independent variables, one at a time.

Cox regression is the regression approach that is most often used when the nominal dependent variable is affected by time and expressed as a rate. The dependent variable in the Cox regression equation is the natural logarithm of the rate.

It is possible to interpret the estimated values of the dependent variable in Cox regression as the rate corresponding to specific values for all the independent variables, but this is a little complicated since the intercept is a function of time. More often, dependent variable values are interpreted as a rate ratio corresponding to the regression coefficient for a specific independent variable.

Both logistic regression and Cox regression rely on the maximum likelihood method for estimating values of regression coefficients and testing hypotheses. In the maximum likelihood method, values for the coefficients are chosen so that the probability of obtaining the sample's observations from a population with those coefficients is as high as possible. Hypothesis testing in logistic and Cox regression uses a likelihood ratio. That likelihood ratio contains the probability of obtaining the sample's observations if the null hypothesis were true in the numerator and the probability of obtaining those observations if the population' coefficients were equal to the sample's estimates of those coefficients in the denominator.

The likelihood ratio can be used to test the omnibus null hypothesis that all the coefficients are equal to 0, or a partial likelihood ratio can be used to test the null hypothesis that a particular coefficient is equal to 0. These likelihood ratios differ in the likelihood used in their numerators. The likelihood ratio for the omnibus null hypothesis has in its numerator the likelihood of obtaining the observed data if all the coefficients were equal to 0. The partial likelihood ratio has in its numerator the likelihood of obtaining the observed data if a particular coefficient were equal to 0 and all the other coefficients were equal to the values estimated from the sample's observations.

Regardless of which null hypothesis is being tested, evaluation of whether or not the likelihood ratio is unusual enough to allow rejection of the null hypothesis involves conversion of the likelihood ratio to a chi-square statistic. That chi-square value has degrees of freedom equal to the difference between the number of coefficients considered in the null hypothesis and the total number of coefficients in the regression equation.

When all the independent variables are nominal, we can still use logistic or Cox regression techniques to analyze them. An alternative to the regression approach for nominal independent variables, however, is the stratified analysis approach. In stratified analysis, we differentiate between one nominal independent variable that is of main interest and other independent variables that represent potential confounders.

We then create a series of 2×2 tables, one for each value of the independent variable(s) representing the confounder(s).

With data that have been stratified, we have a choice of examining the relationship between the dependent variable and the independent variable of main interest within each of the strata separately or over all the strata combined. The choice between these two approaches depends on whether the relationship appears to be consistent over all the strata. When the relationship does not appear to be consistent over the strata, we choose to examine that relationship within each of the strata separately, using the techniques for bivariable analysis of a nominal dependent variable described in Chapter 9. If the relationship between the dependent variable and the main independent variable appears to be the same for all the strata (according to a test of homogeneity), we can facilitate interpretation of the relationship between the dependent variable and the independent variable of main interest by making one summary estimate combining the estimates for each of the strata.

When it is more likely we will observe the nominal dependent variable event the longer we follow individuals and individuals in a study are followed for variable periods of time, we say the dependent variable is affected by time. In previous chapters, we have examined nominal dependent variables that are affected by time by estimating rates rather than probabilities. In this chapter, we examined an alternative approach to nominal dependent variables that are affected by time with a method called life table analysis. In life table analysis, follow-up time is treated like a nominal confounding variable used to create strata. Within each time stratum, the probability of surviving (i.e., avoiding the event) over the time interval is calculated. Of more interest than the probability of surviving (i.e., avoiding the event) a particular time stratum is the cumulative probability of surviving up to and including that time interval.

It is often of interest to compare the survival experience of two groups. Most commonly, entire life tables are compared graphically by examining survival plots. A survival plot graphs time on the abscissa (X-axis) and the cumulative probability of survival (i.e., avoiding the event) on the ordinate (Y-axis).

For both probabilities and rates, methods of interval estimation differ between differences and ratios. That is not true of hypothesis testing. The method we use to test the null hypothesis that the probability difference is equal to 0 or that the probability or odds ratios are equal to 1 is an extension of the Mantel–Haenszel procedure first described in Chapter 9.

The Mantel–Haenszel procedure is also used to test the null hypothesis that two life tables are the same in the population from which the sample was drawn. Although the calculations are the same when a Mantel–Haenszel chi-square is calculated from data stratified by interval of follow-up, there is a feature of hypothesis testing in life-table analysis that is important to keep in mind. That feature is the number of observations in each time stratum becomes smaller as we consider strata for longer time intervals.

EXERCISES

12.1. The Framingham Heart Study (FHS) focused on risk factors for heart disease. Suppose we want to compare the odds of getting heart disease for age, gender (sex = 1 for men, sex = 0 for women), serum cholesterol (scl), diastolic blood pressure (dbp), and body mass index (bmi). We include age and gender to control for their effect. The data for the first 500 persons participating in the FHS is in the Excel file: EXR12_1. Perform a logistic regression analysis on those data with an indicator of heart disease as the dependent variable. From that analysis, do you think the relationship between BMI and heart disease is different for men compared with women?

A. No, they are the same

B. Yes, but they are not significantly different

C. Yes, and they are significantly different

12.2. The FHS focused on risk factors for heart disease. Suppose we want to compare the odds of getting heart disease for age, gender (sex = 1 for men, sex = 0 for women), serum cholesterol (scl), diastolic blood pressure (dbp), and body mass index (bmi). We include age and gender to control for their effect. The data for the first 500 persons participating in the FHS is in the Excel file: EXR12_1. Perform a logistic regression analysis on those data with an indicator of heart disease as the dependent variable. From that analysis, do you think the intercepts of the regression lines for men and women are different?

A. No, they are the same

B. Yes, but they are not significantly different

C. Yes, and they are significantly different

12.3. The FHS focused on risk factors for heart disease. Suppose we want to compare the odds of getting heart disease for age, gender (sex = 1 for men, sex = 0 for women), serum cholesterol (scl), diastolic blood pressure (dbp), and body mass index (bmi). We include age and gender to control for their effect. The data for the first 500 persons participating in the FHS is in the Excel file: EXR12_1. Perform a logistic regression analysis on those data with an indicator of heart disease as the dependent variable. From that analysis, which independent variables are independent risk factors? Select as many as there are correct answers.

A. Serum cholesterol

B. Body mass index

C. Diastolic blood pressure

12.4. The FHS focused on risk factors for heart disease. Suppose we want to compare the odds of getting heart disease for age, gender (sex = 1 for men, sex = 0 for women), serum cholesterol (scl), diastolic blood pressure (dbp), and body mass index (bmi). We include age and gender to control for their effect. The data for the first 500 persons participating in the FHS is in the Excel file: EXR12_1. Perform a logistic regression analysis on those data with an indicator of heart disease as the dependent variable. From that analysis, estimate the odds ratio of heart disease for a five year difference in age. Which of the following is closest to that odds ratio?

A. 1.07

B. 1.20

C. 1.33

D. 2.00

E. 2.66

12.5. The FHS focused on risk factors for heart disease. Suppose we want to compare the odds of getting heart disease for age, gender (sex = 1 for men, sex = 0 for women), serum cholesterol (scl), diastolic blood pressure (dbp), and body mass index (bmi). We include age and gender to control for their effect. The data for the first 500 persons participating in the FHS is in the Excel file: EXR12_1. Perform a logistic regression analysis on those data with an indicator of heart disease as the dependent variable. From that analysis, estimate the odds ratio of heart disease for a two-unit difference in BMI among women. Which of the following is closest to that odds ratio?

A. 1.07

B. 1.20

C. 1.33

D. 2.00

E. 2.66

12.6. Suppose we were to conduct a case–control study to investigate the relationship between exposure to dust produced by a particular industry and development of chronic obstructive pulmonary disease (COPD). Also suppose that we want to control for smoking as a potential confounder. For smokers, 25 out of 50 cases and 10 out of 50 controls were exposed. For nonsmokers, 15 out of 50 cases and 6 out of 50 controls were exposed. Determine the summary odds ratio for those data. Which of the following is closest to your answer?

A. 2.44

B. 2.89

C. 3.22

D. 3.61

E. 3.74

12.7. Suppose we were to conduct a cohort study to investigate the relationship between exposure to cigarette smoke and development of cataracts. Also suppose that we want to control for gender as a potential confounder. For men, 12 out of 50 exposed and 4 out of 50 unexposed persons developed cataracts. For women, 8 out of 50 exposed and 7 out of 50 unexposed persons developed cataracts. Calculate the summary probability ratio for those data. Which of the following is closest to your answer?

A. 1.14

B. 1.82

C. 2.63

D. 3.00

E. 3.22

12.8. Suppose we were to conduct a case–control study to investigate the relationship between exposure to dust produced by a particular industry and development of COPD. Also suppose that we want to control for smoking as a potential confounder. For smokers, 25 out of 50 cases and 10 out of 50 controls were exposed. For nonsmokers, 15 out of 50 cases and 6 out of 50 controls were exposed. Does it make sense to report the summary odds ratio for those data?

A. No, since the strata-specific odds ratios are too different

B. Yes, since the strata-specific odds ratios are not too different

C. Yes, because the test of homogeneity is significant

D. Yes, because the test of homogeneity is not significant

E. No, because the test of homogeneity is significant

F. No, because the test of homogeneity is not significant

12.9. Suppose we were to conduct a cohort study to investigate the relationship between exposure to cigarette smoke and development of cataracts. Also suppose that we want to control for gender as a potential confounder. For men, 12 out of 50 exposed and 4 out of 50 unexposed persons developed cataracts. For women, 8 out of 50 exposed and 7 out of 50 unexposed persons developed cataracts. Test the null hypothesis that the probability ratio is the same among men and women in the population. Which of the following is the best conclusion to draw?

A. Reject both the null and alternative hypotheses

B. Accept both the null and alternative hypotheses

C. Reject the null hypothesis and accept the alternative hypothesis

    D. Accept the null hypothesis and reject the alternative hypothesis

    E. It is best not to draw a conclusion about the null and alternative hypotheses from these data

12.10. Suppose we were to conduct a case–control study to investigate the relationship between exposure to dust produced by a particular industry and development of COPD. Also suppose that we want to control for smoking as a potential confounder. For smokers, 25 out of 50 cases and 10 out of 50 controls were exposed. For nonsmokers, 15 out of 50 cases and 6 out of 50 controls were exposed. Test the null hypothesis that the odds ratio for exposure is equal to 1 in the population versus the alternative that is not equal to 1, allowing a 5% chance of making a type I error. Which of the following is the best conclusion to draw?

    A. Reject both the null and alternative hypotheses

    B. Accept both the null and alternative hypotheses

    C. Reject the null hypothesis and accept the alternative hypothesis

    D. Accept the null hypothesis and reject the alternative hypothesis

    E. It is best not to draw a conclusion about the null and alternative hypotheses from these data

12.11. . Suppose we investigate the rate of cure over a three-week period among persons who received a new treatment for Lyme disease. These data are in the Excel file: EXR12_2. What is the probability that a person who receives the new treatment will be cured within three weeks?

    A. 0.40

    B. 0.49

    C. 0.51

    D. 0.55

    E. 0.60

12.12. Suppose we investigate a new treatment for a particular type of breast cancer by comparing it to the standard treatment in 400 women with stage III breast cancer. The survival over five years appears in the Excel file: EXR12_3. What is the five-year risk of fatality among patients who received the standard treatment?

    A. 0.24

    B. 0.31

    C. 0.36

    D. 0.44

    E. 0.65

12.13. Suppose we investigate the rate of cure over a three-week period among persons who received a new treatment for Lyme disease and among persons who received the standard treatment. These data are in the Excel file: EXR12_2. What is the probability ratio comparing persons who received the new treatment to persons who received the standard treatment?

A. 1.80

B. 2.00

C. 2.33

D. 3.15

E. 4.36

12.14. Suppose we investigate a new treatment for a particular type of breast cancer by comparing it to the standard treatment in 400 women with stage III breast cancer. The survival over five years appears in the Excel file: EXR12_3. What is the five-year probability ratio comparing persons who received the new treatment to persons who received the standard treatment?

A. 1.24

B. 2.19

C. 2.57

D. 2.86

E. 3.22

12.15. Suppose we investigate the rate of cure over a three-week period among persons who received a new treatment for Lyme disease and among persons who received the standard treatment. These data are in the Excel file: EXR12_2. Test the null hypothesis that the three-year probability ratio is equal to 1 in the population versus the alternative that is not equal to 1, allowing a 5% chance of making a type I error. Which of the following is the best conclusion to draw?

A. Reject both the null and alternative hypotheses

B. Accept both the null and alternative hypotheses

C. Reject the null hypothesis and accept the alternative hypothesis

D. Accept the null hypothesis and reject the alternative hypothesis

E. It is best not to draw a conclusion about the null and alternative hypotheses from these data

12.16. Suppose we investigate a new treatment for a particular type of breast cancer by comparing it to the standard treatment in 400 women with stage III breast cancer. The survival over five years appears in the Excel file: EXR12_3. Test the null hypothesis that the five-year probability ratio is equal to 1 in the population versus the alternative that is not equal to 1, allowing a 5% chance of making a type I error. Which of the following is the best conclusion to draw?

A. Reject both the null and alternative hypotheses
B. Accept both the null and alternative hypotheses
C. Reject the null hypothesis and accept the alternative hypothesis
D. Accept the null hypothesis and reject the alternative hypothesis
E. It is best not to draw a conclusion about the null and alternative hypotheses from these data

CHAPTER 13

TESTING ASSUMPTIONS

Introduction to Biostatistical Applications in Health Research with Microsoft Office Excel® and R,
Second Edition. Robert P. Hirsch.
© 2021 John Wiley & Sons, Inc. Published 2021 by John Wiley & Sons, Inc.
Companion website: www.wiley.com/go/hirsch/healthresearch2e

The development by theoretical statisticians of the mathematical methods that serve as the foundation of statistical procedures involves making certain assumptions about the sample and the population from which the sample was obtained. Each time we use one of these procedures, we accept that the assumptions associated with that procedure are true for our sample and its population. In previous chapters, we did not evaluate whether or not all of these assumptions were met since we were more concerned with interpreting the results of statistical analyses rather than performing them. Now, as we think about analyzing our own data, we need to consider these assumptions carefully before we are comfortable using a particular statistical procedure. In this chapter, we will learn what assumptions are associated with which statistical procedures and how we might determine if our sample and its population satisfy those assumptions.

Some of the assumptions associated with statistical procedures can be evaluated using formal (i.e., mathematical or graphical) approaches or accepted rules of thumb. Those assumptions can be evaluated, to some degree, by examination of the sample's observations. We will look more closely at these assumptions in a moment. First, let us consider two assumptions that must be evaluated without the help of examining the sample's observations.

There is one universal assumption applicable to all statistical procedures. That assumption is that the sample is a randomly derived subset of the population (at least as far as values of the dependent variable are concerned). This implies that we have used some method of **probability sampling**. In probability sampling, chance is the final determinant of which sampling units in the population become observational units in the sample. It is this role of chance that interval estimation and statistical hypothesis testing are designed to take into account.

If we know that a sample is, in fact, representative of the population (such as in perfectly performed judgment sampling[1]) then there is no need to use interval estimation or hypothesis testing. In that case, the mean of the sample (for instance) will be equal to the mean of the population. Thus, whenever we employ statistical methods for hypothesis testing or interval estimation, we are assuming that chance has played a role in determining the composition of the sample and, therefore, in determining the sample's estimate(s) of the population's parameter(s) (e.g., the mean).

To evaluate the assumption that the sample was randomly derived from the population, we need to consider the sampling method that has been used to obtain the sample. If probability sampling has been used, the assumption is satisfied. If some other method of sampling has been used (such as systematic or convenience sampling[2]), we need to recognize that, by using statistical procedures to analyze the

---

[1] In judgment sampling, the collection of sampling units in the population selected to be observational units in the sample is specifically chosen because that collection is considered to be representative of the entire population.

[2] Systematic sampling uses a particular algorithm to select sampling units to be included in the sample. For example, we could select patients seen on a particular day of the week. In convenience sampling, those sampling units most available for observation are selected to be in the sample. For example, we could select all patients seen in a convenient practice over a period of time.

sample's data, we are making an assumption. Specifically, we are assuming that this other sampling method has resulted in a sample that is no different than what would have been obtained by using probability sampling. To be valid, this assumption must be based on a thorough understanding of how the sampling method differs from probability sampling and whether those differences could influence the representativeness of the sample.[3]

In this chapter, we will also consider what we can do in the circumstance that an assumption is violated. Unfortunately, there is nothing realistic that can be done to make the distribution of dependent variable values in a sample representative of the population if it is not derived in a way that is essentially random. Instead, we must accept the fact that estimates made from such a sample may not be representative of the population.

A second assumption that is common to most statistical procedures is that the observed persons are statistically independent of one another. This assumption implies that the value of the dependent variable for one observation is not associated with the value of the dependent variable for another observation, except through an association with the independent variable(s).

For example, suppose we were studying the prognostic factors associated with the outcome of a surgical procedure that could be performed on an individual more than once (e.g., cataract extraction). Observations made on two different patients are likely to be independent. Two observations of the procedure on the same patient, however, are not likely to be independent. In the latter case, we might expect to see similar dependent variable values associated with particular independent variable values, even if a biologic association does not exist between the characteristics represented by those variables. This is true because a single patient is likely to have similar values of the dependent variable for many reasons.

Thus, repeated observations on the same patient do not add as much information to our understanding of the relationship between the dependent and independent variables as do observations on different patients. Except for those procedures that are specially designed to take a lack of statistical independence of observations into account, all methods of analysis assume that each observational unit in a sample provides the same amount of information.[4]

As with the assumption of random sampling, the assumption of statistical independence of observations cannot be evaluated by examination of the sample. Rather, concluding that this assumption is satisfied for a particular sample requires understanding of the method of sampling and how elements (e.g., people) in the population might be associated. Sometimes the method of sampling can be assumed to result in observations that are statistically independent. For example, elemental sampling should select statistically independent observations, but cluster sampling is not

---

[3]For instance, in a convenience sample we would have to assume that patients seen at a particular practice are representative of all patients.

[4]Examples of statistical procedures that are designed to take a lack of statistical independence into account are the paired *t*-test described in Chapter 4 and McNemar's test described in Chapter 9.

likely to select independent observations.[5] The situation is more difficult to assess when a systematic or convenience sample is taken. For those methods of sampling, we must have a thorough understanding of the sampling method and the relationships among elements in the population to be convinced that the observations in the sample are statistically independent.

These two assumptions (random sampling and statistical independence) address only the dependent variable. The majority of assumptions made as part of the mathematical development of statistical procedures concern the dependent variable rather than the independent variable(s). The reason for this is that statistical procedures are designed to make estimates of or test hypotheses about the dependent variable in the population. Because of the importance of the dependent variable and, thus, of the assumptions concerning the dependent variable, we will begin our discussion of assumptions made by statistical procedures by focusing on the dependent variable. At the end of this chapter, we will discuss assumptions that are made for the independent variable(s).

There are three other assumptions that are common to the dependent variable in many statistical procedures with which we are familiar. Each of these remaining assumptions can be evaluated by examining the data in the sample. There are different approaches to evaluation of these assumptions for dependent variables that represent different types of data. First, we will look at approaches for continuous dependent variables. Next, we will consider how we can evaluate these assumptions for nominal dependent variables. [6] Further, we will learn what to do if we are concerned about the appropriateness of these assumptions for a particular sample.

13.1 CONTINUOUS DEPENDENT VARIABLES

The most commonly made of the remaining assumptions is that the distribution of point estimates from all samples of a given size (i.e., the sampling distribution) is a Gaussian distribution. This assumption is made for all of the statistical procedures for continuous dependent variables that we have studied. Another common assumption is that the variances of data in the population for each of two or more subgroups of dependent variable values are all equal to the same value. This assumption is applicable to many statistical procedures used to analyze bivariable or multivariable data sets. The third of the remaining assumptions applicable to bivariable and multivariable analyses is that the relationship between the dependent variable and

---

[5]Elemental sampling refers to the situation in which each sampling unit selected from the population consists of one and only one element (e.g., an individual person). Cluster sampling refers to the situation in which sampling units can consist of more than one element (e.g., selecting families rather than individuals).

[6]For ordinal dependent variables, the assumptions made are fewer than the assumptions made for continuous or nominal dependent variables. Even so, ordinal dependent variable values are assumed to be statistically independent and randomly sampled from the population.

the independent variable(s) is an additive (i.e., linear) one. We will see what this implies later. First, let us examine the assumption that all possible point estimates have a Gaussian distribution.

13.1.1 Assuming A Gaussian Distribution

In Chapter 3, we learned that the role of chance in estimation of the value of a population's parameter from a sample's observations is taken into account by considering the (theoretical) distribution of estimates of that parameter from all possible samples of a given size. It is important for us to keep in mind that it is this sampling distribution that is used by statistical procedures to take chance into account. Since this is the distribution that is used by statistical procedures, assumptions about the type of distribution address the distribution of estimates rather than the distribution of data.

The statistical procedures that are used to analyze health research data represented by continuous dependent variables all assume that the sampling distribution is a Gaussian distribution. This is true for univariable, bivariable, and multivariable analyses. To begin, we will consider how this assumption applies to univariable analysis of a continuous dependent variable. Then, we will see how the assumption relates to bivariable and multivariable analyses.

13.1.1.1 Univariable Analyses. When the dependent variable represents continuous data, statistical procedures are usually designed to address the role of chance in estimation of the mean of the distribution of data in the population. Since a single sample allows calculation of only one estimate of the population's mean (for example), we cannot examine a distribution of estimates of that mean when we have only a single sample (which is, essentially, always the case) to determine whether or not the sampling distribution of means is a Gaussian distribution. Thus, we need to rely on our knowledge of what influences the shape of the sampling distribution of means.

In Chapter 3, we learned about two circumstances in which we can expect the sampling distribution of means (or other parameter of location) to be a Gaussian distribution. One of those circumstances is when the population's distribution of data is, itself, a Gaussian distribution. The other is when the sample's size is large enough. We learned that, as samples of larger sizes are considered, this tendency for the sampling distribution of parameters of location (e.g., means) to be a Gaussian distribution, even if the data do not have a Gaussian distribution, is called the central limit theorem.

Thus, we have two ways in which we can evaluate the assumption that the sampling distribution of estimates of location is a Gaussian distribution. The easier of the two is to determine if the sample's size is large enough for us to expect the sampling distribution of estimates to be a Gaussian distribution (because of the central limit theorem). As a rule of thumb, we can use a sample of 30 or more observations for a univariable sample.[7] If we have 30 or more observations in our univariable sample, we can assume that the sampling distribution of estimates (e.g., of the mean) is a Gaussian distribution, and we need not worry further about this assumption.

If the sample if too small for us to rely on the central limit theorem to produce a Gaussian distribution of estimates, we must turn our attention to the distribution of data in the population. If this distribution is a Gaussian distribution, then we can comfortably assume that the sampling distribution of estimates is a Gaussian distribution.[8] Since we cannot examine the population's distribution of data, we need to infer what the population's distribution of data looks like from examination of the sample's distribution of data. There are three general approaches that we can take to evaluate the population's distribution of data from the observations in the sample. These are graphic, numeric, and inferential approaches. Perhaps the most straightforward way is to examine the distribution of data in the sample graphically.

As we begin to think about a graphic display of the data in the sample, we need to recognize that a Gaussian distribution is a distribution of continuous data. This implies that the frequency of any particular data value is virtually 0. This is especially important when we consider a graphic display of data in a sample with a limited number of observations. If we wish to graph the frequency distribution of the data in a sample of limited size, we must display the frequency of data in intervals of values. One way to examine the frequency distribution of the sample's data is using a histogram (see Chapter 2).

A drawback of this approach is that the particular intervals of values we choose to construct the histogram[9] are somewhat arbitrary and can affect the appearance of the frequency distribution. Further, fewer intervals, each of which represent a broader range of values, will be required when constructing a histogram for smaller samples. With fewer intervals in a histogram, it is more difficult to assess the shape of the distribution. This is illustrated in the following example.

■ **EXAMPLE 13.1**

Suppose we are interested in estimating the mean weight and the mean height of children in a certain population. We take a random sample of 20 children from that population and measure their weight (in kg) and their height (in cm). The following table shows the results of those measurements.

---

[7]This is a conservative rule of thumb. Some statisticians suggest that sample with 20 or more observations is large enough to assume that the sampling distribution is a Gaussian distribution.

[8]This process of examining the distribution of data to evaluate an assumption about the distribution of estimates has led many to mistakenly presume that statistical procedures rely on assumptions about the distribution of data in the population. It is well to keep in mind that we are concerned with the distribution of data only because it is the only distribution we are able to examine in a single sample. It is the sampling distribution, rather than the distribution of data, we assume is Gaussian.

[9]Excel refers to these intervals as "bins" which are the middle value of each interval.

Child	Weight	Height	Child	Weight	Height
PL	24	101	CH	31	116
EA	38	135	YO	28	110
SE	47	160	UL	34	123
LE	50	171	IK	25	104
TM	22	98	ET	36	130
EK	12	80	HI	16	86
NO	35	126	SN	40	141
WH	27	107	EW	43	148
OW	32	119	BO	18	91
MU	29	113	OK	20	95

We plan to calculate confidence intervals for the estimates of the means for those two variables using Student's t-distribution. Since Student's t-procedure assumes that estimates of the mean from all possible samples of a given size have a Gaussian distribution,[10] we are concerned about the truth of this assumption for estimates of the mean weight and the mean height in the population that we have sampled. How comfortable should we be in making this assumption?

The first thing we do to answer this question is to consider the size of the sample. We have 20 observations in the sample. Perhaps this is a large enough sample that we can rely on the central limit theorem to ensure that the distribution of estimates of the mean from all possible samples of 20 children is a Gaussian distribution, but we have established a sample with 30 or more observations as the criterion for complete reliance on the central limit theorem. Therefore, we need to examine the distribution of data in the sample to assess the prospect of the data in the population having a Gaussian distribution. If the population's data have a Gaussian distribution, the estimates of the mean from all possible samples of a given size (20 in this case) are guaranteed to have a Gaussian distribution, regardless of the size of the sample.

To examine the distribution of the data in the sample, we can display those data graphically in a histogram. To construct a histogram, we can use Excel's Histogram tool under Data Analysis.[11] The following histograms were drawn using 5-kg intervals starting at 8 kg for weight and 10-cm intervals starting at 71 cm for height.

---

[10]Even though we are converting the sample's mean to a Student's t-value and using Student's t distribution to calculate probabilities, we are not assuming means from all possible samples have a Student's t distribution. Recall from Chapter 4, Student's t distribution is derived from the standard normal distribution by adding degrees of freedom as a third parameter. That parameter takes into account uncertainty about the population's variance of data. The origin of Student's t-distribution and other standard distributions is illustrated in Appendix C.

[11]Although the bars of a histogram should be touching to represent the fact that the data are continuous, Excel's Histogram tool produces graphs that look like bar graphs, rather than histograms.

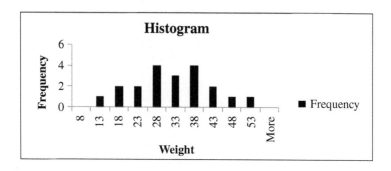

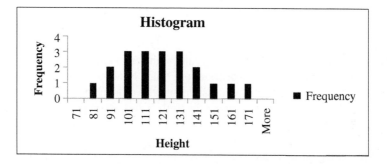

It is not obvious from those histograms whether or not we can be comfortable concluding that the data in the sample appear to have come from a population in which the data have a Gaussian distribution. One of the problems with these histograms is that the sample is so small that histograms must either consist of too few bars, or bars that represent too few observations to allow a Gaussian distribution to be recognized. Further, the intervals of values chosen to correspond to each bar are somewhat arbitrary. Different choices for those intervals might result in histograms that have different appearances. For instance, suppose we keep the same interval widths but change the point at which the intervals begin. In the following histograms, the intervals for weight begin at 12 kg and the intervals for height begin at 80 cm.

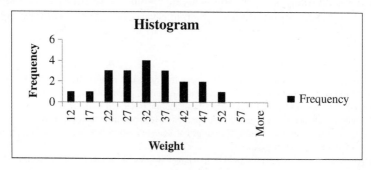

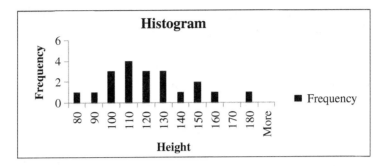

Still, it is difficult to decide whether or not these histograms are suggestive of Gaussian distributions. Changing the point at which the intervals begin has created a histogram for weight that appears more like a Gaussian distribution than our first histogram. That change in the histogram for height, however, resulted in a histogram that seems less symmetric and, therefore, a little less like a Gaussian distribution.   ■

Thus, for small samples, it is difficult to evaluate the distribution of data using a histogram. Unfortunately, it is when we have small samples that we are most concerned about the assumption that the distribution of estimates from all possible samples is a Gaussian distribution. This is the situation in which we are most apt to question the relevance of the central limit theorem to our sample, yet it is also the situation in which our ability to examine the distribution of data in a histogram is the poorest.

Fortunately, there is another approach to displaying the sample's data graphically that does not require creating intervals of values. This approach involves construction of a **cumulative frequency polygon**. In a cumulative frequency polygon, we plot the frequency of data values in the sample (on the ordinate or the Y-axis) that are equal to or less than the corresponding data value on the abscissa. In other words, each point in a cumulative frequency polygon represents the frequency of that data value plus the frequencies of all other data values of a lower magnitude.[12] If data from a Gaussian distribution are presented in a cumulative frequency polygon, the

---

[12]Note that a cumulative frequency polygon is very closely related to the frequency polygon that we encountered in Chapter 2. A frequency polygon results from connecting the tops of the bars in the histogram with a line. As the intervals for the bars gets smaller, the line in the frequency polygon gets smother. The graphic display of the bell-shaped Gaussian distribution is a frequency polygon. The cumulative frequency polygon is based on the same principle except the bars that have been connected in the cumulative frequency polygon represent the frequency with which data are equal to or less than a specific data value rather than the frequency with which data occur within an interval of values.

result is a sigmoid (S-shaped) curve. Construction of a cumulative frequency polygon is illustrated in Example 13.2.

■ EXAMPLE 13.2

In Example 13.1, we examined the distributions of weights and heights in a sample of 20 children, using histograms. In that example, we found that the appearance of the histograms was altered by changing the arbitrary choice of intervals used to construct the histograms. Further, the small size of the sample made evaluation of the shape of the distribution of data from a histogram difficult. Now, let us examine the distributions of those data using cumulative frequency polygons.

To begin, we need to calculate the cumulative frequencies. This is done by arranging the sample's data in order of numeric magnitude, and then counting the number of observations equal to or less than each particular data value. This process is summarized in the following tables. First, we will consider the children's weights.

Weight	Frequency	Cumulative Frequency	Weight	Frequency	Cumulative Frequency
12	1	1	31	1	11
16	1	2	32	1	12
18	1	3	34	1	13
20	1	4	35	1	14
22	1	5	36	1	15
24	1	6	38	1	16
25	1	7	40	1	17
27	1	8	43	1	18
28	1	9	47	1	19
29	1	10	50	1	20

In the cumulative frequency polygon shown, the dots represent the cumulative frequency for each of the 20 observations of weight and the line simply connects each of those cumulative frequencies.[13]

---

[13] This Excel chart is a scatterplot.

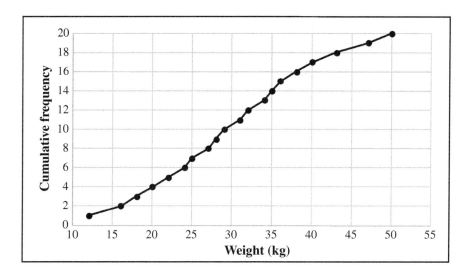

If the weights of the children have a Gaussian distribution in the sample (suggestive of a Gaussian distribution of weight in the population), we expect to see a cumulative frequency polygon that has a balanced, S-shaped appearance. By this, we imply a curve that is shaped like a (often flattened) letter S with the upper curve equal in size to the lower curve. The cumulative frequency polygon for the children's weights seems to have a balanced S shape. Thus, we can be comfortable assuming that the distribution of estimates of the mean weights of children in the population from which our sample was taken is a Gaussian distribution even though the sample is too small for us to be comfortable that the principle in the central limit theorem would produce a Gaussian distribution of estimates.

Now, let us construct a cumulative frequency polygon for the children's heights.

Height	Frequency	Cumulative Frequency	Height	Frequency	Cumulative Frequency
80	1	1	116	1	11
86	1	2	119	1	12
91	1	3	123	1	13
95	1	4	126	1	14
98	1	5	130	1	15
101	1	6	135	1	16
104	1	7	141	1	17
107	1	8	148	1	18
110	1	9	160	1	19
113	1	10	171	1	20

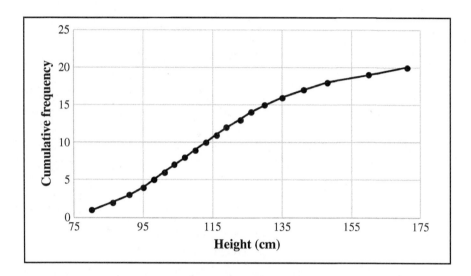

The cumulative frequency polygon for height appears to have a longer curve at the top of its S than at the bottom. This unbalanced appearance suggests that the heights of children in the sample have an asymmetric distribution. Since a Gaussian distribution must be symmetric, we might be concerned that the distribution of heights in the population is not a Gaussian distribution. If the data do not have a Gaussian distribution in the population and the sample's size is too small for us to be comfortable with the principle in the central limit theorem, we might be concerned that the assumption of a Gaussian sampling distribution of estimates of the mean height of children in the population might be violated. ∎

We can see in Example 13.2 that using a cumulative frequency polygon to examine the distribution of data in a sample is easier than using a histogram, in the sense that using cumulative frequency polygons circumvents the requirement of specifying intervals of values to construct a histogram. A disadvantage of cumulative frequency polygons, however, is that their interpretation involves comparison of sigmoid curves: often a difficult task involving quite a bit of subjective judgment. In Example 13.2, we found that an asymmetric distribution can be detected by observation of an unbalanced sigmoid curve. Not all symmetric distributions, however, are Gaussian distributions. For example, a symmetric distribution that is not bell shaped cannot be a Gaussian distribution. Detection of deviations of a symmetric distribution from a Gaussian distribution is more difficult.[14]

There is another, perhaps, better, way to evaluate the distribution of data from a cumulative frequency polygon. That method involves plotting **normalized cumulative proportions** versus the data values. This graphic display is called a

---

[14]This would have to be accomplished by comparing the sigmoid curve representing the data in the sample with a sigmoid curve that we would expect to observe if the data had a Gaussian distribution.

normalized cumulative proportion polygon or, less precisely but more simply, a **normal plot**.[15] We will see in a moment how normalized cumulative proportion polygons aid evaluation of the distribution of data in the sample, but first let us see how to calculate normalized cumulative frequencies.

There are two steps involved in converting cumulative frequencies to normalized cumulative frequencies. The first step is to express the cumulative frequencies as cumulative proportions. A cumulative proportion is calculated by dividing a cumulative frequency (as calculated in Example 13.2) by the total number of observations in the sample. The second step in converting cumulative frequencies into normalized cumulative frequencies is to convert the cumulative proportion to the standard normal deviate that corresponds to that proportion of the standard normal distribution. Since we are considering cumulative proportions, we can represent the cumulative proportion of the sample's distribution using the proportion of the standard normal distribution to the left of a particular standard normal deviate.[16]

For instance, standard normal deviates equal to or less than -1.96 correspond to 0.025 of the standard normal deviates in the standard normal distribution. Thus, if the cumulative proportion for a particular data value is equal to 0.025, the normalized cumulative proportion is -1.96. If, on the other hand, the cumulative proportion is equal to 0.975 ($1 - 0.025$), the normalized cumulative proportion is equal to $+1.96$. This relationship between cumulative proportions and standard normal deviates used as normalized cumulative frequencies is illustrated in Figure 13.1.

The exception to this procedure is the highest data value. That value has a cumulative proportion equal to 1 ($n/n = 1$), and the standard normal deviate that corresponds to a cumulative proportion of 1 is $+\infty$. Since we cannot plot $+\infty$, the normalized cumulative proportion for the highest data value is taken to be equal to the standard normal deviate corresponding to a proportion equal to p' in Equation (13.1).

$$p' = \frac{(2 \cdot n) - 1}{2 \cdot n} \tag{13.1}$$

Now, let us see how normalized cumulative proportion polygons aid in interpretation of the distribution of data in the sample. Interpretation of a normalized cumulative proportion polygon is more straightforward than interpretation of cumulative frequency polygons such as those in Example 13.2. Instead of a sigmoid curve, a Gaussian distribution is represented in a normalized cumulative proportion polygon by a straight line. Thus, deviations of the distribution of data in the sample from a Gaussian distribution can be detected by looking for deviations of the normalized cumulative proportion polygon from a straight line. This is demonstrated in Example 13.3.

---

[15]This plot is the output from the BAHR program "Residual Analysis."
[16]In Excel, you can convert cumulative proportions to a normalized scale by using the "NORM.S.INV(probability)" function ("NORMSINV" in earlier version of Excel).

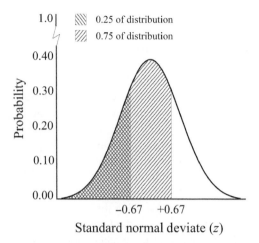

Figure 13.1 An illustration of how standard normal deviates are used to represent normalized cumulative frequencies. The cumulative proportion corresponding to a particular data value is interpreted as the area in the left-hand portion of the standard normal distribution. The standard normal deviate corresponding to the right-hand limit of that area represents the normalized cumulative proportion. Here, we show how the cumulative proportions 0.25 and 0.75 are associated with standard normal deviates that are used to represent normalized cumulative frequencies.

■ EXAMPLE 13.3

Examine normalized cumulative proportion polygons for the data in Example 13.1 to evaluate whether those data appear to have a Gaussian distribution in the sample.

First, we need to express the cumulative frequency as the cumulative proportion. Next, we need to determine the standard normal deviate that corresponds to that proportion of the standard normal distribution. To do this we use the "NORM.S.INV" function in Excel. Those steps are summarized in the following table for the weights of the children in the sample introduced in Example 13.1.

Weight	Cumulative Frequency	Cumulative Proportion	Normalized Value
12	1	0.050	−1.64
16	2	0.100	−1.28
18	3	0.150	−1.04
20	4	0.200	−0.85
22	5	0.250	−0.67
24	6	0.300	−0.52
25	7	0.350	−0.39
27	8	0.400	−0.25

28	9	0.450	−0.13
29	10	0.500	0
31	11	0.550	+0.13
32	12	0.600	+0.25
34	13	0.650	+0.39
35	14	0.700	+0.52
36	15	0.750	+0.67
38	16	0.800	+0.84
40	17	0.850	+1.04
43	18	0.900	+1.28
47	19	0.950	+1.64
50	20	0.975*	+1.96

*Calculated using Equation (13.1).

Next, we use those normalized values in a graphic comparison with the data values, as shown for children's weights. The fact that those normalized cumulative frequencies fall on a straight line[17] indicates that the children's weights have a Gaussian distribution in the sample.

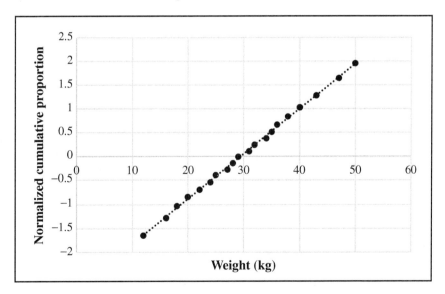

The following table illustrates the calculation of normalized cumulative frequencies for the children's heights in this sample:

[17]Excel calls this a "trendline."

Weight	Cumulative Frequency	Cumulative Proportion	Normalized Value
12	1	0.050	−1.64
16	2	0.100	−1.28
18	3	0.150	−1.04
20	4	0.200	−0.85
22	5	0.250	−0.67
24	6	0.300	−0.52
25	7	0.350	−0.39
27	8	0.400	−0.25
28	9	0.450	−0.13
29	10	0.500	0
31	11	0.550	+0.13
32	12	0.600	+0.25
34	13	0.650	+0.39
35	14	0.700	+0.52
36	15	0.750	+0.67
38	16	0.800	+0.84
40	17	0.850	+1.04
43	18	0.900	+1.28
47	19	0.950	+1.64
50	20	0.975*	+1.96

*Calculated using Equation (13.1).

Those normalized cumulative frequencies are compared to the heights of the children in the sample in the following normalized cumulative proportion polygon:

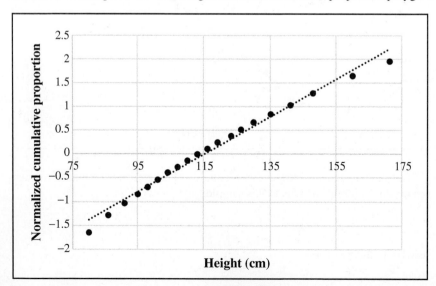

Notice that the normalized cumulative proportion polygon for weight is very close to being a straight line, but the normalized cumulative proportion polygon for height is a curved line (the broken line in that graph shows a straight line for comparison). Weight appears to have a Gaussian distribution, but height does not appear to have a Gaussian distribution in the sample. Thus, we can be comfortable assuming that the sampling distribution of estimates of the mean weight of children is a Gaussian distribution even though the sample is small. We might not be so comfortable making that assumption for the distribution of estimates of the mean height of those children. ■

The distribution of height in Examples 13.1, 13.2, and 13.3 differs from a Gaussian distribution because it is not symmetric. Every Gaussian distribution is a symmetric distribution. A distribution is considered to be symmetric when the half of the distribution above (to the right of) the mean is a mirror image of the half below (to the left of) the mean. An asymmetric distribution is said to be **skewed**. Height in Examples 13.1 and 13.2 has a distribution that is **positively skewed**. A positively skewed distribution is one in which the tail of the histogram or frequency polygon corresponding to higher data values is longer than the tail corresponding to lower data values. A **negatively skewed** distribution has a longer tail corresponding to smaller data values. These two types of skewed distribution are illustrated in Figure 13.2 as they appear in frequency polygons and normalized cumulative proportion polygons.

Even though a distribution is symmetric (i.e., not skewed), it is not necessarily a Gaussian distribution. For example, a uniform distribution[18] is symmetric, but it is not a Gaussian distribution. A Gaussian distribution is a particular type of symmetric distribution that has a certain proportion of data values in the tails of the distribution, a certain proportion of values near the mean, and a certain proportion of values between those in the tails and those near the mean. We refer to a distribution that has proportions of data values in those regions that are the same as the proportions in a Gaussian distribution as **mesokurtic**. A uniform distribution differs from a Gaussian distribution because it has no tails and no peak. In other words, it has too great a proportion of data values between the tails and the area around the mean and too few data values in the tails and near the mean. In a sense, a uniform distribution is too "fat" to be a Gaussian distribution. Distributions of this sort are said to be **platykurtic**. Distributions that are too "skinny" to be a Gaussian distribution have too many data values in the tails and near the mean. These distributions are said to be **leptokurtic**. Figure 13.3 illustrates these types of distributionss.

Thus, to be a Gaussian distribution, a distribution must be mesokurtic and not skewed. An advantage of the normalized cumulative proportion polygon is that it will be a straight line only for a mesokurtic distribution that is not skewed (i.e., only

---

[18]In a uniform distribution, all values occur with the same frequency. A uniform distribution is rectangular rather than bell shaped like a Gaussian distribution.

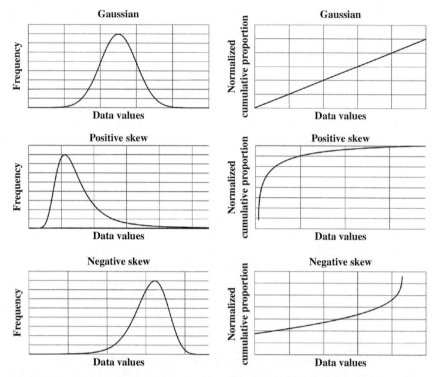

Figure 13.2 Comparison of a symmetric (Gaussian) distribution and distributions that deviate from a symmetric distribution because they are skewed. Each distribution is displayed as a frequency polygon on the left and as a normalized cumulative proportion polygon on the right.

for a Gaussian distribution). Further, we can determine from the normalized cumulative proportion polygon what direction and to what degree a distribution deviates from a mesokurtic distribution that is not skewed.

By looking at the histogram for height in Example 13.1, we can see that the distribution is positively skewed. The normalized cumulative proportion polygon (Example 13.3) deviates from a straight line by being "bowed up" in the middle. A normalized cumulative proportion polygon with this shape indicates a positively skewed distribution. A negatively skewed distribution will be "bowed down" in the middle. A leptokurtic distribution will have a normalized cumulative proportion polygon that is S shaped. A platykurtic distribution can be detected by observing a normalized cumulative proportion polygon that has a reverse S shape. A distribution that is skewed and not mesokurtic will have a normalized cumulative proportion polygon that is both bowed and S shaped (or reverse S shaped). The result will be an S-shaped (or reverse S-shaped) curve that is not symmetric (i.e., with one loop of the S larger than the other).

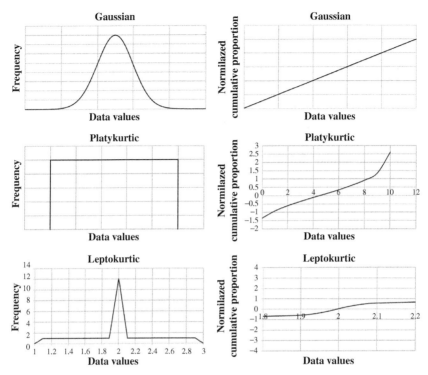

Figure 13.3 Comparison of a mesokurtic (Gaussian) distribution and distributions that deviate from a mesokurtic distribution because they are either platykurtic or leptokurtic. Each distribution is displayed as a frequency polygon on the left and as a normalized cumulative proportion polygon on the right.

Thus, we can examine the normalized cumulative proportion polygon and determine if a distribution is skewed and/or if it is not mesokurtic. This is the graphic approach that is most often used to determine if the data in a sample (that is too small to rely on the central limit theorem) appear to have a Gaussian distribution.[19]

Alternatively, we could use a numeric approach to examine a sample's distribution. This approach involves calculation of numeric values that represent the degree to which a distribution is skewed or the degree to which a distribution is either platykurtic or leptokurtic. To understand these numeric values, it is helpful for us first to understand what are called **moments about the mean** for a distribution. Moments about the mean are the average deviation of data from the mean taken to some specified power (i.e., multiplied times itself a specified number of times). The moments about the mean are symbolized by the Greek letter κ (kappa) and named

---

[19] A normalized cumulative frequency polygon is part of the output of the BAHR program "Residual Analysis."

according to the power to which the difference between the data and the mean is taken. Thus, the first moment about the mean is equal to the following:

$$\kappa_1 = \frac{\sum_{i=1}^{N}(Y_i - \mu)^1}{N} = 0 \tag{13.2}$$

By definition, the mean is the point in a distribution at which the deviations above and below add to 0, as we discussed in Chapter 2. Since the mean is the "center of gravity" of a distribution with an equal "weight" of data above and below it, the first moment about the mean is equal to 0 for any distribution. The second moment about the mean, on the other hand, is not equal to 0 (unless all the data are equal to the mean in a distribution). This is because squaring deviations from the mean creates positive differences for data values that are below the mean as well as data values that are above the mean. The second moment about the mean is shown in Equation (13.3).

$$\kappa_2 = \frac{\sum_{i=1}^{N}(Y_i - \mu)^2}{N} = \sigma^2 \tag{13.3}$$

This second moment about the mean is not new to us. It is the variance of the data in the distribution. The third moment about the mean, however, is something we have yet to encounter (Equation (13.4)).

$$\kappa_3 = \frac{\sum_{i=1}^{N}(Y_i - \mu)^3}{N} \tag{13.4}$$

The third moment about the mean is equal to 0 only if a distribution is symmetric. For positively skewed distributions, the third moment about the mean is greater than 0. For negatively skewed distributions, this moment about the mean is less than 0.[20] The more skewed a distribution is, the larger the value (in either a positive or negative direction) of the third moment about the mean. Thus, we can use the third moment about the mean as a numeric indication of how skewed a distribution is.

There is one drawback of using the third moment about the mean to indicate how skewed a distribution is. The drawback is that, when the moment is not equal to 0, the numeric value of this moment is a function of two things: the degree to which the distribution of data is skewed and the scale of measurement of the data. To create a value that reflects only the degree to which the data are skewed, we need to remove the scale of measurement. A dimensionless value is usually calculated by dividing the third moment about the mean by the cube of the standard deviation of the data

---

[20]This is the origin of the terms "positively" skewed and "negatively" skewed. We use these terms to indicate positivity or negativity of the third moment about the mean.

(Equation (13.5)). This dimensionless form of the third moment about the mean is most often called the **skewness** of the distribution.

$$\text{Skewness} = \frac{\kappa_3}{\sigma^3} \tag{13.5}$$

Equations (13.4) and (13.5) show how the third moment about the mean and the skewness of the distribution would be calculated from the population's data. In practice, we will never make those calculations since we will never be able to observe the entire population. Thus, I have not shown you Equations (13.4) and (13.5) expecting that you will ever use them in a calculation. Rather, those equations help us to understand what is being estimated by the calculations that are actually performed on a sample's data.

If we used Equations (13.4) and (13.5) on the sample's data, we would obtain an estimate of the skewness of the data in the population that is biased. That estimate would be biased for the same reason that the sample's estimate of the variance of the data in the population would be biased if we used the equation for the population's variance in a calculation of the sample's data. We learned in Chapter 3 that the sample's estimate of the variance of the data in the population must be corrected for bias by dividing the sum of the squared differences between the data and the mean by $n - 1$ rather than by n. Dividing by $n - 1$ corrects for a bias that results from the absence of extreme data values in most samples. Likewise, when we estimate the third moment about the mean in the population using data in the sample, we need to correct the bias that would result from the absence of extreme data values in the sample. Since the third moment about the mean is more complicated, the correction for this bias is a little more complicated than the correction used to estimate the variance of the data. Equation (13.6) illustrates the corrected calculation for the third moment about the mean.[21]

$$\kappa_3 \triangleq k_3 = \frac{n \cdot \sum_{i=1}^{n} (Y_i - \overline{Y})^3}{(n - 1) \cdot (n - 2)} \tag{13.6}$$

Then, the sample's estimate of the skewness in the population is calculated by dividing the sample's estimate of the third moment about the mean (from Equation (13.6)) by the cube of the sample's estimate of the standard deviation of data in the population.

$$\widehat{\text{Skewness}} = \frac{k_3}{s^3} \tag{13.7}$$

We will take a look at an example of how to calculate and interpret this numeric value that indicates the degree of asymmetry of a distribution in a moment. Before

[21] Note that the sample's estimate of the third moment about the mean is symbolized by the letter k rather than by κ. This is consistent with the usual convention of using Greek letters to represent the population's parameters and English letters for the sample's estimates.

we do that, however, let us take a look at the fourth moment about the mean (Equation (13.8)).

$$\kappa_4 = \frac{\sum_{i=1}^{N}(Y_i - \mu)^4}{N} \tag{13.8}$$

This fourth moment about the mean is a measure of the degree to which a distribution is mesokurtic. For a mesokurtic distribution, the fourth moment about the mean divided by the fourth power of the standard deviation of the data is equal to 3.[22] To develop a dimensionless measure of **kurtosis**, the fourth moment about the mean is divided by the fourth power of the standard deviation of the data. It is usual to subtract 3 from this dimensionless measure so that a mesokurtic distribution has a kurtosis value of 0 (parallel to a skewness value of 0 for a symmetric distribution). With that adjustment, a negative value for kurtosis indicates a platykurtic distribution and a positive value for kurtosis indicates a leptokurtic distribution.

$$\text{Kurtosis} = \frac{\kappa_4}{\sigma^4} - 3 \tag{13.9}$$

The sample's estimates of the population's fourth moment about the mean and kurtosis are shown in Equations (13.10) and (13.11).

$$\kappa_4 \triangleq k_4 = \frac{\frac{\sum_{i=1}^{n}(Y_i - \overline{Y})^4 \cdot n \cdot (n+1)}{n-1} - \left(\sum_{i=1}^{n}Y_i - \overline{Y})^2\right)^2}{(n-2)\cdot(n-3)} \tag{13.10}$$

$$\widehat{\text{Kurtosis}} = \frac{k_4}{s^4} - 3 \tag{13.11}$$

Now, let us take a look at an example of how we can use skewness and kurtosis to investigate the distribution of data.[23]

■ EXAMPLE 13.4

Estimate the skewness and kurtosis of the distributions of weight and height in the population from which the sample in Example 13.1 was drawn. How do these numeric values compare to the impressions derived from examination of the normalized cumulative proportion polygons in Example 13.3?

To calculate estimates of skewness and kurtosis, we need to calculate the differences between the observations and the mean to the second, third, and fourth powers. These calculations are summarized for weight in the following table:

---

[22] Thus, the mathematic definition of a mesokurtic distribution is one in which the fourth moment about the mean is three times as large as the fourth power of the standard deviation.

[23] Sample estimates of skewness and kurtosis and their confidence intervals are calculated in the BAHR program "Residual Analysis."

Weight (Y)	($Y_i - \overline{Y}$)	($Y_i - \overline{Y})^2$	($Y_i - \overline{Y})^3$	($Y_i - \overline{Y})^4$
12	−18.4	338.56	−6,229.50	114,622.87
16	−14.4	207.36	−2,985.98	42,998.17
18	−12.4	153.76	−1,906.62	23,642.14
20	−9.4	88.36	−830.58	7,807.49
22	−8.4	70.56	−592.70	4,978.71
24	−6.4	40.96	−262.14	1,677.72
25	−5.4	29.16	−157.46	850.31
27	−3.4	11.56	−39.30	133.63
28	−2.4	5.76	−13.82	33.18
29	−1.4	1.96	−2.74	3.84
31	0.6	0.36	0.22	0.13
32	1.6	2.56	4.10	6.55
34	3.6	12.96	46.66	167.96
35	4.6	21.96	97.34	447.75
36	5.6	31.36	175.62	983.45
38	7.6	57.76	438.98	3,336.22
40	9.6	92.16	884.74	8,493.47
43	12.6	158.76	2,000.38	25,204.74
47	16.6	275.56	4,574.30	75,933.31
50	19.6	384.16	7,529.54	147,578.91
Sum 607	0.0	2,004.55	2,730.96	458,900.54

The sample's estimates of the mean and the standard deviation for the children's weights are equal to the following:

$$\overline{Y} = \frac{\sum\limits_{i=1}^{n} Y_i}{n} = \frac{607}{20} = 30.35 \text{ kg}$$

$$s = \sqrt{\frac{\sum\limits_{i=1}^{n} (Y_i - \overline{Y})^2}{n-1}} = \sqrt{\frac{2,004.55}{20-1}} = 10.27 \text{ kg}$$

To estimate the skewness of the distribution of data in the population we use Equations (13.6) and (13.7).

$$k_3 = \frac{n \cdot \sum\limits_{i=1}^{n} (Y_i - \overline{Y})^3}{(n-1) \cdot (n-2)} = \frac{20 \cdot 2,730.96}{(20-1) \cdot (20-2)} = 159.71 \text{ kg}^3$$

$$\widehat{\text{skewness}} = \frac{k_3}{s^3} = \frac{159.71}{10.22^3} = 0.15$$

To estimate the kurtosis of the distribution of data in the population we use Equations (13.10) and (13.11).

$$k_4 = \frac{\dfrac{\sum\limits_{i=1}^{n}(Y_i - \overline{Y})^4 \cdot n \cdot (n+1)}{n-1} - \left(\sum\limits_{i=1}^{n}(Y_i - \overline{Y})^2\right)^2}{(n-2)\cdot(n-3)}$$

$$= \frac{\dfrac{458,900.54 \cdot 20 \cdot (20+1)}{20-1} - 1,984.80^2}{(n-2)\cdot(n-3)} = 20,276.75 \text{ kg}^4$$

$$\widehat{\text{kurtosis}} = \frac{k_4}{s^4} - 3 = \frac{20,276.75}{10.22^4} - 3 = -1.14$$

When we examined the normalized cumulative proportion polygon for weight, we saw a relationship that was very nearly a straight line. If that implies that the distribution of weights is very close to being a Gaussian distribution, then a skewness of 0.15 and a kurtosis of −1.14 must not be sufficiently far from 0 for us to suspect that a distribution is very different from a Gaussian distribution.[24]

Now, let us prepare to estimate the skewness and kurtosis for height.

Height (Y)	$(Y_i - \overline{Y})$	$(Y_i - \overline{Y})^2$	$(Y_i - \overline{Y})^3$	$(Y_i - \overline{Y})^4$
80	−37.7	1,421.29	−53,582.63	2,020,065.26
86	−31.7	1,004.89	−31.855.01	1,009,803.91
91	−26.7	712.89	−19,034.16	508,212.15
95	−22.7	515.29	−11,697.08	265,523.78
98	−19.7	388.09	−7,645.37	150,613.85
101	−16.7	278.89	−4,657.46	77,779.63
104	−13.7	187.69	−2,571.35	35,227.54
107	−10.7	114.49	−1,225.04	13,107.96
110	−7.7	59.29	−456.53	3,515.30
113	−4.7	22.09	−103.82	487.97
116	−1.7	2.89	-4.91	8.35
119	1.3	1.69	2.20	2.86
123	5.3	28.09	148.88	789.05
126	8.3	68.89	571.79	4,745.83
130	12.3	151.29	1,860.87	22,888.66
135	17.3	299.29	5,177.72	89,574.50
141	23.3	542.89	12,649.34	294,729.55
148	30.3	918.09	27,818.13	842,889.25
160	42.3	1,789.29	75,686.97	3,201,558.70
171	53.3	2,840.89	151,419.44	8,070,655.99
Sum 2,354	0.0	11,348.20	142,501.92	16,612,180.11

[24] A rule of thumb for skewness is that values between −1 and +1 indicate a distribution that is essentially symmetric. There is no established rule of thumb for kurtosis.

The sample's estimates of the mean and the standard deviation for the children's height are equal to the following:

$$\overline{Y} = \frac{\sum\limits_{i=1}^{n} Y_i}{n} = \frac{2,354}{20} = 117.7 \, cm$$

$$s = \sqrt{\frac{\sum\limits_{i=1}^{n} (Y_i - Y)^2}{n - 1}} = \sqrt{\frac{11,348.20}{20 - 1}} = 24.44$$

To estimate the skewness of the distribution of data in the population we use Equations (13.6) and (13.7).

$$k_3 = \frac{n \cdot \sum\limits_{i=1}^{n} (Y_i - \overline{Y})^3}{(n-1) \cdot (n-2)} = \frac{20 \cdot 142,501.92}{(20-1) \cdot (20-2)} = 8,333.45 \, cm^3$$

$$\widehat{skewness} = \frac{k_3}{s^3} = \frac{8,333.45}{24.44^3} = 0.57$$

To estimate the kurtosis of the distribution of data in the population we use Equations (13.10) and (13.11).

$$k_4 = \frac{\dfrac{\sum\limits_{i=1}^{n} (Y_i - \overline{Y})^4 \cdot n \cdot (n+1)}{n-1} - \left(\sum\limits_{i=1}^{n} Y_i - \overline{Y})^2\right)^2}{(n-2) \cdot (n-3)}$$

$$= \frac{\dfrac{16,612,180.11 \cdot 20 \cdot (20+1)}{20-1} - 11,348.20^2}{(20-2) \cdot (20-3)} = 779,199.25 \, cm^4$$

$$\widehat{kurtosis} = \frac{k_4}{s^4} - 3 = \frac{779,199.25}{24.44^4} - 3 = -0.82$$

When we examined the histogram and the normalized cumulative proportion polygon for height, we saw a relationship that was positively skewed. Thus, a skewness of 0.57 must be a large enough value to be detectable in a normalized cumulative proportion polygon. The kurtosis of −0.82 is closer to 0 than the value for weight and, therefore, must not be an indication of a distribution that is very different from a mesokurtic distribution.

Now, let us take a look at skewness and kurtosis calculated by Excel. These are part of the output provided by the "Descriptive Statistics" program in "Data Analysis." The following is the output we obtain for these data:

Weight		Height	
Mean	30.35	Mean	117.7
Standard error	2.29676546	Standard error	5.464767535
Median	30	Median	114.5
Mode	#N/A	Mode	#N/A
Standard deviation	10.27144739	Standard deviation	24.43918338
Sample variance	105.5026316	Sample variance	597.2736842
Kurtosis	−0.532319346	Kurtosis	−0.175230042
Skewness	0.147720803	Skewness	0.570905905
Range	38	Range	91
Minimum	12	Minimum	80
Maximum	50	Maximum	171
Sum	607	Sum	2354
Count	20	Count	20

These values are not exactly the same as the ones we calculated. This is because Excel uses the formulae for populations. Thus, the estimates provided by Excel's "Descriptive Statistics" program are biased (underestimated).[25] This bias affects the estimate of skewness much less than the estimate of kurtosis. ∎

In the previous example, we saw how we can calculate and interpret numeric values that indicate the degree of skewness and kurtosis of a distribution. You might have been concerned, however, that the interpretation of skewness and kurtosis in that example was somewhat informal. In fact, you might have that same impression about all the methods that we have used so far to infer from the sample's observations whether or not the population's distribution of data is a Gaussian distribution. If so, you might be pleased to know that it is possible to formally test the null hypothesis that the population's distribution of data is a Gaussian distribution or to test the null hypothesis that the skewness and kurtosis are equal to 0 in the population. This is an example of the third approach to evaluating the assumption of a Gaussian sampling distribution when the sample is too small to rely on the central limit theorem. Next, we will take a look at this approach of hypothesis testing. When we are done, we will examine how these hypothesis tests can aid us in making a decision about the propriety of the assumption that the distribution of estimates of the mean from all possible samples of a given size is a Gaussian distribution.

[25]Skewness and kurtosis calculated by the BAHR program "Residual Analysis" are the sample's estimates and, thus, are unbiased.

One way that we can use the process of statistical hypothesis testing to examine the type of distribution that the data in the population have is by comparing the sample's distribution of data to a theoretical distribution of a known type. The statistical hypothesis testing procedures that are used in this application are called **goodness-of-fit** tests. The theoretical distribution to which we compare the sample's data in a goodness-of-fit test can be any sort of distribution, but we will limit our interest here to the Gaussian distribution.

We have seen previously that we have a choice of which of the representations of the distribution of data in the sample we will compare to a Gaussian distribution. One choice is to compare the data as presented in a histogram (Example 13.1). In this approach, the actual number of data values we observe in the sample corresponding to each interval of values is compared to the number we would have expected to observe in the sample if the population's distribution of data were a Gaussian distribution. The intervals that we use in this comparison are a little bit different from the intervals we might use in a histogram. The reason for a difference is that we want to compare observed and expected frequencies for the entire range of possible values. Thus, the lowest and highest intervals must be open ended. In other words, the lowest interval should include all values equal to or less than a specified value, and the upper interval should include all values equal to or greater than a specified value. Further, the upper and lower limits of all of the intervals should be selected so that no potential values are excluded from the distribution to which we will compare our sample. This is accomplished by specifying the upper limit of one interval as the lower limit of the next interval.[26]

We can calculate the frequencies that we would expect if the distribution of data in the population is a Gaussian distribution, using the estimates of the mean and the standard deviation of the data in the sample. If the sample came from a population with a Gaussian distribution, the expected proportion of data values in any interval can be calculated by finding the difference between the proportions of the standard normal distribution associated with the limits of the interval. This is a procedure that we first encountered in Chapter 2. Recall from that chapter that we can determine the proportion of standard normal deviates equal to or less than a value corresponding to Y, by finding the area in Table B.1 or by using Excel's "NORM.S.DIST" function for the standard normal deviate derived from the following calculation:

$$z = \frac{Y_i - \overline{Y}}{\sigma} \tag{13.12}$$

Once we have calculated the expected proportion of data values in each interval, we can calculate the expected number of values in the sample by multiplying

---

[26] It might appear that this strategy would create overlapping intervals, but recall from Chapter 3 that the probability for any single value in a continuous distribution is virtually 0. Thus, using the same value as the upper limit of one interval and as the lower limit of the next interval does not actually create an overlap.

the expected proportion by the sample's size. Now, we can test the null hypothesis that the sample was drawn from a population with a Gaussian distribution of data by comparing the observed and expected number of data values in the intervals. In Chapter 9, we learned that we can compare observed and expected frequencies in a 2×2 table by using the chi-square procedure. We do the same thing here. One difference is that the calculation of the chi-square statistic in the **chi-square goodness-of-fit test** usually involves more than four comparisons of observed and expected values.

$$\chi^2 = \sum \frac{(\text{Observed} - \text{Expected})^2}{\text{Expected}} \tag{13.13}$$

Another difference between the chi-square procedure for a 2×2 table and the chi-square goodness-of-fit test is in the number of degrees of freedom. The degrees of freedom associated with the chi-square goodness-of-fit test is one less than the number of intervals minus the number of parameters estimated for the theoretical distribution. Since a Gaussian distribution has two parameters (μ and σ), the degrees of freedom for the chi-square goodness-of-fit test, when used to test the null hypothesis that the distribution of data in the population is a Gaussian distribution, is equal to the number of intervals minus three.

For the chi-square goodness-of-fit test to work well, the intervals of data values should not be too narrow. That is to say, the intervals should be wide enough that the corresponding expected frequencies are not too small. None of the intervals should be associated with expected frequencies less than 1. Also, it is best if no more than 20% of the intervals have expected frequencies less than 5.

Now, let us see how the chi-square goodness-of-fit test might be used in the process of testing the assumption that the distribution of means estimated from all possible samples (i.e., the sampling distribution) is a Gaussian distribution.

■ EXAMPLE 13.5

For the observations in Example 13.1, test the null hypotheses that the distribution of weights and the distribution of heights are Gaussian distributions in the population from which the sample of 20 children was drawn. Allow a 5% chance of making a type I error.

First, let us consider the distribution of weight. The following table summarizes the intervals, observed frequencies, and the expected frequencies calculated using Equation (13.12). Since the chi-square goodness-of-fit test works best when all of the expected frequencies are greater than or equal to 1, the lowest interval has been constructed so that it contains the first two bars of the histogram in Example 13.1. There are not enough observations in this sample for us to create intervals so that at least 20% have expected frequencies greater than or equal to 5. For purposes of illustration of the chi-square goodness-of-fit test, we will ignore violation of this criterion here.

Interval	Observed Frequency	Standard Normal Deviate For Limit of Interval		Proportion Equal to or Less Than Limit of Interval		Expected Value for Interval	
		Lower	Upper	Lower	Upper	Proportion	Frequency
≤17	2	−∞	−1.31	0.0000	0.0951	0.0951	1.902
17–22	3	−1.31	−0.82	0.0951	0.2061	0.1110	2.220
22–27	3	−0.82	−0.33	0.2061	0.3707	0.1646	3.292
27–32	4	−0.33	0.16	0.3707	0.5636	0.1929	3.858
32–37	3	0.16	0.65	0.5636	0.7422	0.1786	3.572
37–42	2	0.65	1.13	0.7422	0.8708	0.1286	2.572
42–47	2	1.13	1.62	0.8708	0.9474	0.0766	1.532
≥47	1	1.62	+∞	0.9474	1.0000	0.0526	1.052
Sum	20					1.0000	20.000

Now, we can test the null hypothesis that the distribution of weight in the population is a Gaussian distribution by using the chi-square goodness-of-fit test to compare the observed and expected frequencies. Using Equation (13.13) we get the following result:

$$\chi^2 = \sum \frac{(\text{Observed–Expected})^2}{\text{Expected}}$$
$$= \frac{(2 - 1.902)^2}{1.902} + \frac{(3 - 2.220)^2}{2.220} + \cdots + \frac{(1 - 1.052)^2}{1.052} = 0.675$$

The degrees of freedom associated with this chi-square value are equal to the number of intervals (8) minus 3, or 5 degrees of freedom. From Table B.7, we find that a chi-square value corresponding to 5 degrees of freedom and an α of 0.05 is equal to 11.070. Since 0.675 is less than 11.070, we are unable to reject the null hypothesis that the distribution of weight in the population is a Gaussian distribution.

Next, let us consider the distribution of height. The following table summarizes the intervals, observed frequencies, and the expected frequencies calculated using Equation (13.12). Again, we have combined categories so that all the expected frequencies are at least equal to 1. In this case, the highest interval has been constructed so that it contains the last three bars of the histogram in Example 13.1.

Interval	Observed Frequency	Standard Normal Deviate For Limit of Interval		Proportion Equal to or Less Than Limit of Interval		Expected Value for Interval	
		Lower	Upper	Lower	Upper	Proportion	Frequency
≤80	1	−∞	−1.54	0.0000	0.0618	0.0618	1.236
80–90	1	−1.54	−1.13	0.0618	0.1292	0.0674	1.348
90–100	3	−1.13	−0.72	0.1292	0.2358	0.1066	2.132
100–110	4	−0.72	−0.32	0.2358	0.3745	0.1387	2.774
110–120	3	−0.32	0.09	0.3745	0.5359	0.1614	3.228
120–130	3	0.09	0.50	0.5359	0.6915	0.1556	3.112
130–140	1	0.50	0.91	0.6915	0.8186	0.1271	2.542
140–150	2	0.91	1.32	0.8186	0.9096	0.0880	1.760
≥150	2	1.23	+∞	0.9066	1.0000	0.0934	1.868
Sum	20					1.0000	20.000

Now, we can test the null hypothesis that the distribution of height in the population is a Gaussian distribution by using the chi-square goodness-of-fit test to compare the observed and expected frequencies. Using Equation (13.13) we get the following result:

$$\chi^2 = \sum \frac{(\text{Observed–Expected})^2}{\text{Expected}}$$

$$= \frac{(1 - 1.236)^2}{1.236} + \frac{(1 - 1.384)^2}{1.384} + \cdots + \frac{(2 - 1.868)^2}{1.868} = 2.028$$

The degrees of freedom associated with this chi-square value are equal to the number of intervals (9) minus 3, or 6 degrees of freedom. From Table B.7, we find that a chi-square value corresponding to six degrees of freedom and an α of 0.05 is equal to 12.592. Since 2.028 is less than 12.592, we are unable to reject the null hypothesis that the distribution of height in the population is a Gaussian distribution. ∎

For the same reasons that we were concerned about an informal interpretation of the distribution of data in the sample displayed in a histogram, we might be concerned about a test of statistical hypothesis testing that also relies on creation of intervals of data values by the data analyst. The solution to this concern for graphic representation of the distribution is to use a cumulative frequency polygon. The solution for statistical hypothesis testing is to use a test based on the cumulative frequencies. The most commonly used method to test the null hypothesis that the data in the population have a Gaussian distribution that examines cumulative frequencies is the **Kolmogorov–Smirnov goodness-of-fit test**.[27]

In the Kolmogorov–Smirnov goodness-of-fit test, cumulative frequencies are expressed as cumulative proportions by dividing each cumulative frequency for the sample's observations by the sample's size. These observed cumulative proportions are compared to cumulative proportions that would be expected if the population's data had a Gaussian distribution. To obtain those expected cumulative proportions, we use a process that is similar to the one that we used to obtain normalized cumulative frequencies. In the Kolmogorov–Smirnov procedure, we first convert each observation to the standard normal scale. This is done by using Equation (13.12). Then, we find (in Table B.1) or using Excel's "NORM.S.DIST" function the proportion of the standard normal distribution that corresponds to that standard normal deviate. As in calculation of normalized cumulative frequencies, we are interested in the proportion of the standard normal distribution that corresponds to a particular standard normal deviate or a smaller standard normal deviate. Thus, we are determining the proportion of the standard normal distribution to the left of a particular standard normal deviate.

The calculation of the test statistic for the Kolmogorov–Smirnov goodness-of-fit test involves subtracting expected cumulative proportions from observed cumulative proportions. For each expected cumulative proportion, we perform two subtractions. One of those is the difference between observed and expected cumulative proportions corresponding to a particular data value (symbolized by D').[28] Calculation of those values is shown in Equations (13.14) and (13.15).

$$D = \text{Observed}_i - \text{Expected}_i \qquad (13.14)$$

$$D' = \text{Observed}_{i-1} - \text{Expected}_i \qquad (13.15)$$

From all of the calculated values of D and D' we select the one with the highest absolute (i.e., ignoring the sign) value. That selected value is then compared to a value from Table B.12 corresponding to the selected level of α and the sample's size.[29] If the calculated test statistic is greater than or equal to the value in the table

---

[27]Like the chi-square goodness-of-fit test, the Kolmogorov–Smirnov goodness-of-fit test can be used to compare the observed cumulative proportions to those expected assuming any theoretical distribution. Our interest here is confined to the Gaussian distribution as the expected theoretical distribution.

[28]The reason we make these two calculations is that we are examining a distribution for continuous data (the Gaussian distribution) using discrete information (the cumulative frequency corresponding to a particular data value). As a result, we are not sure which discrete category of observed values is best compared to a particular category of expected values.

[29]If a theoretical distribution other than the Gaussian distribution s compared to the observed distribution, the results of the Kolmogorov–Smirnov goodness-of-fit test must be compared with values in a table that is somewhat different from Table B.12. The values in Table B.12 are particular to tests comparing the Gaussian distribution to the observed distribution. It is designed to maximize the statistical power for this particular comparison.

we can reject the null hypothesis that the distribution of data in the population is a Gaussian distribution. Let us take a look at this procedure in an example.

■ EXAMPLE 13.6

For the observations in Example 13.1, test the null hypothesis that the distribution of data in the population is a Gaussian distribution, using the Kolmogorov–Smirnov goodness-of-fit test. Allow a 5% chance of making a type I error.

To prepare to do the Kolmogorov–Smirnov goodness-of-fit test, we need to convert the cumulative frequencies to cumulative proportions, to calculate the expected cumulative proportions (under the assumption that the population from which the sample was drawn has a Gaussian distribution of data), and to calculate the absolute values of the differences between observed and expected cumulative proportions. Those procedures are summarized in the following table for weight.

Weight	Observed Cumulative Frequency	Observed Cumulative Proportion	Standard Normal Deviate	Expected Cumulative Proportion	$\lvert D \rvert$	$\lvert D' \rvert$
12	1	0.05	−1.787	0.037	0.013	
16	2	0.10	−1.397	0.081	0.019	0.031
18	3	0.15	−1.203	0.115	0.035	0.015
20	4	0.20	−1.008	0.157	0.043	0.007
22	5	0.25	−0.813	0.208	0.042	0.008
24	6	0.30	−0.618	0.268	0.032	0.018
25	7	0.35	−0.521	0.301	0.049	0.001
27	8	0.40	−0.326	0.372	0.028	0.022
28	9	0.45	−0.229	0.410	0.040	0.010
29	10	0.50	−0.131	0.448	0.052	0.002
31	11	0.55	0.063	0.525	0.025	0.025
32	12	0.60	0.161	0.564	0.036	0.014
34	13	0.65	0.355	0.639	0.011	0.039
35	14	0.70	0.453	0.675	0.025	0.025
36	15	0.75	0.550	0.709	0.041	0.009
38	16	0.80	0.745	0.772	0.028	0.022
40	17	0.85	0.940	0.826	0.024	0.026
43	18	0.90	1.232	0.891	0.009	0.041
47	19	0.95	1.621	0.948	0.002	0.048
50	20	1.00	1.913	0.972	0.028	0.022

The maximum value for D is 0.052. The maximum value for D' is 0.048. The Kolmogorov–Smirnov test statistic for weight is the larger of those two values (0.052). In Table B.12, we find the test statistic associated with an α of 0.05 and 20 observations is 0.192. Since 0.052 is smaller than 0.192, we cannot reject the null hypothesis that the distribution of data in the population is a Gaussian distribution.

Next, let us perform the same calculations for height. The following table summarizes those calculations.

Height	Observed Cumulative Frequency	Observed Cumulative Proportion	Standard Normal Deviate	Expected Cumulative Proportion	$|D|$	$|D'|$
80	1	0.05	−1.543	0.061	0.011	
86	2	0.10	−1.297	0.097	0.003	0.047
91	3	0.15	−1.093	0.137	0.013	0.037
95	4	0.20	−0.929	0.176	0.024	0.026
98	5	0.25	−0.806	0.210	0.040	0.010
101	6	0.30	−0.683	0.247	0.053	0.003
104	7	0.35	−0.561	0.288	0.062	0.012
107	8	0.40	−0.438	0.331	0.069	0.019
110	9	0.45	−0.315	0.376	0.074	0.024
113	10	0.50	−0.192	0.424	0.076	0.026
116	11	0.55	−0.070	0.472	0.078	0.028
119	12	0.60	0.053	0.521	0.079	0.029
123	13	0.65	0.217	0.586	0.064	0.014
126	14	0.70	0.340	0.633	0.067	0.017
130	15	0.75	0.503	0.693	0.057	0.007
135	16	0.80	0.708	0.760	0.040	0.010
141	17	0.85	0.953	0.830	0.020	0.030
148	18	0.90	1.240	0.892	0.008	0.042
160	19	0.95	1.731	0.958	0.008	0.058
171	20	1.00	2.181	0.985	0.015	0.035

In this table, the maximum value for D is 0.079 and the maximum value for D' is 0.0.061. The Kolmogorov–Smirnov test statistic for height is the larger of those two values (0.079). In Table B.12, we found that the test statistic associated with an α of 0.05 and 20 observations is equal to 0.192. Since 0.079 is smaller than 0.192, we cannot reject the null hypothesis that the distribution of height in the population is a Gaussian distribution.

This test can also be performed in Excel using the BAHR program "Residual Analysis" and in R using the "ks.test(data,"pnorm",mean,sd)" command where "data" is a vector of data values.[30]

---

[30] See Appendix E for how to create a vector.

```
>ks.test(Weight,"pnorm",30.35,10.27)

 One-sample Kolmogorov-Smirnov test

data:  Weight
D = 0.052291, p-value = 1
alternative hypothesis: two-sided
```

```
>ks.test(Height,"pnorm",117.7,24.44)

 One-sample Kolmogorov-Smirnov test

data:  Height
D = 0.07879, p-value = 0.9986
alternative hypothesis: two-sided
```

Those results are the same as our calculations. We fail to reject the null hypothesis that the distributions of weight and height are Gaussian distributions. Thus, we can be comfortable assuming a Gaussian sampling distribution. ∎

We have seen two different approaches to testing the null hypothesis that the distribution of data in the population is a Gaussian distribution. Both of these methods have been based on a comparison of observed and expected values for the distribution of data in the sample. Another hypothesis testing approach is based on measures of skewness and kurtosis. We will not examine that hypothesis test here, but confidence intervals for skewness and kurtosis are output from the BAHR program "Residual Analysis" that can be used to test hypotheses about skewness and kurtosis.

This brings us to a point at which we need to consider more thoroughly what takes place in tests of hypothesis testing and how they relate to the process of testing the assumption that the sampling distribution (i.e., the distribution of estimates of the mean from all possible samples of a given size) is a Gaussian distribution. The first fact that we should consider is that the null hypothesis in these tests of hypothesis testing is that the population's distribution of data is a Gaussian distribution. If we are unable to reject that null hypothesis, we will analyze the data as if the sampling distribution were a Gaussian distribution. In other words, we will draw the conclusion that the null hypothesis is true when we are unable to reject the null hypothesis. This is risking the type II error (i.e., accepting the null hypothesis as true when the null hypothesis is false). To keep the chance of making a type II error low, we need to maximize the statistical power. One of the most important influences on statistical power is the sample's size. Thus, tests of hypothesis testing that will lead to acceptance of the null hypothesis should be performed on large samples.

Keeping that issue in mind, let us recall why we are interested in testing a null hypothesis about the distribution of data in the population in the first place. A point that should be made clear is that statistical procedures *do not* assume that the data have a Gaussian distribution. Rather, they assume that estimates from all possible samples (of a given size) have a Gaussian distribution. We have been considering the distribution of data as part of our evaluation of the truth of this assumption only because we know that the sampling distribution will be a Gaussian distribution if the population's data have a Gaussian distribution. Further, we know from the central limit theorem that the sampling distribution will be a Gaussian distribution regardless of the distribution of data, if the sample is large enough.

Notice the two issues that are on conflict here. On the one hand, we are interested in evaluating whether or not the distribution of data in the population is a Gaussian distribution only when the sample's size is relatively small. On the other hand, when we use statistical hypothesis testing to evaluate that assumption, we will conclude that the assumption is satisfied when we are unable to reject the null hypothesis. To avoid making a type II error, we should be willing to conclude that the null hypothesis is true only if we have high statistical power. To have high statistical power, we need to have a large sample. When we have a large sample, we do not need to examine the distribution of data. Thus, tests of hypothesis testing about the distribution of data in the population only become helpful under conditions in which they are no longer needed.[31]

Because of this logical antagonism, many statisticians prefer to use the informal graphic approach, rather than the formal inferential approach, when evaluating the assumption that the sampling distribution is a Gaussian distribution. Unfortunately, interpretation of the graphic approach cannot be standardized in the way that statistical hypothesis testing can. Rather, its interpretation relies on an understanding of the central limit theorem and a feeling for how much the data can deviate from a Gaussian distribution, before a statistical procedure becomes invalid.

Our inability to provide specific guidelines for when we need to be concerned about violation of the assumption of a Gaussian sampling distribution might leave you anxious about evaluating this assumption. Unfortunately, this part of statistical analysis remains an art that requires practice. Fortunately, the statistical procedures for continuous dependent variables with which we are familiar can tolerate a fair degree of deviation from a Gaussian distribution.[32] In statistical terminology, we say that those procedures are **robust** as far as the assumption of a Gaussian distribution

---

[31] We need to draw a conclusion about the distribution of data in the population only if our sample's size is small. With small samples, there is a good chance we will be incorrect in concluding from a hypothesis test that the data have a Gaussian distribution. The smaller the sample, the greater the chance of making this mistake. At the same time, smaller samples are in greater danger of violating the assumption that the sampling distribution is a Gaussian distribution. This is because the smaller the sample, the more having a Gaussian distribution depends on the distribution of data in the population.

[32] In other words, the probabilities of making type I and type II errors are nearly the same for distributions that are similar, but not identical, to a Gaussian distribution as the probabilities of those errors would be if the distribution actually were a Gaussian distribution.

is concerned. When a sample suggests too great a violation of the assumption of a Gaussian distribution, there are a number of things we can do. We will discuss those in a little bit, but first let us see how we can apply what we have learned so far to bivariable and multivariable samples.

13.1.1.2 *Bivariable and Multivariable Analyses.* So far, we have considered the assumption of a Gaussian distribution of estimates from all possible samples of a given size only for univariable data sets. Now, let us see how this assumption applies to bivariable and multivariable data sets and how we can evaluate the assumption when we have one or more independent variables. To begin, let us think about a bivariable data set in which the independent variable represents nominal data. In Chapter 7, we learned that a nominal independent variable has the effect of separating dependent variable values into two groups. We also learned that statistical hypothesis testing and interval estimation for this sort of data set involves Student's t-distribution to examine the difference between the means of the dependent variable values in the two groups. Thus, the estimates for which we assume a Gaussian distribution are the differences between means from all possible samples of a given size.

The central limit theorem applies to the distribution of estimates of the difference between means from all possible samples of a given size, in much the same way that it applies to the sampling distribution of estimates of the mean from univariable data sets. Specifically, the sampling distribution of estimates of the differences between means will be a Gaussian distribution if each of the two groups of data (represented by the dependent variable) have a Gaussian distribution, or if the sample's size is sufficiently large. One way in which the central limit theorem is applied differently to differences between means, however, is that a rule of thumb for how large a sample should be to result in a Gaussian sampling distribution is more difficult to specify. To achieve the same level of conservatism that we had when we used a sample's size of 30 for a univariable sample we would need a sample with more than 30 observations in a bivariable sample. How many more observations would be required is not easy to declare.

For a bivariable sample with a nominal independent variable, we would need more than 30 observations overall but not as many as 30 observations in each of the 2 groups specified by values of the independent variable. Which sample's size within this interval of sample's sizes corresponds to a univariable sample with 30 observations depends, in part, on how the number of observations in the bivariable sample are apportioned between the 2 groups. For bivariable samples in which the independent variable represents continuous data, or for multivariable samples, the situation is more complex. One rule of thumb is to require an additional 10 observations for each independent variable.

As we apply the central limit theorem to differences between means, it is important to remember that we do not expect all of the dependent variable values taken together to have a Gaussian distribution. Rather, the distribution of estimates of the difference between means will be a Gaussian distribution if the dependent variable values within each of the two groups have a Gaussian distribution. Therefore, when our sample is too small for us to be comfortable relying on the central limit theorem, we need to think about the distribution of data represented by the dependent variable separately for each value of the independent variable.

This presents a problem. When examining the distribution of data in a univariable sample, we found that a small sample can make interpretation of the distribution difficult.[33] Now, we are suggesting that we must examine two distributions from a small sample. If we truly considered the two distributions of dependent variable values separately, we are likely to have too few observations to evaluate those distributions with any reasonable degree of confidence.

This is not the first time we have faced this problem. In Chapter 7, we were concerned with estimation of the variance of data represented by the dependent variable when we had two groups of dependent variable values in Student's t-test for the difference between means. In that case, we assumed that the variance of data was the same in the two distributions and we used all of the sample's data to calculate a pooled estimate of that variance. We can take a similar approach here. If we assume that the two distributions differ only in their locations,[34] we could adjust the dependent variable values so that their distributions have the same location. Once we do that, we can use all of the dependent variable values in the sample simultaneously to evaluate the distribution of data. A straightforward way to adjust the dependent variable values is to subtract the mean of each group from each of the values in that group. Then, the two distributions will both have an adjusted mean equal to 0. Equation (13.16) shows how adjusted dependent variable values in group j are calculated for observation i in a bivariable sample containing a nominal independent variable.

$$\text{Adjusted } Y_{ij} = Y_{ij} - \overline{Y}_j \tag{13.16}$$

The following example demonstrates that procedure and how all of the dependent variable values in a bivariable sample can be used to evaluate the distribution of data.

---

[33]This is true regardless of which approach to evaluating the assumption of a Gaussian distribution is used. In the recommended graphic approach, smaller samples make it more difficult to conclude that deviations from a Gaussian distribution indicate a distribution in the population that is not a Gaussian distribution rather than solely the result of chance.

[34]This is an assumption we usually make for bivariable or multivariable analysis of a continuous dependent variable. We will discuss this assumption a little later in this chapter.

■ EXAMPLE 13.7

Suppose we measured diastolic blood pressure in a group of 10 untreated and 10 treated persons and observed the following results:

Treated	Untreated
80	94
82	96
85	97
88	98
90	99
91	102
92	103
95	104
96	110
98	112

We plan to test the null hypothesis that the difference between the mean diastolic blood pressure values in those two groups is equal to 0, using Student's *t*-distribution. In doing so, we will be assuming that the distribution of estimates of the difference between those means from all possible samples containing 20 observations is a Gaussian distribution. Evaluate that assumption based on the observations in this sample.

First, we consider the size of the sample to determine if it is large enough that the principle in the central limit theorem will produce a Gaussian distribution of estimates of the difference between the means from all possible samples (i.e., a Gaussian sampling distribution). A total of 20 observations (10 in each group) is too few for us to be able to rely on the central limit theorem. Thus, we need to draw a conclusion about the distribution of data (represented by the dependent variable) to determine if the sampling distribution might be a Gaussian distribution due to a Gaussian distribution of data in the population.

To draw a conclusion about the distribution of data in the population, we examine the distribution of data in the sample. To begin examining the distribution of diastolic blood pressure values in this sample, we calculate the mean diastolic blood pressure for each of the two groups. We find that the mean for the treated group is equal to 89.7 mmHg and that the mean for the untreated group is equal to 101.5 mmHg. Then, we calculate adjusted values for each of the dependent variable values in the sample using Equation (13.16). We do that by subtracting the group's mean from each value in the group. The following table shows those adjusted values:

Treated			Untreated	
Unadjusted	Adjusted		Unadjusted	Adjusted
80	−9.7		94	−7.5
82	−7.7		96	−5.5
85	−4.7		97	−4.5
88	−1.7		98	−3.5
90	0.3		99	−2.5
91	1.3		102	0.5
92	2.3		103	1.5
95	5.3		104	2.5
96	6.3		110	8.5
98	8.3		112	10.5

Now, we can use any of the previously discussed methods for examining the distribution of data to examine the distribution of adjusted dependent variable values in this sample. Most statisticians would do this by constructing a normalized cumulative proportion polygon. The following table summarizes the calculations necessary to construct this graphic display:

Group	Adjusted Value	Cumulative Frequency	Cumulative Proportion	Normalized Value
Treated	−9.7	1	0.050	−1.64
Treated	−7.7	2	0.100	−1.28
Untreated	−7.5	3	0.150	−1.04
Untreated	−5.5	4	0.200	−0.84
Treated	−4.7	5	0.250	−0.67
Untreated	−4.5	6	0.300	−0.52
Untreated	−3.5	7	0.350	−0.39
Untreated	−2.5	8	0.400	−0.25
Treated	−1.7	9	0.450	−0.13
Treated	0.3	10	0.500	0.00
Untreated	0.5	11	0.550	+0.13
Treated	1.3	12	0.600	+0.25
Untreated	1.5	13	0.650	+0.39
Treated	2.3	14	0.700	+0.52
Untreated	2.5	15	0.750	+0.67
Treated	5.3	16	0.800	+0.84
Treated	6.3	17	0.850	+1.04
Treated	8.3	18	0.900	+1.28
Untreated	8.5	19	0.950	+1.64
Untreated	10.5	20	0.975*	+1.96

*Calculated using Equation (13.1).

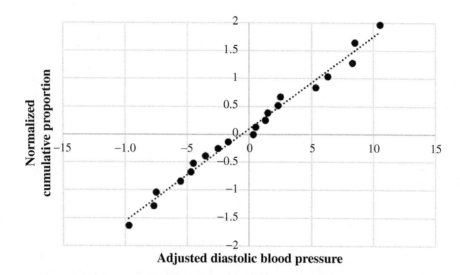

Adjusted diastolic blood pressure

Finally, we use those normalized values is a graphic comparison with the adjusted data values. That normalized cumulative proportion polygon appears to be very close to a straight line. This implies that the distribution of data in the sample is very close to a Gaussian distribution, and, therefore, that the distribution of data in the population is likely to be a Gaussian distribution. If the data in the population have a Gaussian distribution, so will the estimates of differences between means from all possible samples of this size. Thus, we can be comfortable concerning the assumption of Student's t-procedure that the sampling distribution for samples with 20 observations is a Gaussian distribution.   ∎

For bivariable samples that have a continuous independent variable, or for multivariable samples, the distributional assumption is parallel to the one we have just considered for a bivariable sample with a nominal independent variable. Specifically, we assume that estimates from all possible samples of a given size have a Gaussian distribution. This is assumed for continuous dependent variables regardless of whether the estimate is of the slope, intercept, correlation coefficient, or any other measure we have discussed for continuous dependent variables. Also, the central limit theorem applies to distributions of all of these estimates.[35] That implies that we can assume that the distribution of any of those estimates is a Gaussian distribution, if we have a large sample. Further, it implies that, for smaller samples, we need to be concerned about the distribution of data represented by the dependent variable.

---

[35]For some estimates, there are special conditions under which the distribution of estimates is expected to be a Gaussian distribution as a result of the principle in the central limit theorem. For instance, the distribution of estimates of Pearson's correlation is expected to be a Gaussian distribution only if the correlation coefficient in the population is equal to 0.

When we have one or more independent variables representing continuous data it becomes impossible, not just less efficient, to evaluate the distribution of data represented by the dependent variable corresponding to each value of the independent variable(s). Thus, it becomes even more important that we have a method of adjusting the dependent variable values in a sample so that they represent a single distribution of data. Although it might at first seem that we need a different approach for continuous independent variables, the approach is the same for all data sets with a continuous dependent variable regardless of the number of independent variables or the type of data they represent.

To understand why this is true, let us think a little bit more about what we did when we adjusted the dependent variable values in a bivariable data set with a nominal independent variable. By subtracting the mean of each group, we were really subtracting our single best guess for the value of the dependent variable corresponding to a specific value of the independent variable. In regression analysis, a parallel procedure would be to subtract the value of the dependent variable estimated from the regression equation $(\widehat{Y}_i)$ from each observed value of the dependent variable (Y_i). This calculation is illustrated in the following equation:

$$\text{Adjusted } Y_i = Y_i - \widehat{Y}_i \qquad (13.17)$$

If this looks familiar to you, it is because we have encountered this difference before. In regression analysis, this difference is called the **residual**.[36],[37] When we subtracted the group's mean from each observation in the groups specified by values of a nominal independent variable, we actually were calculating the residuals just as we did in previous chapters when performing regression analysis.[38]

Thus, the way that we draw conclusions about the distribution of data in the population is by examining the distribution of residuals in the sample.

This is illustrated for a multivariable data set in the following example.

■ EXAMPLE 13.8

Suppose that the data introduced in Example 13.1 are part of the data collected in a study designed to estimate weight from information on height and age (in years). The following table lists the ages of the children in this sample as well as their weights and heights:

---

[36] In Chapter 7, we found the method of least squares in regression analysis estimated the parameters of the straight line that minimized the squared residuals was called the residual sum of squares.

[37] In regression analysis on Excel, you can get the residuals by checking the "Residuals" box at the bottom of the "regression" dialog box. This will also give you the estimated values.

[38] This should not surprise you if you recall the discussion of the general linear model at the end of Chapter 10. In that discussion, we learned all the procedures we use for continuous dependent variables can be expressed as regression equations.

Child	Weight	Height	Age	Child	Weight	Height	Age
OO	24	101	5	ST	31	116	7
HY	38	135	10	AT	28	110	7
OU	47	160	13	IS	34	123	9
AR	50	171	15	TI	25	104	6
EB	22	98	5	CS	36	130	10
AC	12	80	3	AS	16	86	3
KF	35	126	10	AS	40	141	11
OR	27	107	6	TU	43	148	12
MO	32	119	8	DE	18	91	4
RE	29	113	7	NT	20	95	5

Now, suppose that we performed a multiple regression analysis on these data and obtained the following regression equation:

$$\widehat{WGT} = -15.7769 + (0.367948 \cdot HGT) + (0.361461 \cdot AGE)$$

Evaluate the assumption that estimates from all possible samples of this size would have a Gaussian distribution.

First, let us consider how this assumption applies to multiple regression analysis. The estimates we are making are the regression coefficients. Thus, by using the usual methods to test null hypotheses about those coefficients, we are assuming that the distributions of estimates of the regression coefficients corresponding to each independent variable are Gaussian distributions. That assumption will be satisfied either if we have a large enough sample or if the unexplained portion of the dependent variable (i.e., the residuals) have a Gaussian distribution in the population.

A sample's size of 20 is not large enough for us to be comfortable that the principle in the central limit theorem will ensure that the sampling distribution is a Gaussian distribution. Thus, we need to hope that the distribution of residuals in the population is a Gaussian distribution.

To draw a conclusion about the distribution of residuals in the population, we need to evaluate the distribution of residuals in the sample. We begin this evaluation by calculating the dependent variable values (i.e., the children's weights) that are estimated from values of the independent variables (i.e., heights and ages) by substituting the sample's independent variable values in the regression equation. The residuals are the differences between the estimated values of the children's weights and the observed values of the children's weights. This process is summarized in the following table in which the data have been arranged in increasing order of magnitude of the dependent variable:[39]

Weight (kg)	Height (cm)	Age (yr)	Estimated Weight	Residual
12	80	3	14.9	−2.9
16	86	3	17.0	−1.0
18	91	4	19.2	−1.2
20	95	5	21.1	−0.1
22	98	5	22.2	−0.2
24	101	5	23.2	0.8
25	104	6	24.7	0.3
27	107	6	25.8	1.2
28	110	7	27.3	0.7
29	113	7	28.4	0.6
31	116	7	29.4	1.6
32	119	8	31.0	1.0
34	123	9	32.8	1.2
35	126	10	34.3	0.7
36	130	10	35.7	0.3
38	135	10	37.5	0.5
40	141	11	40.1	−0.1
43	148	12	43.0	0.0
47	160	13	47.7	−0.7
50	171	15	52.5	−2.5

Next, we need to examine the distribution of those residuals. We could use any of the methods we have discussed for this examination. The method we choose is the graphic examination of the normalized cumulative frequencies. To prepare to construct a normalized cumulative proportion polygon, we need to express the cumulative frequencies as cumulative proportions and determine the standard normal deviate that corresponds to that proportion of the standard normal distribution. This process requires that we first sort the residuals in order of their magnitude.

[39]Estimated values and residuals can be obtained in Excel's "Regression" program by checking the "Residuals" box in the "Regression" form.

Residual	Cumulative Frequency	Cumulative Proportion	Normalized Value
−2.9	1	0.050	−1.64
−2.5	2	0.100	−1.28
−1.2	3	0.150	−1.04
−1.0	4	0.200	−0.84
−0.7	5	0.250	−0.67
−0.2	6	0.300	−0.52
−0.1	8	0.400	−0.25
0.0	9	0.450	−0.13
0.3	11	0.550	+0.13
0.5	12	0.600	+0.25
0.6	13	0.650	+0.39
0.7	15	0.750	+0.67
0.8	16	0.800	+0.84
1.0	17	0.850	+1.04
1.2	19	0.950	+1.64
1.6	20	0.975*	+1.96

*Calculated using Equation (13.1).

Finally, we use those normalized values in a graphic comparison with residual value as shown:

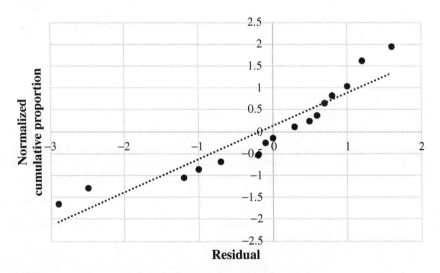

Notice that this normalized cumulative proportion polygon is less suggestive of a Gaussian distribution than the normalized cumulative proportion polygon for the children's weight alone in Example 13.3. Thus, it is possible for a dependent variable that has by itself a Gaussian distribution to have a distribution of its unexplained portion in a multivariable analysis that is not a Gaussian distribution.

This illustrates an important principle. We need to understand that, in bivariable and multivariable analyses, satisfaction of the assumption of a Gaussian distribution of estimates from all possible samples of a given size is not satisfied by a Gaussian distribution of data represented by the dependent variable. Rather, the assumption of a Gaussian distribution of estimates depends, in small samples, on the distribution of residuals in the population. Therefore, we need to examine the distribution of the residuals in small samples to draw a conclusion about the distribution of residuals in the population.   ■

Now, we must ask ourselves what we should do if we have a small sample in which the distribution of continuous dependent variable values (i.e., residuals for bivariable or multivariable data sets) seem to deviate enough from a Gaussian distribution, so that we are concerned about the assumption that the distribution of estimates from all possible samples of that size is a Gaussian distribution. Actually, we have two choices. One choice is to convert the continuous dependent variable into an ordinal dependent variable. Then we could perform a parallel analytic procedure, if one exists, designed for an ordinal dependent variable. The advantage to this approach is that procedures for ordinal dependent variables do not assume a Gaussian distribution (or any particular distribution) for sample's estimates of the population's parameters. In fact, procedures for ordinal dependent variables are not based on a population's parameters at all. This is why they are called nonparametric procedures. We encountered nonparametric procedures in Chapters 5, 8, and 11.

A disadvantage to this approach is that nonparametric procedures generally have lower statistical power than the corresponding procedure for a continuous dependent variable. More importantly, some procedures for continuous dependent variables do not have nonparametric parallels. An important example is regression analysis. Further, a nonparametric procedure that we think of as being parallel to a procedure for a continuous dependent variable generally has important differences in interpretation. Consider, for instance, correlation analysis. We learned in Chapter 8 that Spearman's correlation analysis can be thought of as a nonparametric parallel to Pearson's correlation analysis. The parallel is strained, however, in the interpretation of the coefficients estimated in those two types of correlation analysis. Pearson's correlation coefficient addresses the strength of the linear relationship between two variables while Spearman's correlation coefficient examines a trend.

13.1.2 Transforming Dependent Variables

So, it is not always possible, and sometimes not desirable, to convert continuous data to an ordinal scale and use a nonparametric procedure to circumvent the assumption of a Gaussian sampling distribution. There is an alternative approach, however. This approach involves mathematically expressing the data represented by the dependent variable in a different way. These mathematical manipulations are called **transformations** of the dependent variable.

The logic behind performing transformations of the dependent variable is that if data represented by the dependent variable on its original scale of measurement do not have a Gaussian distribution (or if the residuals do not have a Gaussian distribution), perhaps those data (or residuals) will have a Gaussian distribution if the data represented by the dependent variable are expressed on some other scale of measurement. This often turns out to be true. Then, the data represented by the dependent variable are changed to this other scale of measurement. This change of scale is done only to satisfy the assumptions of a chosen statistical procedure. Usually, the data are analyzed on the transformed scale of measurement, and then the resulting estimates are transformed back to the original scale for interpretation.

We will look more closely at how we use transformations in a moment. Before we do that, let us take some time to step back and see what we have learned about the assumption of a Gaussian sampling distribution. First, we learned that this assumption could be satisfied by having a large sample. If the sample is not very large, the assumption relies on a Gaussian distribution of data (or residuals) in the population. We can evaluate the likelihood that the data (or residuals) have a Gaussian distribution in the population by examining the distribution of the data (or residual) in the sample. This can be done graphically (which I recommend), numerically, or inferentially (which I discourage). If we are concerned about this assumption that the distribution of estimates from all possible samples is a Gaussian distribution, we have two choices that we could make. Those choices and the methods we have discussed for evaluating this assumption are summarized schematically in Flowchart 11.

The trick in using transformations to create a Gaussian distribution of dependent variable values is selecting the appropriate mathematic method to apply to the dependent variable. Theoretically, the ways in which we could transform the dependent variable mathematically are unlimited. Fortunately, a few mathematical methods have been found to work well in the majority of instances.

The one transformation that most often creates a Gaussian distribution of dependent variable values (or a Gaussian distribution of residuals in bivariable or multivariable analyses) is the **log transformation**.[40] As the name implies, the log transformation entails taking the logarithm (the particular log scale used does not matter) of each dependent variable value. Usually one is added to each data value before taking the logarithm as shown in Equation (13.18).[41]

$$Y'_i = \log(Y_i + 1) \tag{13.18}$$

[40]The reason the log transformation works so often is the fact that the most common distribution of data in nature is the **log-normal distribution**. The log-normal distribution is a Gaussian distribution on a log scale.

[41]Adding a value of 1 to each data value before taking the logarithm has been shown, in many instances, to result in a transformed value with better statistical properties than simply taking the logarithm of the data value. A different number could be added to each data value if the data contain values of 0 or less (for which a logarithm cannot be calculated).

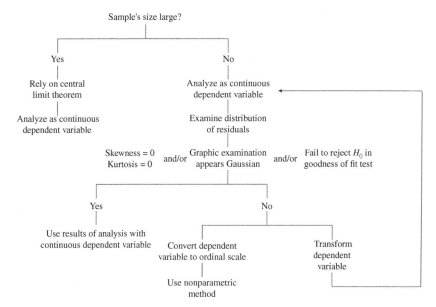

FLOWCHART 11   Summary of the process of evaluating the assumption that estimates for continuous dependent variables from all possible samples of a given size have a Gaussian distribution and dealing with violation of that assumption. The schematic is designed for bivariable or multivariable data sets. For univariable data sets, the distribution of the data rather than the distribution of the residuals can be examined.

The effect of taking the logarithm of numbers is to make larger numbers numerically closer to smaller numbers. Thus, the log transformation is useful for data that are positively skewed. We can see how this works in the following example.

■ EXAMPLE 13.9

In Examples 13.1, 13.2, and 13.3 we found that the children's heights were positively skewed. Let us use a log transformation of height and reexamine its distribution. First, we need to convert each of the height measurements to a logarithmic scale using Equation (13.18). The particular logarithmic scale we use does not matter, so I have used a base 10 scale (called the common log scale).

Now, we could use any of the methods we have learned to evaluate the distribution of the transformed values of height. Let us examine the normalized cumulative proportion polygon. To prepare for this approach, we need to convert the cumulative proportions to normalized values (i.e., standard normal deviates). This is illustrated in the following table.

Height	Log (Height + 1)	Cumulative Proportion	Normalized Value
80	1.91	0.05	−1.64
86	1.94	0.10	−1.28
91	1.96	0.15	−1.04
95	1.98	0.20	−0.84
98	2.00	0.25	−0.67
101	2.01	0.30	−0.52
104	2.02	0.35	−0.39
107	2.03	0.40	−0.25
110	2.05	0.45	−0.13
113	2.06	0.50	0.00
116	2.07	0.55	+0.13
119	2.08	0.60	+0.25
123	2.09	0.65	+0.39
126	2.10	0.70	+0.52
130	2.12	0.75	+0.67
135	2.13	0.80	+0.84
141	2.15	0.85	+1.04
148	2.17	0.90	+1.28
160	2.21	0.95	+1.64
171	2.24	0.975*	+1.96

*Calculated using Equation (13.1).

Finally, we can compare the log-transformed values of height to their corresponding normalized cumulative frequencies.

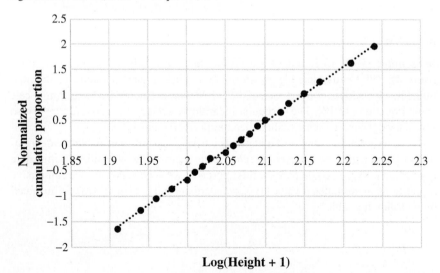

Log(Height + 1)

Examining the normalized cumulative proportion polygon reveals a relationship that is very nearly a straight line. Therefore, the log transformation appears to have corrected the positive skewness of the distribution of height. ∎

Thus, a possible solution to a positively skewed distribution is to perform a logarithmic transformation of the dependent variable. In other words, we would add 1 to each dependent variable value and take the logarithm of each of those sums (Equation (13.18)). Those transformed values are used in place of the dependent variable values in any further statistical calculations if the transformed values seem to satisfy the assumptions of the statistical procedure better than do the dependent variable values in their original form.

When we perform statistical procedures on transformed values of the dependent variable, the results of that analysis relate to the transformed scale rather than the original scale. For instance, if we are calculating means on data that have been subjected to a logarithmic transformation, then the means we obtain are the means of the logarithms of the data rather than the means of the data on its original scale. Often, it is desirable to convert back to the original scale after statistical analyses are completed so that the results of the analysis can be interpreted on a scale that is familiar. This can be accomplished for means that have been calculated from the transformed form of the data by performing a mathematical operation that is the reverse of the operation that was used in transforming the data. For a logarithmic transformation, the opposite operation is to use the mean of the transformed data as the exponent of the base of the log scale that was employed in the transformation.[42] This operation is called taking the **antilog** of the mean. This is illustrated for a mean that has been calculated using a common logarithm transformation in Equation (13.19).

$$\overline{Y} = \text{antilog}(\overline{Y}') - 1 = 10^{\overline{Y}'} - 1 \tag{13.19}$$

The following example illustrates this process of performing statistical calculations on transformed data and converting back to the original scale.

∎ EXAMPLE 13.10

Let us calculate a 95%, two-tailed confidence interval for the height of children in the population from which the sample in Example 13.1 was drawn.

As we have discussed previously, a sample containing 20 observations is not large enough for us to be confident that the sampling distribution will be a Gaussian distribution. Therefore, we need to examine the distribution of data in the sample out of concern about the distribution of data in the population. In Example 13.2, we found that the distribution of height in the sample appeared to differ from a Gaussian distribution. Although this difference is probably not great enough to interfere

---

[42] A mean that has been calculated on a logarithmic scale and then transformed back to its original scale is called a **geometric mean**.

with the assumption of a Gaussian sampling distribution, we found (in 13.8) that a logarithmic transformation of height created transformed data that was closer to a Gaussian distribution. Thus, let us calculate the confidence interval using the transformed data. The following table summarizes the calculations that will be used to estimate the mean and the standard error required by Student's t-procedure (see Chapter 4).

	Height Y_i	Log(Height + 1) Y_i'	$(Y_i' - \overline{Y}')$	$(Y_i' - \overline{Y}')^2$
	80	1.91	−0.157	0.02479
	86	1.94	−0.126	0.01598
	91	1.96	−0.102	0.01043
	95	1.98	−0.084	0.00700
	98	2.00	−0.070	0.00494
	101	2.01	−0.057	0.00329
	104	2.02	−0.045	0.00200
	107	2.03	−0.032	0.00106
	110	2.05	−0.021	0.00042
	113	2.06	−0.009	0.00008
	116	2.07	0.002	0.00001
	119	2.08	0.013	0.00018
	123	2.09	0.028	0.00076
	126	2.10	0.038	0.00144
	130	2.12	0.051	0.00264
	135	2.13	0.068	0.00457
	141	2.15	0.086	0.00746
	148	2.17	0.107	0.01151
	160	2.21	0.141	0.01985
	171	2.24	0.170	0.02877
Sum	2, 354	41.32	0.000	0.14715

Thus, the mean and variance of the logarithmic transformation of height are equal to the following:

$$\overline{Y}' = \frac{\sum_{i=1}^{n} Y_i'}{n} = \frac{41.32}{20} = 2.07$$

$$s_{Y'}^2 = \frac{\sum_{i=1}^{n} (Y_i' - Y)^2}{n - 1} = \frac{0.14715}{20 - 1} = 0.00774$$

The standard error for the mean of the logarithmic transformation of height is calculated in the usual way:

$$s_{\overline{Y}'} = \sqrt{\frac{s_{Y'}^2}{n}} = \sqrt{\frac{0.00774}{20}} = 0.01968$$

Now, we can calculate a 95%, two-tailed confidence interval for the log of height using Student's t-distribution. Student's t-value that we use in that calculation is the value from Table B.2 that corresponds to an α of 0.05 split between the two tails of Student's t-distribution, and $20 - 1 = 19$ degrees of freedom.

$$\mu' \triangleq \overline{Y}' \pm (t_{0.05/2} \cdot s_{\overline{Y}'}) = 2.07 \pm (2.093 \cdot 0.01968) = 2.02\text{–}2.11$$

The mean (2.07) and the confidence interval (2.02–2.11) we have calculated are for the log of height (plus 1), rather than for height. Interpretation of these values is somewhat awkward for us since their units are the log of centimeters. Thus, it is helpful for us to find the antilog of these values. To do that, we use Equation (13.19) for the mean and similar calculations for the limits of the confidence interval.

$$\overline{Y} = \text{antilog}(\overline{Y}') - 1$$

Thus, we estimate the mean of height to be equal to 115.4 cm and, with 95% confidence, between 104.9 and 127.0 cm. These values are different from the ones we would have obtained if we had not performed our statistical calculations on log-transformed dependent variable values (in Example 13.3, we found the mean to be equal to 117.7 cm). Further, the relationship between the estimated mean and the confidence interval is different when calculated on a log scale that when calculated on the original scale. Normally, the mean is in the center of the confidence interval. Notice here, however, that the mean (when converted back to its original scale) is closer to the lower limit of the confidence interval than it is to the upper limit of that interval. This will always be true when calculations are performed on a logarithmic scale and converted back to the original scale. ∎

The logarithmic transformation is the most important transformation in analysis of health research data, simply because the most common distribution encountered for biologic data that do not have a Gaussian distribution can be transformed to a Gaussian distribution by taking the logarithm of the data.[43] The next most common deviation of health research data from a Gaussian distribution is a distribution with positive skewness that does not become a Gaussian distribution, when we take logarithms of the data.

---

[43] Biologic data often come from a **log-normal** distribution. This is a distribution in which the log of the data values has a Gaussian distribution.

There are two ways in which the logarithmic transformation might be inadequate in correcting a distribution with positive skewness. First, the degree of skewness might be greater than can be corrected by taking logarithms of the data. In this case, the **square root transformation** might be effective in creating a symmetric distribution. This transformation is usually performed by taking the square root of each dependent variable value plus 0.5 (Equation (13.20)).[44]

$$Y_i' = \sqrt{Y_i + 0.5} \tag{13.20}$$

Alternatively, the logarithmic transformation might overcorrect the degree of positive skewness of the data, creating a degree of negative skewness. In this case, the **inverse transformation** might be better at correcting for positive skewness. To use the inverse transformation, each dependent variable value is divided into one as shown in Equation (13.21).[45] If values of 0 exist among the dependent variable values, 1 (or any other value) can be added to each dependent variable value before performing the division, to avoid dividing by 0.

$$Y_i' = \frac{1}{Y_i} \tag{13.21}$$

Data that are positively skewed are by far the most commonly encountered deviation from a Gaussian distribution (at least among health research data). Occasionally, however, we might encounter data that are negatively skewed. A transformation that is often effective in creating a symmetric distribution from a negatively skewed distribution is the **power transformation.** This transformation is performed by taking each dependent variable value to some power. Negative skewness can be corrected by making this power a positive integer.[46] The positive integer that is used most often is 2. Then, the type of power transformation used is called the **square transformation** (Equation (13.22)).

$$Y_i' = Y_i^2 \tag{13.22}$$

Distributions of continuous data that are not mesokurtic are less frequently encountered than skewed distributions. Most often, problems of kurtosis result from using statistical procedures for continuous dependent variables on data that are not really continuous. For example, we might wish to perform an analysis of variance (ANOVA) on data that are proportions. One solution to problems

---

[44]If the dependent variable consists of negative values less than −0.5, the absolute value of the minimum dependent variable value can be added to each dependent variable value before taking the square root.

[45]When means are calculated on data transformed with the inverse transformation and then converted back to their original scale, we refer to the mean on its original scale as the **harmonic mean**.

[46]Actually, the square root and the inverse transformations can be considered special types of power transformation in which the power is less than 1. The square root transformation corresponds to a power of 0.5 and the inverse transformation corresponds to a power of −1.

of kurtosis is to use an **angular transformation.** For data such as proportions, however, it is probably better to use statistical procedures that are designed to analyze nominal dependent variables.

For continuous dependent variables with problems with kurtosis (especially platykurtic distributions), an angular transformation that is often successful in creating a Gaussian sampling distribution is the **arcsine transformation**. To use an arcsine transformation on continuous data, each dependent variable value is divided by its maximum absolute value (to make all the values between −1 and +1). Then, the arcsine is found for each fraction.

13.1.3 Assuming Equal Variances

The procedures we investigated in previous chapters for bivariable and multivariable analysis of a continuous dependent variable all assumed that the variance of data represented by the dependent variable was the same regardless of the value of the independent variable(s). We first encountered this assumption when we studied Student's t-procedure for comparing means between two groups of dependent variable values. In that procedure, we calculated a pooled estimate of the variance of the data as the weighted average of the variance estimates in each group. This calculation makes sense only if we believe that the distributions of data represented by the dependent variable in the two groups have the same variance in the population.[47] We calculated a similar pooled variance (called the within mean square) in ANOVA. Perhaps less obviously, we did the same in regression analysis when we calculated the residual mean square.

Thus, another assumption that we need to consider when analyzing continuous dependent variables is the assumption that the variation of data represented by the dependent variable is the same in the population for dependent variable values corresponding to all values of the independent variable(s). We mentioned this assumption in previous chapters. At that time, we pointed out that this is known as the assumption of **homoscedasticity**, or as the assumption of **homogeneity of variances.**

Unlike the assumption that the distribution of estimates from all possible samples of a given size is a Gaussian distribution, the assumption of homoscedasticity cannot be satisfied by having a large sample. The central limit theorem applies only to the shape of the distribution of estimates, not to the variance of the data. Therefore, we need to consider the appropriateness of the assumption of homoscedasticity in the population by examining the sample's observations regardless of the size of the sample.

The approaches we take in examining the sample's observations to evaluate the assumption of homoscedasticity in the population are parallel to the approaches we encountered when examining the sample's distribution of data to evaluate the

---

[47]That is, any differences in the variance estimates in the sample are due to chance rather than to differences in the variances of the data in the population.

distribution of data in the population. Namely, we can take a graphic, numeric, or inferential approach.

The graphic approach to examination of the variance of data in the sample is more straightforward than the graphic approach to examination of the distribution of the sample's data. There are only two issues we need to discuss, and the first is one with which we are familiar. The first issue is that we need to consider the variance of the residuals rather than the variance of the dependent variable values themselves. The reason for this is the same reason that we were interested in the distribution of the residuals rather than the distribution of dependent variable values. To compare distributions or to compare variances, we need to adjust the locations of the distributions of the dependent variable values that correspond to different values of the independent variable(s).

The second issue is most important when we are examining a multivariable sample, and concerns to what we want to compare the variation in residuals. The assumption is that the variation is the same for dependent variable values corresponding to each value of each independent variable. If we create a graphic display of residuals versus values of the independent variables, our display becomes unwieldy if we have more than one continuous independent variable. There is a way that we can represent dependent variable values corresponding to specific values of each of the independent variable with a single set of dependent variable values, however. That set of values consists of the estimated values of the dependent variable. Since each of the independent variables contributes to those estimated values, each estimated value of the dependent variable corresponds to a specific set of independent variable values.[48]

Thus, the graphic approach we use to evaluate the assumption of homoscedasticity compares values of the residual (on the ordinate) to corresponding estimated values of the dependent variable (on the abscissa).[49] If the assumption of homoscedasticity is valid, we expect to see approximately the same amount of dispersion of residual values for all estimated values of the dependent variable. The most commonly encountered deviation from homoscedasticity in health research data is an increase in the dispersion of the residual values as the estimated values of the dependent variable increase. More rarely, the dispersion of the residual values might decrease as the estimated values of the dependent variable increase. The appearance of these two violations of the assumption of homoscedasticity in this graphic approach is illustrated in Figure 13.5.

---

[48]To calculate these estimated values, we first need to perform the analysis. Thus, we often need to use a selected statistical method before we are able to determine whether or not the assumptions for that method are satisfied. This is true whenever we need to calculate residuals or estimated values of the dependent variable.

[49]This is easy to do in regression analysis in Excel. Checking the "Residuals" box in the "Regression" dialog box gives you the estimated values and the residuals. The plot is output from the BAHR program "Residual Analysis."

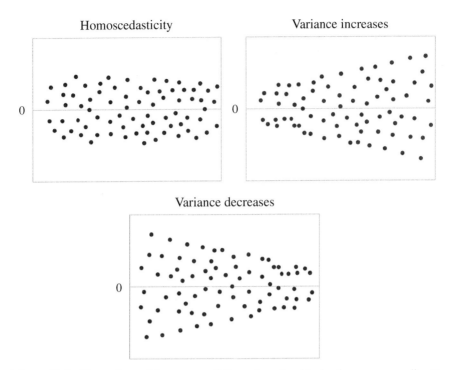

Figure 13.5   Illustrations of the pattern of dispersion of residual values corresponding to estimated values of the dependent variable ($\widehat{Y}_i$) when the assumption of homoscedasticity is valid and when it is violated.

   This graphic approach to evaluation of the assumption of homoscedasticity is most useful when we have one or more continuous independent variables. When the independent variables are nominal, we can, if we choose, take a numeric approach. That approach involves comparison of the estimates of the variance of dependent variable values that correspond to each group specified by the values of the independent variable(s). We can make that comparison informally by calculating those variance estimates and determining that their values are close together. Alternatively, we can make that comparison formally by testing the null hypothesis that those variances are equal in the population from which the sample was drawn.

   When we considered an inferential approach to evaluating the assumption that estimates from all possible samples of a given size have a Gaussian distribution, we explained that the approach had a logical flaw. That flaw was related to the reduction in our ability to reject the null hypothesis that the data have a Gaussian distribution as the sample's size decreased. This was especially serious when we evaluated the assumption of a Gaussian sampling distribution, since the distribution of data (or residuals) is relevant to the sampling distribution only when the sample contains few observations.

We do not have quite the same problem with a test of the null hypothesis that the variance of data is the same for all values of the independent variable(s). The difference is that larger samples are not immune to heteroscedasticity (i.e., a lack of homoscedasticity). Still, our ability to reject the null hypothesis that the variances are the same decreases as the sample's size decreases. Therefore, an inferential approach to the assumption of homoscedasticity applies a less rigorous criterion to conclude that the assumption is valid for smaller samples than it does for larger samples. For this reason, most statisticians rely on either the graphic or the numeric approaches to evaluate the assumption of homoscedasticity. The advantage of these approaches is that they are not as influenced by the sample's size as is the inferential approach. Their disadvantage is that they do not provide a standard criterion for decision-making like the inferential approach does.

Actually, we looked at the inferential approach to evaluating the assumption of homoscedasticity in bivariable analysis on the computer in Chapter 4. This approach uses an F-test. It is illustrated in Example 7.11.

For multivariable analysis, we need a different approach. A commonly used method is called **Bartlett's test**. The test statistic is approximately a chi-square with degrees of freedom equal to $k - 1$ (the number of variances compared minus 1). It is calculated as in Equation (13.23)

$$\chi^2_{k-1\mathrm{df}} = \left[(\ln(s_\mathrm{p}^2) \cdot \sum_{i=1}^{k}(n_i - 1) \right] - \left[\sum_{i=1}^{k}((n_i - 1) \cdot \ln(s_i^2)) \right] \qquad (13.23)$$

where
$s_\mathrm{p}^2 =$ pooled variance estimate (i.e., within mean square)
$k =$ number of variances compared

We will take a look at an example in which we examine the assumption of homoscedasticity in a moment, but first let us consider the options available to us if we believe this assumption is not valid. When we are concerned that our sample might violate the assumption of homoscedasticity, we can take any of three possible approaches to analysis of that sample. Two of those approaches are the same as the ones we considered when we were concerned about the assumption that estimates from all possible samples of a given size have a Gaussian distribution. Namely, we can use a nonparametric parallel procedure on the continuous data, converted to an ordinal scale, or we can transform the dependent variable using some mathematical operation that creates homoscedasticity.

The drawbacks of using a nonparametric procedure to circumvent the assumption of homoscedasticity are the same as the drawbacks to circumventing the assumption of a Gaussian sampling distribution. Specifically, nonparametric methods have lower statistical power and the interpretation of the results of nonparametric methods often has important differences from the interpretation of methods for continuous dependent variable. Further, some statistical procedures for continuous dependent variables do not have nonparametric parallels (e.g., regression analysis).

So, it is usually better to find a transformation for the dependent variable that will create homoscedasticity than to use a nonparametric method to circumvent the assumption of homoscedasticity. The transformations that are used most often are the same ones we considered for small samples from populations in which the data do not have a Gaussian distribution. The transformations we examined for distributions that are positively skewed (i.e., the logarithmic, square root, and inverse transformations) are often effective in creating homoscedasticity in data sets that have an increase in the dispersion of residuals as the estimated value of the dependent variable increases. The square root transformation can correct heteroscedasticity that is less severe, and the inverse transformation can correct heteroscedasticity that is more severe, than the degree of heteroscedasticity corrected by the logarithmic transformation.[50]

An increase in the dispersion of the residuals as the estimated value of the dependent variable increases is the most common type of violation of the assumption of homoscedasticity in health research data. Evan so, we can sometimes see the opposite type of relationship. That is to say, we occasionally observe the dispersion of the residuals decreasing as the estimated value of the dependent variable increases. In this case, we might try the square transformation that we used previously to create asymmetric distribution from a negatively skewed distribution. Other patterns of heteroscedasticity are more difficult to overcome using transformation of dependent variable values. Usually, patterns of change in the dispersion of the residuals that are not monotonic increases or decreases are best resolved by some approach other than transformation of the dependent variable.[51]

Now, let us take a look at an example of how we can detect a violation of the assumption of homoscedasticity and how we might use a transformation to correct this problem.

■ EXAMPLE 13.11

Suppose we were interested in comparing serum glutamic transaminase (AST) among 4 groups of 10 patients, and we observed the following AST measurements (units/mL).

---

[50] The logarithmic transformation is most effective when the standard deviation of the residuals (e.g., the square root of the within mean square in ANOVA or the square root of the residual mean square in regression analysis) increases proportionally to estimated values of the dependent variable. The square root transformation can create homoscedasticity when the standard deviation of the residuals increases proportionally to the square root of the estimated values of the dependent variable. The inverse transformation works best when the standard deviation of the residuals increases proportionally to the square of the estimated values of the dependent variable.

[51] When the dispersion of the residuals increases (or more rarely, decreases) toward the middle of the interval of estimated values of the dependent variable, compared to either extreme of the interval, an angular transformation might be effective.

Group I	Group II	Group III	Group IV
36	23	57	30
22	36	42	26
31	44	36	42
19	33	39	23
37	42	42	21
29	48	43	43
32	24	29	39
23	28	52	32
25	34	60	39
31	40	51	31

Let us evaluate the assumption of homoscedasticity for these data and, if necessary, transform the data to achieve homoscedasticity.

To begin, we need to apply the appropriate analysis to these data. Since we have a continuous dependent variable and three nominal independent variables representing one factor, the appropriate analysis is a one-way ANOVA. Using Excel's "ANOVA: Single Factor" procedure, we get the following output:

Anova: Single Factor						
SUMMARY						
Groups	*Count*	*Sum*	*Average*	*Variance*		
Group I	10	285	28.5	36.5		
Group II	10	352	35.2	71.51111111		
Group III	10	451	45.1	94.32222222		
Group IV	10	326	32.6	62.04444444		
ANOVA						
Source of Variation	*SS*	*df*	*MS*	*F*	*P-valve*	*F crit*
Between groups	1,495.7	3	498.5666667	7.543246197	0.00048614	2.866265551
Within groups	2,379.4	36	66.09444444			
Total	3,875.1	39				

The most straightforward way to examine the assumption of homoscedasticity in a data set such as this is to estimate the variance of the data for each group of dependent variable values and determine, by inspection, whether or not those estimates are close to the same value. Those estimates are summarized in the first table of the output. We can see from that table that the variance of the data increases as the estimated value of the dependent variable increases. This is even more striking in a graphic evaluation of the dispersion of the residuals.

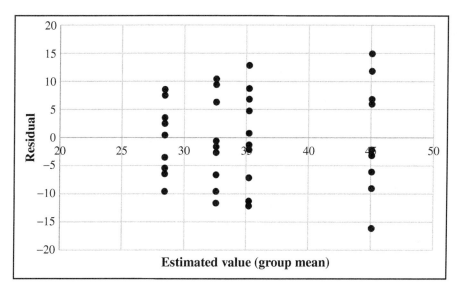

To examine this inferentially, we use Bartlett's test. To do this, we use Equation (13.23).

$$\chi^2_{k-1\,df} = \left[(\ln(s_s^2)) \cdot \sum_{i=1}^{k}(n_i - 1) \right] - \left[\sum_{i=1}^{k}((n_i - 1) \cdot \ln(s_i^2)) \right]$$

$$= [(\ln(66.094) \cdot (9 + 9 + 9 + 9)] - [(9 \cdot \ln(36.5)) + (9 \cdot \ln(71.51))$$

$$+ (9 \cdot \ln(94.32)) + (9 \cdot \ln(62.04))]$$

$$= 150.88 - 148.88 = 2.00$$

We compare that calculated value to a critical value from Table B.7 corresponding to an α of 0.05 and three degrees of freedom. That value is 7.815. Since the calculated value is less than the critical value, we fail to reject the null hypothesis that the variances are equal to the same value in the population. From this result, we conclude that the assumption of homoscedasticity is satisfied.

Even though the inferential approach concluded the assumption is satisfied, we might be concerned that the relatively small sample did not have sufficient power to detect the systematic differences in variances we observed graphically. For illustration, let us use a log (base 10) transformation on these data and re-examine the residual plot. With the log-transformed data, we get the following ANOVA output:

Anova: Single Factor						
SUMMARY						
Groups	*Count*	*Sum*	*Average*	*Variance*		
Group I	10	14.61186289	1.461186289	0.008573137		
Group II	10	15.47395884	1.547395884	0.011275871		
Group III	10	16.5468096	1.65468096	0.008922225		
Group IV	10	15.15006441	1.515006441	0.011256428		
ANOVA						
Source of Variation	*SS*	*df*	*MS*	*F*	*P-valve*	*F crit*
Between groups	0.199592563	3	0.066530854	6.64848788	0.00109157	2.866265551
Within groups	0.360248947	36	0.010006915			
Total	0.55984151	39				

When we inspect the dispersion of the residuals graphically, we get the following result:

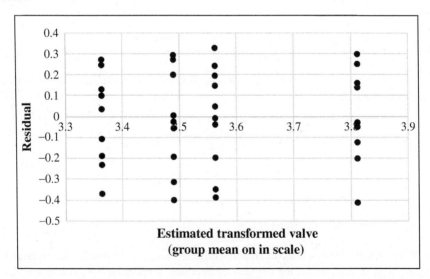

The logarithmic transformation appears to have created variances of transformed data that are much more similar than the variances of the data on its original scale. Thus, we can be comfortable with the assumption of homoscedasticity if we perform statistical analyses on the transformed data as long as the transformation does not create a problem with other assumptions (like the assumption of a Gaussian sampling distribution). ∎

Transformation of the dependent variable is a useful tool for either distributions of data in small samples or for heteroscedasticity. It is important to realize, however, that use of a transformation to correct heteroscedasticity of residuals that have a Gaussian distribution will create a skewed distribution of residuals. Likewise, transforming the dependent variable to create a Gaussian distribution can also create heteroscedasticity, if the dispersion of residuals was uniform before the transformation. Therefore, we cannot consider these two assumptions separately. If we do, we run the risk of creating problems for one while we are attempting to solve problems for the other.

Fortunately, positively skewed distributions of residuals calculated from health research data are most often associated with dispersion of those residuals that increase as estimated values of the dependent variable increase. This implies that, if a particular transformation solves a problem with the distribution of the residuals, it is likely, at the same time, to solve a problem with the dispersion of the residuals. To be certain this is the case for a particular data set, however, it is wise to reexamine both the assumption of a Gaussian sampling distribution and the assumption of homoscedasticity, whenever a transformation is used.

Earlier, I said that there are three possible approaches to analysis of data that appear to violate the assumption of homoscedasticity. So far, we have discussed only two: nonparametric procedures and transformation of the dependent variable. The third approach is to use a method of statistical analysis that is designed for a continuous dependent variable but does not assume homoscedasticity. We saw one of these in Chapter 7 when we considered the *t*-test for unequal variances. Other methods are beyond to scope of this text.[52]

In summary, we have seen some similarities and some differences between the methods to evaluate appropriateness and to correct discrepancies for the assumption of homoscedasticity (Flowchart 12) and the assumption of a Gaussian distribution of estimates from all possible samples of a given size (Flowchart 11). The similarities are that both assumptions can be evaluated by graphic, numeric, or inferential examination of the sample's observations, and both often can be corrected by using a transformation of the dependent variable or circumvented by using a nonparametric procedure. The most important difference between these assumptions is that the assumption of homoscedasticity is not satisfied by having a large sample.[53]

---

[52] An example of such a method is a weighted regression analysis. Since these methods are rarely used in analysis of health research data, I will not address them in this text.

[53] Another difference is the existence of statistical procedures for continuous dependent variables that do not assume homoscedasticity. As mentioned, most of these procedures are difficult and rarely used.

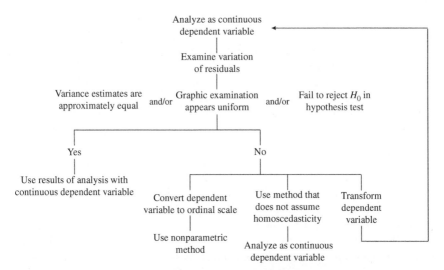

FLOWCHART 12   Summary of the process of evaluating the assumption of homoscedasticity and correcting for violation of that assumption. This assumption is applicable only for bivariable or multivariable analyses of a continuous dependent variable.

13.1.4   Assuming Additive Relationships

In the last part of Chapter 10, I pointed out that all the procedures that we had discussed for continuous dependent variables could be expressed as regression equations. This was known as the principle of the **general linear model.** An implication of this fact is that all these statistical methods assume that we can represent the relationship between the dependent variable and the independent variable(s) in a linear or additive model. There are two situations in which we might be concerned about this assumption of **additivity.**

For continuous independent variables, an additive model implies a straight-line relationship with values of the dependent variable. In bivariable regression or correlation analysis, we assume that values of the dependent variable change in a consistent direction and by a consistent amount for each unit change in the value of the independent variable. If the amount that the dependent variable changes is inconsistent for each unit change in the value of the independent variable, the amount of variation in dependent variable values that is explained by the regression equation or that is reflected in the correlation coefficient will be lower than it would be if the amount of change in dependent variable values were consistent.

In multivariable regression or correlation analysis, we make a parallel assumption. In the multivariable case, however, we assume a straight-line relationship between each particular independent variable and the variation in the dependent variable that is not explained by the other independent variables.[54] The reason that we make this assumption in multivariable analyses is related to the way in which coefficients are estimated and hypotheses are tested in multiple regression. The processes involve comparison of full and reduced models as we discussed in Chapter 10.

For nominal independent variables, an additive model becomes distinct from other sorts of models only when the data set contains more than one nominal independent variable and those independent variables represent more than one characteristic or factor (e.g., in factorial ANOVA). An additive model, in this case, implies that the effect of one factor can be added to the effect of another factor and that the effect of the interaction(s) can be added to the effects of the factors. Deviations from an additive relationship among those factors and/or interaction(s) can produce misleading results (such as spurious interactions) when the data are analyzed using a method that assumes additivity.

The best way to detect violations of the assumption that the relationships between the dependent and independent variables are additive is a graphic approach. One such approach might be to examine a scatterplot (see Chapter 7). This approach becomes difficult, however, when there is more than one independent variable, especially if some of those independent variables represent continuous data.

A more universally applicable graphic approach is to examine the same graph used to evaluate the assumption of homoscedasticity. In that graph we compared estimated values of the dependent variable[55] (on the abscissa) to the residuals (on the ordinate). If an additive model fits the data, we expect to see the residual centered on zero throughout the range of estimated values of the dependent variable. If, on the other hand, relationships are not additive, we would see a predominance of negative residuals corresponding to some estimated values and a predominance of positive residuals corresponding to other estimated values of the dependent variable. Let us see how that graphic approach can help us detect violation of the assumption of additivity in the following example.

■ EXAMPLE 13.12

In Chapter 10, we considered as an example (Example 10.1) an experiment to investigate the relationship between the dose of a particular drug and the associated change in diastolic blood pressure among hypertensive patients. The data set we examined provided observations on 10 patients each of whom had been randomly assigned to receive a different dose of the drug in 5-mg intervals from 5 to 50 mg. The following data were observed:

---

[54] That is, we make the assumption of additivity for the relationship between each independent variable and the residuals from an analysis that takes all other independent variables into account.

[55] These estimated values of the dependent variable are from the results of the analysis for which we are evaluating the assumption of additivity.

Dose	Blood Pressure Change
5	0.5
10	0.5
15	0.6
20	1.5
25	1.3
30	5.2
35	5.8
40	14.3
45	18.7
50	41.0

When we performed a regression analysis on these data, we estimated the following regression equation for the change in blood pressure (BPC) as a function of dose (DOSE):

$$BPC = -10.3 + (0.7 \cdot DOSE)$$

Let us evaluate the assumption of additivity (linearity) for these data.

Since this is a bivariable data set, we could use a scatterplot to determine if there seems to be a straight-line relationship between the change in blood pressure and dose (as we did in Example 10.1).

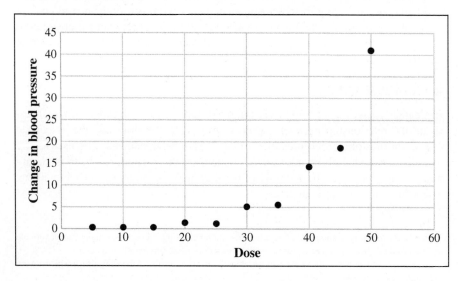

We can see from the scatterplot that the assumption of additivity does not seem appropriate for this data set. That is to say, this is not a straight-line relationship.

If we had more than one independent variable, the scatterplot would not be a very useful way to evaluate the assumption of additivity. Rather, we could evaluate the assumption of additivity by examining a graphic display of the residual values corresponding to the estimated values of the dependent variable. To see how this graphic approach can be used to detect violation of the assumption of additivity, let us use that approach on these data.

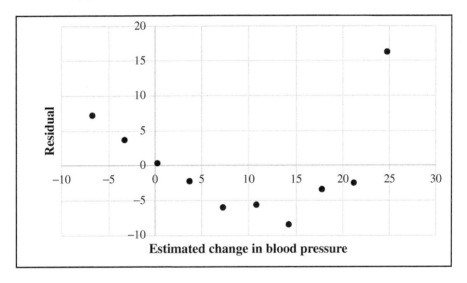

Estimated change in blood pressure

If the assumption of additivity were satisfied by these data, we would see a balance of positive and negative residuals corresponding to the estimated values of the dependent variable throughout the range of estimated values. That is to say, there would be no predominance of positive or negative residuals corresponding to some of the estimated values.

Here, we see positive residual values corresponding to the lowest and highest estimated values and negative residual values corresponding to the intermediate estimated values. That pattern implies that the straight line that regression analysis fits to these data deviates in a systematic way from the observed values. Specifically, the straight line underestimates low and high dependent variable values and overestimates intermediate dependent variable values. Any systematic discrepancy between observed and estimated dependent variable values will result in an unbalanced pattern of residual values, compared to estimated values of the dependent variable such as we see here. ■

As an alternative to the graphic approach to evaluate the assumption of additivity, we might use an inferential approach. One inferential approach that can be used in regression analysis is restricted to data sets in which several dependent variable values have been observed for each value of the independent variable.[56] This is an unusual type of data set in health research.

Another inferential approach is one in which polynomial regression analysis is performed. Polynomial regression model contain powers of the same independent variable are included as if they were separate independent variables. Equation (13.24) shows a simple polynomial regression equation:[57]

$$\widehat{Y}_i = a + (b_1 \cdot X_i) + (b_2 \cdot X_i^2) \tag{13.24}$$

Deviations from linearity are tested in polynomial regression analysis by testing the null hypotheses that the regression coefficients associated with higher powers of the independent variable are equal to 0 in the population.[58] This approach can be used for any continuous independent variable.

Even so, we need to be mindful of the fact that inferential approaches to evaluating assumptions involves accepting the null hypothesis as true when we believe that the assumption has been satisfied. Accepting the null hypothesis is a conclusion that we usually try to avoid in statistical hypothesis testing. When we accept the null hypothesis as true, we are in danger of making a type II error. Therefore, the statistical power of the test of hypothesis testing is important when we accept the null hypothesis. In other words, the degree to which the data violate an assumption must be greater for smaller samples than for larger samples, to result in rejection of the null hypothesis. Because of this feature of statistical hypothesis testing, most statisticians use graphic approaches, rather than inferential approaches, to evaluate the propriety of assumptions.

When we are concerned about the assumption of additivity, there are three possible solutions we can consider. These are the same three solutions we discussed for violations of the assumption of homoscedasticity. Namely, we can use a nonparametric procedure that is parallel to the procedure for a continuous dependent variable (if one exists), we can transform the dependent variable, or we can use a method for the continuous dependent variable that takes nonadditivity into account. One such procedure is polynomial regression analysis. These solutions and the process we follow to evaluate the assumption of additivity are summarized in Flowchart 13.

The transformations of the dependent variable that are most often used to contend with nonadditivity are the same as the transformations that are used for distributions of data that are not Gaussian distributions, and for heteroscedasticity. The

[56]In this approach, the regression sum of squares is compared to a between sum of squares from an ANOVA in which each continuous independent variable value is considered a category specified by a collection of nominal independent variables. The greater the difference between those sums of squares, the greater the deviation from linearity.

[57]This is known as a second-order or quadratic regression equation. Additional powers of the independent variable can be added to the polynomial regression equation, but a quadratic equation is usually sufficient to evaluate the assumption of additivity

[58]As we will see soon, polynomial regression analysis can be used not only to evaluate the assumption of additivity, but also as a solution to violation of this assumption.

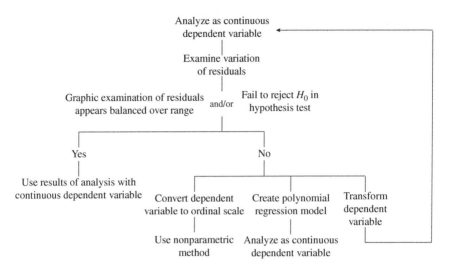

FLOWCHART 13   Summary of the process of evaluating the assumption of additivity and correcting for violation of that assumption. This assumption is applicable only for bivariable or multivariable analyses.

transformation that is most often effective is the logarithmic transformation. The logarithmic transformation is useful when a relationship is multiplicative rather than additive.[59] If positive residuals are associated with low and high estimated values and negative residuals are associated with intermediate estimated values of the dependent variable (such as in Example 13.11), the first type of transformation to try with health research data is the logarithmic transformation. Alternatively, the square root of inverse transformations might be effective in creating additivity in this situation. If the opposite pattern of residuals is observed (i.e., negative residuals associated with low and high estimated values and positive residuals associated with intermediate estimated values of the dependent variable), a power (e.g., square) transformation might be useful.

It is important to keep in mind that transformation of the dependent variable can effect three separate assumptions in analysis of continuous dependent variable. This implies that use of a transformation to solve one problem has the potential of creating other problems. Fortunately, violations of the assumptions of a Gaussian distribution, homoscedasticity, and additivity tend to occur together in the same set of data. The reason for this is that many types of data in health research have a distribution called a **log-normal distribution.**

A log-normal distribution is a positively skewed distribution. Positively skewed distributions tend to have greater dispersion of values as higher values are considered. Further, relationships among log-normal distributions tend to be multiplicative rather than linear. Thus, it is common in health research to encounter a positively

---

[59]The reason for this is the fact that addition on a log scale is the same as multiplication on a linear scale.

skewed distribution with variances that increase as estimated values increase, and positive residual values associated with low and high estimated values of the dependent variable. By definition, taking the logarithm of data in a log-normal distribution results in a Gaussian distribution (this is the origin of the name of the log-normal distribution). This is why the logarithmic transformation is so often effective in solving problems with these assumptions in health research.

Even though violations of one assumption are frequently associated with particular types of violations of other assumptions for analysis of continuous dependent

TABLE 13.1. The Five Most Commonly Employed Transformations for Continuous Dependent Variables and the Types of Violations of Assumptions for Which They Can Be Effective

Type of Transform	Assumption Violated		
	Gaussian Distribution	Homoscedasticity	Additivity
Logarithmic	Positive skewness (moderate)	Standard deviation proportional to the estimated value of the dependent variable	Positive residuals associated with low and high estimated values of the dependent variable
Square root	Positive skewness (severe)	Variance proportional to the estimated value of the dependent variable	Positive residuals associated with low and high estimated values of the dependent variable
Inverse	Positive skewness	Standard deviation proportional to square of estimated value of the dependent variable	Positive residuals associated with low and high estimated values of the dependent variable
Power (e.g., square)	Negative skewness	Standard deviation decreases as the estimated value of the dependent variable increases	Negative residuals associated with low and high estimated values of the dependent variable
Angular	Not mesokurtic	Various patterns, but often standard deviation greatest for intermediate estimated values of the dependent variable	Sigmoid pattern of residuals

variables, it is good practice to reevaluate each of these testable assumptions whenever a transformation is used. Table 13.1 lists the most commonly used transformations and the types of violations of assumptions they can correct.

Although data that are positively skewed and heteroscedastic are most often involved in multiplicative, rather than additive, relationships, it is not uncommon to encounter nonadditive (**curvilinear**) relationships without violation of the assumptions of a Gaussian distribution or homoscedasticity, especially in regression analysis. In addition, some curvilinear relationships are too complex to be corrected by transformation of the dependent variable. In these circumstances, it is better to use an analytic method that takes curvilinearity into account. For regression analysis, such a method is polynomial regression. The next example compares transformation of the dependent variable and polynomial regression analysis as solutions to nonadditivity.

■ EXAMPLE 13.13

Let us compare a logarithmic transformation of the dependent variable to polynomial regression as solutions to nonadditivity (curvilinearity) of the relationship between the change in blood pressure and dose for the data presented in Example 13.12.

First, let us see what happens to the pattern of residual values if we were to perform a regression analysis on log-transformed values (Equation (13.18)) of the change in blood pressure as the dependent variable and dose as the independent variable. The regression equation that we would obtain from that analysis is as follows:

$$\log(\text{BPC} + 1) = -0.212 + (0.033 \cdot \text{Dose})$$

Using that regression equation to estimate values of the dependent variable, we obtain the following residuals:

Dose	Log-Transformed Blood Pressure Change	Estimated Value	Residual
5	0.176	−0.045	0.221
10	0.176	0.121	0.055
15	0.204	0.288	−0.084
20	0.398	0.454	−0.056
25	0.362	0.621	−0.259
30	0.792	0.788	0.004
35	0.833	0.954	−0.121
40	1.185	1.121	0.064
45	1.294	1.287	0.007
50	1.623	1.454	0.169

Now, let us examine graphically how those residuals are related to the estimated dependent variable values.

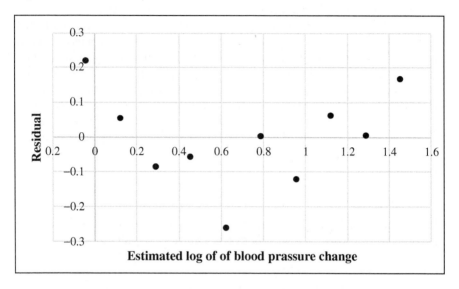

From the graphic display, we can see that the logarithmic transformation has some effect on the pattern of residual values, but those residuals do not seem to be balanced around 0 throughout the range of estimated values of the transformed dependent variable. Rather, there appears to be a pattern in which residuals tend to be positive for the lower estimated values, negative for the middle estimated values, and positive for the higher estimated values of the transformed dependent variable.

Next, let us compare the results from using a logarithmic transformation to a polynomial regression approach. We find that the following third-order polynomial regression equation fits the observed data well.[60]

$$BPC = -4.693 + (1.154 \cdot Dose) - (0.067 \cdot Dose^2) + (0.001 \cdot Dose^3)$$

Using that polynomial equation to estimate blood pressure changes, we acquire the following residual values:

[60]This is evident since $Dose^3$ is statistically significant and adding $Dose^4$ does not have a statistically significant regression coefficient. The latter implies $Dose^4$ does not add important information to the estimation of dependent variable values.

Dose	Blood Pressure Change	Estimated Value	Residual
5	0.5	−0.443	0.943
10	0.5	1.382	−0.882
15	0.6	1.700	−1.100
20	1.5	1.426	0.074
25	1.3	1.476	−0.176
30	5.2	2.769	2.431
35	5.8	6.219	−0.419
40	14.3	12.744	1.556
45	18.7	23.260	−4.560
50	41.0	38.684	2.316

Now, let us examine graphically how those residuals are related to the estimated dependent variable values.

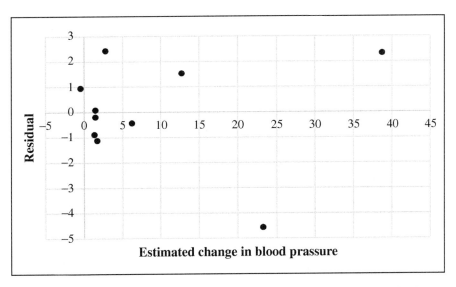

Estimated change in blood prassure

We can see that the polynomial regression approach is more effective, for these data, in solving the problem of nonadditivity (or curvilinearity). We draw this conclusion because of the balance of positive and negative residuals throughout the range of estimated values for the change in blood pressure. This does not appear to be a perfect solution, however. Even though we have solved the nonadditivity problem, we seem to have a problem with heteroscedasticity (the dispersion of the residual values appears to increase as the estimated value of the dependent variable increases). For this reason, it might be necessary to use both the log transformation and a polynomial function. ■

Example 13.13 illustrates the necessity to reexamine each of the assumptions we make when we employ statistical methods designed to analyze continuous dependent variables. In that example, a solution to a problem with the assumption of additivity led to concern about the assumption of homoscedasticity. To be entirely comfortable with regression analysis applied to these data, we need to continue our search for a method that will satisfy all the assumptions made by that method of analysis. As we continue that search, we should keep in mind that statistical methods for continuous dependent variables are robust. That is to say, these methods can tolerate a fair degree of divergence from these assumptions. Even so, we should use transformations and/or other methods to come as close as possible to satisfying the assumptions of a Gaussian sampling distribution, homoscedasticity, and additivity. The next example illustrates how we might proceed for the data introduced in Example 13.12.

■ EXAMPLE 13.14

In Example 13.13, we found that a polynomial regression analysis solves the problem of nonadditivity, but that solution creates heteroscedasticity for the data introduced in Example 13.12. Let us investigate a combination of solutions to solve both problems simultaneously. Specifically, let us see what happens when we perform a polynomial regression analysis on log-transformed values for blood pressure changes.

First, let us perform a polynomial regression analysis on blood pressure changes that have been transformed using Equation (13.18). We find that the following second-order polynomial regression equation is the best fit to the sample's observations.[61]

$$\log(\text{BPC} + 1) = 0.12470 - (0.00034 \cdot \text{Dose}) + (0.00061 \cdot \text{Dose}^2)$$

Using that regression equation to estimate values of the dependent variable, we obtain the following residuals:

Dose	Log-Transformed Blood Pressure Change	Estimated Value	Residual
5	0.176	0.138	+0.038
10	0.176	0.182	−0.006
15	0.204	0.257	−0.053
20	0.398	0.362	+0.035
25	0.362	0.498	−0.137
30	0.792	0.665	+0.127
35	0.833	0.862	−0.030
40	1.185	1.090	+0.094
45	1.294	1.348	−0.054
50	1.623	1.637	−0.014

[61] That is to say, Dose^2 is statistically significant, but adding Dose^3 does not add statistically significant information.

Now, let us examine graphically how those residuals are related to the estimated dependent variable values.

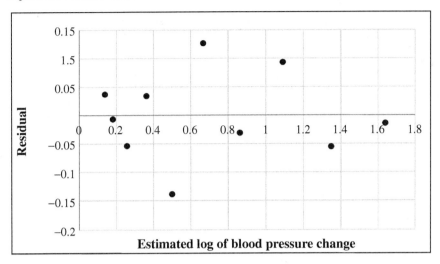

From that graphic display, we can see that the residuals are more uniformly balanced around zero throughout the range of estimated values of the dependent variable. Thus, it appears that the logarithmic transformation has helped to correct the heteroscedasticity and that the polynomial regression approach has corrected the nonadditivity. Now, we need to consider the assumption of a Gaussian distribution of estimates from all possible samples containing 10 observations. This sample's size is not sufficiently large for us to be comfortable that estimates of the regression coefficients, etc., will have a Gaussian distribution regardless of the distribution of the data. Therefore, we need to examine the distribution of the data. We can do that by constructing a normalized cumulative proportion polygon for the residual values. The next table shows the normalized cumulative frequencies that were used to construct the following polygon.

Residual (ordered)	Cumulative Frequency	Cumulative Proportion	Normalized Value
−0.137	1	0.10	−1.28
−0.054	2	0.20	−0.84
−0.053	3	0.30	−0.52
−0.030	4	0.40	−0.25
−0.014	5	0.50	0.00
−0.006	6	0.60	0.25
+0.035	7	0.70	0.52
+0.038	8	0.80	0.84
+0.095	9	0.90	1.28
+0.127	10	0.95*	1.64

*Calculated using Equation (13.1).

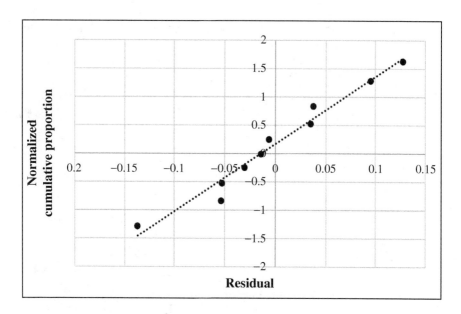

That normalized cumulative proportion polygon suggests that the distribution of residual values might be slightly leptokurtic. This is probably not sufficiently different from a Gaussian distribution, however, to cause us to abandon regression analysis. Further, trial and error investigation of other transformations, etc., does not result in a more Gaussian-type polygon. Thus, we can accept polynomial regression using the log transformation as a reasonable analytic approach to these data. ■

13.1.5 Dealing With Outliers

Outliers are data points that do not seem to fit the pattern suggested by other data points. When examining residuals while evaluating assumptions, it is not uncommon to observe a data point with a large residual compared to other data points. For instance, in Example 13.13 when using a polynomial function, the data point that corresponds to a dose of 45 mg has a residual of −4.560, substantially more than the residuals for other data points. This realization might lead us to suspect that something is wrong with that observation.

There are several rules of thumb intended to determine whether a particular data point is sufficiently unusual to be considered an outlier. The better ones use the interquartile range (see Chapter 2). When applied to residuals, the interquartile range is the interval centered on 0 that includes 50% of the values. For the polynomial model in Example 13.13, the interquartile range is 1.900. Then, residuals that are more than two interquartile ranges from zero are considered to be outliers. Thus, a residual less than −3.800 or greater than 3.800 is considered to be an outlier. The residual of −4.560 falls outside the interval and can be considered an outlier.

Once we have identified an outlier, what should we do? We definitely *do not* want to remove the outlier from the dataset based solely on the fact that it is an outlier. Instead, we want to go back to the data collection process and determine whether or not an error in measurement was made. If that is the case and the error cannot be corrected, then the outlier can be removed.

A reason we do not want to remove outliers without identifying an error is that the outlier may be an indication that we are trying to fit the wrong model to the data. In Example 13.14, a log transformation is applied to the polynomial equation. With that model, the residual for a dose of 45 mg is no longer an outlier and removing it would have been a mistake.

13.2 NOMINAL DEPENDENT VARIABLES

The assumptions we need to consider for analysis of nominal dependent variables are similar to those we make for analysis of continuous dependent variables. The ways in which we evaluate the appropriateness of those assumptions, however, is quite different from the ways we have just discussed for continuous dependent variables. Also, the solutions to suspected violation of those assumptions differ in some ways from the solutions for continuous dependent variables. Most notably, we cannot convert nominal variables to an ordinal scale and use a nonparametric method of analysis. The reason for this is that ordinal data contain more information than do nominal data (see Chapter 5). We can ignore information (as we do when converting continuous data to an ordinal scale), but we cannot create information (as a conversion from nominal data to an ordinal scale would require). Thus, we need to find other sorts of solutions to violation of assumptions for data sets containing a nominal dependent variable.

13.2.1 Assuming a Gaussian Distribution

Almost all of the statistical methods we encountered in previous chapters for interval estimation or hypothesis testing with nominal dependent variables rely on the assumption that estimates of a population's parameter (or some other, related value) calculated from all possible samples of a given size (i.e., the sampling distribution) have a Gaussian distribution.[62] This assumption is violated by every sample containing a nominal dependent variable. The reason that we can be sure that this assumption is always incorrect is because nominal data (and, therefore, anything calculated from nominal data) is discrete. In other words, we can choose two values for nominal data between which it is even theoretically impossible for another value to exist. The Gaussian distribution, on the other hand, is a distribution of continuous data. Between any two values of continuous data it is, at least theoretically, necessary that other values exist.

---

[62] An exception to this is Fisher's Exact Test.

Even though estimates for parameters of distributions of nominal data calculated from all possible samples of a given size can never truly have a Gaussian distribution, the sampling distribution of estimates gets closer to a Gaussian distribution as the sample's size increases. Part of the reason for this is due to the same principle in the central limit theorem that informed us that the distribution of estimates of the mean tends toward a Gaussian distribution as the size of the samples increases. Another part of the reason for this is the fact that estimates calculated from nominal data get more like estimates calculated from continuous data as the sample's size increases.

As an illustration, let us consider a nominal dependent variable representing data with two categories: cured and not cured. The parameter of the distribution of data in which we are most likely to have an interest in estimating is the probability of cure. If we were to imagine the distribution of estimates of that probability from samples with, say, 10 observations each, that distribution would include frequencies of only 11 different estimates. For samples with 20 observations, 21 different estimates are possible. As the size of the sample increases, the number of possible values for an estimate of a parameter of a distribution of nominal data increases and thus, becomes more like a distribution of estimates for continuous data.

There are three things we can conclude from these characteristics of nominal data and estimates of parameters of distributions of nominal data. First, the sampling distribution can never really be a Gaussian distribution. This is why we refer to methods for nominal dependent variables that are based on the Gaussian distribution as **normal approximations** (see Chapter 6). Second, the size of the sample has an important influence on how close the sampling distribution is to being a Gaussian distribution. Thus, part of our consideration of the appropriateness of a statistical method for a nominal dependent variable (based on a Gaussian sampling distribution) is how large the sample is. This also is an issue for continuous dependent variables, but the reasons for the sample's size being important are a little more complicated for nominal dependent variables.

The third thing that we can conclude from the characteristics of nominal data is that the population's distribution of data will never even be close to a Gaussian distribution. Consider, for instance, our previous illustration of nominal data with the categories of cured and not cured. The distribution of data could be represented graphically as the frequency of persons who are cured and the frequency of persons who are not cured. There are only two possible values for nominal data represented by a single nominal dependent variable (see Chapter 2). A distribution with only two possible data values cannot be a Gaussian distribution. Therefore, we cannot rely on the principle in the central limit theorem which states that the distribution of estimates from all possible samples of a given size will be a Gaussian distribution if the data have a Gaussian distribution, since nominal data never have a Gaussian distribution.

In the process of evaluating assumptions in the analysis of nominal dependent variables, therefore, examination of the sample's distribution of data for smaller samples can never be part of the process of speculation about the distribution of estimates from all possible samples (i.e., the sampling distribution). If the size of the sample containing a nominal dependent variable is too small for us to be comfortable with the assumption of a Gaussian sampling distribution, we must conclude that the assumption has not been satisfied. Unlike with continuous dependent variables, we cannot consider the population's distribution of nominal data as an indication that this assumption has been satisfied.

One of the implications of this distinction between the assumptions of a Gaussian distribution for nominal versus continuous dependent variables is that evaluation of the assumption for nominal dependent variables is much less complicated than evaluation of that assumption for continuous dependent variables. For nominal dependent variables, we need to only consider the size of the sample. In Chapter 6, we provided some rules of thumb for the sizes of samples required to use statistical procedures based on a Gaussian distribution. In univariable and bivariable analysis, normal approximations should be used only if the number of observations in the sample with the condition and without the condition specified by a nominal dependent variable are either equal to or greater than 5.[63]

Notice that this rule of thumb implies that larger samples are required when more extreme probabilities (i.e., further from 0.5) are considered. This is true for all normal approximations for nominal data. The further probabilities are from 0.5, the larger the sample's size that is required to use a normal approximation. Thus, it is not just the sample's size that is the issue. Rather, the issue is the sample's size and how the observations in the sample are apportioned between categories.

That rule of thumb for univariable procedures with nominal dependent variables is based on the expectation that we are using a normal approximation to calculate a confidence interval. That is the most likely circumstance, since interest in most univariable samples is in estimation rather than in hypothesis testing (see Chapter 6). When we wish to use a normal approximation approach for interval estimation, we examine the actual division of observations in the sample between the nominal categories. When we wish to use a normal approximation for statistical hypothesis testing, however, we consider the division of the observations in the sample dictated by the null hypothesis.[64] In other words, we are concerned about the number of observations we would expect to observe in each nominal category if the null hypothesis were true, rather than the number we have observed in each category. If the null hypothesis for a univariable sample stated that the probability of each category is equal to 0.5, then the sample's size required for the normal approximation

---

[63] This is probably the most commonly encountered rule of thumb; however, some statisticians suggest a more conservative criterion. R.A. Fisher, for instance, suggested a minimum of 15 observations in each category. Although this is likely to be too restrictive, we need to realize the assumption of a Gaussian distribution is seldom completely satisfied, but the larger the sample, the closer we get to satisfying that assumption.

[64] The reason for this distinction between interval estimation and hypothesis testing in terms of how we evaluate the size of the sample, is statistical hypothesis testing is always performed under the assumption that the null hypothesis is true. If the null hypothesis is true, the value of the population's parameter stated in the null hypothesis is assumed to be the value of the parameter in the population. In interval estimation, on the other hand, the sample's point estimate is our best guess of the value of the population's parameter.

would be 10 or more observations. This would be true regardless of the number of observations in each nominal category actually contained in the sample. For statistical hypothesis testing, the important issue is that the null hypothesis that the probability is equal to 0.5 in the population tells us to expect 5 observations in each nominal category when the sample consists of 10 observations.

In bivariable analyses of a nominal dependent variable, the size of the sample (and apportionment of the sample among categories) required for a normal approximation is much like the requirement for univariable analysis. When using the normal approximation for the difference between two probabilities, the chi-square test, or the Mantel–Haenszel test for statistical hypothesis testing, none of the expected frequencies in the corresponding 2×2 table should be no fewer than 5. The chi-square test for trend is a little bit more complicated, for that procedure will involve more than the four categories we have in a 2×2 table. With more than four categories, statistical hypothesis testing using a normal approximation requires 80% of the categories to have expected frequencies greater than or equal to 5, and none of the expected frequencies less than 1.

It becomes more difficult to supply rules of thumb for multivariable analyses of nominal dependent variables. The greatest degree of complication is encountered when some of the independent variables represent continuous data (such as in most logistic and Cox regression analyses). Rather than attempt rules of thumb, we will simply point out that these procedures for nominal dependent variables also involve the size of the sample. The overall sample's size that is required for a normal approximation in multivariable analyses is larger than the sample's size for bivariable or univariable analyses. It is not necessary, however, that the number of observations corresponding to each independent variable value (e.g., the number of observations in each stratum in a stratified analysis) be large.

When we are concerned about the assumption of a Gaussian distribution for a normal approximation procedure, there is only one solution that is commonly employed. That solution is to abandon the normal approximation and to use a procedure that is specifically designed for the actual sampling distribution. These procedures are called **exact tests**.

13.2.2   Assuming Equal Variances

In the previous discussion, we came to understand that sampling distributions of estimates for nominal dependent variables never really are Gaussian distributions. Now, we will consider the fact that variances for groups of nominal data are never equal unless the probabilities associated with those groups are equal. As we learned in Chapter 6, the variance of nominal data is equal to the probability of the event multiplied by the probability of the complement of the event.[65] Any time we are considering different probabilities, the variances of data that those probabilities

---

[65]This is not true for the normal approximation to the Poisson in which the variance is a constant.

represent must be different.[66] Therefore, procedures for nominal dependent variables do not assume homoscedasticity.

13.2.3 Assuming Additive Relationships

All normal approximations for bivariable or multivariable analyses of a nominal dependent variable assume an additive relationship, as did analyses for continuous dependent variables. Relationships involving nominal dependent variables, however, very often do not meet this assumption, unless the dependent variable is transformed. We encountered some of these transformations in previous chapters, for example, we used a logarithmic transformation of probability ratios when we calculated summary estimates over all strata in stratified analysis. We did this to satisfy the assumption of additivity in calculation of a weighted average. Also, we found that a logarithmic transformation of rates in Cox regression and a logit transformation of probabilities in logistic regression were required to satisfy the assumption of additivity.

The following table provides a quick reference to what assumptions are made about the dependent variable by most statistical procedures.

Dependent Variable	Independent Variables?	Procedure	Random Sample	Independence	Gaussian Distribution	Homoscedasticity	Additivity
Continuous	No	All	X	X	X	–	–
Ordinal	No	All	X	X	–	–	–
Nominal	No	Approximation	X	X	X	–	–
Nominal	No	Exact	X	X	–	–	–
Continuous	Yes	All	X	X	X	X	X
Ordinal	Yes	All	X	X	–	–	—
Nominal	Yes	Approximation	X	X	X	–	X
Nominal	Yes	Exact	X	X	–	–	X

13.3 INDEPENDENT VARIABLES

There is one assumption that we make for all independent variables regardless of the type of data that they represent. That assumption is that the values of the independent variables in the sample are measured with perfect precision (i.e., without random error). To see why we make this assumption and what happens if it is violated, imagine a clinical trial in which we randomize some persons to receive a drug and other persons to receive a placebo. Suppose that the dependent variable represents diastolic blood pressure. Thus, the data from this study consist of two groups of diastolic blood pressure values: one for persons who received the drug and one

---

[66] An exception to this rule is when the different probabilities are complements of one another.

for persons who received the placebo. Those two groups are specified by the two values of the nominal independent variable representing the treatment. Most likely, we would analyze these data by comparing the means of diastolic blood pressure between the two groups of persons. If the drug is efficacious in lowering diastolic blood pressure, we would expect the mean of the diastolic blood pressure vales to be lower for persons who received the drug than the mean for persons who received the placebo.

If we did not measure values of the independent variable in that example with perfect precision, some of the persons who received the placebo would have their diastolic blood pressure values listed among the values for persons who received the drug and vice versa, The effect of that imprecision would be to increase the mean diastolic blood pressure in the group that is thought to contain measurements for persons who received the drug and to decrease that mean in the group that is thought to contain measurements for persons who received the placebo. In other words, the difference between the means of the two groups would be closer to 0 that it would have been if we specified, without error, to which group a person belongs.

This example illustrates the general effect of measuring an independent variable with less than perfect precision. Regardless of what type of point estimate is used to summarize relationships among dependent variable values (differences between means, correlation coefficients, regression coefficients, odds ratios, etc.), measuring independent variable values imprecisely will cause point estimates to be closer, on the average, to the value usually stated in the null hypothesis (i.e., 0 for differences, correlation coefficients, and regression coefficients, and 1 for ratios) than the corresponding value in the population.[67] That is to say, point estimates for dependent variable values will be biased[68] toward the null value when independent variables are imprecisely measured.

For independent variables that are included in a data set because they represent characteristics for which we wish to control (i.e., confounding variables), the problem of imprecise measurement leads to an additional concern. As for all independent variables, any point estimate for dependent variable values corresponding to various values of a confounding variable will be closer to the null value, on the average, than the population's value. Consequently, less of the variation in dependent variable values associated with the confounding variable will be accounted for in the analysis. That implies that including the confounding variable in the analysis will be less effective in controlling for confounding by the characteristic that it represents that it would if the confounding variable were measured precisely. Thus, imprecision in measurement of confounding variables results in incomplete control of confounding.

---

[67] Here, we are assuming that imprecision in measuring independent variable is random and equal for all the observational units. This is sometimes called **nondifferential impression**.

[68] Recall that bias is a directional deviation from the truth. This is an example of random error in the measurement of independent variable values that result in a biased estimate. We consider the estimate to be biased since it deviates from the population's value in a specific direction (i.e., toward the value in the null hypothesis).

Evaluation of this assumption that independent variable values have been measured with perfect precision is like evaluation of the assumptions of a random sample and of statistical independence of dependent variable values. That is to say, this assumption cannot be evaluated by examining the sample's data. Rather, we need to understand the way in which independent variable values have been measured. For most independent variables, our evaluation will not be to determine whether or not those independent variables have been measured with perfect precision, since it is virtually impossible to measure most data in health research perfectly. Instead, the issue more often is to determine the degree of imprecision in our measurements. The greater the degree of imprecision, the greater the effect of that imprecision.

Another assumption sometimes made about independent variables is that they have been sampled naturalistically. That is so that their distribution in the sample represents their distribution in the population. This assumption is made only when interpreting the strength of the association between the dependent variable and the independent variable(s). A parameter that does this is the correlation coefficient. This assumption was discussed in Chapter 7. Like the assumptions of a random sample or statistical independence of measurements, this assumption can only be evaluated by understanding the sampling method. There is no remedy if the assumption is violated.

CHAPTER SUMMARY

There is one assumption made by all statistical procedures of estimation and hypothesis testing. That is the assumption of a random sample. The way in which we evaluate this assumption is by understanding the method of sampling and determination if it results in a sample that is essentially random. If this assumption is violated, there is nothing we can do to make a sample representative of the population.

A second assumption that is nearly as universal as the assumption of a random sample is the assumption that the dependent variable values have been sample in such a way that they are independent of one another. Evaluation of this assumption, like the first, relies on an understanding of the sampling process to determine if each observation of the dependent variable provides independent information about the dependent variable in the population. If this assumption is violated, special statistical methods that take the lack of independence into account must be used. Two such methods discussed in this text are the paired t-test and McNemar's test.

A third assumption that is made for continuous and nominal dependent variables is that the sampling distribution is a Gaussian distribution. This is probably the most misunderstood assumption, for people often believe it is the distribution of data that is assumed to be Gaussian. It is not. That impression results from the fact that, if the sample is too small to rely on the central limit theorem to produce a Gaussian sampling distribution, we examine the distribution of continuous data. That is because that sampling distribution will be Gaussian if the data are Gaussian regardless of the sample's size.

We looked at three ways in which to evaluate the distribution of data in the sample. They were graphic, numeric, and inferential approaches. The best graphic approach is examination of a normalized cumulative proportion plot which is often called a normal plot. Here, a Gaussian distribution is represented as a straight line. The numeric approach involves estimating the skewness and kurtosis of the distribution. A Gaussian distribution will have a skewness equal to 0 and a kurtosis equal to 0. The best inferential approach is a Kolmogorov–Smirnov test.

A problem with the inferential approach is that it has low statistical power for small samples and it is only when we have small samples that we are interested in the distribution of data. For this reason, many statisticians prefer the graphic approach when evaluating the distribution of data in a small sample.

When the assumption of a Gaussian sampling distribution is applied to bivariable and multivariable datasets, it is not the distribution of data we examine when we have a small sample, but rather the distribution of residuals. A residual is the difference between an observed and an estimated value of the dependent variable. The same graphic, numeric, and inferential approaches to evaluating the distribution of data can be applied to the distribution of residuals.

If there is a problem with the assumption of a Gaussian sampling distribution, there are two possible solutions. One is to convert the data to an ordinal scale and use a nonparametric method. A problem with that solution is that there is no nonparametric regression analysis.

The second solution is to transform the dependent variable values. That is to put the dependent variable values on a different scale. The most commonly successful transformation is the log transformation. It is effective in solving a problem with a positive skew. Other transformations for a positive skew are the square root and the inverse transformation. Power transformations can solve problems with a negative skew and angular transformations can solve problems with kurtosis.

Another assumption for bivariable and multivariable datasets with continuous dependent variables is the assumption of homoscedasticity. Here, we are assuming that the variance of the dependent variable is the same regardless of the value(s) of the independent variable(s). The assumption of homoscedasticity can be evaluated graphically, numerically, or inferentially.

When there are continuous independent variables, the graphic approach is the best choice. In this approach, the residuals are plotted against the estimated values of the dependent variable. If there is homoscedasticity, the points in that graph will be evenly spread around 0 throughout the range of estimated values. In the case of heteroscedasticity, the spread will be uneven, usually increasing as the estimate value increases.

When there are only nominal independent variables, either the numeric or inferential approach can be used. The numeric approach involves looking at the variance estimates in each group and judging whether they appear to be close together. The inferential approach involves an F-test in bivariable analysis and Bartlett's test in multivariable analysis.

Problems with the assumption of homoscedasticity can be solved either by converting the data to an ordinal scale and using a nonparametric analysis or by transforming the dependent variable. The same transformations used for problems with the assumption of a Gaussian sampling distribution can be used to solve problems with homoscedasticity. Another solution is to use statistical methods that do not assume homoscedasticity like the t-test for unequal variances.

Another assumption for bivariable and multivariable data sets with a continuous dependent variable is the assumption of additivity or linearity. In this assumption, we assume that the relationship between the dependent variable and independent variable(s) is a linear one. This implies that, for instance, means are compared as differences and the relationship with a continuous independent variable can be described by a straight line.

Linearity can be assessed graphically or inferentially. The graph that is used is the same one that was used to evaluate homoscedasticity. This is a graph of residuals compared to estimated values of the dependent variable. If the relationship is linear, the residual will be uniformly spread around 0 throughout the range of estimated values. If the assumption of linearity is violated, there will be a predominance of positive residuals in some regions and negative residuals in other regions. The inferential approach involves polynomial functions. If there is linearity, these polynomial functions will not be statistically significant.

If the assumption of linearity has been violated, we can transform the dependent variable looking for a scale in which there is linearity. Alternatively, we can include polynomial functions of the independent variable(s). In the case of binomial correlation analysis, we also have the option of converting the continuous variables to an ordinal scale.

Sometimes, a dataset contains an observation or two that do not seem to fit in with the rest of the observations. These unusual observations are often called outliers. The temptation is to assume something is wrong with those observations and remove them from the dataset. We should resist this temptation. Instead, we should go back to the data collection process and see if anything unusual happened. If not, the presence of outliers might be an indication we are using the wrong model.

For a nominal dependent variable, we make the assumption that the sampling distribution can be represented as a Gaussian distribution whenever we use a normal approximation. Nothing can be done to make the distribution of data Gaussian, so we must rely on the sample's size to satisfy this assumption. The univariable rule of thumb is that we need at least five events and five nonevents to be comfortable with the normal approximation. The bivariable rule of thumb is that there should be at least five expected events for each value in a 2×2 table. More are needed in multivariable analysis, although no accepted rule of thumb exists.

Methods for nominal dependent variable do not assume homoscedasticity. Most method do not calculate a pooled variance estimate. When a pooled variance estimate is calculated, it is done assuming unequal variances.

All bivariable and multivariable procedures for a nominal dependent variable assume additivity or linearity. This is solved, however, with built-in transformations.

For example, ratio measures are analyzed on a log scale. Division is subtraction on a log scale solving the problem of additivity. Logistic and Cox regression analyses have built-in transformations as well.

There is one universal assumption for independent variables. That is, they are measured with perfect precision. Violation of this assumption will cause associations to be underestimated and confounding to be incompletely controlled. There is no solution to violation of this assumption. The best that can be done is to consider this effect when interpreting results of analyses.

A second assumption for independent variables is made when performing correlation analysis. This is that the independent variable has been sampled naturalistically. This can only be evaluated by understanding the sampling method. Nothing can be done to fix it if this assumption is violated.

EXERCISES

13.1. Suppose we are interested in the relationship between dietary sodium intake (NA) and diastolic blood pressure (DBP). To investigate this relationship, we measure both for a sample of 40 persons. Because DBP and NA both increase with age, we decide to control for age in our analysis. The data for this question are in the Excel file: EXR10_1 on the website accompanying this textbook. Evaluate the assumption of a Gaussian sampling distribution. Which of the following is the best conclusion?

A. Based on the sample's size, the assumption is satisfied

B. Based on the distribution of data, the assumption is satisfied

C. The assumption is violated

13.2. Suppose we are interested in which blood chemistry measurements are predictive of urine creatinine. To investigate this, we identify 100 persons and measure their urine creatinine levels. We also measure serum creatinine, blood urea nitrogen (BUN), and serum potassium. These data are in the Excel file: EXR10_2 on the website accompanying this textbook. Use Excel or R to perform a regression with urine creatinine as the dependent variable and serum creatinine, BUN, and serum potassium as the independent variables. Evaluate the assumption of a Gaussian sampling distribution. Which of the following is the best conclusion?

A. Based on the sample's size, the assumption is satisfied

B. Based on the distribution of data, the assumption is satisfied

C. The assumption is violated

13.3. Suppose we are interested in the relationship between dietary sodium intake (NA) and diastolic blood pressure (DBP). To investigate this relationship, we measure both for a sample of 40 persons. Because DBP and NA both increase with age, we decide to control for age in our analysis. The data for this question are in the Excel file: EXR10_1 on the website accompanying this textbook. Evaluate the assumption of homoscedasticity. Which of the following is the best conclusion?

A. The assumption is satisfied
B. The assumption is violated

13.4. Suppose we are interested in which blood chemistry measurements are predictive of urine creatinine. To investigate this, we identify 100 persons and measure their urine creatinine levels. We also measure serum creatinine, blood urea nitrogen (BUN), and serum potassium. These data are in the Excel file: EXR10_2 on the website accompanying this textbook. Use Excel or R to perform a regression with urine creatinine as the dependent variable and serum creatinine, BUN, and serum potassium as the independent variables. Evaluate the assumption of homoscedasticity. Which of the following is the best conclusion?

A. The assumption is satisfied
B. The assumption is violated

13.5. Suppose we are interested in the relationship between dietary sodium intake (NA) and diastolic blood pressure (DBP). To investigate this relationship, we measure both for a sample of 40 persons. Because DBP and NA both increase with age, we decide to control for age in our analysis. The data for this question are in the Excel file: EXR10_1 on the website accompanying this textbook. Evaluate the assumption of linearity. Which of the following is the best conclusion?

A. The assumption is satisfied
B. The assumption is violated

13.6. Suppose we are interested in which blood chemistry measurements are predictive of urine creatinine. To investigate this, we identify 100 persons and measure their urine creatinine levels. We also measure serum creatinine, blood urea nitrogen (BUN), and serum potassium. These data are in the Excel file called EXR10_2 on the website accompanying this textbook. Use Excel or R to perform a regression with urine creatinine as the dependent variable and serum creatinine, BUN, and serum potassium as the independent variables. Evaluate the assumption of linearity. Which of the following is the best conclusion?

A. The assumption is satisfied
B. The assumption is violated

13.7. Suppose we are interested in the relationship between dietary sodium intake (NA) and diastolic blood pressure (DBP). To investigate this relationship, we measure both for a sample of 40 persons. Because DBP and NA both increase with age, we decide to control for age in our analysis. The data for this question are in the Excel file: EXR10_1 on the website accompanying this textbook. Perform a log transformation on DBP then evaluate the assumption of homoscedasticity. Which of the following is the best conclusion?

A. The assumption is satisfied

B. The assumption is violated

13.8. Suppose we are interested in which blood chemistry measurements are predictive of urine creatinine. To investigate this, we identify 100 persons and measure their urine creatinine levels. We also measure serum creatinine, blood urea nitrogen (BUN), and serum potassium. These data are in the Excel file called EXR10_2 on the website accompanying this textbook. Use Excel or R to perform a regression with the log of urine creatinine as the dependent variable and serum creatinine, BUN, and serum potassium as the independent variables. Evaluate the assumption of homoscedasticity. Which of the following is the best conclusion?

A. The assumption is satisfied

B. The assumption is violated

13.9. In a study of clinical depression, patients were randomly assigned to one of four drug groups (three active drugs and a placebo) and to a cognitive therapy group (active versus placebo). The dependent variable is a difference between scores on a depression questionnaire. The results are in the Excel file: EXR10_5 on the website accompanying this textbook. Evaluate the assumption that the sampling distribution is Gaussian. Which of the following is the best conclusion to draw?

A. Based on the sample's size, the assumption is satisfied

B. Based on the distribution of data, the assumption is satisfied

C. The assumption is violated

13.10. In a multicenter study of a new treatment for hypertension, patients at nine centers were randomly assigned to a new treatment or standard treatment. The dependent variable is a difference in diastolic blood pressure from a pretreatment value. The results are in the Excel file: EXR10_6 on the website accompanying this textbook. Evaluate the assumption that the sampling distribution is Gaussian. Which of the following is the best conclusion to draw?

A. Based on the sample's size, the assumption is satisfied

B. Based on the distribution of data, the assumption is satisfied

C. The assumption is violated

13.11. In a study of clinical depression, patients were randomly assigned to one of four drug groups (three active drugs and a placebo) and to a cognitive therapy group (active versus placebo). The dependent variable is a differ-ence between scores on a depression questionnaire. The results are in the Excel file: EXR10_5 on the website accompanying this textbook. Evaluate the assumption homoscedasticity. Which of the following is the best conclu-sion to draw?

A. The assumption is satisfied

B. The assumption is violated

13.12. In a multicenter study of a new treatment for hypertension, patients at nine centers were randomly assigned to a new treatment or standard treatment. The dependent variable is a difference in diastolic blood pressure from a pretreatment value. The results are in the Excel file: EXR10_6 on the website accompanying this textbook. Evaluate the assumption of homoscedasticity. Which of the following is the best conclusion to draw?

A. The assumption is satisfied

B. The assumption is violated

APPENDIX A

FLOWCHARTS

Chapters 4 through 12 are structured to reflect the thinking process of statisticians when choosing a statistical method to analyze a particular set of data. At the beginning of each of these chapters, the methods discussed in that chapter appear in a flowchart that summarizes statisticians' thinking process. In this appendix, we have brought these flowcharts together so that they are easier to use. As explained in the introduction to Part Two, you should start by using the master flowchart (designated as Flowchart A.1 in the text) that appears below. Following the steps in this flowchart will lead to the chapter of the text that discusses the types of statistical methods that might be used to analyze a particular set of data. The flowcharts following the master flowchart in this appendix are labeled according to the chapter in which they are discussed (A.2–A.10). Examining these flowcharts will reveal the most commonly used statistical methods to analyze your data.

In each of the subsequent flowcharts, the estimate that is most often used to describe the dependent variable is in bold, the common name of the statistical test is enclosed in a box, the standard distribution (or approach) that is used to test hypotheses and/or calculate confidence intervals is in bold and underlined.

Introduction to Biostatistical Applications in Health Research with Microsoft Office Excel® and R,
Second Edition. Robert P. Hirsch.
© 2021 John Wiley & Sons, Inc. Published 2021 by John Wiley & Sons, Inc.
Companion website: www.wiley.com/go/hirsch/healthresearch2e

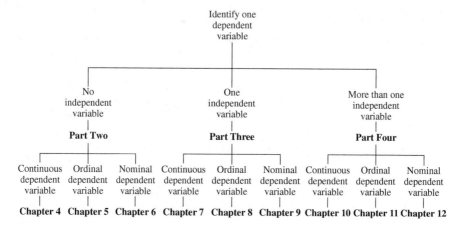

FLOWCHART A.1   Master flowchart.

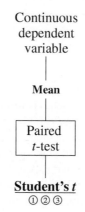

FLOWCHART A.2   Chapter 4: univariable analysis of a continuous dependent variable.

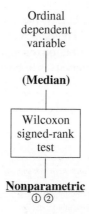

FLOWCHART A.3   Chapter 5: univariable analysis of an ordinal dependent variable.

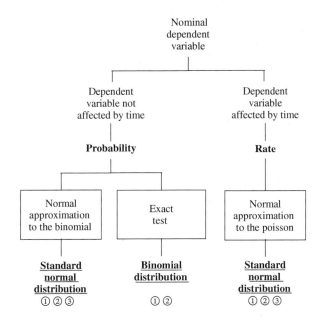

FLOWCHART A.4   Chapter 6: univariable analysis of a nominal dependent variable.

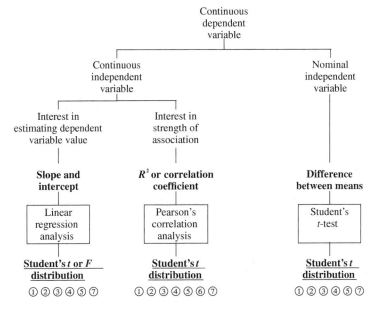

FLOWCHART A.5   Chapter 7: bivariable analysis of a continuous dependent variable.

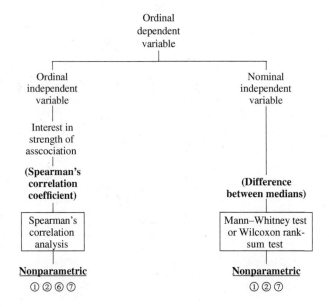

FLOWCHART A.6 Chapter 8: bivariable analysis of an ordinal dependent variable.

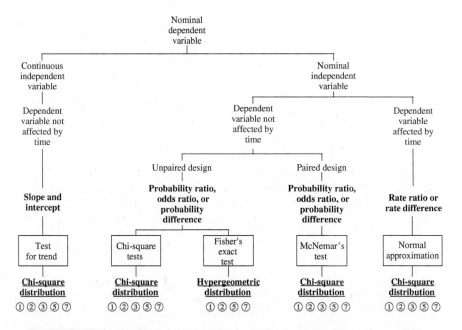

FLOWCHART A.7 Chapter 9: bivariable analysis of a nominal dependent variable.

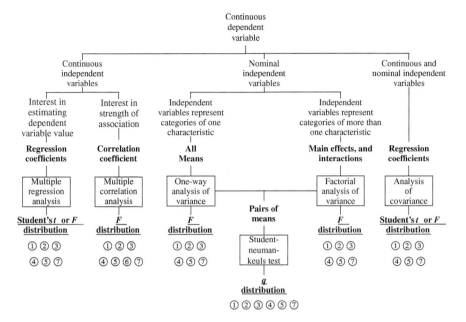

FLOWCHART A.8 Chapter 10: multivariable analysis of a continuous dependent variable.

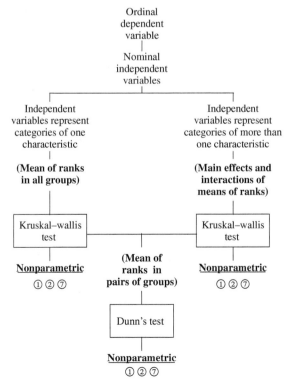

FLOWCHART A.9 Chapter 11: multivariable analysis of an ordinal dependent variable.

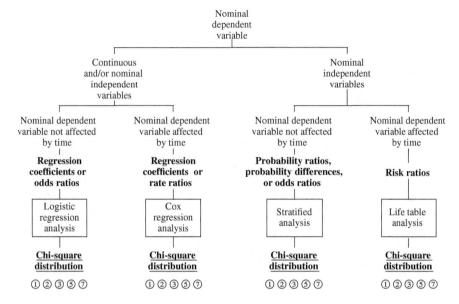

FLOWCHART A.10   Chapter 12: multivariable analysis of a nominal dependent variable.

Added to these flowcharts are indicators of the assumptions made by each test. These numbers stand for the following assumptions:

1. Random sample of dependent variable values
2. Independence of observations of the dependent variable
3. Gaussian sampling distribution
4. Homoscedasticity (homogeneity of variances)
5. Additivity (linearity)
6. Naturalistic sample of independent variable values
7. Independent variable measured with perfect precision

APPENDIX B

STATISTICAL TABLES

Introduction to Biostatistical Applications in Health Research with Microsoft Office Excel® and R,
Second Edition. Robert P. Hirsch.
© 2021 John Wiley & Sons, Inc. Published 2021 by John Wiley & Sons, Inc.
Companion website: www.wiley.com/go/hirsch/healthresearch2e

TABLE B.1. Area in One Tail of the Standard Normal Distribution*

z	0	1	2	3	4	5	6	7	8	9
0.0	0.5000	0.4960	0.4920	0.4880	0.4840	0.4801	0.4761	0.4721	0.4681	0.4641
0.1	0.4602	0.4562	0.4522	0.4483	0.4443	0.4404	0.4364	0.4325	0.4286	0.4247
0.2	0.4207	0.4168	0.4129	0.4090	0.4052	0.4013	0.3974	0.3936	0.3897	0.3859
0.3	0.3821	0.3783	0.3745	0.3707	0.3669	0.3632	0.3594	0.3557	0.3520	0.3483
0.4	0.3446	0.3409	0.3372	0.3336	0.3300	0.3264	0.3228	0.3192	0.3156	0.3121
0.5	0.3085	0.3050	0.3015	0.2981	0.2946	0.2912	0.2877	0.2843	0.2810	0.2776
0.6	0.2743	0.2709	0.2676	0.2643	0.2611	0.2578	0.2546	0.2514	0.2483	0.2451
0.7	0.2420	0.2389	0.2358	0.2327	0.2297	0.2266	0.2236	0.2207	0.2177	0.2148
0.8	0.2119	0.2090	0.2061	0.2033	0.2005	0.1977	0.1949	0.1922	0.1894	0.1867
0.9	0.1841	0.1814	0.1788	0.1762	0.1736	0.1711	0.1685	0.1660	0.1635	0.1611
1.0	0.1587	0.1562	0.1539	0.1515	0.1492	0.1469	0.1446	0.1423	0.1401	0.1379
1.1	0.1357	0.1335	0.1314	0.1292	0.1271	0.1251	0.1230	0.1210	0.1190	0.1170
1.2	0.1151	0.1131	0.1112	0.1093	0.1075	0.1056	0.1038	0.1020	0.1003	0.0985
1.3	0.0968	0.0951	0.0934	0.0918	0.0901	0.0885	0.0869	0.0853	0.0838	0.0823
1.4	0.0808	0.0793	0.0778	0.0764	0.0749	0.0735	0.0721	0.0708	0.0694	0.0681
1.5	0.0668	0.0655	0.0643	0.0630	0.0618	0.0606	0.0594	0.0582	0.0571	0.0559
1.6	0.0548	0.0537	0.0526	0.0516	0.0505	0.0495	0.0485	0.0475	0.0465	0.0455
1.7	0.0446	0.0436	0.0427	0.0418	0.0409	0.0401	0.0392	0.0384	0.0375	0.0367
1.8	0.0359	0.0351	0.0344	0.0336	0.0329	0.0322	0.0314	0.0307	0.0301	0.0294
1.9	0.0287	0.0281	0.0274	0.0268	0.0262	0.0256	0.0250	0.0244	0.0239	0.0233

z	0	1	2	3	4	5	6	7	8	9
2.0	0.0228	0.0222	0.0217	0.0212	0.0207	0.0202	0.0197	0.0192	0.0188	0.0183
2.1	0.0179	0.0174	0.0170	0.0166	0.0162	0.0158	0.0154	0.0150	0.0146	0.0143
2.2	0.0139	0.0136	0.0132	0.0129	0.0125	0.0122	0.0119	0.0116	0.0113	0.0110
2.3	0.0107	0.0104	0.0102	0.0099	0.0096	0.0094	0.0091	0.0089	0.0087	0.0084
2.4	0.0082	0.0080	0.0078	0.0075	0.0073	0.0071	0.0069	0.0068	0.0066	0.0064
2.5	0.0062	0.0060	0.0059	0.0057	0.0055	0.0054	0.0052	0.0051	0.0049	0.0048
2.6	0.0047	0.0045	0.0044	0.0043	0.0041	0.0040	0.0039	0.0038	0.0037	0.0036
2.7	0.0035	0.0034	0.0033	0.0032	0.0031	0.0030	0.0029	0.0028	0.0027	0.0026
2.8	0.0026	0.0025	0.0024	0.0023	0.0023	0.0022	0.0021	0.0021	0.0020	0.0019
2.9	0.0019	0.0018	0.0018	0.0017	0.0016	0.0016	0.0015	0.0015	0.0014	0.0014
3.0	0.0013	0.0013	0.0013	0.0012	0.0012	0.0011	0.0011	0.0011	0.0010	0.0010
3.1	0.0010	0.0009	0.0009	0.0009	0.0008	0.0008	0.0008	0.0008	0.0007	0.0007
3.2	0.0007	0.0007	0.0006	0.0006	0.0006	0.0006	0.0006	0.0005	0.0005	0.0005
3.3	0.0005	0.0005	0.0005	0.0004	0.0004	0.0004	0.0004	0.0004	0.0004	0.0003
3.4	0.0003	0.0003	0.0003	0.0003	0.0003	0.0003	0.0003	0.0003	0.0003	0.0002
3.5	0.0002	0.0002	0.0002	0.0002	0.0002	0.0002	0.0002	0.0002	0.0002	0.0002
3.6	0.0002	0.0002	0.0001	0.0001	0.0001	0.0001	0.0001	0.0001	0.0001	0.0001
3.7	0.0001	0.0001	0.0001	0.0001	0.0001	0.0001	0.0001	0.0001	0.0001	0.0001
3.8	0.0001	0.0001	0.0001	0.0001	0.0001	0.0001	0.0001	0.0001	0.0001	0.0001

*To determine the area in one tail of the standard normal distribution, calculate a standard normal deviate (z) to two decimal places. Find the first two digits of that deviate (units and tenths) in the left-hand column. Find the third digit (hundredths) in the top row. The corresponding area is at the intersection of that column and that row.

TABLE B.2. Critical Values of Student's t-Distribution*

$\alpha(2)$	0.50	0.20	0.10	0.05	0.02	0.01	0.005	0.002	0.001
$\alpha(1)$	0.25	0.10	0.05	0.025	0.01	0.005	0.0025	0.001	0.0005
df									
1	1.000	3.078	6.314	12.71	31.82	63.66	127.3	318.3	636.6
2	0.816	1.886	2.920	4.303	6.965	9.925	14.09	22.33	31.60
3	0.765	1.638	2.353	3.182	4.541	5.841	7.453	10.22	12.92
4	0.741	1.533	2.132	2.776	3.747	4.604	5.598	7.173	8.610
5	0.727	1.476	2.015	2.571	3.365	4.032	4.773	5.893	6.869
6	0.718	1.440	1.943	2.447	3.143	3.707	4.317	5.208	5.959
7	0.711	1.415	1.895	2.365	2.998	3.499	4.029	4.785	5.408
8	0.706	1.397	1.860	2.306	2.896	3.355	3.833	4.501	5.041
9	0.703	1.383	1.833	2.262	2.821	3.250	3.690	4.297	4.781
10	0.700	1.372	1.812	2.228	2.764	3.169	3.581	4.144	4.587
11	0.697	1.363	1.796	2.201	2.718	3.106	3.497	4.025	4.437
12	0.695	1.356	1.782	2.179	2.681	3.055	3.428	3.930	4.318
13	0.694	1.350	1.771	2.160	2.650	3.012	3.372	3.852	4.221
14	0.692	1.345	1.761	2.145	2.624	2.977	3.326	3.787	4.140
15	0.691	1.341	1.753	2.131	2.602	2.947	3.286	3.733	4.073
16	0.690	1.337	1.746	2.120	2.583	2.921	3.252	3.686	4.015
17	0.689	1.333	1.740	2.110	2.567	2.898	3.222	3.646	3.965
18	0.688	1.330	1.734	2.101	2.552	2.878	3.197	3.610	3.922

α(2)	0.50	0.20	0.10	0.05	0.02	0.01	0.005	0.002	0.001
α(1)	0.25	0.10	0.05	0.025	0.01	0.005	0.0025	0.001	0.0005
df									
19	0.688	1.328	1.729	2.093	2.539	2.861	3.174	3.579	3.883
20	0.687	1.325	1.725	2.086	2.528	2.845	3.153	3.552	3.850
22	0.686	1.321	1.717	2.074	2.508	2.819	3.119	3.505	3.792
24	0.685	1.318	1.711	2.064	2.492	2.797	3.091	3.467	3.745
26	0.684	1.315	1.706	2.056	2.479	2.779	3.067	3.435	3.707
28	0.683	1.313	1.701	2.048	2.467	2.763	3.047	3.408	3.674
30	0.683	1.310	1.697	2.042	2.457	2.750	3.030	3.385	3.646
32	0.682	1.309	1.694	2.037	2.449	2.738	3.015	3.365	3.622
34	0.682	1.307	1.691	2.032	2.441	2.728	3.002	3.348	3.601
36	0.681	1.306	1.688	2.028	2.434	2.719	2.990	3.333	3.582
38	0.681	1.304	1.686	2.024	2.429	2.712	2.980	3.319	3.566
40	0.681	1.303	1.684	2.021	2.423	2.704	2.971	3.307	3.551
45	0.680	1.301	1.679	2.014	2.412	2.690	2.952	3.281	3.520
50	0.679	1.299	1.676	2.009	2.403	2.678	2.937	3.261	3.496
55	0.679	1.297	1.674	2.004	2.396	2.668	2.925	3.245	3.477
60	0.679	1.296	1.671	2.000	2.390	2.660	2.915	3.232	3.460
65	0.678	1.295	1.669	1.997	2.385	2.654	2.906	3.221	3.447

(Continued)

TABLE B.2. (*Continued*)

70	0.678	1.294	1.667	1.994	2.381	2.648	2.899	3.211	3.435
75	0.678	1.293	1.665	1.992	2.377	2.643	2.893	3.203	3.425
80	0.678	1.292	1.664	1.990	2.374	2.639	2.887	3.195	3.416
85	0.677	1.291	1.663	1.988	2.371	2.635	2.882	3.189	3.409
90	0.677	1.291	1.662	1.987	2.368	2.632	2.878	3.183	3.402
100	0.677	1.290	1.660	1.984	2.364	2.626	2.871	3.174	3.390
150	0.676	1.287	1.655	1.976	2.351	2.609	2.849	3.145	3.357
200	0.676	1.286	1.653	1.972	2.345	2.601	2.839	3.131	3.340
500	0.675	1.283	1.648	1.965	2.334	2.586	2.820	3.107	3.310
∞	0.674	1.282	1.645	1.960	2.326	2.576	2.807	3.090	3.290

*To locate Student's t-value, find the degrees of freedom in the leftmost column and the appropriate α at the top of the table ($\alpha(2)$ indicates a two-tailed value and $\alpha(1)$ indicates a one-tailed value). The number in the body of the table where this row and column intersect is Student's t-value from a distribution with that number of degrees of freedom and that corresponds to an area equal to α.

TABLE B.3. Critical Values of Wilcoxon's *T* Statistic*

$\alpha(2)$	0.50	0.20	0.10	0.05	0.02	0.01	0.005	0.001
$\alpha(1)$	0.25	0.10	0.05	0.025	0.01	0.005	0.0025	0.0005
n								
4	2	0						
5	4	2	0					
6	6	3	2	0				
7	9	5	3	2	0			
8	12	8	5	3	1	0		
9	16	10	8	5	3	1	0	
10	20	14	10	8	5	3	1	
11	24	17	13	10	7	5	3	0
12	29	21	17	13	9	7	5	1
13	35	26	21	17	12	9	7	2
14	40	31	25	21	15	12	9	4
15	47	36	30	25	19	15	12	6
16	54	42	35	29	23	19	15	8
17	61	48	41	34	27	23	19	11
18	69	55	47	40	32	27	23	14
19	77	62	53	46	37	32	27	18
20	86	69	60	52	43	37	32	21

(Continued)

TABLE B.3. (Continued)

	95	77	67	58	49	42	37	25
21	95	77	67	58	49	42	37	25
22	104	86	75	65	55	48	42	30
23	114	94	83	73	62	54	48	35
24	125	104	91	81	69	61	54	40
25	136	113	100	89	76	68	60	45
26	148	124	110	98	84	75	67	51
27	160	134	119	107	92	83	74	57
28	172	145	130	116	101	91	82	64
29	185	157	140	126	110	100	90	71
30	198	169	151	137	120	109	98	78
32	226	194	175	159	140	128	116	94
34	257	221	200	182	162	148	136	111
36	289	250	227	208	185	171	157	130
38	323	281	256	235	211	194	180	150
40	358	313	286	264	238	220	204	172
42	396	348	319	294	266	247	230	195
44	436	384	353	327	296	276	258	220

$\alpha(2)$	0.50	0.20	0.10	0.05	0.02	0.01	0.005	0.001
$\alpha(1)$	0.25	0.10	0.05	0.025	0.01	0.005	0.0025	0.0005
n								
46	477	422	389	361	328	307	287	246
48	521	462	426	396	362	339	318	274
50	566	503	466	434	397	373	350	304
55	688	615	573	536	493	465	438	385
60	822	739	690	648	600	567	537	476
65	968	875	820	772	718	681	647	577
70	1,126	1,022	960	907	846	805	767	689
75	1,296	1,181	1,112	1,053	986	940	898	811
80	1,478	1,351	1,276	1,211	1,136	1,086	1,039	943
85	1,672	1,533	1,451	1,380	1,298	1,242	1,191	1,086
90	1,878	1,727	1,638	1,560	1,471	1,410	1,355	1,240
95	2,097	1,933	1,836	1,752	1,655	1,589	1,529	1,404
100	2,327	2,151	2,045	1,955	1,850	1,779	1,714	1,578

*To locate Wilcoxon's T value, find the sample's size in the leftmost column and the appropriate α at the top of the table ($\alpha(2)$ indicates a two-tailed value and $\alpha(1)$ indicates a one-tailed value). A calculated T value is statistically significant (i.e., the null hypothesis can be rejected) if it is equal to or less than the value in the table.

TABLE B.4. Critical Values of the F Distribution[*]

					Numerator df = 1					
$\alpha(1)$	0.25	0.10	0.05	0.025	0.01	0.005	0.0025	0.001	0.0005
Denom df									
1	5.83	39.9	161.	648.	4,050.	16,200.	64,800.	$4 \cdot 10^5$	$2 \cdot 10^6$
2	2.57	8.53	18.5	385	98.5	199.	399.	999.0	2,000.
3	2.02	5.54	10.1	17.4	34.1	55.6	89.6	167.	267.
4	1.81	4.54	7.71	12.2	21.2	31.3	45.7	74.1	106.
5	1.69	4.06	6.61	10.0	16.3	22.8	31.4	47.2	63.6
6	1.62	3.78	5.99	8.81	13.7	18.6	24.8	35.5	46.1
7	1.57	3.59	5.59	8.07	12.2	16.2	21.1	29.2	37.0
8	1.54	3.46	5.32	7.57	11.3	14.7	18.8	25.4	31.6
9	1.51	3.36	5.12	7.21	10.6	13.6	17.2	22.9	28.0
10	1.49	3.29	4.96	6.94	10.0	12.8	16.0	21.0	25.5
11	1.47	3.23	4.84	6.72	9.65	12.2	15.2	19.7	23.7
12	1.46	3.18	4.75	6.55	9.33	11.8	14.5	18.6	22.2
13	1.45	3.14	4.67	6.41	9.07	11.4	13.9	17.8	21.1
14	1.44	3.10	4.60	6.30	8.86	11.1	13.5	17.1	20.2
15	1.43	3.07	4.54	6.20	8.68	10.8	13.1	16.6	19.5
16	1.42	3.05	4.49	6.12	8.53	10.6	12.8	16.1	18.9
17	1.42	3.03	4.45	6.04	8.40	10.4	12.6	15.7	18.4
18	1.41	3.01	4.41	5.98	8.29	10.2	12.3	15.4	17.9

19	1.41	2.99	4.38	5.92	8.18	10.1	12.1	15.1	17.5
20	1.40	2.97	4.35	5.87	8.10	9.94	11.9	14.8	17.2
21	1.40	2.96	4.32	5.83	8.02	9.83	11.8	14.6	16.9
22	1.40	2.95	4.30	5.79	7.95	9.73	11.6	14.4	16.6
23	1.39	2.94	4.28	5.75	7.88	9.63	11.5	14.2	16.4
24	1.39	2.93	4.26	5.72	7.82	9.55	11.4	14.0	16.2
25	1.39	2.92	4.24	5.69	7.77	9.48	11.3	13.9	16.0
26	1.38	2.91	4.23	5.66	7.72	9.41	11.2	13.7	15.8
27	1.38	2.90	4.21	5.63	7.68	9.34	11.1	13.6	15.6
28	1.38	2.89	4.20	5.61	7.64	9.28	11.0	13.5	15.5
29	1.38	2.89	4.18	5.59	7.60	9.23	11.0	13.4	15.3
30	1.38	2.88	4.17	5.57	7.56	9.18	10.9	13.3	15.2
35	1.37	2.85	4.12	5.48	7.42	8.98	10.6	12.9	14.7
40	1.36	2.84	4.08	5.42	7.31	8.83	10.4	12.6	14.4
45	1.36	2.82	4.06	5.38	7.23	8.71	10.3	12.4	14.1
50	1.35	2.81	4.03	5.34	7.17	8.63	10.1	12.2	13.9
60	1.35	2.79	4.00	5.29	7.08	8.49	9.96	12.0	13.5
70	1.35	2.78	3.98	5.25	7.01	8.40	9.84	11.8	13.3
80	1.34	2.77	3.96	5.22	6.96	8.33	9.75	11.7	13.2
90	1.34	2.76	3.95	5.20	6.93	8.28	9.68	11.6	13.0

(Continued)

TABLE B.4. (*Continued*)

				Numerator df = 1					
α(1)	0.25	0.10	0.05	0.025	0.01	0.005	0.0025	0.001	0.0005
Denom df									
100	1.34	2.76	3.94	5.18	6.90	8.24	9.62	11.5	12.9
200	1.33	2.73	3.89	5.10	6.76	8.06	9.38	11.2	12.5
500	1.33	2.72	3.86	5.05	6.69	7.95	9.23	11.0	12.3
∞	1.32	2.71	3.84	5.02	6.64	7.88	9.14	10.8	12.1

				Numerator df = 2					
α(1)	0.25	0.10	0.05	0.025	0.01	0.005	0.0025	0.001	0.0005
Denom df									
1	7.50	49.5	200.	800.	5,000.	20,000.	80,000.	$5 \cdot 10^5$	$2 \cdot 10^6$
2	3.00	9.00	19.0	39.0	99.0	199.	399.	999.	2,000.
3	2.28	5.46	9.55	16.0	30.8	49.8	79.0	149.	237.
4	2.00	4.32	6.94	10.6	18.0	26.3	38.0	61.2	87.4
5	1.85	3.78	5.79	8.43	13.3	18.3	25.0	37.1	49.8
6	1.76	3.46	5.14	7.26	10.9	14.5	19.1	27.0	34.8
7	1.70	3.26	4.74	6.54	9.55	12.4	15.9	21.7	27.2
8	1.66	3.11	4.46	6.06	8.65	11.0	13.9	18.5	22.7
9	1.62	3.01	4.26	5.71	8.02	10.1	12.5	16.4	19.9
10	1.60	2.92	4.10	5.46	7.56	9.43	11.6	14.9	17.9
11	1.58	2.86	3.98	5.26	7.21	8.91	10.8	13.8	16.4

12	1.56	2.81	3.89	5.10	6.93	8.51	10.3	13.0	15.3
13	1.55	2.76	3.81	4.97	6.70	8.19	9.84	12.3	14.4
14	1.53	2.73	3.74	4.86	6.51	7.92	9.47	11.8	13.7
15	1.52	2.70	3.68	4.77	6.36	7.70	9.17	11.3	13.2
16	1.51	2.67	3.63	4.69	6.23	7.51	8.92	11.0	12.7
17	1.51	2.64	3.59	4.62	6.11	7.35	8.70	10.7	12.3
18	1.50	2.62	3.55	4.56	6.01	7.21	8.51	10.4	11.9
19	1.49	2.61	3.52	4.51	5.93	7.09	8.35	10.2	11.6
20	1.49	2.59	3.49	4.46	5.85	6.99	8.21	9.95	11.4
21	1.48	2.57	3.47	4.42	5.78	6.89	8.08	9.77	11.2
22	1.48	2.56	3.44	4.38	5.72	6.81	7.96	9.61	11.0
23	1.47	2.55	3.42	4.35	5.66	6.73	7.86	9.47	10.8
24	1.47	2.54	3.40	4.32	5.61	6.66	7.77	9.34	10.6
25	1.47	2.53	3.39	4.29	5.57	6.60	7.69	9.22	10.5
26	1.46	2.52	3.37	4.27	5.53	6.54	7.61	9.12	10.3
27	1.46	2.51	3.35	4.24	5.49	6.49	7.54	9.02	10.2
28	1.46	2.50	3.34	4.22	5.45	6.44	7.48	8.93	10.1
29	1.45	2.50	3.33	4.20	5.42	6.40	7.42	8.85	9.99
30	1.45	2.49	3.32	4.18	5.39	6.35	7.36	8.77	9.90
35	1.44	2.46	3.27	4.11	5.27	6.19	7.14	8.47	9.52
40	1.44	2.44	3.23	4.05	5.18	6.07	6.99	8.25	9.25

(Continued)

539

TABLE B.4. (Continued)

Numerator df = 2

α(1)	0.25	0.10	0.05	0.025	0.01	0.005	0.0025	0.001	0.0005
Denom df									
45	1.43	2.42	3.20	4.01	5.11	5.97	6.86	8.09	9.04
50	1.43	2.41	3.18	3.97	5.06	5.90	6.77	7.96	8.88
60	1.42	2.39	3.15	3.93	4.98	5.79	6.63	7.77	8.65
70	1.41	2.38	3.13	3.89	4.92	5.72	6.53	7.64	8.49
80	1.41	2.37	3.11	3.86	4.88	5.67	6.46	7.54	8.37
90	1.41	2.36	3.10	3.84	4.85	5.62	6.41	7.47	8.28
100	1.41	2.36	3.09	3.83	4.82	5.59	6.37	7.41	8.21
200	1.40	2.33	3.04	3.76	4.71	5.44	6.17	7.15	7.90
500	1.39	2.31	3.01	3.72	4.65	5.35	6.06	7.00	7.72
∞	1.39	2.30	3.00	3.69	4.61	5.30	5.99	6.91	7.60

Numerator df = 3

α(1)	0.25	0.10	0.05	0.025	0.01	0.005	0.0025	0.001	0.0005
Denom df									
1	8.20	53.6	216.	864.	5,400.	21,600.	86,500.	$5 \cdot 10^5$	$2 \cdot 10^6$
2	3.15	9.16	19.2	39.2	99.2	199.	399.	999.	2,000.
3	2.36	5.39	9.28	15.4	29.5	47.5	76.1	141.	225.
4	2.05	4.19	6.59	9.98	16.7	24.3	35.0	56.2	80.1
5	1.88	3.62	5.41	7.76	12.1	16.5	22.4	33.2	44.4

6	1.78	3.29	4.76	6.60	9.78	12.9	16.9	23.7	30.5
7	1.72	3.07	4.35	5.89	8.45	10.9	13.8	18.8	23.5
8	1.67	2.92	4.07	5.42	7.59	9.60	12.0	15.8	19.4
9	1.63	2.81	3.86	5.08	6.99	8.72	10.7	13.9	16.8
10	1.60	2.73	3.71	4.83	6.55	8.08	9.83	12.6	15.0
11	1.58	2.66	3.59	4.63	6.22	7.60	9.17	11.6	13.7
12	1.56	2.61	3.49	4.47	5.95	7.23	8.65	10.8	12.7
13	1.55	2.56	3.41	4.35	5.74	6.93	8.24	10.2	11.9
14	1.53	2.52	3.34	4.24	5.56	6.68	7.91	9.73	11.3
15	1.52	2.49	3.29	4.15	5.42	6.48	7.63	9.34	10.8
16	1.51	2.46	3.24	4.08	5.29	6.30	7.40	9.01	10.3
17	1.50	2.44	3.20	4.01	5.19	6.16	7.21	8.73	9.99
18	1.49	2.42	3.16	3.95	5.09	6.03	7.04	8.49	9.69
19	1.49	2.40	3.13	3.90	5.01	5.92	6.89	8.28	9.42
20	1.48	2.38	3.10	3.86	4.94	5.82	6.76	8.10	9.20
21	1.48	2.36	3.07	3.82	4.87	5.73	6.64	7.94	8.99
22	1.47	2.35	3.05	3.78	4.82	5.65	6.54	7.80	8.82
23	1.47	2.34	3.03	3.75	4.76	5.58	6.45	7.67	8.66
24	1.46	2.33	3.01	3.72	4.72	5.52	6.36	7.55	8.51
25	1.46	2.32	2.99	3.69	4.68	5.46	6.29	7.45	8.39
26	1.45	2.31	2.98	3.67	4.64	5.41	6.22	7.36	8.27

(Continued)

TABLE B.4. (*Continued*)

Numerator df = 3

α(1)	0.25	0.10	0.05	0.025	0.01	0.005	0.0025	0.001	0.0005
Denom df									
27	1.45	2.30	2.96	3.65	4.60	5.36	6.16	7.27	8.16
28	1.45	2.29	2.95	3.63	4.57	5.32	6.10	7.19	8.07
29	1.45	2.28	2.93	3.61	4.54	5.28	6.05	7.12	7.98
30	1.44	2.28	2.92	3.59	4.51	5.24	6.00	7.05	7.89
35	1.43	2.25	2.87	3.52	4.40	5.09	5.80	6.79	7.56
40	1.42	2.23	2.84	3.46	4.31	4.98	5.66	6.59	7.33
45	1.42	2.21	2.81	3.42	4.25	4.89	5.55	6.45	7.15
50	1.41	2.20	2.79	3.39	4.20	4.83	5.47	6.34	7.01
60	1.41	2.18	2.76	3.34	4.13	4.73	5.34	6.17	6.81
70	1.40	2.16	2.74	3.31	4.07	4.66	5.26	6.06	6.67
80	1.40	2.15	2.72	3.28	4.04	4.61	5.19	5.97	6.57
90	1.39	2.15	2.71	3.26	4.01	4.57	5.14	5.91	6.49
100	1.39	2.14	2.70	3.25	3.98	4.54	5.11	5.86	6.43
200	1.38	2.11	2.65	3.18	3.88	4.41	4.94	5.63	6.16
500	1.37	2.09	2.62	3.14	3.82	4.33	4.84	5.51	6.01
∞	1.37	2.08	2.62	3.12	3.78	4.28	4.77	5.42	5.91

$\alpha(1)$	0.25	0.10	0.05	0.025	0.01	0.005	0.0025	0.001	0.0005
Denom df									
1	8.58	55.8	225.	900.	5,620.	22,500.	90,000.	$6 \cdot 10^5$	$2 \cdot 10^6$
2	3.23	9.24	19.2	39.2	99.2	199.	399.	999.	2,000.
3	2.39	5.34	9.12	15.1	28.7	46.2	73.9	137.	218.
4	2.06	4.11	6.39	9.60	16.0	23.2	33.3	53.4	76.1
5	1.89	3.52	5.19	7.39	11.4	15.6	21.0	31.1	41.5
6	1.79	3.18	4.53	6.23	9.15	12.0	15.7	21.9	28.1
7	1.72	2.96	4.12	5.52	7.85	10.1	12.7	17.2	21.4
8	1.66	2.81	3.84	5.05	7.01	8.81	10.9	14.4	17.6
9	1.63	2.69	3.63	4.72	6.42	7.96	9.74	12.6	15.1
10	1.59	2.61	3.48	4.47	5.99	7.34	8.89	11.3	13.4
11	1.57	2.54	3.36	4.28	5.67	6.88	8.25	10.3	12.2
12	1.55	2.48	3.26	4.12	5.41	6.52	7.76	9.63	11.2
13	1.53	2.43	3.18	4.00	5.21	6.23	7.37	9.07	10.5
14	1.52	2.39	3.11	3.89	5.04	6.00	7.06	8.62	9.95
15	1.51	2.36	3.06	3.80	4.89	5.80	6.80	8.25	9.48
16	1.50	2.33	3.01	3.73	4.77	5.64	6.58	7.94	9.08
17	1.49	2.31	2.96	3.66	4.67	5.50	6.39	7.68	8.75
18	1.48	2.29	2.93	3.61	4.58	5.37	6.23	7.46	8.47

Numerator df = 4

(Continued)

TABLE B.4. (*Continued*)

Numerator df = 4

α(1)	0.25	0.10	0.05	0.025	0.01	0.005	0.0025	0.001	0.0005
Denom df									
19	1.47	2.27	2.90	3.56	4.50	5.27	6.09	7.27	8.23
20	1.47	2.25	2.87	3.51	4.43	5.17	5.97	7.10	8.02
21	1.46	2.23	2.84	3.48	4.37	5.09	5.86	6.95	7.83
22	1.45	2.22	2.82	3.44	4.31	5.02	5.76	6.81	7.67
23	1.45	2.21	2.80	3.41	4.26	4.95	5.67	6.70	7.52
24	1.44	2.19	2.78	3.38	4.22	4.89	5.60	6.59	7.39
25	1.44	2.18	2.76	3.35	4.18	4.84	5.53	6.49	7.27
26	1.44	2.17	2.74	3.33	4.14	4.79	5.46	6.41	7.16
27	1.43	2.17	2.73	3.31	4.11	4.74	5.40	6.33	7.06
28	1.43	2.16	2.71	3.29	4.07	4.70	5.35	6.25	6.97
29	1.43	2.15	2.70	3.27	4.04	4.66	5.30	6.19	6.89
30	1.42	2.14	2.69	3.25	4.02	4.62	5.25	6.12	6.82
35	1.41	2.11	2.64	3.18	3.91	4.48	5.07	5.88	6.51
40	1.40	2.09	2.61	3.13	3.83	4.37	4.93	5.70	6.30
45	1.40	2.07	2.58	3.09	3.77	4.29	4.83	5.56	6.13
50	1.39	2.06	2.56	3.05	3.72	4.23	4.75	5.46	6.01
60	1.38	2.04	2.53	3.01	3.65	4.14	4.64	5.31	5.82
70	1.38	2.03	2.50	2.97	3.60	4.08	4.56	5.20	5.70

	0.25	0.10	0.05	0.025	0.01	0.005	0.0025	0.001	0.0005
80	1.38	2.02	2.49	2.95	3.56	4.03	4.50	5.12	5.60
90	1.37	2.01	2.47	2.93	3.53	3.99	4.45	5.06	5.53
100	1.37	2.00	2.46	2.92	3.51	3.96	4.42	5.02	5.48
200	1.36	1.97	2.42	2.85	3.41	3.84	4.26	4.81	5.23
500	1.35	1.96	2.39	2.81	3.36	3.76	4.17	4.69	5.09
∞	1.35	1.94	2.37	2.79	3.32	3.72	4.11	4.62	5.00

Numerator df = 5

$\alpha(1)$:	0.25	0.10	0.05	0.025	0.01	0.005	0.0025	0.001	0.0005
Denom df									
1	8.82	57.2	230.	922.	5,760.	23,100.	92,200.	$6 \cdot 10^5$	$2 \cdot 10^6$
2	3.28	9.29	19.3	39.3	99.3	199.	399.	999.	2,000.
3	2.41	5.31	9.01	14.9	28.2	45.4	72.6	135.	214.
4	2.07	4.05	6.26	9.36	15.5	22.5	32.3	51.7	73.6
5	1.89	3.45	5.05	7.15	11.0	14.9	20.2	29.8	39.7
6	1.79	3.11	4.39	5.99	8.75	11.5	14.9	20.8	26.6
7	1.71	2.88	3.97	5.29	7.46	9.52	12.0	16.2	20.2
8	1.66	2.73	3.69	4.82	6.63	8.30	10.3	13.5	16.4
9	1.62	2.61	3.48	4.48	6.06	7.47	9.12	11.7	14.1
10	1.59	2.52	3.33	4.24	5.64	6.87	8.29	10.5	12.4
11	1.56	2.45	3.20	4.04	5.32	6.42	7.67	9.58	11.2
12	1.54	2.39	3.11	3.89	5.06	6.07	7.20	8.89	10.4

(Continued)

TABLE B.4. (Continued)

				Numerator df = 5						
α(1)	0.25	0.10	0.05	0.025	0.01	0.005	0.0025	0.001	0.0005
Denom df									
13	1.52	2.35	3.03	3.77	4.86	5.79	6.82	8.35	9.66
14	1.51	2.31	2.96	3.66	4.69	5.56	6.51	7.92	9.11
15	1.49	2.27	2.90	3.58	4.56	5.37	6.26	7.57	8.66
16	1.48	2.24	2.85	3.50	4.44	5.21	6.05	7.27	8.29
17	1.47	2.22	2.81	3.44	4.34	5.07	5.87	7.02	7.98
18	1.46	2.20	2.77	3.38	4.25	4.96	5.72	6.81	7.71
19	1.46	2.18	2.74	3.33	4.17	4.85	5.58	6.62	7.48
20	1.45	2.16	2.71	3.29	4.10	4.76	5.46	6.46	7.27
21	1.44	2.14	2.68	3.25	4.04	4.68	5.36	6.32	7.10
22	1.44	2.13	2.66	3.22	3.99	4.61	5.26	6.19	6.94
23	1.43	2.11	2.64	3.18	3.94	4.54	5.18	6.08	6.80
24	1.43	2.10	2.62	3.15	3.90	4.49	5.11	5.98	6.68
25	1.42	2.09	2.60	3.13	3.85	4.43	5.04	5.89	6.56
26	1.42	2.08	2.59	3.10	3.82	4.38	4.98	5.80	6.46
27	1.42	2.07	2.57	3.08	3.78	4.34	4.92	5.73	7.37
28	1.41	2.06	2.56	3.06	3.75	4.30	4.87	5.66	6.28
29	1.41	2.06	2.55	3.04	3.73	4.26	4.82	5.59	6.21
30	1.41	2.05	2.53	3.03	3.70	4.23	4.78	5.53	6.13

	0.25	0.10	0.05	0.025	0.01	0.005	0.0025	0.001	0.0005
35	1.40	2.02	2.49	2.96	3.59	4.09	4.60	5.30	5.85
40	1.39	2.00	2.45	2.90	3.51	3.99	4.47	5.13	5.64
45	1.38	1.98	2.42	2.86	3.45	3.91	4.37	5.00	5.49
50	1.37	1.97	2.40	2.83	3.41	3.85	4.30	4.90	5.37
60	1.37	1.95	2.37	2.79	3.34	3.76	4.19	4.76	5.20
70	1.36	1.93	2.35	2.75	3.29	3.70	4.11	4.66	5.08
80	1.36	1.92	2.33	2.73	3.26	3.65	4.05	4.58	4.99
90	1.35	1.91	2.32	2.71	3.23	3.62	4.01	4.53	4.92
100	1.35	1.91	2.31	2.70	3.21	3.59	3.97	4.48	4.87
200	1.34	1.88	2.26	2.63	3.11	3.47	3.82	4.29	4.64
500	1.33	1.86	2.23	2.59	3.05	3.40	3.73	4.18	4.51
∞	1.33	1.85	2.22	2.57	3.02	3.35	3.68	4.10	4.42

Numerator df = 6

$\alpha(1)$	0.25	0.10	0.05	0.025	0.01	0.005	0.0025	0.001	0.0005
Denom df									
1	8.98	58.2	234.	937.	5,860.	23,400.	93,700.	$6 \cdot 10^5$	$2 \cdot 10^6$
2	3.31	9.33	19.3	39.3	99.3	199.	399.	999.	2,000.
3	2.42	5.28	8.94	14.7	27.9	44.8	71.7	133.	211.9
4	2.08	4.01	6.16	9.20	15.2	22.0	31.5	50.5	71.9
5	1.89	3.40	4.95	6.98	10.7	14.5	19.6	28.8	38.5
6	1.78	3.05	4.28	5.82	8.47	11.1	14.4	20.0	25.6

(*Continued*)

TABLE B.4. (*Continued*)

Numerator df = 6

α(1)	0.25	0.10	0.05	0.025	0.01	0.005	0.0025	0.001	0.0005
Denom df									
7	1.71	2.83	3.87	5.12	7.19	9.16	11.5	15.5	19.3
8	1.65	2.67	3.58	4.65	6.37	7.95	9.83	12.9	15.7
9	1.61	2.55	3.37	4.32	5.80	7.13	8.68	11.1	13.3
10	1.58	2.46	3.22	4.07	5.39	6.54	7.87	9.93	11.7
11	1.55	2.39	3.09	3.88	5.07	6.10	7.27	9.05	10.6
12	1.53	2.33	3.00	3.73	4.82	5.76	6.80	8.38	9.74
13	1.51	2.28	2.92	3.60	4.62	5.48	6.44	7.86	9.07
14	1.50	2.24	2.85	3.50	4.46	5.26	6.14	7.44	8.53
15	1.48	2.21	2.79	3.41	4.32	5.07	5.89	7.09	8.10
16	1.47	2.18	2.74	3.34	4.20	4.91	5.68	6.80	7.74
17	1.46	2.15	2.70	3.28	4.10	4.78	5.51	6.56	7.43
18	1.45	2.13	2.66	3.22	4.01	4.66	5.36	6.35	7.18
19	1.44	2.11	2.63	3.17	3.94	4.56	5.23	6.18	6.95
20	1.44	2.09	2.60	3.13	3.87	4.47	5.11	6.02	6.76
21	1.43	2.08	2.57	3.09	3.81	4.39	5.01	5.88	6.59
22	1.42	2.06	2.55	3.05	3.76	4.32	4.92	5.76	6.44
23	1.42	2.05	2.53	3.02	3.71	4.26	4.84	5.65	6.30
24	1.41	2.04	2.51	2.99	3.67	4.20	4.76	5.55	6.18

25	1.41	2.02	2.49	2.97	3.63	4.15	4.70	5.46	6.07
26	1.41	2.01	2.47	2.94	3.59	4.10	4.64	5.38	5.98
27	1.40	2.00	2.46	2.92	3.56	4.06	4.58	5.31	5.89
28	1.40	2.00	2.45	2.90	3.53	4.02	4.53	5.24	5.80
29	1.40	1.99	2.43	2.88	3.50	3.98	4.48	5.18	5.73
30	1.39	1.98	2.42	2.87	3.47	3.95	4.44	5.12	5.66
35	1.38	1.95	2.37	2.80	3.37	3.81	4.27	4.89	5.39
40	1.37	1.93	2.34	2.74	3.29	3.71	4.14	4.73	5.19
45	1.36	1.91	2.31	2.70	3.23	3.64	4.05	4.61	5.04
50	1.36	1.90	2.29	2.67	3.19	3.58	3.98	4.51	4.93
60	1.35	1.87	2.25	2.63	3.12	3.49	3.87	4.37	4.76
70	1.34	1.86	2.23	2.59	3.07	3.43	3.79	4.28	4.64
80	1.34	1.85	2.21	2.57	3.04	3.39	3.74	4.20	4.56
90	1.33	1.84	2.20	2.55	3.01	3.35	3.70	4.15	4.50
100	1.33	1.83	2.19	2.54	2.99	3.33	3.66	4.11	4.45
200	1.32	1.80	2.14	2.47	2.89	3.21	3.52	3.92	4.22
500	1.31	1.79	2.12	2.43	2.84	3.14	3.43	3.81	4.10
∞	1.31	1.77	2.10	2.41	2.80	3.09	3.37	3.74	4.02

(Continued)

TABLE B.4. (*Continued*)

Numerator df = 7

α(1)	0.25	0.10	0.05	0.025	0.01	0.005	0.0025	0.001	0.0005
Denom df									
1	9.10	58.9	237.	948.	5,930.	23,700.	94,900.	$6 \cdot 10^5$	$2 \cdot 10^6$
2	3.34	9.35	19.4	39.4	99.4	199.	399.	999.	2,000.
3	2.43	5.27	8.89	14.6	27.7	44.4	71.0	132.	209.
4	2.08	3.98	6.09	9.07	15.0	21.6	31.0	49.7	70.7
5	1.89	3.37	4.88	6.85	10.5	14.2	19.1	28.2	37.6
6	1.78	3.01	4.21	5.70	8.26	10.8	14.0	19.5	24.9
7	1.70	2.78	3.79	4.99	6.99	8.89	11.2	15.0	18.7
8	1.64	2.62	3.50	4.53	6.18	7.69	9.49	12.4	15.1
9	1.60	2.51	3.29	4.20	5.61	6.88	8.36	10.7	12.8
10	1.57	2.41	3.14	3.95	5.20	6.30	7.56	9.52	11.2
11	1.54	2.34	3.01	3.76	4.89	5.86	6.97	8.66	10.1
12	1.52	2.28	2.91	3.61	4.64	5.52	6.51	8.00	9.28
13	1.50	2.23	2.83	3.48	4.44	5.25	6.15	7.49	8.63
14	1.49	2.19	2.76	3.38	4.28	5.03	5.86	7.08	8.11
15	1.47	2.16	2.71	3.29	4.14	4.85	5.62	6.74	7.68
16	1.46	2.13	2.66	3.22	4.03	4.69	5.41	6.46	7.33
17	1.45	2.10	2.61	3.16	3.93	4.56	5.24	6.22	7.04
18	1.44	2.08	2.58	3.10	3.84	4.44	5.09	6.02	6.78
19	1.43	2.06	2.54	3.05	3.77	4.34	4.96	5.85	6.57
20	1.43	2.04	2.51	3.01	3.70	4.26	4.85	5.69	6.38

21	6.21	5.56	4.75	4.18	3.64	2.97	2.49	2.02	1.42
22	6.07	5.44	4.66	4.11	3.59	2.93	2.46	2.01	1.41
23	5.94	5.33	4.58	4.05	3.54	2.90	2.44	1.99	1.41
24	5.82	5.23	4.51	3.99	3.50	2.87	2.42	1.98	1.40
25	5.71	5.15	4.44	3.94	3.46	2.85	2.40	1.97	1.40
26	5.62	5.07	4.38	3.89	3.42	2.82	2.39	1.96	1.39
27	5.53	5.00	4.33	3.85	3.39	2.80	2.37	1.95	1.39
28	5.45	4.93	4.28	3.81	3.36	2.78	2.36	1.94	1.39
29	5.38	4.87	4.24	3.77	3.33	2.76	2.35	1.93	1.38
30	5.31	4.82	4.19	3.74	3.30	2.75	2.33	1.93	1.38
35	5.04	4.59	4.02	3.61	3.20	2.68	2.29	1.90	1.37
40	4.85	4.44	3.90	3.51	3.12	2.62	2.25	1.87	1.36
45	4.71	4.32	3.81	3.43	3.07	2.58	2.22	1.85	1.35
50	4.60	4.22	3.74	3.38	3.02	2.55	2.20	1.84	1.34
60	4.44	4.09	3.63	3.29	2.95	2.51	2.17	1.82	1.33
70	4.32	3.99	3.56	3.23	2.91	2.47	2.14	1.80	1.33
80	4.24	3.92	3.50	3.19	2.87	2.45	2.13	1.79	1.32
90	4.18	3.87	3.46	3.15	2.84	2.43	2.11	1.78	1.32
100	4.13	3.83	3.43	3.13	2.82	2.42	2.10	1.78	1.32
200	3.92	3.65	3.29	3.01	2.73	2.35	2.06	1.75	1.30
500	3.80	3.54	3.20	2.94	2.68	2.31	2.03	1.73	1.30
∞	3.72	3.47	3.15	2.90	2.64	2.29	2.01	1.72	1.29

(Continued)

TABLE B.4. (*Continued*)

Numerator df = 8

α(1)	0.25	0.10	0.05	0.025	0.01	0.005	0.0025	0.001	0.0005
Denom df									
1	9.19	59.4	239.	957.	5,980.	23,900.	95,700.	$6 \cdot 10^5$	$2 \cdot 10^6$
2	3.35	9.37	19.4	39.4	99.4	199.	399.	999.	2,000.
3	2.44	5.25	8.85	14.5	27.5	44.1	70.5	131.	208.
4	2.08	3.95	6.04	8.98	14.8	21.4	30.6	49.0	69.7
5	1.89	3.34	4.82	6.76	10.3	14.0	18.8	27.6	36.9
6	1.78	2.98	4.15	5.60	8.10	10.6	13.7	19.0	24.3
7	1.70	2.75	3.73	4.90	6.84	8.68	10.9	14.6	18.2
8	1.64	2.59	3.44	4.43	6.03	7.50	9.24	12.0	14.6
9	1.60	2.47	3.23	4.10	5.47	6.69	8.12	10.4	12.4
10	1.56	2.38	3.07	3.85	5.06	6.12	7.33	9.20	10.9
11	1.53	2.30	2.95	3.66	4.74	5.68	6.74	8.35	9.76
12	1.51	2.24	2.85	3.51	4.50	5.35	6.29	7.71	8.94
13	1.49	2.20	2.77	3.39	4.30	5.08	5.93	7.21	8.29
14	1.48	2.15	2.70	3.29	4.14	4.86	5.64	6.80	7.78
15	1.46	2.12	2.64	3.20	4.00	4.67	5.40	6.47	7.37
16	1.45	2.09	2.59	3.12	3.89	4.52	5.20	6.19	7.02
17	1.44	2.06	2.55	3.06	3.79	4.39	5.03	5.96	6.73
18	1.43	2.04	2.51	3.01	3.71	4.28	4.89	5.76	6.48
19	1.42	2.02	2.48	2.96	3.63	4.18	4.76	5.59	6.27
20	1.42	2.00	2.45	2.91	3.56	4.09	4.65	5.44	6.09

21	5.92	5.31	4.55	4.01	3.51	2.87	2.42	1.98	1.41
22	5.78	5.19	4.46	3.94	3.45	2.84	2.40	1.97	1.40
23	5.65	5.09	4.38	3.88	3.41	2.81	2.37	1.95	1.40
24	5.54	4.99	4.31	3.83	3.36	2.78	2.36	1.94	1.39
25	5.43	4.91	4.25	3.78	3.32	2.75	2.34	1.93	1.39
26	5.34	4.83	4.19	3.73	3.29	2.73	2.32	1.92	1.38
27	5.25	4.76	4.14	3.69	3.26	2.71	2.31	1.91	1.38
28	5.18	4.69	4.09	3.65	3.23	2.69	2.29	1.90	1.38
29	5.11	4.64	4.04	3.61	3.20	2.67	2.28	1.89	1.37
30	5.04	4.58	4.00	3.58	3.17	2.65	2.27	1.88	1.37
35	4.78	4.36	3.83	3.45	3.07	2.58	2.22	1.85	1.36
40	4.59	4.21	3.71	3.35	2.99	2.53	2.18	1.83	1.35
45	4.45	4.09	3.62	3.28	2.94	2.49	2.15	1.81	1.34
50	4.34	4.00	3.55	3.22	2.89	2.46	2.13	1.80	1.33
60	4.19	3.86	3.45	3.13	2.82	2.41	2.10	1.77	1.32
70	4.08	3.77	3.37	3.08	2.78	2.38	2.07	1.76	1.32
80	4.00	3.70	3.32	3.03	2.74	2.35	2.06	1.75	1.31
90	3.94	3.65	3.28	3.00	2.72	2.34	2.04	1.74	1.31
100	3.89	3.61	3.25	2.97	2.69	2.32	2.03	1.73	1.30
200	3.68	3.43	3.11	2.86	2.60	2.26	1.98	1.70	1.29
500	3.56	3.33	3.03	2.79	2.55	2.22	1.96	1.68	1.28
∞	3.48	3.27	2.97	2.74	2.51	2.19	1.94	1.67	1.28

(Continued)

TABLE B.4. (*Continued*)

Numerator df = 9

$\alpha(1)$	0.25	0.10	0.05	0.025	0.01	0.005	0.0025	0.001	0.0005
Denom df									
1	9.26	59.9	241.	963.	6,020.	24,100.	96,400.	$6 \cdot 10^5$	$2 \cdot 10^6$
2	3.37	9.38	19.4	39.4	99.4	199	399.	999.	2,000.
3	2.44	5.24	8.81	14.5	27.3	43.9	70.1	130.	207.
4	2.08	3.94	6.00	8.90	14.7	21.1	30.3	48.5	69.0
5	1.89	3.32	4.77	6.68	10.2	13.8	18.5	27.2	36.3
6	1.77	2.96	4.10	5.52	7.98	10.4	13.4	18.7	23.9
7	1.69	2.72	3.68	4.82	6.72	8.51	10.7	14.3	17.8
8	1.63	2.56	3.39	4.36	5.91	7.34	9.03	11.8	14.3
9	1.59	2.44	3.18	4.03	5.35	6.54	7.92	10.1	12.1
10	1.56	2.35	3.02	3.78	4.94	5.97	7.14	8.96	10.6
11	1.53	2.27	2.90	3.59	4.63	5.54	6.56	8.12	9.48
12	1.51	2.21	2.80	3.44	4.39	5.20	6.11	7.48	8.66
13	1.49	2.16	2.71	3.31	4.19	4.94	5.76	6.98	8.03
14	1.47	2.12	2.65	3.21	4.03	4.72	5.47	6.58	7.52
15	1.46	2.09	2.59	3.12	3.89	4.54	5.23	6.26	7.11
16	1.44	2.06	2.54	3.05	3.78	4.38	5.04	5.98	6.77
17	1.43	2.03	2.49	2.98	3.68	4.25	4.87	5.75	6.49
18	1.42	2.02	2.46	2.93	3.60	4.14	4.72	5.56	6.24
19	1.41	1.98	2.42	2.88	3.52	4.04	4.60	5.39	6.03
20	1.41	1.96	2.39	2.84	3.46	3.96	4.49	5.24	5.85

21	5.69	5.11	4.39	3.88	3.40	2.80	2.37	1.95	1.40
22	5.55	4.99	4.30	3.81	3.35	2.76	2.34	1.93	1.39
23	5.43	4.89	4.22	3.75	3.30	2.73	2.32	1.92	1.39
24	5.31	4.80	4.15	3.69	3.26	2.70	2.30	1.91	1.38
25	5.21	4.71	4.09	3.64	3.22	2.68	2.28	1.89	1.38
26	5.12	4.64	4.03	3.60	3.18	2.65	2.27	1.88	1.37
27	5.04	4.57	3.98	3.56	3.15	2.63	2.25	1.87	1.37
28	4.96	4.50	3.93	3.52	3.12	2.61	2.24	1.87	1.37
29	4.89	4.45	3.89	3.48	3.09	2.59	2.22	1.86	1.36
30	4.82	4.39	3.85	3.45	3.07	2.57	2.21	1.85	1.36
35	4.57	4.18	3.68	3.32	2.96	2.50	2.16	1.82	1.35
40	4.38	4.02	3.56	3.22	2.89	2.45	2.12	1.79	1.34
45	4.25	3.91	3.47	3.15	2.83	2.41	2.10	1.77	1.33
50	4.14	3.82	3.40	3.09	2.78	2.38	2.07	1.76	1.32
60	3.98	3.69	3.30	3.01	2.72	2.33	2.04	1.74	1.31
70	3.88	3.60	3.23	2.95	2.67	2.30	2.02	1.72	1.31
80	3.80	3.53	3.17	2.91	2.64	2.28	2.00	1.71	1.30
90	3.74	3.48	3.13	2.87	2.61	2.26	1.99	1.70	1.30
100	3.69	3.44	3.10	2.85	2.59	2.24	1.97	1.69	1.29
200	3.49	3.26	2.96	2.73	2.50	2.18	1.93	1.66	1.28
500	3.37	3.16	2.88	2.66	2.44	2.14	1.90	1.64	1.27
∞	3.30	3.10	2.83	2.62	2.41	2.11	1.88	1.63	1.27

(Continued)

TABLE B.4. (*Continued*)

Numerator df = 10

α(1) Denom df	0.25	0.10	0.05	0.025	0.01	0.005	0.0025	0.001	0.0005
1	9.32	60.2	242.	969.	6,060.	24,200.	96,900.	$6 \cdot 10^5$	$2 \cdot 10^6$
2	3.38	9.39	19.4	39.4	99.4	199.	399.	999.	2,000.
3	2.44	5.23	8.79	14.4	27.2	437	69.8	129.	206.
4	2.08	3.92	5.96	8.84	14.5	21.0	30.0	48.1	68.3
5	1.89	3.30	4.74	6.62	10.1	13.6	18.3	26.9	35.9
6	1.77	2.94	4.06	5.46	7.87	10.3	13.2	18.4	23.5
7	1.69	2.70	3.64	4.76	6.62	8.38	10.5	14.1	17.5
8	1.63	2.54	3.35	4.30	5.81	7.21	8.87	11.5	14.0
9	1.59	2.42	3.14	3.96	5.26	6.42	7.77	9.89	11.8
10	1.55	2.32	2.98	3.72	4.85	5.85	6.99	8.75	10.3
11	1.52	2.25	2.85	3.53	4.54	5.42	6.41	7.92	9.24
12	1.50	2.19	2.75	3.37	4.30	5.09	5.97	7.29	8.43
13	1.48	2.14	2.67	3.25	4.10	4.82	5.62	6.80	7.81
14	1.46	2.10	2.60	3.15	3.94	4.60	5.33	6.40	7.31
15	1.45	2.06	2.54	3.06	3.80	4.42	5.10	6.08	6.91
16	1.44	2.03	2.49	2.99	3.69	4.27	4.90	5.81	6.57
17	1.43	2.00	2.45	2.92	3.59	4.14	4.73	5.58	6.29
18	1.42	1.98	2.41	2.87	3.51	4.03	4.59	5.39	6.05
19	1.41	1.96	2.38	2.82	3.43	3.93	4.46	5.22	5.81
20	1.40	1.94	2.35	2.77	3.37	3.85	4.35	5.08	5.66

21	1.39	1.92	2.32	2.73	3.31	3.77	4.26	4.95	5.50
22	1.39	1.90	2.30	2.70	3.26	3.70	4.17	4.83	5.36
23	1.38	1.89	2.27	2.67	3.21	3.64	4.09	4.73	5.24
24	1.38	1.88	2.25	2.64	3.17	3.59	4.03	4.64	5.13
25	1.37	1.87	2.24	2.61	3.13	3.54	3.96	4.56	5.03
26	1.37	1.86	2.22	2.59	3.09	3.49	3.91	4.48	4.94
27	1.36	1.85	2.20	2.57	3.06	3.45	3.85	4.41	4.86
28	1.36	1.84	2.19	2.55	3.03	3.41	3.81	4.35	4.78
29	1.35	1.83	2.18	2.53	3.00	3.38	3.76	4.29	4.71
30	1.35	1.82	2.16	2.51	2.98	3.34	3.72	4.24	4.65
35	1.34	1.79	2.11	2.44	2.88	3.21	3.56	4.03	4.39
40	1.33	1.76	2.08	2.39	2.80	3.12	3.44	3.87	4.21
45	1.32	1.74	2.05	2.35	2.74	3.04	3.35	3.76	4.08
50	1.31	1.73	2.03	2.32	2.70	2.99	3.28	3.67	3.97
60	1.30	1.71	1.99	2.27	2.63	2.90	3.18	3.54	3.82
70	1.30	1.69	1.97	2.24	2.59	2.85	3.11	3.45	3.71
80	1.29	1.68	1.95	2.21	2.55	2.80	3.05	3.39	3.64
90	1.29	1.67	1.94	2.19	2.52	2.77	3.01	3.34	3.58
100	1.28	1.66	1.93	2.18	2.50	2.74	2.98	3.30	3.53
200	1.27	1.63	1.88	2.11	2.41	2.63	2.84	3.12	3.33
500	1.26	1.61	1.85	2.07	2.36	2.56	2.76	3.02	3.22
∞	1.25	1.60	1.83	2.05	2.32	2.52	2.71	2.96	3.14

(*Continued*)

TABLE B.4. (*Continued*)

α(1)	0.25	0.10	0.05	0.025	0.01	0.005	0.0025	0.001	0.0005
Denom df									
1	9.41	60.7	244.	977.	6,110.	24,400.	97,700.	$6 \cdot 10^5$	$2 \cdot 10^6$
2	3.39	9.41	19.4	39.4	99.4	199.	399.	999.	2,000.
3	2.45	5.22	8.74	14.3	27.1	43.4	69.3	128.	204.
4	2.08	3.90	5.91	8.75	14.4	20.7	29.7	47.4	67.4
5	1.89	3.27	4.68	6.52	9.89	13.4	18.0	26.4	35.2
6	1.77	2.90	4.00	5.37	7.72	10.0	12.9	18.0	23.0
7	1.68	2.67	3.57	4.67	6.47	8.18	10.3	13.7	17.0
8	1.62	2.50	3.28	4.20	5.67	7.01	8.61	11.2	13.6
9	1.58	2.38	3.07	3.87	5.11	6.23	7.52	9.57	11.4
10	1.54	2.28	2.91	3.62	4.71	5.66	6.75	8.45	9.94
11	1.51	2.21	2.79	3.43	4.40	5.24	6.18	7.63	8.88
12	1.49	2.15	2.69	3.28	4.16	4.91	5.74	7.00	8.09
13	1.47	2.10	2.60	3.15	3.96	4.64	5.40	6.52	7.48
14	1.45	2.05	2.53	3.05	3.80	4.43	5.12	6.13	6.99
15	1.44	2.02	2.48	2.96	3.67	4.25	4.88	5.81	6.59
16	1.43	1.99	2.42	2.89	3.55	4.10	4.69	5.55	6.26
17	1.41	1.96	2.38	2.82	3.46	3.97	4.52	5.32	5.98
18	1.40	1.93	2.34	2.77	3.37	3.86	4.38	5.13	5.75
19	1.40	1.91	2.31	2.72	3.30	3.76	4.26	4.97	5.55

Numerator df = 12

20	1.39	1.89	2.28	2.68	3.23	3.68	4.15	4.82	5.37
21	1.38	1.87	2.25	2.64	3.17	3.60	4.06	4.70	5.21
22	1.37	1.86	2.23	2.60	3.12	3.54	3.97	4.58	5.08
23	1.37	1.84	2.20	2.57	3.07	3.47	3.89	4.48	4.96
24	1.36	1.83	2.18	2.54	3.03	3.42	3.83	4.39	4.85
25	1.36	1.82	2.16	2.51	2.99	3.37	3.76	4.31	4.75
26	1.35	1.81	2.15	2.49	2.96	3.33	3.71	4.24	4.66
27	1.35	1.80	2.13	2.47	2.93	3.28	3.66	4.17	4.58
28	1.34	1.79	2.12	2.45	2.90	3.25	3.61	4.11	4.51
29	1.34	1.78	2.10	2.43	2.87	3.21	3.56	4.05	4.44
30	1.34	1.77	2.09	2.41	2.84	3.18	3.52	4.00	4.38
35	1.32	1.74	2.04	2.34	2.74	3.05	3.36	3.79	4.13
40	1.31	1.71	2.00	2.29	2.66	2.95	3.25	3.64	3.95
45	1.30	1.70	1.97	2.25	2.61	2.88	3.16	3.53	3.82
50	1.30	1.68	1.95	2.22	2.56	2.82	3.09	3.44	3.71
60	1.29	1.66	1.92	2.17	2.50	2.74	2.99	3.32	3.57
70	1.28	1.64	1.89	2.14	2.45	2.68	2.92	3.23	3.46
80	1.27	1.63	1.88	2.11	2.42	2.64	2.87	3.16	3.39
90	1.27	1.62	1.86	2.09	2.39	2.61	2.83	3.11	3.33
100	1.27	1.61	1.85	2.08	2.37	2.58	2.80	3.07	3.28
200	1.25	1.58	1.80	2.01	2.27	2.47	2.66	2.90	3.09
500	1.24	1.56	1.77	1.97	2.22	2.40	2.58	2.81	2.97
∞	1.24	1.55	1.75	1.94	2.18	2.36	2.53	2.74	2.90

(Continued)

TABLE B.4. (Continued)

				Numerator df = 14						
α(1)	0.25	0.10	0.05	0.025	0.01	0.005	0.0025	0.001	0.0005	
Denom df										
1	9.47	61.1	245.	983.	6,140.	24,600.	98,300.	$6 \cdot 10^5$	$2 \cdot 10^6$	
2	3.41	9.42	19.4	39.4	99.4	199.	399.	999.	2,000.	
3	2.45	5.20	8.71	14.3	26.9	43.2	69.0	128.	203.	
4	2.08	3.88	5.87	8.68	14.2	20.5	29.4	46.9	66.8	
5	1.89	3.25	4.64	6.46	9.77	13.2	17.8	26.1	34.7	
6	1.76	2.88	3.96	5.30	7.60	9.88	12.7	17.7	22.6	
7	1.68	2.64	3.53	4.60	6.36	8.03	10.1	13.4	16.6	
8	1.62	2.48	3.24	4.13	5.56	6.87	8.43	10.9	13.3	
9	1.57	2.35	3.03	3.80	5.01	6.09	7.35	9.33	11.1	
10	1.54	2.26	2.86	3.55	4.60	5.53	6.58	8.22	9.67	
11	1.51	2.18	2.74	3.36	4.29	5.10	6.02	7.41	8.62	
12	1.48	2.12	2.64	3.21	4.05	4.77	5.58	6.79	7.84	
13	1.46	2.07	2.55	3.08	3.86	4.51	5.24	6.31	7.23	
14	1.44	2.02	2.48	2.98	3.70	4.30	4.96	5.93	6.75	
15	1.43	1.99	2.42	2.89	3.56	4.12	4.73	5.62	6.36	
16	1.42	1.95	2.37	2.82	3.45	3.97	4.54	5.35	6.03	
17	1.41	1.93	2.33	2.75	3.35	3.84	4.37	5.13	5.76	
18	1.40	1.90	2.29	2.70	3.27	3.73	4.23	4.94	5.53	
19	1.39	1.88	2.26	2.65	3.19	3.64	4.11	4.78	5.33	
20	1.38	1.86	2.22	2.60	3.13	3.55	4.00	4.64	5.15	

21	1.37	1.84	2.20	2.56	3.07	3.48	3.91	4.51	5.00
22	1.36	1.83	2.17	2.53	3.02	3.41	3.82	4.40	4.87
23	1.36	1.81	2.15	2.50	2.97	3.35	3.75	4.30	4.75
24	1.35	1.80	2.13	2.47	2.93	3.30	3.68	4.21	4.64
25	1.35	1.79	2.11	2.44	2.89	3.25	3.62	4.13	4.54
26	1.34	1.77	2.09	2.42	2.86	3.20	3.56	4.06	4.46
27	1.34	1.76	2.08	2.39	2.82	3.16	3.51	3.99	4.38
28	1.33	1.75	2.06	2.37	2.79	3.12	3.46	3.93	4.30
29	1.33	1.75	2.05	2.36	2.77	3.09	3.42	3.88	4.24
30	1.33	1.74	2.04	2.34	2.74	3.06	3.38	3.82	4.18
35	1.31	1.70	1.99	2.27	2.64	2.93	3.22	3.62	3.93
40	1.30	1.68	1.95	2.21	2.56	2.83	3.10	3.47	3.76
45	1.29	1.66	1.92	2.17	2.51	2.76	3.02	3.36	3.63
50	1.28	1.64	1.89	2.14	2.46	2.70	2.95	3.27	3.52
60	1.27	1.62	1.86	2.09	2.39	2.62	2.85	3.15	3.38
70	1.27	1.60	1.84	2.06	2.35	2.56	2.78	3.06	3.28
80	1.26	1.59	1.82	2.03	2.31	2.52	2.73	3.00	3.20
90	1.26	1.58	1.80	2.02	2.29	2.49	2.69	2.95	3.14
100	1.25	1.57	1.79	2.00	2.27	2.46	2.65	2.91	3.10
200	1.24	1.54	1.74	1.93	2.17	2.35	2.52	2.74	2.91
500	1.23	1.52	1.71	1.89	2.12	2.28	2.44	2.64	2.79
∞	1.22	1.50	1.69	1.87	2.08	2.24	2.39	2.58	2.72

(Continued)

TABLE B.4. (*Continued*)

Numerator df = 16

$\alpha(1)$	0.25	0.10	0.05	0.025	0.01	0.005	0.0025	0.001	0.0005
Denom df									
1	9.52	61.3	246.	987.	6,170.	24,700.	98,700.	$6 \cdot 10^5$	$2 \cdot 10^6$
2	3.41	9.43	19.4	39.4	99.4	199.	399.	999.	2,000.
3	2.46	5.20	8.69	14.2	26.8	43.0	68.7	127.	202.
4	2.08	3.86	5.84	8.63	14.2	20.4	29.2	46.6	66.2
5	1.88	3.23	4.60	6.40	9.68	13.1	17.6	25.8	34.3
6	1.76	2.86	3.92	5.24	7.52	9.76	12.6	17.4	22.3
7	1.68	2.62	3.49	4.54	6.28	7.91	9.91	13.2	16.4
8	1.62	2.45	3.20	4.08	5.48	6.76	8.29	10.8	13.0
9	1.57	2.33	2.99	3.74	4.92	5.98	7.21	9.15	10.9
10	1.53	2.23	2.83	3.50	4.52	5.42	6.45	8.05	9.46
11	1.50	2.16	2.70	3.30	4.21	5.00	5.89	7.24	8.43
12	1.48	2.09	2.60	3.15	3.97	4.67	5.46	6.63	7.65
13	1.46	2.04	2.51	3.03	3.78	4.41	5.11	6.16	7.05
14	1.44	2.00	2.44	2.92	3.62	4.20	4.84	5.78	6.57
15	1.42	1.96	2.38	2.84	3.49	4.02	4.61	5.46	6.18
16	1.41	1.93	2.33	2.76	3.37	3.87	4.42	5.20	5.86
17	1.40	1.90	2.29	2.70	3.27	3.75	4.25	4.99	5.59
18	1.39	1.87	2.25	2.64	3.19	3.64	4.11	4.80	5.36
19	1.38	1.85	2.21	2.59	3.12	3.54	3.99	4.64	5.16
20	1.37	1.83	2.18	2.55	3.05	3.46	3.89	4.49	4.99

21	4.84	4.37	3.79	3.38	2.99	2.51	2.16	1.81	1.36
22	4.71	4.26	3.71	3.31	2.94	2.47	2.13	1.80	1.36
23	4.59	4.16	3.63	3.25	2.89	2.44	2.11	1.78	1.35
24	4.48	4.07	3.56	3.20	2.85	2.41	2.09	1.77	1.34
25	4.39	3.99	3.50	3.15	2.81	2.38	2.07	1.76	1.34
26	4.30	3.92	3.45	3.11	2.78	2.36	2.05	1.75	1.33
27	4.22	3.86	3.40	3.07	2.75	2.34	2.04	1.74	1.33
28	4.15	3.80	3.35	3.03	2.72	2.32	2.02	1.73	1.32
29	4.08	3.74	3.31	2.99	2.69	2.30	2.01	1.72	1.32
30	4.02	3.69	3.27	2.96	2.66	2.28	1.99	1.71	1.32
35	3.78	3.48	3.11	2.83	2.56	2.21	1.94	1.67	1.30
40	3.61	3.34	2.99	2.74	2.48	2.15	1.90	1.65	1.29
45	3.48	3.23	2.90	2.66	2.43	2.11	1.87	1.63	1.28
50	3.38	3.14	2.84	2.61	2.38	2.08	1.85	1.61	1.27
60	3.23	3.02	2.74	2.53	2.31	2.03	1.82	1.59	1.26
70	3.13	2.93	2.67	2.47	2.27	2.00	1.79	1.57	1.26
80	3.06	2.87	2.62	2.43	2.23	1.97	1.77	1.56	1.25
90	3.00	2.82	2.58	2.39	2.21	1.95	1.76	1.55	1.25
100	2.96	2.78	2.55	2.37	2.19	1.94	1.75	1.54	1.24
200	2.76	2.61	2.41	2.25	2.09	1.87	1.69	1.51	1.23
500	2.65	2.52	2.33	2.19	2.04	1.83	1.66	1.49	1.22
∞	2.58	2.45	2.28	2.14	2.00	1.80	1.64	1.47	1.21

(*Continued*)

TABLE B.4. (Continued)

Numerator df = 18

$\alpha(1)$	0.25	0.10	0.05	0.025	0.01	0.005	0.0025	0.001	0.0005
Denom df									
1	9.55	61.6	247.	990.	6,190.	24,800.	99,100.	$6 \cdot 10^5$	$2 \cdot 10^6$
2	3.42	9.44	19.4	39.4	99.4	199.	399.	999.	2,000.
3	2.46	5.19	8.67	14.2	26.8	42.9	68.5	127.	202.
4	2.08	3.85	5.82	8.59	14.1	20.3	29.0	46.3	65.8
5	1.88	3.22	4.58	6.36	9.61	13.0	17.4	25.6	34.0
6	1.76	2.85	3.90	5.20	7.45	9.66	12.4	17.3	22.0
7	1.67	2.61	3.47	4.50	6.21	7.83	9.79	13.1	16.2
8	1.61	2.44	3.17	4.03	5.41	6.68	8.18	10.6	12.8
9	1.56	2.31	2.96	3.70	4.86	5.90	7.11	9.01	10.7
10	1.53	2.22	2.80	3.45	4.46	5.34	6.35	7.91	9.30
11	1.50	2.14	2.67	3.26	4.15	4.92	5.79	7.11	8.27
12	1.47	2.08	2.57	3.11	3.91	4.59	5.36	6.51	7.50
13	1.45	2.02	2.48	2.98	3.72	4.33	5.02	6.03	6.90
14	1.43	1.98	2.41	2.88	3.56	4.12	4.74	5.66	6.43
15	1.42	1.94	2.35	2.79	3.42	3.95	4.51	5.35	6.04
16	1.40	1.91	2.30	2.72	3.31	3.80	4.32	5.09	5.72
17	1.39	1.88	2.26	2.65	3.21	3.67	4.16	4.87	5.45
18	1.38	1.85	2.22	2.60	3.13	3.56	4.02	4.68	5.23
19	1.37	1.83	2.18	2.55	3.05	3.46	3.90	4.52	5.03
20	1.36	1.81	2.15	2.50	2.99	3.38	3.79	4.38	4.86

21	4.71	4.26	3.70	3.31	2.93	2.46	2.12	1.79	1.36
22	4.58	4.15	3.62	3.24	2.88	2.43	2.10	1.78	1.35
23	4.46	4.05	3.54	3.18	2.83	2.39	2.08	1.76	1.34
24	4.35	3.96	3.47	3.12	2.79	2.36	2.05	1.75	1.34
25	4.26	3.88	3.41	3.08	2.75	2.34	2.04	1.74	1.33
26	4.17	3.81	3.36	3.03	2.72	2.31	2.02	1.72	1.33
27	4.10	3.75	3.31	2.99	2.68	2.29	2.00	1.71	1.32
28	4.02	3.69	3.26	2.95	2.65	2.27	1.99	1.70	1.32
29	3.96	3.63	3.22	2.92	2.63	2.25	1.97	1.69	1.31
30	3.90	3.58	3.18	2.89	2.60	2.23	1.96	1.69	1.31
35	3.66	3.38	3.02	2.76	2.50	2.16	1.91	1.65	1.29
40	3.49	3.23	2.90	2.66	2.42	2.11	1.87	1.62	1.28
45	3.36	3.12	2.82	2.59	2.36	2.07	1.84	1.60	1.27
50	3.26	3.04	2.75	2.53	2.32	2.03	1.81	1.59	1.27
60	3.11	2.91	2.65	2.45	2.25	1.98	1.78	1.56	1.26
70	3.01	2.83	2.58	2.39	2.20	1.95	1.75	1.55	1.25
80	2.94	2.76	2.53	2.35	2.17	1.92	1.73	1.53	1.24
90	2.88	2.71	2.49	2.32	2.14	1.91	1.72	1.52	1.24
100	2.84	2.68	2.46	2.29	2.12	1.89	1.71	1.52	1.23
200	2.65	2.51	2.32	2.18	2.03	1.82	1.66	1.48	1.22
500	2.54	2.41	2.24	2.11	1.97	1.78	1.62	1.46	1.21
∞	2.47	2.35	2.19	2.06	1.93	1.75	1.60	1.44	1.20

(Continued)

TABLE B.4. (*Continued*)

					Numerator df = 20				
$\alpha(1)$	0.25	0.10	0.05	0.025	0.01	0.005	0.0025	0.001	0.0005
Denom df									
1	9.58	61.7	248.	993.	6,210.	24,800.	99,300.	$6 \cdot 10^5$	$2 \cdot 10^6$
2	3.43	9.44	19.4	39.4	99.4	199.	399.	999.	2,000.
3	2.46	5.18	8.66	14.2	26.7	42.8	683	126.	201.
4	2.08	3.84	5.80	8.56	14.0	20.2	28.9	46.1	65.5
5	1.88	3.21	4.56	6.33	9.55	12.9	17.3	25.4	33.8
6	1.76	2.84	3.87	5.17	7.40	9.59	12.3	17.1	21.8
7	1.67	2.59	3.44	4.47	6.16	7.75	9.70	12.9	16.0
8	1.61	2.42	3.15	4.00	5.36	6.61	8.09	10.5	12.7
9	1.56	2.30	2.94	3.67	4.81	5.83	7.02	8.90	10.6
10	1.52	2.20	2.77	3.42	4.41	5.27	6.27	7.80	9.17
11	1.49	2.12	2.65	3.23	4.10	4.86	5.71	7.01	8.14
12	1.47	2.06	2.54	3.07	3.86	4.53	5.28	6.40	7.37
13	1.45	2.01	2.46	2.95	3.66	4.27	4.94	5.93	6.78
14	1.43	1.96	2.39	2.84	3.51	4.06	4.66	5.56	6.31
15	1.41	1.92	2.33	2.76	3.37	3.88	4.44	5.25	5.93
16	1.40	1.89	2.28	2.68	3.26	3.73	4.25	4.99	5.61
17	1.39	1.86	2.23	2.62	3.16	3.61	4.09	4.78	5.34
18	1.38	1.84	2.19	2.56	3.08	3.50	3.95	4.59	5.12
19	1.37	1.81	2.16	2.51	3.00	3.40	3.83	4.43	4.92
20	1.36	1.79	2.12	2.46	2.94	3.32	3.72	4.29	4.75

21	4.60	4.17	3.63	3.24	2.88	2.42	2.10	1.78	1.35
22	4.47	4.06	3.54	3.18	2.83	2.39	2.07	1.76	1.34
23	4.36	3.96	3.47	3.12	2.78	2.36	2.05	1.74	1.34
24	4.25	3.87	3.40	3.06	2.74	2.33	2.03	1.73	1.33
25	4.16	3.79	3.34	3.01	2.70	2.30	2.01	1.72	1.33
26	4.07	3.72	3.28	2.97	2.66	2.28	1.99	1.71	1.32
27	3.99	3.66	3.23	2.93	2.63	2.25	1.97	1.70	1.32
28	3.92	3.60	3.19	2.89	2.60	2.23	1.96	1.69	1.31
29	3.86	3.54	3.14	2.86	2.57	2.21	1.94	1.68	1.31
30	3.80	3.49	3.11	2.82	2.55	2.20	1.93	1.67	1.30
35	3.56	3.29	2.95	2.69	2.44	2.12	1.88	1.63	1.29
40	3.39	3.14	2.83	2.60	2.37	2.07	1.84	1.61	1.28
45	3.26	3.04	2.74	2.53	2.31	2.03	1.81	1.58	1.27
50	3.16	2.95	2.68	2.47	2.27	1.99	1.78	1.57	1.26
60	3.02	2.83	2.58	2.39	2.20	1.94	1.75	1.54	1.25
70	2.92	2.74	2.51	2.33	2.15	1.91	1.72	1.53	1.24
80	2.85	2.68	2.46	2.29	2.12	1.88	1.70	1.51	1.23
90	2.79	2.63	2.42	2.25	2.09	1.86	1.69	1.50	1.23
100	2.75	2.59	2.38	2.23	2.07	1.85	1.68	1.49	1.23
200	2.56	2.42	2.25	2.11	1.97	1.78	1.62	1.46	1.21
500	2.45	2.33	2.17	2.04	1.92	1.74	1.59	1.44	1.20
∞	2.37	2.27	2.12	2.00	1.88	1.71	1.57	1.42	1.19

(Continued)

TABLE B.4. (*Continued*)

Numerator df = ∞

α(1)	0.25	0.10	0.05	0.025	0.01	0.005	0.0025	0.001	0.0005
Denom df									
1	9.85	63.3	254.	1,020.	6,370.	25,500.	$1 \cdot 10^5$	$6 \cdot 10^5$	$3 \cdot 10^6$
2	3.48	9.49	19.5	39.5	99.5	199.	399.	999.	2,000.
3	2.47	5.13	8.53	13.9	26.1	41.8	66.8	123.	196.
4	2.08	3.76	5.63	8.26	13.5	19.3	27.6	44.0	62.6
5	1.87	3.11	4.37	6.02	9.02	12.1	16.3	23.8	31.6
6	1.74	2.72	3.67	4.85	6.88	8.88	114	15.7	20.0
7	1.65	2.47	3.23	4.14	5.65	7.08	8.81	11.7	14.4
8	1.58	2.29	2.93	3.67	4.86	5.95	7.25	9.33	11.3
9	1.53	2.16	2.71	3.33	4.31	5.19	6.21	7.81	9.26
10	1.48	2.06	2.54	3.08	3.91	4.64	5.47	6.76	7.91
11	1.45	1.97	2.40	2.88	3.60	4.23	4.93	6.00	6.93
12	1.42	1.90	2.30	2.72	3.36	3.90	4.51	5.42	6.20
13	1.40	1.85	2.21	2.60	3.17	3.65	4.18	4.97	5.64
14	1.38	1.80	2.13	2.49	3.00	3.44	3.91	4.60	5.19
15	1.36	1.76	2.07	2.40	2.87	3.26	3.69	4.31	4.83
16	1.34	1.72	2.01	2.32	2.75	3.11	3.50	4.06	4.52
17	1.33	1.69	1.96	2.25	2.65	2.98	3.34	3.85	4.27
18	1.32	1.66	1.92	2.19	2.57	2.87	3.20	3.67	4.05
19	1.30	1.63	1.88	2.13	2.49	2.78	3.08	3.51	3.87
20	1.29	1.61	1.84	2.09	2.42	2.69	2.97	3.38	3.71

21	1.28	1.59	1.81	2.04	2.36	2.61	2.88	3.26	3.56
22	1.28	1.57	1.78	2.00	2.31	2.55	2.80	3.15	3.43
23	1.27	1.55	1.76	1.97	2.26	2.48	2.72	3.05	3.32
24	1.26	1.53	1.73	1.94	2.21	2.43	2.65	2.97	3.22
25	1.25	1.52	1.71	1.91	2.17	2.38	2.59	2.89	3.13
26	1.25	1.50	1.69	1.88	2.13	2.33	2.54	2.82	3.05
27	1.24	1.49	1.67	1.85	2.10	2.29	2.48	2.75	2.97
28	1.24	1.48	1.65	1.83	2.06	2.25	2.44	2.69	2.90
29	1.23	1.47	1.64	1.81	2.03	2.21	2.39	2.64	2.84
30	1.23	1.46	1.62	1.79	2.01	2.18	2.35	2.59	2.78
35	1.20	1.41	1.56	1.70	1.89	2.04	2.18	2.38	2.54
40	1.19	1.38	1.51	1.64	1.80	1.93	2.06	2.23	2.37
45	1.18	1.35	1.47	1.59	1.74	1.85	1.97	2.12	2.23
50	1.16	1.33	1.44	1.55	1.68	1.79	1.89	2.03	2.13
60	1.15	1.29	1.39	1.48	1.60	1.69	1.78	1.89	1.98
70	1.13	1.27	1.35	1.44	1.54	1.62	1.69	1.79	1.87
80	1.12	1.24	1.32	1.40	1.49	1.56	1.63	1.72	1.79
90	1.12	1.23	1.30	1.37	1.46	1.52	1.58	1.66	1.72
100	1.11	1.21	1.28	1.35	1.43	1.49	1.54	1.62	1.67
200	1.07	1.14	1.19	1.23	1.28	1.31	1.35	1.39	1.42
500	1.05	1.09	1.11	1.14	1.16	1.18	1.20	1.23	1.24
∞	1.00	1.00	1.00	1.00	1.00	1.00	1.00	1.00	1.00

*To locate an *F* value, first find the table that is headed by the degrees of freedom in the numerator of your *F* ratio. Then, find the degrees of freedom in the denominator of your *F* ratio in the leftmost column. Finally, find the appropriate α at the top of the table. The number in the body of the table where this row and column intersect is the *F* statistic from a distribution with those numerator and denominator degrees of freedom and that corresponds to an area of α in one tail of the *F* distribution.

TABLE B.5. Critical Values of Spearman's Correlation Coefficient*

$\alpha(2)$	0.50	0.20	0.10	0.05	0.02	0.01	0.005	0.002	0.001
$\alpha(1)$	0.25	0.10	0.05	0.025	0.01	0.005	0.0025	0.001	0.0005
n									
4	0.600	1.000	1.000						
5	0.500	0.800	0.900	1.000	1.000				
6	0.371	0.657	0.829	0.886	0.943	1.000	1.000		
7	0.321	0.571	0.714	0.786	0.893	0.929	0.964	1.000	1.000
8	0.310	0.524	0.643	0.738	0.833	0.881	0.905	0.952	0.976
9	0.267	0.483	0.600	0.700	0.783	0.833	0.867	0.917	0.933
10	0.248	0.455	0.564	0.648	0.745	0.794	0.830	0.879	0.903
11	0.236	0.427	0.536	0.618	0.709	0.755	0.800	0.845	0.873
12	0.217	0.406	0.503	0.587	0.678	0.727	0.769	0.818	0.846
13	0.209	0.385	0.484	0.560	0.648	0.703	0.747	0.791	0.824
14	0.200	0.367	0.464	0.538	0.626	0.679	0.723	0.771	0.802
15	0.189	0.354	0.446	0.521	0.604	0.654	0.700	0.750	0.779
16	0.182	0.341	0.429	0.503	0.582	0.635	0.679	0.729	0.762
17	0.176	0.328	0.414	0.485	0.566	0.615	0.662	0.713	0.748
18	0.170	0.317	0.401	0.472	0.550	0.600	0.643	0.695	0.728
19	0.165	0.309	0.391	0.460	0.535	0.584	0.628	0.677	0.712
20	0.161	0.299	0.380	0.447	0.520	0.570	0.612	0.662	0.696
21	0.156	0.292	0.370	0.435	0.508	0.556	0.599	0.648	0.681
22	0.152	0.284	0.361	0.425	0.496	0.544	0.586	0.634	0.667
23	0.148	0.278	0.353	0.415	0.486	0.532	0.573	0.622	0.654
24	0.144	0.271	0.344	0.406	0.476	0.521	0.562	0.610	0.642
25	0.142	0.265	0.337	0.398	0.466	0.511	0.551	0.598	0.630

TABLE B.5. (*Continued*)

$\alpha(2)$	0.50	0.20	0.10	0.05	0.02	0.01	0.005	0.002	0.001
$\alpha(1)$	0.25	0.10	0.05	0.025	0.01	0.005	0.0025	0.001	0.0005
n									
26	0.138	0.259	0.331	0.390	0.457	0.501	0.541	0.587	0.619
27	0.136	0.255	0.324	0.382	0.448	0.491	0.531	0.577	0.608
28	0.133	0.250	0.317	0.375	0.440	0.483	0.522	0.567	0.598
29	0.130	0.245	0.312	0.368	0.433	0.475	0.513	0.558	0.589
30	0.128	0.240	0.306	0.362	0.425	0.467	0.504	0.549	0.580
35	0.118	0.222	0.283	0.335	0.394	0.433	0.468	0.510	0.539
40	0.110	0.207	0.264	0.313	0.368	0.405	0.439	0.479	0.507
45	0.103	0.194	0.248	0.294	0.347	0.382	0.414	0.453	0.479
50	0.097	0.184	0.235	0.279	0.329	0.363	0.393	0.430	0.456
55	0.093	0.175	0.224	0.266	0.314	0.346	0.375	0.411	0.435
60	0.089	0.168	0.214	0.255	0.300	0.331	0.360	0.394	0.418
65	0.085	0.161	0.206	0.244	0.289	0.318	0.346	0.379	0.402
70	0.082	0.155	0.198	0.235	0.278	0.307	0.333	0.365	0.388
75	0.079	0.150	0.191	0.227	0.269	0.297	0.322	0.353	0.375
80	0.076	0.145	0.185	0.220	0.260	0.287	0.312	0.342	0.363
85	0.074	0.140	0.180	0.213	0.252	0.279	0.303	0.332	0.353
90	0.072	0.136	0.174	0.207	0.245	0.271	0.294	0.323	0.343
95	0.070	0.133	0.170	0.202	0.239	0.264	0.287	0.314	0.334
100	0.068	0.129	0.165	0.197	0.233	0.257	0.279	0.307	0.326

*To find Spearman's correlation coefficient that is associated with a certain chance of making a type I error, find the column corresponding with that value of α at the top of table ($\alpha(2)$ indicates a two-tailed value and $\alpha(1)$ indicates a one-tailed value) and the row corresponding to the sample's size in the leftmost column. The value in the body of the table where that column and row intersect is the absolute value of Spearman's correlation coefficient that is expected to occur in α of the samples when Spearman's correlation coefficient is equal to 0 in the population.

TABLE B.6. Critical Values of the Mann–Whitney U Statistic*

	$\alpha(2)$	0.20	0.10	0.05	0.02	0.01	0.005	0.002	0.001
	$\alpha(1)$	0.10	0.05	0.025	0.01	0.005	0.0025	0.001	0.0005
n_S	n_L								
1	1	–	–	–	–	–	–	–	–
	2	–	–	–	–	–	–	–	–
	3	–	–	–	–	–	–	–	–
	4	–	–	–	–	–	–	–	–
	5	–	–	–	–	–	–	–	–
	6	–	–	–	–	–	–	–	–
	7	–	–	–	–	–	–	–	–
	8	–	–	–	–	–	–	–	–
	9	9	–	–	–	–	–	–	–
	10	10	–	–	–	–	–	–	–
	12	12	–	–	–	–	–	–	–
	14	14	–	–	–	–	–	–	–
	16	16	–	–	–	–	–	–	–
	18	18	–	–	–	–	–	–	–
	20	19	20	–	–	–	–	–	–
	22	21	22	–	–	–	–	–	–
	24	23	22	–	–	–	–	–	–
	26	25	26	–	–	–	–	–	–
	28	27	28	–	–	–	–	–	–
	30	28	30	–	–	–	–	–	–
	32	30	32	–	–	–	–	–	–
	34	32	34	–	–	–	–	–	–
	36	34	36	–	–	–	–	–	–
	38	36	38	–	–	–	–	–	–
1	40	37	39	40	–	–	–	–	–
2	2	–	–	–	–	–	–	–	–
	3	6	–	–	–	–	–	–	–
	4	8	–	–	–	–	–	–	–
	5	9	10	–	–	–	–	–	–
	6	11	12	–	–	–	–	–	–
	7	10	14	–	–	–	–	–	–

TABLE B.6. (*Continued*)

n_S	n_L	0.20	0.10	0.05	0.02	0.01	0.005	0.002	0.001
$\alpha(2)$		**0.20**	**0.10**	**0.05**	**0.02**	**0.01**	**0.005**	**0.002**	**0.001**
$\alpha(1)$		**0.10**	**0.05**	**0.025**	**0.01**	**0.005**	**0.0025**	**0.001**	**0.0005**
	8	14	15	16	–	–	–	–	–
	9	16	17	18	–	–	–	–	–
	10	17	19	20	–	–	–	–	–
	12	20	22	23	–	–	–	–	–
	14	23	25	27	28	–	–	–	–
	16	27	29	31	32	–	–	–	–
	18	30	32	34	36	–	–	–	–
	20	33	36	38	39	40	–	–	–
	22	36	39	41	43	44	–	–	–
	24	39	42	45	47	48	–	–	–
	26	42	46	48	51	52	–	–	–
	28	45	49	52	54	55	56	–	–
	30	48	53	55	58	59	60	–	–
	32	51	56	59	62	63	64	–	–
	34	55	59	63	65	67	68	–	–
	36	58	63	66	69	71	72	–	–
	38	61	66	70	73	75	76	–	–
	40	64	69	73	77	78	79	–	–
$\alpha(2)$		**0.20**	**0.10**	**0.05**	**0.02**	**0.01**	**0.005**	**0.002**	**0.001**
$\alpha(1)$		**0.10**	**0.05**	**0.025**	**0.01**	**0.005**	**0.0025**	**0.001**	**0.0005**
n_S	n_L								
2	**32**	51	56	59	62	63	64	–	–
	34	55	59	63	65	67	68	–	–
	36	58	63	66	69	71	72	–	–
	38	61	66	70	73	75	76	–	–
	40	64	69	73	77	78	79	–	–
3	**3**	8	9	–	–	–	–	–	–
	4	11	12	–	–	–	–	–	–
	5	13	14	15	–	–	–	–	–
	6	15	16	17	–	–	–	–	–
	7	15	19	20	21	–	–	–	–
	8	19	21	22	24	–	–	–	–

(*Continued*)

TABLE B.6. (*Continued*)

	$\alpha(2)$	0.20	0.10	0.05	0.02	0.01	0.005	0.002	0.001
	$\alpha(1)$	0.10	0.05	0.025	0.01	0.005	0.0025	0.001	0.0005
n_S	n_L								
	9	22	23	25	26	27	–	–	–
	10	24	26	27	29	30	–	–	–
	12	28	31	32	34	35	36	–	–
	14	32	35	37	40	41	42	–	–
	16	37	40	42	45	46	47	–	–
	18	41	45	47	50	52	53	54	–
	20	45	49	52	55	57	58	60	–
	22	50	54	57	60	62	64	65	66
	24	54	59	62	66	68	69	71	72
	26	58	63	67	71	73	75	77	78
	28	63	68	72	76	79	80	82	83
	30	67	73	77	81	84	86	88	89
	32	71	77	82	87	89	91	94	95
	34	76	82	87	92	95	97	99	101
	36	80	87	92	97	100	103	105	106
	38	84	91	97	102	105	108	111	112
3	40	89	96	102	107	111	114	116	118
4	4	13	15	16	–	–	–	–	–
	5	16	18	19	20	–	–	–	–
	6	19	21	22	23	24	–	–	–
	7	20	24	25	27	28	–	–	–
	8	25	27	28	30	31	32	–	–
	9	27	30	32	33	35	36	–	–
	10	30	33	35	37	38	39	40	–
	12	36	39	41	43	45	46	48	–
	14	41	45	47	50	52	53	55	56
	16	47	50	53	57	59	60	62	63
	18	52	56	60	63	66	67	69	71
	20	58	62	66	70	72	75	77	78
	22	63	68	72	77	79	82	84	85
	24	69	74	79	83	86	89	91	93
	26	74	80	85	90	93	96	98	100
	28	80	86	91	96	100	103	106	108
4	30	85	92	97	103	107	110	113	115

TABLE B.6. (*Continued*)

n_S	n_L	$\alpha(2)$ 0.20 $\alpha(1)$ 0.10	0.10 0.05	0.05 0.025	0.02 0.01	0.01 0.005	0.005 0.0025	0.002 0.001	0.001 0.0005
4	32	91	98	104	110	114	117	120	122
	34	96	104	110	116	120	124	127	130
	36	102	110	116	123	127	131	135	137
	38	107	116	122	130	134	138	142	144
4	40	113	121	129	136	141	145	149	152
5	5	20	21	23	24	25	–	–	–
	6	23	25	27	28	29	30	–	–
	7	24	29	30	32	34	35	–	–
	8	30	32	34	36	38	39	40	–
	9	33	36	38	40	42	43	44	45
	10	37	39	42	44	46	47	49	50
	12	43	47	49	52	54	56	58	59
	14	50	54	57	60	63	64	67	68
	16	57	61	65	68	71	73	75	77
	18	63	68	72	76	79	81	84	86
	20	70	75	80	84	87	90	93	95
	22	77	82	97	92	96	98	102	104
	24	84	90	95	100	104	107	110	113
	26	90	97	102	108	112	115	119	121
	28	97	104	110	116	120	124	128	130
	30	104	111	117	124	128	132	136	139
	32	110	118	125	132	137	141	145	148
	34	117	125	132	140	145	149	154	157
	36	124	132	140	148	153	158	163	166
	38	130	140	147	156	161	166	171	175
5	40	137	147	155	164	169	174	180	184
6	6	27	29	31	33	34	35	–	–
	7	29	34	36	38	39	40	42	–
	8	35	38	40	42	44	45	47	48
	9	39	42	44	47	49	50	52	53
	10	43	46	49	52	54	55	57	58
	12	51	55	58	61	63	65	68	69

(*Continued*)

TABLE B.6. (*Continued*)

n_S	n_L	0.20	0.10	0.05	0.02	0.01	0.005	0.002	0.001
		0.10	0.05	0.025	0.01	0.005	0.0025	0.001	0.0005
	14	59	63	67	71	73	75	78	79
	16	67	71	75	80	83	85	88	90
	18	74	80	84	89	92	95	98	100
	20	82	88	93	98	102	105	108	111
	22	90	96	102	108	111	115	119	121
	24	98	105	111	117	121	125	129	132
	26	106	113	119	126	131	134	139	142
	28	114	122	128	135	140	144	149	152
6	30	122	130	137	145	150	154	159	163
n_S	n_L	0.20	0.10	0.05	0.02	0.01	0.005	0.002	0.001
		0.10	0.05	0.025	0.01	0.005	0.0025	0.001	0.0005
6	32	129	138	146	154	159	164	169	173
	34	137	147	154	163	169	174	179	183
	36	145	155	163	172	178	184	190	194
	38	153	163	172	182	188	193	200	204
6	40	161	172	181	191	197	203	210	214
7	7	36	38	41	43	45	46	48	49
	8	40	43	46	49	50	52	54	55
	9	45	48	51	54	56	58	60	61
	10	49	53	56	59	61	63	65	67
	12	58	63	66	70	72	75	77	79
	14	67	72	76	81	83	86	89	91
	16	76	82	86	91	94	97	101	103
	18	85	91	96	102	105	108	112	115
	20	94	101	106	112	116	120	124	126
	22	103	110	116	123	127	131	135	138
	24	112	120	126	133	138	142	147	150
	26	121	129	136	144	149	153	158	162
	28	130	139	146	154	160	164	170	174
	30	139	149	156	165	170	176	181	185

TABLE B.6. (*Continued*)

n_S	n_L	$\alpha(2)$ 0.20	0.10	0.05	0.02	0.01	0.005	0.002	0.001
		$\alpha(1)$ 0.10	0.05	0.025	0.01	0.005	0.0025	0.001	0.0005
	32	148	158	166	175	181	187	193	197
	34	157	168	176	186	192	198	204	209
	36	166	177	186	196	203	209	216	221
	38	175	187	196	207	214	220	227	232
7	40	184	196	206	217	225	231	239	244
8	8	45	49	51	55	57	58	60	62
	9	50	54	57	61	63	65	67	68
	10	56	60	63	67	69	71	74	75
	12	66	70	74	79	81	84	87	89
	14	76	81	86	90	94	96	100	102
	16	86	92	97	102	106	109	113	115
	18	96	103	108	114	118	122	126	129
	20	106	113	119	126	130	134	139	142
	22	117	124	131	138	142	147	152	155
	24	127	135	142	150	155	159	165	168
	26	137	146	153	161	167	172	177	181
	28	147	156	164	173	179	184	190	195
	30	157	167	175	185	191	197	203	208
	32	167	178	187	197	203	209	216	221
	34	177	188	198	208	215	222	229	234
	36	188	199	209	220	228	234	242	247
	38	198	210	220	232	240	247	255	260
8	40	208	221	231	244	252	259	268	273
n_S	n_L	$\alpha(2)$ 0.20 / $\alpha(1)$ 0.10	0.10 / 0.05	0.05 / 0.025	0.02 / 0.01	0.01 / 0.005	0.005 / 0.0025	0.002 / 0.001	0.001 / 0.0005
9	9	56	60	64	67	70	72	74	76
	10	62	66	70	74	77	79	82	83
	12	73	78	82	87	90	93	96	98
	14	85	90	95	100	104	107	111	113
	16	96	102	107	113	117	121	125	128
	18	107	114	120	126	131	135	139	142

(*Continued*)

TABLE B.6. (*Continued*)

n_S	n_L	α(2) 0.20	0.10	0.05	0.02	0.01	0.005	0.002	0.001
		α(1) 0.10	0.05	0.025	0.01	0.005	0.0025	0.001	0.0005
	20	118	126	132	140	144	149	154	157
	22	130	138	145	153	158	162	168	172
	24	141	150	157	166	171	176	182	186
	26	152	162	170	179	185	190	196	201
	28	164	174	182	192	198	204	211	215
	30	175	185	194	205	212	218	225	230
	32	186	197	207	218	225	231	239	244
	34	197	209	219	231	238	245	253	259
	36	209	221	232	244	252	259	267	273
	38	220	233	244	257	265	273	282	288
9	40	231	245	257	270	279	286	296	302
10	10	68	73	77	81	84	87	90	92
	12	81	86	91	96	99	102	106	108
	14	93	99	104	110	114	117	121	124
	16	106	112	118	124	129	133	137	140
	18	118	125	132	139	143	148	153	156
	20	130	138	145	153	158	163	168	172
	22	143	152	159	167	173	178	184	188
	24	155	165	173	182	188	193	200	204
	26	168	178	186	196	202	208	215	220
	28	180	191	200	210	217	223	231	236
	30	192	204	213	224	232	238	246	252
	32	205	217	227	239	246	253	262	267
	34	217	230	241	253	261	268	277	283
	36	229	243	254	267	276	284	293	299
	38	242	256	268	281	290	299	308	315
10	40	254	269	281	296	305	314	324	331

*To find a Mann–Whitney U statistic that is associated with a certain chance of making a type I error, find the column corresponding with that value of α at the top of table (α(2) indicates a two-tailed value and α(1) indicates a one-tailed value) and the row corresponding to the sample's size in the leftmost column. The value in the body of the table where that column and row intersect is the value of the Mann–Whitney U statistic that is expected to occur in α of the samples when there is no association between the groups in the population.

TABLE B.7. Critical Values of the Chi-Square Distribution[*]

$\alpha(1)$	0.50	0.25	0.10	0.05	0.025	0.01	0.005	0.001
df								
1	0.455	1.323	2.706	3.841	5.024	6.635	7.879	10.828
2	1.386	2.773	4.605	5.991	7.378	9.210	10.597	13.816
3	2.366	4.108	6.251	7.815	9.348	11.345	12.838	16.266
4	3.357	5.385	7.779	9.488	11.143	13.277	14.860	18.467
5	4.351	6.626	9.236	11.070	12.833	15.086	16.750	20.515
6	5.348	7.841	10.645	12.592	14.449	16.812	18.548	22.458
7	6.346	9.037	12.017	14.067	16.013	18.475	20.278	24.322
8	7.344	10.219	13.362	15.507	17.535	20.090	21.955	26.124
9	8.343	11.389	14.684	16.919	19.023	21.666	23.589	27.877
10	9.342	12.549	15.987	18.307	20.483	23.209	25.188	29.588
11	10.341	13.701	17.275	19.675	21.920	24.725	26.757	31.264
12	11.340	14.845	18.549	21.026	23.337	26.217	28.300	32.909
13	12.340	15.984	19.812	22.362	24.736	27.688	29.819	34.528
14	13.339	17.117	21.064	23.685	26.119	29.141	31.319	36.123
15	14.339	18.245	22.307	24.996	27.488	30.578	32.801	37.697
16	15.338	19.369	23.542	26.296	28.845	32.000	34.267	39.252
17	16.338	20.489	24.769	27.587	30.191	33.409	35.718	40.790
18	17.338	21.605	25.989	28.869	31.526	34.805	37.156	42.312
19	18.338	22.718	27.204	30.144	32.852	36.191	38.582	43.820
20	19.337	23.828	28.412	31.410	34.170	37.566	39.997	45.315
21	20.337	24.935	29.615	32.671	35.479	38.932	41.401	46.797
22	21.337	26.039	30.813	33.924	36.781	40.289	42.796	48.268
23	22.337	27.141	32.007	35.172	38.076	41.638	44.181	49.728
24	23.337	28.241	33.196	36.415	39.364	42.980	45.559	51.179

(*Continued*)

TABLE B.7. (*Continued*)

$\alpha(1)$	0.50	0.25	0.10	0.05	0.025	0.01	0.005	0.001
df								
25	24.337	29.339	34.382	37.652	40.646	44.314	46.928	52.620
26	25.336	30.435	35.563	38.885	41.923	45.642	48.290	54.052
27	26.336	31.528	36.741	40.113	43.195	46.963	49.645	55.476
28	27.336	32.620	37.916	41.337	44.461	48.278	50.993	56.892
29	28.336	33.711	39.087	42.557	45.722	49.588	52.336	58.301
30	29.336	34.800	40.256	43.773	46.979	50.892	53.672	59.703
35	34.336	40.223	46.059	49.802	53.203	57.342	60.275	66.619
40	39.335	45.616	51.805	55.758	59.342	63.691	66.766	73.402
45	44.335	50.985	57.505	61.656	65.410	69.957	73.166	80.077
50	49.335	56.334	63.167	67.505	71.420	76.154	79.490	86.661
55	54.335	61.665	68.796	73.311	77.380	82.292	85.749	93.168
60	59.335	66.981	74.397	79.082	83.298	88.379	91.952	99.607
65	64.335	72.285	79.973	84.821	89.177	94.422	98.105	105.99
70	69.334	77.577	85.527	90.531	95.023	100.43	104.22	112.32
75	74.334	82.858	91.061	96.217	100.84	106.39	110.29	118.60
80	79.334	88.130	96.578	101.88	106.63	112.33	116.32	124.84
85	84.334	93.394	102.08	107.52	112.39	118.24	122.33	131.04
90	89.334	98.650	107.57	113.15	118.14	124.12	128.30	137.21
95	94.334	103.90	113.04	118.75	123.86	129.97	134.25	143.34
100	99.334	109.14	118.50	124.34	129.56	135.81	140.17	149.45

*To locate a chi-square value, find the degrees of freedom in the leftmost column and the appropriate α at the top of the table (only one-tailed α are appropriate in the chi-square distribution). The number in the body of the table where this row and column intersect is the value from the chi-square distribution with that number of degrees of freedom and that corresponds to an area equal to α in the upper tail.

TABLE B.8. Critical Values of the q Distribution*

				$\alpha(2) = 0.10$					
k	2	3	4	5	6	7	8	9	10
df									
1	8.929	13.44	16.36	18.49	20.15	21.51	22.64	23.62	24.48
2	4.130	5.733	6.773	7.538	8.139	8.633	9.049	9.409	9.725
3	3.328	4.467	5.199	5.738	6.162	6.511	6.806	7.062	7.287
4	3.015	3.976	4.586	5.035	5.388	5.679	5.926	6.139	6.327
5	2.850	3.717	4.264	4.664	4.979	5.238	5.458	5.648	5.816
6	2.748	3.559	4.065	4.435	4.726	4.966	5.168	5.344	5.499
7	2.680	3.451	3.931	4.280	4.555	4.780	4.972	5.137	5.283
8	2.630	3.374	3.843	4.169	4.431	4.646	4.829	4.987	5.126
9	2.592	3.316	3.761	4.084	4.337	4.545	4.721	4.873	5.007
10	2.563	3.270	3.704	4.018	4.264	4.465	4.636	4.783	4.913
11	2.540	3.234	3.658	3.965	4.205	4.401	4.568	4.711	4.838
12	2.521	3.204	3.621	3.922	4.156	4.349	4.511	4.652	4.776
13	2.505	3.179	3.589	3.885	4.116	4.305	4.464	4.602	4.724
14	2.491	3.158	3.563	3.854	4.081	4.267	4.424	4.560	4.680
15	2.479	3.140	3.540	3.828	4.052	4.235	4.390	4.524	4.641
16	2.469	3.124	3.520	3.804	4.026	4.207	4.360	4.492	4.608
17	2.460	3.110	3.503	3.784	4.004	4.183	4.334	4.464	4.579
18	2.452	3.098	3.488	3.767	30,984	4.161	4.311	4.440	4.554
19	2.455	3.087	3.474	3.751	3.966	4.142	4.290	4.418	4.531
20	2.439	3.078	3.462	3.736	3.950	4.124	4.271	4.398	4.510
30	2.400	3.017	3.648	3.648	3.851	4.016	4.155	4.275	4.381
40	2.381	2.988	3.349	3.605	3.803	3.963	4.099	4.215	4.317
50	2.372	2.974	3.584	3.584	3.586	3.937	4.071	4.185	4.286
60	2.363	2.959	3.562	3.562	3.562	3.911	4.042	4.155	4.254
∞	2.326	2.902	3.478	3.478	3.478	3.808	4.931	4.037	4.129

(*Continued*)

TABLE B.8. (*Continued*)

k	11	12	13	14	15	16	17	18	19
df									
1	25.24	25.92	26.54	27.10	27.62	28.10	28.54	28.96	29.35
2	10.01	10.26	10.49	10.70	10.89	11.07	11.24	11.39	11.54
3	7.487	7.667	7.832	7.982	8.120	8.249	8.368	8.479	8.584
4	6.495	6.645	6.783	6.909	7.025	7.133	7.233	7.327	7.414
5	5.966	6.101	6.223	6.336	6.440	6.536	6.626	6.710	6.789
6	5.637	5.762	5.875	5.979	6.075	6.164	6.247	6.325	6.398
7	5.413	5.530	5.637	5.735	5.826	5.910	5.988	6.061	6.130
8	5.250	5.362	5.464	5.558	5.644	5.274	5.799	5.869	5.935
9	5.127	5.234	5.333	5.423	5.506	5.583	5.655	5.723	5.786
10	5.029	5.134	5.229	5.317	5.397	5.472	5.542	5.607	5.668
11	4.951	5.053	5.146	5.231	5.309	5.382	5.450	5.514	5.573
12	4.886	4.986	5.077	5.160	5.236	5.308	5.374	5.436	4.495
13	4.832	4.930	5.019	5.100	5.176	5.245	5.311	5.372	5.429
14	4.786	4.882	4.970	5.050	5.124	5.192	5.256	5.316	5.373
15	4.746	4.841	4.927	5.006	5.079	5.147	5.209	5.269	5.324
16	4.712	4.805	4.890	4.968	5.040	5.107	5.169	5.227	5.282
17	4.682	4.774	4.858	4.935	5.005	5.071	5.133	5.190	5.244
18	4.655	4.746	4.829	4.905	4.975	5.040	5.101	5.158	5.211
19	4 631	4.721	4.803	4.879	4.948	5.012	5.073	5.129	5.182
20	4.609	4.699	4.780	4.855	4.924	4.987	5.047	5.103	5.155
30	4.474	4.559	4.635	4.706	4.770	4.830	4.866	4.939	4.988
40	4.408	4.490	4.564	4.632	4.695	4.752	4.807	4.857	4.905
50	4.375	4.456	4.519	4.595	4.657	4.714	4.767	4.816	4.863
60	4.342	4.421	4.493	4.558	4.619	4.675	4.727	4.775	4.821
∞	4.211	4.285	4.351	4.412	4.468	4.519	4.568	4.612	4.654

TABLE B.8. (*Continued*)

				$\alpha(2) = 0.05$					
k	**2**	**3**	**4**	**5**	**6**	**7**	**8**	**9**	**10**
df									
1	17.97	26.98	32.82	37.08	40.17	43.12	45.40	47.36	49.07
2	6.085	8.331	9.798	10.88	11.74	12.44	13.03	13.54	13.99
3	4.501	5.910	6.825	7.502	8.037	8.478	8.853	9.177	9.462
4	3.927	5.040	5.757	6.287	6.707	7.053	7.347	7.602	7.826
5	3.635	4.602	5.218	5.673	6.033	6.330	6.582	6.802	6.995
6	3.461	4.339	4.896	5.305	5.628	5.895	6.122	6.319	6.493
7	3.344	4.165	4.681	5.060	5.359	5.606	5.815	5.998	6.158
8	3.261	4.041	4.529	4.886	5.167	5.399	5.597	5 767	5.918
9	3.199	3.949	4.415	4.756	5.024	5.244	5.432	5.595	5.739
10	3.151	3.877	4.327	4.654	5.912	5.124	5.305	5.461	5.599
11	3.133	3.820	4.256	4.574	4.823	5.028	5.202	5.353	5.487
12	3.082	3.773	4.199	4.508	4.751	4.950	5.119	5.265	5.395
13	3.055	3.735	4.151	4.453	4.690	4.885	5.049	5.192	5.318
14	3.033	3.702	4.111	4.407	4.639	4.829	4.990	5.131	5.254
15	3.014	3.674	4.076	4.367	4.595	4.782	4.940	5.077	5.198
16	2.998	3.649	4.046	4.333	4.557	4.741	4.897	5.031	5.150
17	2.984	3.628	4.020	4.303	4.524	4.705	4.858	4.991	5.108
18	2.971	3.609	3.997	4.277	4.495	4.673	4.824	4.956	5.071
19	2.960	3.593	3.977	4.253	4.469	4.645	4.794	4.924	5.038
20	2.950	3.578	3.958	4.232	4.445	4.620	4.768	4.896	5.008
30	2.888	3.486	3.845	4.102	4.302	4.464	4.602	4.720	4.824
40	2.858	3.442	3.791	4.039	4.232	4.389	4.521	4.635	4.735
50	2.844	4.423	3.764	4.008	4.196	4.352	4.481	4.593	4.691
60	2.829	3.399	3.399	3.977	4.163	4.314	4.441	4.550	4.646
∞	2.772	3.314	3.633	3.858	4.030	4.170	4.286	4.387	4.474

(*Continued*)

TABLE B.8. (*Continued*)

k	11	12	13	14	15	16	17	18	19
df									
1	50.59	51.96	53.20	54.33	55.36	56.32	57.22	58.04	58.83
2	14.39	14.75	15.08	15.38	15.65	15.91	16.14	16.37	16.57
3	9.717	9.946	10.15	10.35	10.53	10.69	10.84	10.98	11.11
4	8.027	8.208	8.373	8.525	8.664	8.794	8.914	9.028	9.134
5	7.168	7.324	7.466	7.596	7.717	7.828	7.932	8.030	8.122
6	6.649	6.789	6.917	7.034	7.143	7.244	7.338	7.426	7.508
7	6.302	6.431	6.550	6.658	6.759	6.852	6.939	7.020	7.097
8	6.054	6.175	6.287	6.389	6.483	6.571	6.653	6.729	6.802
9	5.867	5.983	6.089	6.186	6.276	6.359	6.437	6.510	6.579
10	5.722	5.833	5.935	6.028	6.114	6.194	6.269	6.339	6.405
11	5.605	5.713	5.811	5.901	6.984	6.062	6.134	6.202	6.265
12	5.511	5.615	5.710	5.798	5.878	5.953	6.023	6.089	6.151
13	5.431	5.533	5.625	5.711	5.789	5.862	5.931	5.995	6.055
14	5.364	5.463	5.554	5.637	5.714	5.786	5.852	5.915	5.974
15	5.306	5.404	5.493	5.574	5.649	5.720	5.785	5.846	5.904
16	5.256	5.352	5.439	5.520	5.593	5.662	5.727	5.786	5.843
17	5.212	5.307	5.392	5.471	5.544	5.612	5.675	5.734	5.790
18	5.174	5.267	5.352	5.429	5.501	5.568	5.630	5.688	5.743
19	5.140	5.231	5.315	5.391	5.462	5.528	5.589	5.647	5.701
20	5.108	5.199	5.282	5.357	5.427	5.493	5.553	5.610	5.663
30	4.917	5.001	5.077	5.147	5.211	5.271	5.327	5.379	5.429
40	4.824	4.904	4.977	5.044	5.106	5.163	5.216	5.266	5.313
50	4.778	4.856	4.928	4.993	5.054	5.110	5.162	5.210	5.256
60	4.732	4.808	4.878	4.942	5.001	5.056	5.107	5.154	5.199
∞	4.552	4.622	4.685	4.743	4.796	4.845	4.891	4.934	4.974

TABLE B.8. (*Continued*)

				$\alpha(2) = 0.01$					
k	**2**	**3**	**4**	**5**	**6**	**7**	**8**	**9**	**10**
df									
1	90.03	135.0	164.3	185.6	202.2	215.8	227.2	237.0	245.6
2	14.04	19.02	22.29	24.72	26.63	28.20	29.53	30.68	31.69
3	8.261	10.62	12.17	13.33	14.24	15.00	15.64	16.20	16.69
4	6.512	8.120	9.173	9.958	10.58	11.10	11.55	11.93	12.27
5	5.702	6.976	7.804	8.421	8.913	9.321	9.669	9.972	10.24
6	5.243	6.331	7.033	7.556	7.973	8.318	8.613	8.869	9.097
7	4.949	5.919	6.543	7.005	7.373	7.679	7.939	8.166	8.368
8	4.746	5.635	6.204	6.625	6.960	7.237	7.474	7.681	7.863
9	4.596	5.428	5.957	6.348	6.658	6.915	7.134	7.325	7.495
10	4.482	5.270	5.769	6.163	6.428	6.669	6.875	7.055	7.213
11	4.392	5.146	5.621	5.970	6.247	6.476	6.672	6.842	6.992
12	4.320	5.046	5 502	5.836	6.101	6.321	6.507	6.670	6.814
13	4.260	4.964	5.404	5.727	5.981	6.192	6.372	6.528	6.667
14	4.210	4.895	5.322	5.634	5.881	6.085	6.258	6.409	6.543
15	4.168	4.836	5.252	5.556	5.796	5.994	6.162	6.309	6.439
16	4.131	4.786	5.192	5.489	5.722	5.915	6.079	6.022	6.349
17	4.099	4.742	5.140	5.430	5.659	5.847	6.007	6.147	6.270
18	4.071	4.703	5.094	5.379	5.603	5.788	5.944	6.081	6.201
19	4.046	4.670	5.054	5.334	5.554	5.735	5.889	6.022	6.141
20	4.024	4.639	5.018	5.294	5.510	5.688	5.839	5.970	6.087
30	3.889	4.455	4.799	5.048	5.242	5.401	5.536	5.653	5.756
40	3.825	4.367	4.696	4.931	5.114	5.265	5.392	5.502	5.559
50	3.794	4.325	4.645	4.874	5.014	5.198	5.322	5.429	5.503
60	3.762	4.282	4.595	4.818	4.991	5.133	5.253	5.356	5.447
∞	3.643	4.120	4.403	4.603	4.757	4.882	4.987	5.078	5.157

(*Continued*)

TABLE B.8. (*Continued*)

k	11	12	13	14	15	16	17	18	19
df									
1	253.2	260.0	266.2	271.8	277.0	281.8	286.3	290.4	294.3
2	32.59	33.40	34.13	34.81	35.43	36.00	36.53	37.03	37.50
3	17.13	17.53	17.89	18.22	18.52	18.81	19.07	19.32	19.55
4	12.57	12.84	13.09	13.32	13.53	13.73	13.91	14.08	14.24
5	10.48	10.70	10.89	11.08	11.24	11.40	11.55	11.68	11.81
6	9.301	9.485	9.653	9.808	9.951	10.08	10.21	10.32	10.43
7	8.548	8.711	8.860	8.997	9.124	9.242	9.353	9.456	9.554
8	8.027	8.176	8.312	8.436	8.552	8.659	8.760	8.854	8.943
9	7.647	7.784	7.910	8.025	8.132	8.232	8.325	8.412	8.495
10	7.356	7.485	7.603	7.712	7.812	7.906	7.993	8.076	8.153
11	7.128	7.250	7.362	7.465	7.560	7.649	7.732	7.809	7.883
12	6.943	7.060	7.167	7.265	7.356	7.441	7.520	7.594	7.665
13	6.791	6.903	7.006	7.101	7.188	7.269	7.345	7.417	7.485
14	6.664	6.772	6.871	6.962	7.047	7.126	7.199	7.268	7.333
15	6.555	6.660	6.757	6.845	6.927	7.003	7.074	7.142	7.204
16	6.462	6.564	6.658	6.744	6.823	6.898	6.967	7.032	7.093
17	6.381	6.480	6.572	6.656	6.734	6.806	6.873	6.937	6.997
18	6.310	6.407	6.497	6.579	6.655	6.725	6.792	6.854	6.912
19	6.247	6.342	6.430	6.510	6.585	6.654	6.719	6.780	6.837
20	6.191	6.285	6.371	6.450	6.523	6.591	6.654	6.714	6.771
30	5.849	5.932	6.008	6.078	6.143	6.203	6.259	6.311	6.361
40	5.686	5.764	5.835	5.900	5.961	6.017	6.069	6.119	6.165
50	5.607	5.682	5.751	5.814	5.873	5.927	5.978	6.025	6.060
60	5.528	5.601	5.667	5 728	5.785	5.837	5.886	6.931	5.974
∞	5.227	5.290	5.348	5.400	5.448	5.493	5.535	5.611	5.611

TABLE B.8. (*Continued*)

k	2	3	4	5	6	7	8	9	10
				$\alpha(2) = 0.001$					
df									
1	900.3	1,351.	1,643.	1,856.	2,022	2,158.	2,272.	2,370.	2,455.
2	44.69	60.42	70.77	78.43	84.49	89.46	93,067	97.30	100.5
3	18.28	23.32	26.65	29.13	31.11	32.74	34.12	35.33	36.39
4	12.18	14.99	16.84	18.23	19.34	20.26	21.04	21.73	22.33
5	9.714	11.67	12.96	13.93	14.71	15.35	15.90	16.38	16.81
6	8.427	9.960	10.97	11.72	12.32	12.83	13.26	13.63	13.97
7	7.648	8.930	9.763	10.40	10.90	11.32	11.68	11.99	12.27
8	7.130	8.250	8.978	9.522	9.958	10.32	10.64	10.91	11.15
9	6.762	7.768	8.419	8.906	9.295	9.619	9.897	10.14	10.36
10	6.487	7.411	8.006	8.450	8.804	9.099	9.352	9.573	9.769
11	6.275	7.136	7.687	8.098	8.426	8.699	8.933	9.138	9.319
12	6.106	6.917	7.436	7.821	8.127	8.383	8.601	8.793	8.962
13	5.970	6.740	7.231	7.595	7.885	8.126	8.333	8.513	8.673
14	5.856	6.594	7.062	7.409	7.685	7.195	8.110	8.282	8.434
15	5.760	6.470	6.290	7.252	7.517	7.736	7.925	8.088	8.234
16	5.678	6.365	6.799	7.119	7.374	7.585	7.766	7.923	8.063
17	5.608	6.275	6.695	7.005	7.250	7.454	7.629	7.781	7.916
18	5.546	6.196	6.604	6.905	7.143	7.341	7.510	7.657	7.788
19	5.492	6.127	6.525	6.817	7.049	7.242	7.405	7.549	7.676
20	5.444	6.065	6.454	6.740	6.966	7.154	7.313	7.453	7.577
30	5.156	5.698	6.033	6.278	6.470	6.628	6.763	6.880	6.984
40	5.022	5.528	5.838	6.063	6.240	6.386	6.509	6.616	6.711
50	4.958	5.447	5.746	5.902	6.131	6.271	6.389	6.491	6.581
60	4.894	5.365	5.653	5.860	6.022	6.155	6.268	6.366	6.451
∞	4.654	5.063	5.309	5.619	5.619	5.730	5.823	5.093	5.973

(*Continued*)

TABLE B.8. (*Continued*)

k	11	12	13	14	15	16	17	18	19
df									
1	2,532.	2,600.	2,662.	2,718.	2,770.	28.18	2,863.	2,904.	2,943.
2	103.3	105.9	108.2	110.4	112.3	114.2	115.9	117.4	118.9
3	37.34	38.20	38.98	39.69	40.35	40.97	41.54	42.07	42.58
4	22.87	23.36	23.81	24.21	24.59	24.94	25.27	25.58	25.87
5	17.18	17.53	17.85	18.13	18.41	18.66	18.89	19.10	19.31
6	14.27	14.54	14.79	15.01	15.22	15.42	15.60	15 78	15.94
7	12.52	12.74	12.95	13.14	13.32	13.48	13.64	13.78	13.92
8	11.36	11.56	11.74	11.91	12.06	12.21	12.34	12 47	12.59
9	10.55	10.73	10.89	11.03	11.08	11.30	11.42	11.54	11.64
10	9.946	10.11	10.25	10.39	10.52	10.64	10.75	10.85	10.95
11	9.482	9.630	9.766	9.892	10.01	10.12	10.22	10.31	10.41
12	9.115	9.254	9.381	9.489	9.606	9.707	9.802	9.891	9.975
13	8.817	8.948	9.068	9.178	9.281	9.376	9.466	9.550	9.629
14	8.571	8.696	8.809	8.914	9.012	9.103	9.188	9.267	9.343
15	8.365	8.483	8.592	8.693	8.786	8.872	8.954	9.030	9.102
16	8.189	8.303	8.407	8.504	8.593	8.676	8.755	8.828	8.897
17	8.037	8.148	8.248	8.342	8.427	8.508	8.583	8.654	8.720
18	7.906	8.012	8.110	8.199	8.283	8.361	8.434	8.502	8.567
19	7.790	7.893	7.988	8.075	8.156	8.232	8.303	8.369	8.432
20	7.688	7.788	7.880	7.966	8.044	8.118	8.186	8.251	8.312
30	7.077	7.162	7.239	7.310	7.375	7.437	7.494	7.548	7.599
40	6.796	6.872	6.942	7.007	7.067	7.122	7.174	7.223	7.269
50	6.762	6.735	6.802	6.864	6.871	6.973	7.023	7.069	7.113
60	6.528	6.598	6.661	6.720	6.774	6.824	6.871	6.914	6.965
∞	6.036	6.092	6.144	6.191	6.234	6.274	6.312	6.347	6.380

*To find a value of q, first locate the table headed by the appropriate value of α. Then, find the degrees of freedom in the leftmost column and the number of means involved in the comparison (k) in the top row of the table. Where this row and column intersect is the value of q corresponding to an area of α in the q distribution with that number of degrees of freedom and k means.

TABLE B.9. Critical Values of Kruskal–Wallis H Statistics*

n_1	n_2	n_3	n_4	n_5	$\alpha(2)$ 0.10	0.05	0.02	0.01	0.005	0.002	0.001
2	2	2			4.571						
3	2	1			4.286						
3	2	2			4.500	4.714					
3	3	1			4.571	5.143					
3	3	2			4.556	5.361	6.250				
3	3	3			4.622	5.600	6.489	(7.200)	7.200		
4	2	1			4.500						
4	2	2			4.458	5.333	6.000				
4	3	1			4.056	5.208					
4	3	2			4.511	5.444	6.144	6.444	7.000		
4	3	3			4.709	5.791	6.564	6.745	7.318	8.018	
4	4	1			4.167	4.967	(6.667)	6.667			
4	4	2			4.555	5.455	6.600	7.036	7.282	7.855	
4	4	3			4.545	5.598	6.712	7.144	7.598	8.227	8.909
4	4	4			4.654	5.692	6.962	7.654	8.000	8.654	9.269
5	2	1			4.200	5.000					
5	2	2			4.373	5.160	6.000	6.533			
5	3	1			4.018	4.960	6.044				
5	3	2			4.651	5.251	6.124	6.909	7.182		
5	3	3			4.533	5.648	6.533	7.079	7.636	8.048	8.727
5	4	1			3.987	4.985	6.431	6.955	7.364		
5	4	2			4.541	5.273	6.505	7.205	7.573	8.114	8.591
5	4	3			4.549	5.656	6.676	7.445	7.927	8.481	8.795
5	4	4			4.619	5.657	6.953	7.760	8.189	8.868	9.168
5	5	1			4.109	5.127	6.145	7.309	8.182		
5	5	2			4.623	5.338	6.446	7.338	8.131	6.446	7.338
5	5	3			4.545	5.705	6.866	7.578	8.316	8.809	9.521
5	5	4			4.523	5.666	7.000	7.823	8.523	9.163	9.606
5	5	5			4.940	5.780	7.220	8.000	8.780	9.620	9.920
6	1	1									
6	2	1			4.200	4.822					
6	2	2			4.545	5.345	6.182	6.982			
6	3	1			3.909	4.855	6.236				
6	3	2			4.682	5.348	6.227	6.970	7.515	8.182	
6	3	3			4.538	5.615	6.590	7.410	7.872	8.628	9.346
6	4	1			4.038	4.947	6.174	7.106	7.614		

(Continued)

TABLE B.9. (*Continued*)

n_1	n_2	n_3	n_4	n_5	$\alpha(2)$ 0.10	0.05	0.02	0.01	0.005	0.002	0.001
6	4	2			4.494	5.340	6.571	7.340	7.846	8.494	8.827
6	4	3			4.604	5.610	6.725	7.500	8.033	8.918	9.170
6	4	4			4.595	5.681	6.900	7.795	8.381	9.167	9.861
6	5	1			4.128	4.990	6.138	7.182	8.077	8.515	
6	5	2			4.596	5.338	6.585	7.376	8.196	8.967	9.189
6	5	3			4.535	5.602	6.829	7.590	8.314	9.150	9.669
6	5	4			4.522	5.661	7.018	7.936	8.643	9.458	9.960
6	5	5			4.547	5.729	7.110	8.028	8.859	9.771	10.271
6	6	1			4.000	4.945	6.286	7.121	8.165	9.077	9.692
6	6	2			4.438	5.410	6.667	7.467	8.210	9.219	9.752
6	6	3			4.558	5.625	6.900	7.725	8.458	9.458	10.150
6	6	4			4.548	5.724	7.107	8.000	8.754	9.662	10.342
6	6	5			4.542	5.765	7.152	8.124	8.987	9.948	10.524
6	6	6			4.643	5.801	7.240	8.222	9.170	10.187	10.889
7	7	7			4.594	5.819	7.332	8.378	9.373	10.516	11.310
8	8	8			4.595	5.805	7.355	8.465	9.495	10.805	11.705
2	2	1	1		—						
2	2	2	1		5.357	5.679					
2	2	2	2		5.667	6.167	(6.667)	6.667			
3	1	1	1		—						
3	2	1	1		5.143						
3	2	2	1		5.556	5.833	6.500				
3	2	2	2		5.644	6.333	6.978	7.133	7.533		
3	3	1	1		5.333	6.333					
3	3	2	1		5.689	6.244	6.689	7.200	7.400		
3	3	2	2		5.745	6.527	7.182	7.636	7.873	8.018	8.455
3	3	3	1		5.655	6.600	7.109	7.400	8.055	8.345	
3	3	3	2		5.879	6.727	7.636	8.105	8.379	8.803	9.030
3	3	3	3		6.026	7.000	7.872	8.538	8.897	9.462	9.513
4	1	1	1		—						
4	2	1	1		5.250	5.833					
4	2	2	1		5.533	6.133	6.667	7.000			
4	2	2	2		5.755	6.545	7.091	7.391	7.964	8.291	
4	3	1	1		5.067	6.178	6.711	7.067			
4	3	2	1		5.591	6.309	7.018	7.455	7.773	8.182	
4	3	2	2		5.750	6.621	7.530	7.871	8.273	8.689	8.909

TABLE B.9. (*Continued*)

	$\alpha(2)$				0.10	0.05	0.02	0.01	0.005	0.002	0.001
n_1	n_2	n_3	n_4	n_5							
4	3	3	1		5.689	6.545	7.485	7.758	8.212	8.697	9.182
4	3	3	2		5.872	6.795	7.763	8.333	8.718	9.167	8.455
4	3	3	3		6.016	6.984	7.995	8.659	9.253	9.709	10.016
4	4	1	1		5.182	5.945	7.091	7.909	7.909		
4	4	2	1		5.568	6.386	7.364	7.886	8.341	8.591	8.909
4	4	2	2		5.808	6.731	7.750	8.346	8.692	9.269	9.462
4	4	3	1		5.692	6.635	7.660	8.231	8.583	9.038	9.327
4	4	3	2		5.901	6.874	7.951	8.621	9.165	9.615	9.945
4	4	3	3		6.019	7.038	8.181	8.876	9.495	10.105	10.467
4	4	4	1		5.564	6.725	7.879	8.588	9.000	9.478	9.758
4	4	4	2		5.914	6.957	8.157	8.871	9.486	10.043	10.429
4	4	4	3		6.042	7.142	8.350	9.075	9.742	10.542	10.929
4	4	4	4		6.088	7.235	8.515	9.287	9.971	10.809	11.338
2	1	1	1	1	—						
2	2	1	1	1	5.786						
2	2	2	1	1	6.250	6.750					
2	2	2	2	1	6.600	7.133	(7.533)	7.533			
2	2	2	2	2	6.982	7.418	8.073	8.291	(8.727)	8.727	
3	1	1	1	1							
3	2	1	1	1	6.139	6.583					
3	2	2	1	1	6.511	6.800	7.400	7.600			
3	2	2	2	1	6.709	7.309	7.836	8.127	8.327	8.618	
3	2	2	2	2	6.955	7.682	8.303	8.682	8.985	9.273	9.364
3	3	1	1	1	6.311	7.111	7.467				
3	3	2	1	1	6.600	7.200	7.892	8.073	8.345		
3	3	2	2	1	6.788	7.591	8.258	8.576	8.924	9.167	9.303
3	3	2	2	2	7.026	7.910	8.667	9.115	9.474	9.769	10.026
3	3	3	1	1	6.788	7.576	8.242	8.424	8.848	(9.455)	9.455
3	3	3	2	1	6.910	7.769	8.590	9.051	9.410	9.769	9.974
3	3	3	2	2	7.121	8.044	9.011	9.505	9.890	10.330	10.637
3	3	3	3	1	7.077	8.000	8.879	9.451	9.846	10.286	10.549
3	3	3	3	2	7.210	8.200	9.267	9.876	10.333	10.838	11.171
3	3	3	3	3	7.333	8.333	9.467	10.200	10.733	10.267	11.667

*To find a value of H, find the numbers of observations in each of the groups of dependent variable values in the leftmost column. It does not matter which group is considered group 1. Where this row and column intersect is the value of H that is expected to occur in α of the samples when there are differences between the groups in the population.

TABLE B.10. Critical Values of Dunn's Q Statistics*

$\alpha(2)$	0.50	0.20	0.10	0.05	0.02	0.01	0.005	0.002	0.001
k									
2	0.674	1.282	1.645	1.960	2.327	2.576	2.807	3.091	3.291
3	1.383	1.834	2.128	2.394	2.713	2.936	3.144	3.403	3.588
4	1.732	2.128	2.394	2.639	2.936	3.144	3.342	3.588	3.765
5	1.960	2.327	2.576	2.807	3.091	3.291	3.481	3.719	3.891
6	2.128	2.475	2.713	2.936	3.209	3.403	3.588	3.820	3.988
7	2.261	2.593	2.823	3.038	3.304	3.494	3.675	3.902	4.067
8	2.369	2.690	2.914	3.124	3.384	3.570	3.748	3.972	4.134
9	2.461	2.773	2.992	3.197	3.453	3.635	3.810	4.031	4.191
10	2.540	2.845	3.059	3.261	3.512	3.692	3.865	4.083	4.241
11	2.609	2.908	3.119	3.317	3.565	3.743	3.914	4.129	4.286
12	2.671	2.965	3.172	3.368	3.613	3.789	3.957	4.171	4.326
13	2.726	3.016	3.220	3.414	3.656	3.830	3.997	4.209	4.363
14	2.777	3.062	3.264	3.456	3.695	3.868	4.034	4.244	4.397
15	2.823	3.105	3.304	3.494	3.731	3.902	4.067	4.276	4.428
16	2.866	3.144	3.342	3.529	3.765	3.935	4.098	4.305	4.456
17	2.905	3.181	3.376	3.562	3.796	3.965	4.127	4.333	4.483
18	2.942	3.215	3.409	3.593	3.825	3.993	4.154	4.359	4.508
19	2.976	3.246	3.439	3.622	3.852	4.019	4.179	4.383	4.532
20	3.008	3.276	3.467	3.649	3.878	4.044	4.203	4.406	4.554
21	3.038	3.304	3.494	3.675	3.902	4.067	4.226	4.428	4.575
22	3.067	3.331	3.519	3.699	3.925	4.089	4.247	4.448	4.595
23	3.094	3.356	3.543	3.722	3.947	4.110	4.268	4.468	4.614
24	3.120	3.380	3.566	3.744	3.968	4.130	4.287	4.486	4.632
25	3.144	3.403	3.588	3.765	3.988	4.149	4.305	4.504	4.649

*To find a value of Q, find the number of means of ranks in the comparison interval in the leftmost column, then locate the desired α value in the top row of the table. Where this column and row intersect is the value of Q that is expected to occur in α of the samples from a population in which there is no association between the groups.

TABLE B.11. Ranks Associated with the Limits of a Confidence Interval for the Median*

n	90% Interval		95% Interval		99% Interval	
	Lower	Upper	Lower	Upper	Lower	Upper
7	1	7	–	–	–	–
8	1	8	1	8	–	–
9	2	8	1	9	–	–
10	2	9	1	10	–	–
11	2	10	2	10	1	11
12	3	10	2	11	1	12
13	3	11	2	12	1	13
14	3	12	3	12	2	13
15	4	12	3	13	2	14
16	4	13	4	13	2	15
17	5	13	4	14	3	15
18	5	14	4	15	3	16
19	5	15	5	15	3	17
20	6	15	5	16	4	17
21	6	16	6	16	4	18
22	7	16	6	17	4	19
23	7	17	6	18	5	19
24	7	18	7	18	5	20
25	8	18	7	19	6	20
26	8	19	8	19	6	21
27	9	19	8	20	6	22
28	9	20	8	21	7	22
29	10	20	9	21	7	23
30	10	21	9	22	7	24
31	10	22	10	22	8	24
32	11	22	10	23	8	25
33	11	23	10	24	9	25
34	12	23	11	24	9	26
35	12	24	11	25	9	27
36	13	24	12	25	10	27
37	13	25	12	26	10	28
38	13	26	12	27	11	28
39	14	26	13	27	11	29
40	14	27	13	28	11	30

*To determine a confidence interval for a median, rank the data according to numeric magnitude. Then, locate the sample's size in the left-most column and the level of confidence in the top row. Where those two intersect, you will find the ranks of the data that correspond to the lower and upper limits of the confidence interval.

TABLE B.12. Critical Values of Kolmogorov–Smirnov D Statistic for Goodness-of-Fit Test*

$\alpha(1)$	0.15	0.10	0.05	0.025	0.01
n					
1	0.421	0.445	0.486	0.519	0.562
2	0.386	0.408	0.446	0.476	0.516
3	0.350	0.370	0.404	0.432	0.468
4	0.321	0.339	0.371	0.395	0.429
5	0.297	0.314	0.343	0.366	0.397
6	0.278	0.294	0.321	0.343	0.371
7	0.262	0.277	0.303	0.323	0.350
8	0.248	0.263	0.287	0.360	0.332
9	0.237	0.250	0.273	0.292	0.316
10	0.227	0.239	0.262	0.279	0.303
11	0.218	0.230	0.251	0.268	0.290
12	0.209	0.221	0.242	0.258	0.280
13	0.202	0.214	0.234	0.249	0.270
14	0.196	0.207	0.226	0.241	0.261
15	0.190	0.201	0.219	0.234	0.254
16	0.184	0.195	0.213	0.227	0.246
17	0.179	0.190	0.207	0.221	0.240
18	0.175	0.185	0.202	0.215	0.233
19	0.171	0.180	0.197	0.210	0.228
20	0.167	0.176	0.192	0.205	0.222
22	0.159	0.168	0.184	0.196	0.213
24	0.153	0.162	0.177	0.189	0.204
26	0.147	0.156	0.170	0.182	0.197
28	0.142	0.150	0.164	0.175	0.190
30	0.138	0.146	0.159	0.170	0.184
32	0.134	0.141	0.154	0.165	0.179
34	0.130	0.137	0.150	0.160	0.173
36	0.126	0.134	0.146	0.156	0.169
38	0.123	0.130	0.142	0.152	0.164
40	0.120	0.127	0.139	0.148	0.160
45	0.114	0.120	0.131	0.140	0.152
50	0.108	0.114	0.125	0.123	0.144
55	0.103	0.109	0.119	0.127	0.138

TABLE B.12. (*Continued*)

$\alpha(1)$	0.15	0.10	0.05	0.025	0.01
n					
60	0.099	0.104	0.114	0.122	0.132
65	0.095	0.100	0.110	0.117	0.127
70	0.092	0.097	0.106	0.113	0.122
75	0.088	0.094	0.102	0.109	0.118
80	0.086	0.091	0.099	0.106	0.115
85	0.084	0.088	0.096	0.102	0.112
90	0.081	0.086	0.094	0.100	0.108
100	0.077	0.081	0.089	0.095	0.103
110	0.073	0.078	0.085	0.090	0.098
120	0.070	0.074	0.081	0.087	0.094
130	0.068	0.071	0.078	0.083	0.090
140	0.065	0.069	0.075	0.080	0.087
150	0.063	0.067	0.073	0.078	0.084

*To find a critical value for D, find the sample's size in the left-most column and the one-tailed value of α in the top row. For a two-tailed α, double the one-tailed α. Where that row and column intersect is the critical value of D.

APPENDIX C

STANDARD DISTRIBUTIONS

Standard distributions are used to take chance into account for estimation of parameters of distributions of continuous and nominal dependent variables. These standard distributions belong to two families: Gaussian family and binomial family.

C.1 GAUSSIAN FAMILY

The distributions of the Gaussian family are derived from the standard normal (z) distribution. Other members of the family arise from the addition of parameters to the standard normal distribution. There are two parameters that are called degrees of freedom. The first (df_1) represents the amount of information the sample contains to estimate the variance. The second (df_2) represents the number of independent variables. Another parameter (k) represents the number of means involved in a hypothesis test. Three of the distributions are symmetric around 0 $(z, t,$ and $q)$ and two are asymmetric with 0 as the lower limit of possible values $(F$ and $\chi^2)$. Standard distributions in the Gaussian family are used either for continuous dependent variables or for nominal dependent variables when a normal approximation is used to take chance into account. The distributions to the right of the broken line are for continuous dependent variables and the distributions to the left of the broken line are for nominal dependent variables.

Introduction to Biostatistical Applications in Health Research with Microsoft Office Excel® and R,
Second Edition. Robert P. Hirsch.
© 2021 John Wiley & Sons, Inc. Published 2021 by John Wiley & Sons, Inc.
Companion website: www.wiley.com/go/hirsch/healthresearch2e

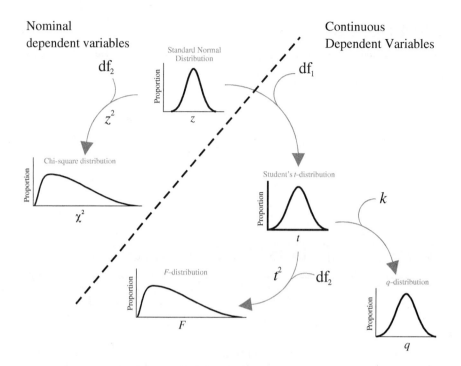

C.2 BINOMIAL FAMILY

The distributions of the binomial family are discrete distributions derived from the binomial distribution. These are the sampling distributions we used while conducting exact tests or calculating exact confidence intervals for a nominal dependent variable. We encountered three members of this family. The binomial and Poisson distributions are for univariable samples and the hypergeometric distribution is for a bivariable sample. The Poisson distribution represents what happens to the binomial distribution as the number of events (a) approaches 0 and the number of observations (n) approaches infinity. The parameter of the Poisson distribution is equal to the number of events. The hypergeometric represents two binomial distributions combined. The parameter of the hypergeometric distribution is any value that describes a 2×2 table with a given set of marginal frequencies.

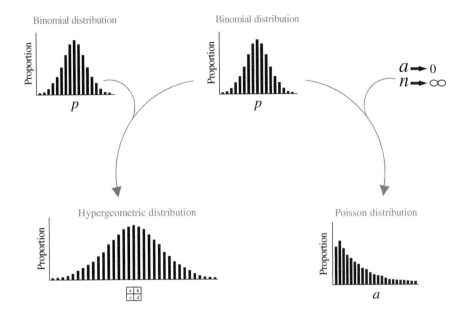

APPENDIX D

EXCEL PRIMER

Excel is a spreadsheet. At the minimum, a spreadsheet provides for organization of data into rows and columns. Most spreadsheets provide tools that can be used to work with the data. Excel has many such tools, but for our purpose we only need to know about a few.

This primer is intended for those who have little or no experience using Excel. It provides a foundation upon which the methods discussed in the text can be built.

D.1 TOPOGRAPHY

The basic unit in a spreadsheet is the cell. It is the cell that contains a data item. Each cell is defined by its column (usually specified by letters) and its row (usually specified by numbers). Each cell has an "address" that can be used to refer to the cell. For example, the upper left-hand cell is "A1." This tells us that it is in the "A" column and the first row of the spreadsheet.

A "page" of cells is called a "sheet" and an Excel file is called a "workbook." A workbook consists of one or more sheets. Often, new sheets are generated to display the output from a particular procedure. Alternatively, they can be generated by the users (Figure D.1).

Introduction to Biostatistical Applications in Health Research with Microsoft Office Excel® and R,
Second Edition. Robert P. Hirsch.
© 2021 John Wiley & Sons, Inc. Published 2021 by John Wiley & Sons, Inc.
Companion website: www.wiley.com/go/hirsch/healthresearch2e

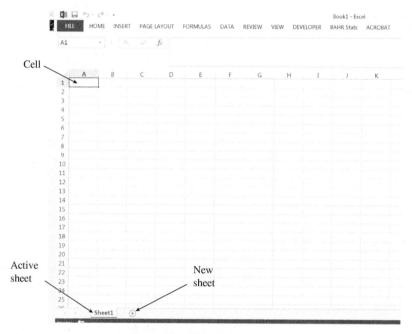

Figure D.1 Excel spreadsheet.

D.2 DATA, NAMES, AND FORMULAS

A cell can contain a datum, name, formula, or a function. We will save functions for the next section.

There are several types of data that are recognized by Excel. By default, cells are set to contain the "general" format. This format interprets numbers as numbers and any other types of characters as an alphanumeric string. This format can be changed to have a number with a fixed number of decimal places, scientific numbering (eq. 1.5E1 is the same as 15), currency, time, dates, percentages, or fractions. For most purposes, the general format is fine.

Another powerful feature of Excel is the ability to have a cell represent a calculation. This could be a numeric calculation, such as $19 + 23$, or a calculation that references cells. An example of the latter would be $A1^*B1$ in which the cell will contain the product of the values in the A1 cell and the B1 cell. For Excel to recognize a formula and distinguish it from an alphanumeric string, the first character in the cell must be an equal sign.[1] So, $19 + 23$ becomes $=19 + 23$ and $A1^*B1$ becomes $= A1^*B1$.

Something you are bound to do sooner or later is to copy and paste a cell's content into another cell. There are a couple of useful ways to do that. If you paste a cell

---

[1]Other characters can be used, but it is a good idea to form the habit of using an equal sign.

TABLE D.1. Table of Excel Functions Commonly Used in Statistics[2]

Function	Description
=ABS(ref)[3]	Absolute value of a number
=AVERAGE(range)	Average of numbers in the range
=BINOM.DIST(ref)	Binomial distribution probability
=CHISQ.DIST (ref,df,cumulative)[4]	Right-tailed probability for the chi-square distribution
=COUNT(range)	Number of numeric cells in a range
=EXP(ref)	e To the specified power
=F.DIST(ref,df1,df2,cumulative)	Left-tailed probability of the F-distribution
=FISHER(ref),=FISHERINV(ref)	Fisher's transformation
=HYPERGEOMETRIC(ref,ref,ref,ref)	Probability from the hypergeometric distribution
=INT(ref)	Rounds number down to next integer
=KURT(range)	Provides the kurtosis of data
=LN(ref)	Natural logarithm of a number
=LOG(ref,base)	Logarithm to the specified base
=MAX(range)	Selects the largest value in a range
=MEDIAN(range)	Median of a range
=MIN(range)	Selects the smallest value in a range
=MODE(range)	Mode of a range
=NORM.DIST(ref,mean,,sd,cumulative)	Probability from a normal distribution
=NORM.S.DIST(z,cumulative)	Probability from standard normal distribution
=NORM.S.INV(probability)	z-Value corresponding to a probability
=POISSON.DIST(ref,mean,cumulative	Probability from the Poisson distribution
=PRODUCT(range)	Product of a range of cells
=RAND()	A random number between 0 and 1
=RANDBETWEEN(bottom,top)	A random number between bottom and top
=RANK.AVG(ref,range,order)	Ranks a specific number relative to a range
=SKEW(range)	Provides the skewness of data
=SQRT(ref)	Square root of a value
=STDEV.S(range)	Standard deviation of a data set
=SUM(range)	Sum of a range of numbers
=T.DIST(ref,mean,stdev)	Probability from Student's t-distribution
=VAR.S(range)	Variance of a data set

[2]Not all of these will be used in this text.
[3]"ref" could be a reference to a cell or a number.
[4]"df" stands for degrees of freedom.

with the right mouse button, you will get several choices, if there is anything on the clipboard. One is just a simple paste. That takes the contents of one cell and puts it in another cell. If the cell contains a formula that references other cells, those referenced cells will change. For instance, if we were to copy a cell with $=A1^*B1$ to the cell below it, the formula will become $= A2^*B2$. This is convenient if want to perform a calculation on each member of a column, but it is inconvenient if we do not want to have some or all of the cell references changed. You can keep a cell reference the same by using $ signs. Place a $ in front of a column reference and/or a row reference to specify that the address is not to change. For example, $=\$A\$1^*\$B\$1$ will always multiply A1 by B1, regardless of where it is pasted.

Sometimes, it is the result of a calculation that we want to copy, rather than the formula. You can do this by right-clicking on a cell and selecting the paste option that appears as a clipboard with "123." This will paste the result of the calculation, rather than the formula.

D.3   BUILT-IN FUNCTIONS

An even more powerful feature of Excel is that it provides hundreds of functions that can be referenced. An example is "=SUM(A1:A12)." This tells Excel to take the sum of the contents of cells A1 through A12. Useful functions in statistics are listed in Table D.1. Many of these might not make sense to you now, but as you study statistics, their utility becomes clearer.

D.3.1   Menu Bar

Under the "Home" tab of the menu bar, there a couple of useful features. They are both in the "Format" item. The first is "Autofit column width." This adjusts the width of selected columns to match the cells' content. This is especially useful when interpreting output from Excel's procedures. The second is "Format cells." This allows you to change the type of data in a cell.

Under the "Data" tab of the menu bar is where we find Excel's statistical procedures. The preface to this text describes how to activate these.

APPENDIX E

R PRIMER

R is a free collection of programs for data analysis. To access it, open a browser and go to "cran.r-project.org/bin/windows/bases/:\" if you work in Windows or "cran.r-project.org/bin/macosx" if you work on a Mac. Click on "Download R" This will download the installation file. Run that file and follow the instructions.

R is easier to use if you download and install "RStudio." Do this after you have installed R as described above. To download RStudio, go to www.rstudio.com/products/rstudio/download and click on "DOWNLOAD" under "RStudio Desktop, Open Source License." Pick your operating system from the list and click on the download file. Run that file and follow the instructions. Now, you should have RStudio on your desktop. When you want to run R, just double click the RStudio icon.

When you run RStudio, you will see a screen divided into four quadrants (Figure E.1). The lower left quadrant is where you enter your commands and receive your output. These are entered under the "Console" tab. The commands are entered at the ">" prompt. The output will appear below the command. Previous commands can be viewed, edited, and resubmitted using the up-arrow key.

The lower-right quadrant lists the packages (collections of programs) that have been installed under the "Packages" tab. There will be a checkmark in the box to the left of packages that are already loaded. To load a package, simply click on its box. To install new packages, click on "Install" in the upper left-hand corner of this tab.

Introduction to Biostatistical Applications in Health Research with Microsoft Office Excel® and R, Second Edition. Robert P. Hirsch.
© 2021 John Wiley & Sons, Inc. Published 2021 by John Wiley & Sons, Inc.
Companion website: www.wiley.com/go/hirsch/healthresearch2e

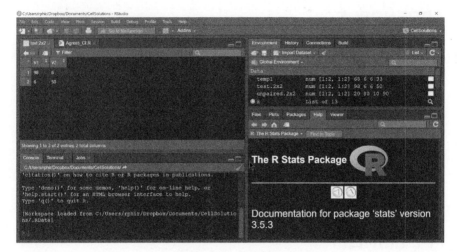

Figure E.1 RStudio.

This quadrant is also where you will get help with programs under the "Help" tab. You can access help by clicking on a package name or by typing a command in the help search window in the upper right-hand corner of the window. This quadrant is also where plots you generate will appear.

The upper left-hand quadrant is where you can view your data files or write a program. The data files are listed in the upper right-hand quadrant. Just click on the name of the file to view it. To import a new data file (e.g., from Excel), click on "Import" in the upper left-hand corner of the upper right-hand quadrant.

Most of the datasets you use in R will probably be imported from Excel. Excel is an easier environment to create and manage datasets than is R. If you want to create a simple dataset in R, you can start by creating a vector of data values called "Age" as follows:

>Age<-c(45,48,51,54,57,59,62,65)

Vectors can be combined using the "cbind" command. The following creates a dataset called "Data1" with two variables, Age and Sex:

>Data1<-cbind(Age,Sex)

The "merge" command requires two vectors with the same number of elements. If you have vectors of different lengths, you can create missing values in the shorter vector using "NA" to stand for missing data.

For some statistical analyses, we need to construct a matrix of data values. A matrix is a dataset that had a defined number of rows and columns. A commonly used matrix is a 2×2 matrix. That is one with two rows and two columns. To create such a matrix, we first create a vector of data values. Enter the data first for one column and then for the next column of the matrix.

>My2x2<-c(20,10,80,90)

Then, dimension the matrix.

>dim(My2x2)<-c(2,2)

This creates the following matrix:

20	80
10	90

APPENDIX F

ANSWERS TO ODD EXERCISES

Chapter 1	Chapter 4	Chapter 7
1.1 D	4.1 B	7.1 E
1.3 B	4.3 E	7.3 E
1.5 D	4.5 A	7.5 C
1.7 E	4.7 C	7.7 D
		7.9 B
		7.11 E
		7.13 C
Chapter 2	**Chapter 5**	**Chapter 8**
2.1 B	5.1 E	8.1 E
2.3 D	5.3 B	8.3 D
2.5 C		8.5 C
Chapter 3	**Chapter 6**	**Chapter 9**
3.1 D	6.1 D	9.1 A
3.3 C	6.3 B	9.3 E
3.5 E	6.5 C	9.5 C
3.7 D	6.7 C	9.7 D
3.9 C	6.9 D	9.9 C

Introduction to Biostatistical Applications in Health Research with Microsoft Office Excel® and R,
Second Edition. Robert P. Hirsch.
© 2021 John Wiley & Sons, Inc. Published 2021 by John Wiley & Sons, Inc.
Companion website: www.wiley.com/go/hirsch/healthresearch2e

Chapter 10	Chapter 12	Chapter 13
10.1 C	12.1 C	13.1 C
10.3 C	12.3 A,B	13.3 B
10.5 E	12.5 A	13.5 A
10.7 A	12.7 B	13.7 A
10.9 C	12.9 C	13.9 B
10.11 E	12.11 C	13.11 B
10.13 E	12.13 A	
10.15 C	12.15 C	
10.17 E		
10.19 B		
Chapter 11		
11.1 E		
11.3 C		
11.5 E		

INDEX

Introduction to Biostatistical Applications in Health Research with Microsoft Office Excel® and R,
Second Edition. Robert P. Hirsch.
© 2021 John Wiley & Sons, Inc. Published 2021 by John Wiley & Sons, Inc.
Companion website: www.wiley.com/go/hirsch/healthresearch2e